Imaging in Ophthalmology—Volume I

Imaging in Ophthalmology—Volume I

Editors

Vito Romano
Yalin Zheng
Mariantonia Ferrara

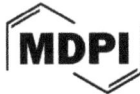

Basel • Beijing • Wuhan • Barcelona • Belgrade • Novi Sad • Cluj • Manchester

Editors

Vito Romano
Eye Unit, ASST Spedali Civili
di Brescia
Piazzale Spedali Civili
Brescia
Italy

Yalin Zheng
University of Liverpool
Liverpool
UK

Mariantonia Ferrara
School of Medicine
University of Malaga
Malaga
Spain

Editorial Office
MDPI
St. Alban-Anlage 66
4052 Basel, Switzerland

This is a reprint of articles from the Special Issue published online in the open access journal *Journal of Clinical Medicine* (ISSN 2077-0383) (available at: https://www.mdpi.com/journal/jcm/special_issues/ophthalmic_imaging).

For citation purposes, cite each article independently as indicated on the article page online and as indicated below:

Lastname, A.A.; Lastname, B.B. Article Title. *Journal Name* **Year**, *Volume Number*, Page Range.

ISBN 978-3-7258-0785-7 (Hbk)
ISBN 978-3-7258-0786-4 (PDF)
doi.org/10.3390/books978-3-7258-0786-4

© 2024 by the authors. Articles in this book are Open Access and distributed under the Creative Commons Attribution (CC BY) license. The book as a whole is distributed by MDPI under the terms and conditions of the Creative Commons Attribution-NonCommercial-NoDerivs (CC BY-NC-ND) license.

Contents

Mariantonia Ferrara, Yalin Zheng and Vito Romano
Editorial: Imaging in Ophthalmology
Reprinted from: *J. Clin. Med.* **2022**, *11*, 5433, doi:10.3390/jcm11185433 1

Min-Su Kim, Hyung-Bin Lim, Woo-Hyuk Lee, Yeo-Kyoung Won, Ki-Yup Nam and Jung-Yeul Kim
Wide-Field Swept-Source OCT Analysis of Interocular Symmetry of Choroidal Thickness in Subjects with Uncomplicated Pachychoroid
Reprinted from: *J. Clin. Med.* **2021**, *10*, 4253, doi:10.3390/jcm10184253 6

Cheng Wan, Han Li, Guo-Fan Cao, Qin Jiang and Wei-Hua Yang
An Artificial Intelligent Risk Classification Method of High Myopia Based on Fundus Images
Reprinted from: *J. Clin. Med.* **2021**, *10*, 4488, doi:10.3390/jcm10194488 16

Sandrine Anne Zweifel, Nastasia Foa, Maximilian Robert Justus Wiest, Adriano Carnevali, Katarzyna Zaluska-Ogryzek, Robert Rejdak and Mario Damiano Toro
Differences between *Mycobacterium chimaera* and *tuberculosis* Using Ocular Multimodal Imaging: A Systematic Review
Reprinted from: *J. Clin. Med.* **2021**, *10*, 4880, doi:10.3390/jcm10214880 29

Francisco Pérez-Bartolomé, Carlos Rocha-De-Lossada, José-María Sánchez-González, Silvia Feu-Basilio, Josep Torras-Sanvicens and Jorge Peraza-Nieves
Anterior-Segment Swept-Source Ocular Coherence Tomography and Scheimpflug Imaging Agreement for Keratometry and Pupil Measurements in Healthy Eyes
Reprinted from: *J. Clin. Med.* **2021**, *10*, 5789, doi:10.3390/jcm10245789 41

Jooyoung Yoon, Kyung Rim Sung and Joong Won Shin
Changes in Peripapillary and Macular Vessel Densities and Their Relationship with Visual Field Progression after Trabeculectomy
Reprinted from: *J. Clin. Med.* **2021**, *10*, 5862, doi:10.3390/jcm10245862 50

Alvin Wei Jun Teo, Hassan Mansoor, Nigel Sim, Molly Tzu-Yu Lin and Yu-Chi Liu
In Vivo Confocal Microscopy Evaluation in Patients with Keratoconus
Reprinted from: *J. Clin. Med.* **2022**, *11*, 393, doi:10.3390/jcm11020393 60

Alfredo Niro, Giancarlo Sborgia, Luisa Lampignano, Gianluigi Giuliani, Fabio Castellana, Roberta Zupo, et al.
Association of Neuroretinal Thinning and Microvascular Changes with Hypertension in an Older Population in Southern Italy
Reprinted from: *J. Clin. Med.* **2022**, *11*, 1098, doi:10.3390/jcm11041098 78

Pasquale Napolitano, Fausto Tranfa, Luca D'Andrea, Ciro Caruso, Michele Rinaldi, Alberto Mazzucco, et al.
Topographic Outcomes in Keratoconus Surgery: Epi-on versus Epi-off Iontophoresis Corneal Collagen Cross-Linking
Reprinted from: *J. Clin. Med.* **2022**, *11*, 1785, doi:10.3390/jcm11071785 91

Sujin Hoshi, Kuniharu Tasaki, Kazushi Maruo, Yuta Ueno, Haruhiro Mori, Shohei Morikawa, et al.
Improvement in Dacryoendoscopic Visibility after Image Processing Using Comb-Removal and Image- Sharpening Algorithms
Reprinted from: *J. Clin. Med.* **2022**, *11*, 2073, doi:10.3390/jcm11082073 100

Zuhui Zhang, Xiaolei Lin, Xinxin Yu, Yana Fu, Xiaoyu Chen, Weihua Yang and Qi Dai
Meibomian Gland Density: An Effective Evaluation Index of Meibomian Gland Dysfunction Based on Deep Learning and Transfer Learning
Reprinted from: *J. Clin. Med.* **2022**, *11*, 2396, doi:10.3390/jcm11092396 . . . . **108**

Rita Mencucci, Michela Cennamo, Ludovica Alonzo, Carlotta Senni, Aldo Vagge, Lorenzo Ferro Desideri, et al.
Corneal Findings Associated to Belantamab-Mafodotin (Belamaf) Use in a Series of Patients Examined Longitudinally by Means of Advanced Corneal Imaging
Reprinted from: *J. Clin. Med.* **2022**, *11*, 2884, doi:10.3390/jcm11102884 . . . . **121**

Thibaud Garcin, Emmanuel Crouzet, Chantal Perrache, Thierry Lepine, Philippe Gain and Gilles Thuret
Specular Microscopy of Human Corneas Stored in an Active Storage Machine
Reprinted from: *J. Clin. Med.* **2022**, *11*, 3000, doi:10.3390/jcm11113000 . . . . **128**

Dragana Drobnjak Nes, Pål Berg-Hansen, Sigrid A. de Rodez Benavent, Einar A. Høgestøl, Mona K. Beyer, Daniel A. Rinker, et al.
Exploring Retinal Blood Vessel Diameters as Biomarkers in Multiple Sclerosis
Reprinted from: *J. Clin. Med.* **2022**, *11*, 3109, doi:10.3390/jcm11113109 . . . . **139**

Zhengwei Zhang, Jinhan Yao, Shuimiao Chang, Piotr Kanclerz, Ramin Khoramnia, Minghui Deng and Xiaogang Wang
Incidence and Risk Factors for Berger's Space Development after Uneventful Cataract Surgery: Evidence from Swept-Source Optical Coherence Tomography
Reprinted from: *J. Clin. Med.* **2022**, *11*, 3580, doi:10.3390/jcm11133580 . . . . **147**

Jiawei Ren, Xinbo Gao, Liming Chen, Huishan Lin, Yao Liu, Yuying Zhou, et al.
Characteristics of the Ciliary Body in Healthy Chinese Subjects Evaluated by Radial and Transverse Imaging of Ultrasound Biometric Microscopy
Reprinted from: *J. Clin. Med.* **2022**, *11*, 3696, doi:10.3390/jcm11133696 . . . . **158**

Alfonso Savastano, Matteo Ripa, Maria Cristina Savastano, Tomaso Caporossi, Daniela Bacherini, Raphael Kilian, et al.
Retromode Imaging Modality of Epiretinal Membranes
Reprinted from: *J. Clin. Med.* **2022**, *11*, 3936, doi:10.3390/jcm11143936 . . . . **169**

Alberto Morelli, Rosangela Ferrandina, Eleonora Favuzza, Michela Cennamo and Rita Mencucci
3D Visualization System in Descemet Membrane Endothelial Keratoplasty (DMEK): A Six-Month Comparison with Conventional Microscope
Reprinted from: *J. Clin. Med.* **2022**, *11*, 4312, doi:10.3390/jcm11154312 . . . . **178**

Davide Allegrini, Diego Vezzola, Alfredo Borgia, Raffaele Raimondi, Tania Sorrentino, Domenico Tripepi, et al.
OCT Analysis of Retinal Pigment Epithelium in Myopic Choroidal Neovascularization: Correlation Analysis with Different Treatments
Reprinted from: *J. Clin. Med.* **2022**, *11*, 5023, doi:10.3390/jcm11175023 . . . . **187**

Luca Pagano, Haider Shah, Kunal Gadhvi, Mohammad Ahmad, Nardine Menassa, Giulia Coco, et al.
Assessment of Corneal Angiography Filling Patterns in Corneal Neovascularization
Reprinted from: *J. Clin. Med.* **2023**, *12*, 633, doi:10.3390/jcm12020633 . . . . **195**

Alessandro Ruzza, Stefano Ferrari, Matteo Airaldi, Vito Romano and Diego Ponzin
Effect of Low-Temperature Preservation in Optisol-GS on Preloaded, Endothelium-Out DMEK Grafts
Reprinted from: *J. Clin. Med.* **2023**, *12*, 1026, doi:10.3390/jcm12031026 204

Alberto Barros, Javier Lozano-Sanroma, Juan Queiruga-Piñeiro, Luis Fernández-Vega Cueto, Eduardo Anitua, Ignacio Alcalde and Jesús Merayo-Lloves
Recovery of Corneal Innervation after Treatment in Dry Eye Disease: A Confocal Microscopy Study
Reprinted from: *J. Clin. Med.* **2023**, *12*, 1841, doi:10.3390/jcm12051841 215

Pablo Arlanzon-Lope, Miguel Angel. Campos, Ivan Fernandez-Bueno and Rosa M. Coco-Martin
Does PLEX® Elite 9000 OCT Identify and Characterize Most Posterior Pole Lesions in Highly Myopic Patients?
Reprinted from: *J. Clin. Med.* **2023**, *12*, 1846, doi:10.3390/jcm12051846 231

Matilde Buzzi, Guglielmo Parisi, Paola Marolo, Francesco Gelormini, Mariantonia Ferrara, Raffaele Raimondi, et al.
The Short-Term Results of Autologous Platelet-Rich Plasma as an Adjuvant to Re-Intervention in the Treatment of Refractory Full-Thickness Macular Holes
Reprinted from: *J. Clin. Med.* **2023**, *12*, 2050, doi:10.3390/jcm12052050 248

Magdalena Kal, Mateusz Winiarczyk, Dorota Zarębska-Michaluk, Dominik Odrobina, Elżbieta Cieśla, Bernadetta Płatkowska-Adamska, et al.
Long-Term Effect of SARS-CoV-2 Infection on the Retinal and Choroidal Microvasculature
Reprinted from: *J. Clin. Med.* **2023**, *12*, 2528, doi:10.3390/jcm12072528 259

Sarah Hammadi, Nikolaos Tzoumas, Mariantonia Ferrara, Ingrid Porpino Meschede, Katharina Lo, Claire Harris, et al.
Bruch's Membrane: A Key Consideration with Complement-Based Therapies for Age-Related Macular Degeneration
Reprinted from: *J. Clin. Med.* **2023**, *12*, 2870, doi:10.3390/jcm12082870 270

Antonio Moramarco, Natalie di Geronimo, Matteo Airaldi, Lorenzo Gardini, Francesco Semeraro, Danilo Iannetta, et al.
Intraoperative OCT for Lamellar Corneal Surgery: A User Guide
Reprinted from: *J. Clin. Med.* **2023**, *12*, 3048, doi:10.3390/jcm12093048 305

Muhannd El Faouri, Naseer Ally, Myrta Lippera, Siddharth Subramani, George Moussa, Tsveta Ivanova, et al.
Long-Term Safety and Efficacy of Pars Plana Vitrectomy for Uveitis: Experience of a Tertiary Referral Centre in the United Kingdom
Reprinted from: *J. Clin. Med.* **2023**, *12*, 3252, doi:10.3390/jcm12093252 319

Agnieszka M. Zbrzezny and Andrzej E. Grzybowski
Deceptive Tricks in Artificial Intelligence: Adversarial Attacks in Ophthalmology
Reprinted from: *J. Clin. Med.* **2023**, *12*, 3266, doi:10.3390/jcm12093266 331

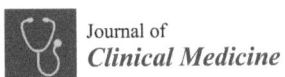

Editorial

Editorial: Imaging in Ophthalmology

Mariantonia Ferrara [1], Yalin Zheng [2,3] and Vito Romano [4,5,*]

1. Manchester Royal Eye Hospital, Oxford Road, Manchester M13 9WL, UK
2. Department of Eye and Vision Science, University of Liverpool, Liverpool L69 3BX, UK
3. St Paul's Eye Unit, Royal Liverpool University Hospital, Liverpool L69 3BX, UK
4. Eye Clinic, Department of Medical and Surgical Specialties, Radiological Sciences, and Public Health, University of Brescia, 25121 Brescia, Italy
5. ASST Civil Hospital of Brescia, 25123 Brescia, Italy
* Correspondence: vito.romano@gmail.com

Over the last decade, ophthalmology has significantly benefited from advances in vivo non-invasive ophthalmic imaging techniques that play currently a fundamental role in the clinical assessment, diagnosis, management, and monitoring of a wide variety of conditions involving both the anterior and posterior segment [1–6]. Imaging technologies, including anterior and posterior segment optical coherence tomography (OCT), OCT angiography, wide-field retinal imaging, specular and confocal microscopy, corneal topography, and ocular ultrasound, have dramatically improved the morphological and functional evaluation of ocular structures, both in healthy and pathological eyes [1–11].

The detection of tissue microstructural changes, even at the subclinical level, can improve our ability to not only make an appropriate diagnosis, but also to elucidate pathogenetic mechanisms and to plan an appropriate management strategy for several pathological conditions. In this regard, for instance, an analysis of the retinal and corneal changes associated with SO tamponade provided important information on the potential effects of this compound on ocular tissues and facilitated the early detection of complications [12–15]. This aspect is of great clinical relevance, especially when considering that SO-related complications can be severe and potentially sight-threatening [16]. Furthermore, imaging techniques allow the identification of new biomarkers with different potential applications, including the detection and prediction of progression or responses to the treatment of common ocular diseases (e.g., age-related macular degeneration, AMD, diabetic retinopathy, DR, and myopic choroidal neovascularization) [17–19]; the early detection of systemic diseases, including hypertension [20] and multiple sclerosis [21]; the prediction of functional outcomes after surgical procedures [22]; or the detection of potential complications associated with systemic dugs [23].

With regard to the anterior segment, corneal topography and tomography have an established role in the accurate evaluation of the corneal shape as well as in the preoperative assessment for refractive and cataract surgery [24]. They are also relevant in the diagnosis, surgical planning, and long-term monitoring of various corneal pathologies, including keratoconus [25–27], ectatic corneal diseases, and pterygium or corneal scars [28,29]. It worth noting that keratometry measurements may significantly differ on the basis of the methodology used (e.g., anterior segment-OCT vs. Pentacam) [30]. Specular microscopy is a fundamental tool in the assessment of corneal and diagnosis and in the management of corneal endothelial disorders [31]. This technique can be also used to assess corneas stored in cold storage or in organoculture using an active storage machine [32]. Confocal microscopy allows for the detailed analysis of corneal nerves as well as for understanding their important role in the corneal structure and function in common corneal diseases such as keratoconus [33] but also as early markers of ocular involvement in systemic diseases, such as type 2 diabetes [34].

Citation: Ferrara, M.; Zheng, Y.; Romano, V. Editorial: Imaging in Ophthalmology. *J. Clin. Med.* **2022**, *11*, 5433. https://doi.org/10.3390/jcm11185433

Received: 5 September 2022
Accepted: 13 September 2022
Published: 15 September 2022

Publisher's Note: MDPI stays neutral with regard to jurisdictional claims in published maps and institutional affiliations.

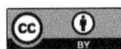

Copyright: © 2022 by the authors. Licensee MDPI, Basel, Switzerland. This article is an open access article distributed under the terms and conditions of the Creative Commons Attribution (CC BY) license (https://creativecommons.org/licenses/by/4.0/).

With regard to posterior segment, the advent of OCT and OCTA and their recent developments has dramatically improved the assessment of retinal and choroidal disorders. The diagnosis and the management of medical retinal diseases, including AMD, DR, and retinal vein occlusion, has been optimized by the use of these techniques, and the need for more invasive investigations, such as fluorescein angiography, has decreased [35–37]. This shift has also been seen in the anterior segment [38–42]. The evaluation and management of vitreoretinal interface diseases have particularly benefited from these imaging techniques, which allow for detailed structural analysis of the retinal tissues and the identification of multiple anatomical findings for classification [43,44], differential diagnosis [45–47], surgical planning [48–50], prognosis [45,49,51], and long-term monitoring [50,52]. It has been recently suggested that retromode imaging modalities, which rely on confocal scanning laser ophthalmoscopic technology, may be a promising additional tool for the assessment of ERMs [53].

The possibility of combining different imaging modalities can optimize the processes of differential diagnosis, particularly in diseases sharing multiple common clinical aspects, including macular oedema of different etiologies [54] or inflammatory pathologies [55–57], as shown for chorioretinal lesions associated with Mycobacterium (M.) chimaera, M. tuberculosis, and other ocular granulomatous infectious diseases [58].

Finally, there is a growing interest in the use of artificial intelligence (AI) and deep learning in ophthalmology due to the promising results achieved in the detection of common ocular diseases such as AMD, diabetic retinopathy, and glaucoma, and the potential applications for screening, diagnosis, and monitoring of these conditions [59]. The high accuracy of a computer-aided diagnosis algorithm using deep convolutional neural networks in recognizing and classifying high levels of myopia through fundus images has also been reported [60]. Interestingly, an AI system based on transfer learning and deep learning has been successfully applied for meibography analysis [61].

In this issue, we aimed to highlight the multiple potential applications of imaging techniques in ophthalmology, and we hope that this will be appreciated by readers.

Funding: This research received no external funding.

Conflicts of Interest: The authors declare no conflict of interest.

References

1. Fogel-Levin, M.; Sadda, S.R.; Rosenfeld, P.J.; Waheed, N.; Querques, G.; Freund, B.K.; Sarraf, D. Advanced retinal imaging and applications for clinical practice: A consensus review. *Surv. Ophthalmol.* **2022**, *67*, 1373–1390, Online ahead of print. [CrossRef] [PubMed]
2. Romano, V.; Steger, B.; Ahmad, M.; Coco, G.; Pagano, L.; Ahmad, S.; Zhao, Y.; Zheng, Y.; Kaye, S.B. Imaging of vascular abnormalities in ocular surface disease. *Surv. Ophthalmol.* **2021**, *67*, 31–51. [CrossRef] [PubMed]
3. Hood, D.C.; La Bruna, S.; Tsamis, E.; Thakoor, K.A.; Rai, A.; Leshno, A.; de Moraes, C.G.V.; Cioffi, G.A.; Liebmann, J.M. Detecting glaucoma with only OCT: Implications for the clinic, research, screening and AI development. *Prog. Retin. Eye Res.* **2022**, *90*, 101052. [CrossRef] [PubMed]
4. Romano, V.; Tey, A.; Hill, N.M.; Ahmad, S.; Britten, C.; Batterbury, M.; Willoughby, C.; Kaye, S.B. Influence of graft size on graft survival following Descemet stripping automated endothelial keratoplasty. *Br. J. Ophthalmol.* **2015**, *99*, 784–788. [CrossRef]
5. Borroni, D.; Romano, V.; Kaye, S.B.; Somerville, T.; Napoli, L.; Fasolo, A.; Gallon, P.; Ponzin, D.; Esposito, A.; Ferrari, S. Metagenomics in ophthalmology: Current findings and future prospectives. *BMJ Open Ophthalmol.* **2019**, *4*, e000248. [CrossRef]
6. Liu, S.; Romano, V.; Steger, B.; Kaye, S.B.; Hamill, K.J.; Willoughby, C.E. Gene-based antiangiogenic applications for corneal neovascularization. *Surv. Ophthalmol.* **2018**, *63*, 193–213. [CrossRef]
7. Ren, J.; Gao, X.; Chen, L.; Lin, H.; Liu, Y.; Zhou, Y.; Liao, Y.; Xie, C.; Zuo, C.; Lin, M. Characteristics of the Ciliary Body in Healthy Chinese Subjects Evaluated by Radial and Transverse Imaging of Ultrasound Biometric Microscopy. *J. Clin. Med.* **2022**, *11*, 3696. [CrossRef]
8. Kim, M.-S.; Lim, H.-B.; Lee, W.-H.; Won, Y.-K.; Nam, K.-Y.; Kim, J.-Y. Wide-Field Swept-Source OCT Analysis of Interocular Symmetry of Choroidal Thickness in Subjects with Uncomplicated Pachychoroid. *J. Clin. Med.* **2021**, *10*, 4253. [CrossRef]
9. Zhang, Z.; Yao, J.; Chang, S.; Kanclerz, P.; Khoramnia, R.; Deng, M.; Wang, X. Incidence and Risk Factors for Berger's Space Development after Uneventful Cataract Surgery: Evidence from Swept-Source Optical Coherence Tomography. *J. Clin. Med.* **2022**, *11*, 3580. [CrossRef]

10. Parekh, M.; Leon, P.; Ruzza, A.; Borroni, D.; Ferrari, S.; Ponzin, D.; Romano, V. Graft detachment and rebubbling rate in Descemet membrane endothelial keratoplasty. *Surv. Ophthalmol.* **2018**, *63*, 245–250. [CrossRef]
11. Romano, V.; Steger, B.; Myneni, J.; Batterbury, M.; Willoughby, C.E.; Kaye, S.B. Preparation of ultrathin grafts for Descemet-stripping endothelial keratoplasty with a single microkeratome pass. *J. Cataract Refract. Surg.* **2017**, *43*, 12–15. [CrossRef] [PubMed]
12. Ferrara, M.; Coco, G.; Sorrentino, T.; Jasani, K.M.; Moussa, G.; Morescalchi, F.; Dhawahir-Scala, F.; Semeraro, F.; Steel, D.H.W.; Romano, V.; et al. Retinal and corneal changes associated with intraocular silicone oil tamponade. *J. Clin. Med.* **2022**, *11*, 5234. [CrossRef] [PubMed]
13. Romano, V.; Angi, M.; Scotti, F.; del grosso, R.; Romano, D.; Semeraro, F.; Vinciguerra, P.; Costagliola, C.; Romano, M.R. Inflammation and macular oedema after pars plana vitrectomy. *Mediat. Inflamm.* **2013**, *2013*, 971758. [CrossRef]
14. Morescalchi, F.; Costagliola, C.; Duse, S.; Gambicorti, E.; Parolini, B.; Arcidiacono, B.; Romano, M.R.; Semeraro, F. Heavy silicone oil and intraocular inflammation. *BioMed Res. Int.* **2014**, *2014*, 574825. [CrossRef] [PubMed]
15. Romano, M.R.; Vallejo-Garcia, J.L.; Parmeggiani, F.; Romano, V.; Vinciguerra, P. Interaction between perfluorcarbon liquid and heavy silicone oil: Risk factor for 'sticky oil' formation. *Curr. Eye Res.* **2012**, *37*, 563–566. [CrossRef]
16. Romano, M.R.; Ferrara, M.; Nepita, I.; D'Amato Tothova, J.; Giacometti Schieroni, A.; Reami, D.; Mendichi, R.; Liggieri, L.; Repetto, R. Biocompatibility of intraocular liquid tamponade agents: An update. *Eye* **2021**, *35*, 2699–2713. [CrossRef] [PubMed]
17. Schreur, V.; de Breuk, A.; Venhuizen, F.G.; Sánchez, C.I.; Tack, C.J.; Klevering, B.J.; de Jong, E.K.; Hoyng, C.B. Retinal Hyperreflective Foci in Type 1 Diabetes Mellitus. *Retina* **2020**, *40*, 1565–1573. [CrossRef]
18. Sitnilska, V.; Enders, P.; Cursiefen, C.; Fauser, S.; Altay, L. Association of Imaging Biomarkers and Local Activation of Complement in Aqueous Humor of Patients with Early Forms of Age-Related Macular Degeneration. *Graefes Arch. Clin. Exp. Ophthalmol.* **2021**, *259*, 623–632. [CrossRef]
19. Allegrini, D.; Vezzola, D.; Borgia, A.; Raimondi, R.; Sorrentino, T.; Tripepi, D.; Stradiotto, E.; Alì, M.; Montesano, G.; Romano, M.R. OCT Analysis of Retinal Pigment Epithelium in Myopic Choroidal Neovascularization: Correlation Analysis with Different Treatments. *J. Clin. Med.* **2022**, *11*, 5023. [CrossRef]
20. Niro, A.; Sborgia, G.; Lampignano, L.; Giuliani, G.; Castellana, F.; Zupo, R.; Bortone, I.; Puzo, P.; Pascale, A.; Pastore, V.; et al. Association of Neuroretinal Thinning and Microvascular Changes with Hypertension in an Older Population in Southern Italy. *J. Clin. Med.* **2022**, *11*, 1098. [CrossRef]
21. Drobnjak Nes, D.; Berg-Hansen, P.; de Rodez Benavent, S.A.; Høgestøl, E.A.; Beyer, M.K.; Rinker, D.A.; Veiby, N.; Karabeg, M.; Petrovski, B.; Celius, E.G.; et al. Exploring Retinal Blood Vessel Diameters as Biomarkers in Multiple Sclerosis. *J. Clin. Med.* **2022**, *11*, 3109. [CrossRef] [PubMed]
22. Yoon, J.; Sung, K.R.; Shin, J.W. Changes in Peripapillary and Macular Vessel Densities and Their Relationship with Visual Field Progression after Trabeculectomy. *J. Clin. Med.* **2021**, *10*, 5862. [CrossRef] [PubMed]
23. Mencucci, R.; Cennamo, M.; Alonzo, L.; Senni, C.; Vagge, A.; Ferro Desideri, L.; Scorcia, V.; Giannaccare, G. Corneal Findings Associated to Belantamab-Mafodotin (Belamaf) Use in a Series of Patients Examined Longitudinally by Means of Advanced Corneal Imaging. *J. Clin. Med.* **2022**, *11*, 2884. [CrossRef] [PubMed]
24. Kanclerz, P.; Khoramnia, R.; Wang, X. Current Developments in Corneal Topography and Tomography. *Diagnostics* **2021**, *11*, 1466. [CrossRef] [PubMed]
25. Napolitano, P.; Tranfa, F.; D'Andrea, L.; Caruso, C.; Rinaldi, M.; Mazzucco, A.; Ciampa, N.; Melenzane, A.; Costagliola, C. Topographic Outcomes in Keratoconus Surgery: Epi-on versus Epi-off Iontophoresis Corneal Collagen Cross-Linking. *J. Clin. Med.* **2022**, *11*, 1785. [CrossRef]
26. Gasser, T.; Romano, V.; Seifarth, C.; Bechrakis, N.E.; Kaye, S.B.; Steger, B. Morphometric characterisation of pterygium associated with corneal stromal scarring using high-resolution anterior segment optical coherence tomography. *Br. J. Ophthalmol.* **2017**, *101*, 660–664. [CrossRef]
27. Brunner, M.; Czanner, G.; Vinciguerra, R.; Romano, V.; Ahmad, S.; Batterbury, M.; Britten, C.; Willoughby, C.E.; Kaye, S.B. Improving precision for detecting change in the shape of the cornea in patients with keratoconus. *Sci Rep.* **2018**, *8*, 12345. [CrossRef]
28. Vinciguerra, P.; Mencucci, R.; Romano, V.; Spoerl, E.; Camesasca, F.I.; Favuzza, E.; Azzolini, C.; Mastropasqua, R.; Vinciguerra, R. Imaging mass spectrometry by matrix-assisted laser desorption/ionization and stress-strain measurements in iontophoresis transepithelial corneal collagen cross-linking. *BioMed Res Int.* **2014**, *2014*, 404587. [CrossRef]
29. Lanza, M.; Cennamo, M.; Iaccarino, S.; Romano, V.; Bifani, M.; Irregolare, C.; Lanza, A. Evaluation of corneal deformation analyzed with a Scheimpflug based device. *Cont. Lens Anterior Eye* **2015**, *38*, 89–93. [CrossRef]
30. Pérez-Bartolomé, F.; Rocha-De-Lossada, C.; Sánchez-González, J.-M.; Feu-Basilio, S.; Torras-Sanvicens, J.; Peraza-Nieves, J. Anterior-Segment Swept-Source Ocular Coherence Tomography and Scheimpflug Imaging Agreement for Keratometry and Pupil Measurements in Healthy Eyes. *J. Clin. Med.* **2021**, *10*, 5789. [CrossRef]
31. Chaurasia, S.; Vanathi, M. Specular microscopy in clinical practice. *Indian J. Ophthalmol.* **2021**, *69*, 517–524. [CrossRef]
32. Garcin, T.; Crouzet, E.; Perrache, C.; Lepine, T.; Gain, P.; Thuret, G. Specular Microscopy of Human Corneas Stored in an Active Storage Machine. *J. Clin. Med.* **2022**, *11*, 3000. [CrossRef]
33. Teo, A.W.J.; Mansoor, H.; Sim, N.; Lin, M.T.-Y.; Liu, Y.-C. In Vivo Confocal Microscopy Evaluation in Patients with Keratoconus. *J. Clin. Med.* **2022**, *11*, 393. [CrossRef] [PubMed]

34. dell'Omo, R.; Cifariello, F.; De Turris, S.; Romano, V.; Di Renzo, F.; Di Taranto, D.; Coclite, G.; Agnifili, L.; Mastropasqua, L.; Costagliola, C. Confocal microscopy of corneal nerve plexus as an early marker of eye involvement in patients with type 2 diabetes. *Diabetes Res. Clin. Pract.* **2018**, *142*, 393–400. [CrossRef] [PubMed]
35. Tran, K.; Pakzad-Vaezi, K. Multimodal imaging of diabetic retinopathy. *Curr. Opin. Ophthalmol.* **2018**, *29*, 566–575. [CrossRef] [PubMed]
36. Guymer, R.; Wu, Z. Age-related macular degeneration (AMD): More than meets the eye. The role of multimodal imaging in today's management of AMD-A review. *Clin. Exp. Ophthalmol.* **2020**, *48*, 983–995. [CrossRef]
37. Tsai, G.; Banaee, T.; Conti, F.F.; Singh, R.P. Optical Coherence Tomography Angiography in Eyes with Retinal Vein Occlusion. *J. Ophthalmic Vis. Res.* **2018**, *13*, 315–332. [CrossRef]
38. Duker, J.S.; Kaiser, P.K.; Binder, S.; de Smet, M.D.; Gaudric, A.; Reichel, E.; Sadda, S.R.; Sebag, J.; Spaide, R.F.; Stalmans, P. The International Vitreomacular Traction Study Group classification of vitreomacular adhesion, traction, and macular hole. *Ophthalmology* **2013**, *120*, 2611–2619. [CrossRef]
39. Brunner, M.; Romano, V.; Steger, B.; Vinciguerra, R.; Lawman, S.; Williams, B.; Hicks, N.; Czanner, G.; Zheng, Y.; Willoughby, C.E.; et al. Imaging of Corneal Neovascularization: Optical Coherence Tomography Angiography and Fluorescence Angiography. *Investig. Ophthalmol. Vis. Sci.* **2018**, *59*, 1263–1269. [CrossRef]
40. Brunner, M.; Steger, B.; Romano, V.; Hodson, M.; Zheng, Y.; Heimann, H.; Kaye, S.B. Identification of Feeder Vessels in Ocular Surface Neoplasia Using Indocyanine Green Angiography. *Curr. Eye Res.* **2018**, *43*, 163–169. [CrossRef]
41. Romano, V.; Steger, B.; Brunner, M.; Ahmad, S.; Willoughby, C.E.; Kaye, S.B. Method for Angiographically Guided Fine-Needle Diathermy in the Treatment of Corneal Neovascularization. *Cornea* **2016**, *35*, 1029–1032. [CrossRef] [PubMed]
42. Romano, V.; Steger, B.; Zheng, Y.; Ahmad, S.; Willoughby, C.E.; Kaye, S.B. Angiographic and In Vivo Confocal Microscopic Characterization of Human Corneal Blood and Presumed Lymphatic Neovascularization: A Pilot Study. *Cornea* **2015**, *34*, 1459–1465. [CrossRef] [PubMed]
43. Palme, C.; Wanner, A.; Romano, V.; Franchi, A.; Haas, G.; Kaye, S.B.; Steger, B. Indocyanine Green Angiographic Assessment of Conjunctival Melanocytic Disorders. *Cornea* **2021**, *40*, 1519–1524. [CrossRef] [PubMed]
44. Hubschman, J.P.; Govetto, A.; Spaide, R.F.; Schumann, R.; Steel, D.; Figueroa, M.S.; Sebag, J.; Gaudric, A.; Staurenghi, G.; Haritoglou, C.; et al. Optical coherence tomography-based consensus definition for lamellar macular hole. *Br. J. Ophthalmol.* **2020**, *104*, 1741–1747. [CrossRef] [PubMed]
45. Romano, M.R.; Allegrini, D.; Della Guardia, C.; Schiemer, S.; Baronissi, I.; Ferrara, M.; Cennamo, G. Vitreous and intraretinal macular changes in diabetic macular edema with and without tractional components. *Graefes Arch. Clin. Exp. Ophthalmol.* **2019**, *257*, 1–8. [CrossRef]
46. Romano, M.R.; Ilardi, G.; Ferrara, M.; Cennamo, G.; Allegrini, D.; Pafundi, P.C.; Costagliola, C.; Staibano, S.; Cennamo, G. Intraretinal changes in idiopathic versus diabetic epiretinal membranes after macular peeling. *PLoS ONE* **2018**, *13*, e0197065. [CrossRef]
47. Govetto, A.; Sarraf, D.; Hubschman, J.P.; Tadayoni, R.; Couturier, A.; Chehaibou, I.; Au, A.; Grondin, C.; Virgili, G.; Romano, M.R. Distinctive Mechanisms and Patterns of Exudative Versus Tractional Intraretinal Cystoid Spaces as Seen With Multimodal Imaging. *Am. J. Ophthalmol.* **2020**, *212*, 43–56. [CrossRef]
48. Govetto, A.; Hubschman, J.P.; Sarraf, D.; Figueroa, M.S.; Bottoni, F.; dell'Omo, R.; Curcio, C.A.; Seidenari, P.; Delledonne, G.; Gunzenhauser, R.; et al. The role of Müller cells in tractional macular disorders: An optical coherence tomography study and physical model of mechanical force transmission. *Br. J. Ophthalmol.* **2020**, *104*, 466–472. [CrossRef]
49. Chua, P.Y.; Sandinha, M.T.; Steel, D.H. Idiopathic epiretinal membrane: Progression and timing of surgery. *Eye* **2022**, *36*, 495–503. [CrossRef]
50. Yang, J.M.; Choi, S.U.; Kim, Y.J.; Kim, R.; Yon, D.K.; Lee, S.W.; Shin, J.I.; Lee, J.Y.; Kim, J.G. Association between epiretinal membrane, epiretinal proliferation, and prognosis of full-thickness macular hole closure. *Retina* **2022**, *42*, 46–54. [CrossRef]
51. Romano, M.R.; Rossi, T.; Borgia, A.; Catania, F.; Sorrentino, T.; Ferrara, M. Management of refractory and recurrent macular holes: A comprehensive review. *Surv. Ophthalmol.* **2022**, *67*, 908–931. [CrossRef] [PubMed]
52. Romano, M.R.; Comune, C.; Ferrara, M.; Cennamo, G.; De Cillà, S.; Toto, L.; Cennamo, G. Retinal Changes Induced by Epiretinal Tangential Forces. *J. Ophthalmol.* **2015**, *2015*, 372564. [CrossRef] [PubMed]
53. Savastano, A.; Ripa, M.; Savastano, M.C.; Caporossi, T.; Bacherini, D.; Kilian, R.; Rizzo, C.; Rizzo, S. Retromode Imaging Modality of Epiretinal Membranes. *J. Clin. Med.* **2022**, *11*, 3936. [CrossRef]
54. Dysli, M.; Rückert, R.; Munk, M.R. Differentiation of Underlying Pathologies of Macular Edema Using Spectral Domain Optical Coherence Tomography (SD-OCT). *Ocul. Immunol. Inflamm.* **2019**, *27*, 474–483. [CrossRef]
55. Baharani, A.; Errera, M.H.; Jhingan, M.; Samanta, A.; Agarwal, A.; Singh, S.R.; Reddy, P.R.R.; Grewal, D.S.; Chhablani, J. Choroidal imaging in uveitis: An update. *Surv. Ophthalmol.* **2022**, *67*, 965–990. [CrossRef]
56. Ferrara, M.; Eggenschwiler, L.; Stephenson, A.; Montieth, A.; Nakhoul, N.; Araùjo-Miranda, R.; Foster, C.S. The Challenge of Pediatric Uveitis: Tertiary Referral Center Experience in the United States. The Challenge of Pediatric Uveitis: Tertiary Referral Center Experience in the United States. *Ocul. Immunol. Inflamm.* **2019**, *27*, 410–417. [CrossRef] [PubMed]
57. Thomas, A.S.; Lin, P. Multimodal imaging in infectious and noninfectious intermediate, posterior and panuveitis. *Curr. Opin. Ophthalmol.* **2021**, *32*, 169–182. [CrossRef]

58. Zweifel, S.A.; Foa, N.; Wiest, M.R.J.; Carnevali, A.; Zaluska-Ogryzek, K.; Rejdak, R.; Toro, M.D. Differences between Mycobacterium chimaera and tuberculosis Using Ocular Multimodal Imaging: A Systematic Review. *J. Clin. Med.* **2021**, *10*, 4880. [CrossRef]
59. Williams, B.M.; Borroni, D.; Liu, R.; Zhao, Y.; Zhang, J.; Lim, J.; Ma, B.; Romano, V.; Qi, H.; Ferdousi, M.; et al. An artificial intelligence-based deep learning algorithm for the diagnosis of diabetic neuropathy using corneal confocal microscopy: A development and validation study. *Diabetologica* **2020**, *63*, 419–430. [CrossRef]
60. Wan, C.; Li, H.; Cao, G.-F.; Jiang, Q.; Yang, W.-H. An Artificial Intelligent Risk Classification Method of High Myopia Based on Fundus Images. *J. Clin. Med.* **2021**, *10*, 4488. [CrossRef]
61. Zhang, Z.; Lin, X.; Yu, X.; Fu, Y.; Chen, X.; Yang, W.; Dai, Q. Meibomian Gland Density: An Effective Evaluation Index of Meibomian Gland Dysfunction Based on Deep Learning and Transfer Learning. *J. Clin. Med.* **2022**, *11*, 2396. [CrossRef] [PubMed]

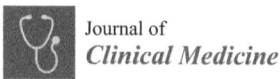

Article

Wide-Field Swept-Source OCT Analysis of Interocular Symmetry of Choroidal Thickness in Subjects with Uncomplicated Pachychoroid

Min-Su Kim [1], Hyung-Bin Lim [1], Woo-Hyuk Lee [2], Yeo-Kyoung Won [1], Ki-Yup Nam [3] and Jung-Yeul Kim [1,*]

[1] Department of Ophthalmology, Chungnam National University College of Medicine, Daejeon 35015, Korea; kms1406@naver.com (M.-S.K.); cromfans@hanmail.net (H.-B.L.); wyk900105@hanmail.net (Y.-K.W.)
[2] Department of Ophthalmology, Gyeongsang National University College of Medicine, Changwon 51472, Korea; lwhyuk@naver.com
[3] Department of Ophthalmology, Chungnam National University College of Medicine, Sejong 30099, Korea; oksnam1231@hanmail.net
* Correspondence: kimjy@cnu.ac.kr; Tel.: +82-42-280-8433; Fax: +82-42-255-3745

Abstract: Background: We aimed to study the bilateral choroidal thickness (CT) symmetry and difference in uncomplicated pachychoroid subjects using wide-field swept-source optical coherence tomography (SS-OCT). Methods: All subjects underwent a wide-field 16-mm one-line scan using SS-OCT. Bilateral CT was measured at, and compared among, the following 12 points: three points at 900-μm intervals from the nasal optic disc margin (nasal peripapillary area), one point at the subfovea, six points at 900-μm intervals from the fovea to the nasal and temporal areas (macular area), and two peripheral points 5400 and 8100 μm from the fovea (peripheral area). Results: There were no statistically significant differences in CT between the right and left eyes in any area (all $p > 0.05$); they all showed significant positive correlations (all $p < 0.01$). However, the correlation coefficients (ρ) were smaller for the nasal peripapillary and peripheral areas compared to the macular area. Conclusions: The CTs in each region were bilaterally symmetrical in subjects with uncomplicated pachychoroid. However, interocular difference in CT increased from the center to the periphery, indicating that the anatomical variation of the nasal peripapillary and peripheral choroid was greater than that of the macula.

Keywords: choroidal thickness; interocular symmetry; uncomplicated pachychoroid; wide-field swept-source optical coherence tomography

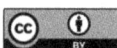

1. Introduction

The rapid development of optical coherence tomography (OCT) has shed light on the morphological and pathophysiological features of various chorioretinal diseases [1]. In particular, enhanced depth image (EDI)- and swept source (SS)-OCT enable more accurate qualitative and quantitative analyses of the choroid than conventional SD-OCT [2–4]. Detailed analysis of the choroid using these state-of-the-art imaging techniques has led to new concepts, such as "pachychoroid" and "pachychoroid disease spectrum".

The pachychoroid disease spectrum, first introduced by Warrow et al. [5], is characterized by increased focal or diffuse choroidal thickening, a pathologically dilated vein in Haller's layer (pachyvessel) and thinning in Sattler's layer and the choriocapillary layer [6–8]. The pachychoroid disease spectrum includes pachychoroid pigment epitheliopathy (PPE), central serous chorioretinopathy (CSC), pachychoroid neovasculopathy (PNV), polypoidal choroidal vasculopathy (PCV), focal choroidal excavation, and peripapillary pachychoroid syndrome [7]. An abnormally thick choroid without these specific findings on retinal imaging is referred to as uncomplicated pachychoroid [7–10]. Several studies have proposed cutoff choroidal thickness (CT) values to define a thick choroid. However, CT can be affected by various factors, including age [11,12], sex [13], axial length

(AL) [13,14], spherical equivalent (SE) [11], intraocular pressure (IOP) [15], mean arterial pressure [16], and diurnal variation [17]. There is no consensus regarding the cutoff value for thick choroid, but many studies defined pachychoroid as CT > 300 μm [7,10,18].

The recently developed swept-source OCT (SS-OCT) uses a wavelength of 1040–1060 μm, which enables deeper penetration. Therefore, SS-OCT can be used to obtain more detailed and clearer images of deeper structures (e.g., the choroid and choroidoscleral junction) than previous imaging modalities. The scan rate of commercially available SS-OCT is nearly twofold higher than that of conventional SD-OCT, thus reducing motion artifacts and enabling acquisition of wide-field B-scan images [19]. A number of studies on peripheral retinal and choroidal morphology have been conducted using wide-field OCT [20–22].

In most healthy individuals, both eyes are not anatomically or functionally identical, but have a generally similar appearance. Therefore, if there is a change in interocular symmetry, the physician should seek to determine whether it is due to disease or constitutes asymmetry within the normal range, as this has important implications for treatment planning. To our knowledge, there have been no studies on the interocular symmetry of CT in uncomplicated pachychoroid. In this study, we compared bilateral CT values among the macular, nasal peripapillary, and peripheral areas using wide-field (16-mm) SS-OCT in subjects with uncomplicated pachychoroid.

2. Materials and Methods

This retrospective, observational study was approved by the Institutional Review Board of Chungnam National University Hospital (Daejeon, Republic of Korea). Informed consent was obtained from all participants, and the study protocol adhered to the tenets of the Declaration of Helsinki.

2.1. Participants

The study population consisted of young, healthy adults with uncomplicated pachychoroid, all of whom visited the retina clinic of Chungnam National University Hospital for retina and vitreous evaluation between March 2018 and June 2020. Information on age, sex, medical history, and history of previous ocular surgery were collected; all subjects underwent comprehensive assessments of best-corrected visual acuity (BCVA), IOP (CT-80; Topcon Corporation, Tokyo, Japan), SE (KR-1; Topcon Corporation), and AL (IOL Master®; Carl Zeiss Meditec, Jena, Germany), as well as dilated fundus examinations. SS-OCT (PLEX Elite 9000; Carl Zeiss Meditec, Dublin, CA, USA) was performed to evaluate baseline ocular findings and measure CT. As in previous studies [7–10,18], uncomplicated pachychoroid was defined as eyes with thick choroid (subfoveal CT > 300 μm or and extrafoveal focus that exceeded subfoveal CT by at least 50 μm), pachyvessels (dilated choroidal vessels), inner choroidal attenuation, and no abnormal findings (e.g., PPE, CSC, PNV, and PCV) on OCT imaging. We also defined pachyvessels as dilated outer choroidal vessels observed on SS-OCT en face slabs of outer choroid, which correlated with the areas of maximal CT with increased Haller's layer in cross-sectional OCT.

This study included subjects with bilateral uncomplicated pachychoroid and BCVA of 20/20 or better, none of whom had any medical history (e.g., diabetes or hypertension). Subjects with unilateral uncomplicated pachychoroid, SE < −6.0 D, AL > 26.5 mm, anisometropia > 3.0 D, IOP > 21 mmHg, chorioretinal disease, glaucoma, optic nerve disease, or previous ocular surgery history (including refractive surgery) were excluded.

2.2. Image Acquisition

The Zeiss PLEX® Elite 9000 instrument is based on SS-OCT and uses a swept-source tunable laser with a center wavelength between 1040 nm and 1060 nm as a light source. In addition, it has a speed of 100,000 A-scans/s and, in tissue, provides an A-scan depth of 3.0 mm, an optical axial resolution of 6.3 μm, a digital axial resolution of 1.95 μm, and a transverse resolution of 20 μm.

The Zeiss PLEX® Elite 9000 instrument offers a variety of scan types. In this study, the HD spotlight 1 (16 mm) (magnification, 10×–100×) scan was used. This provides a single, high-definition scan with a depth of 3.0 mm, 100 B-scans, 1024 A-scans, and a length of 16 mm anywhere on the fundus image. The examiner can set the number of scan frames (scan repetitions) to 10–100 (10-scan interval). In this study, the HD spotlight 1 scan (length of 16 mm, 100 scan frames) set the scan angle to 0 degrees to take a horizontal scan including fovea, and it was performed twice for all participants by an experienced examiner. The best scan with a signal strength ≥9 was selected for the analysis. The results of individuals with an OCT scan signal strength <9 or scan artifacts were excluded.

2.3. CT Measurements

CT measurements were conducted in the same manner as described in our previous report [23]. For the 16-mm HD spotlight scan, CT was measured from the outer part of the hyperreflective line (corresponding to the retinal pigment epithelium RPE) to the inner surface of the sclera, using a caliper and built-in review software. Measurements were made at 12 points: 3 points at 900-μm intervals from the nasal optic disc margin (nasal points 1–3; nasal peripapillary area), 1 point at the subfovea, 6 points at 900-μm intervals from the fovea to the nasal and temporal areas (nasal points 4–6; temporal points 1–3; macular area), and 2 points at 2700-μm intervals from temporal point 3 (temporal points 4 and 5; peripheral area) (Figure 1). All scans were assessed by two investigators (M.S.K. and Y.K.W.). The reproducibility of the measurements was evaluated based on the coefficient of variation (CV) and intraclass correlation coefficient (ICC). Mean values of two measurements were used for the analysis.

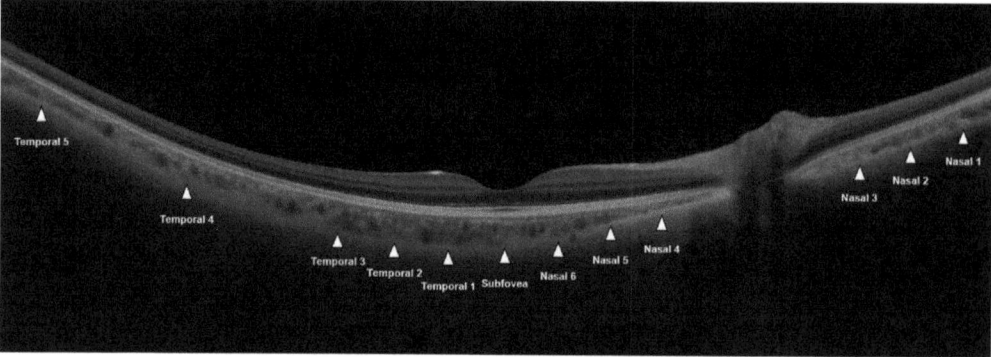

Figure 1. A 16-mm wide-field (16-mm) optical coherence tomography image of a healthy individual. Choroidal thickness was measured with a caliper at 12 points, i.e., at 900-μm intervals from the nasal optic disc margin (nasal points 1–3), at the subfovea, at 900-μm intervals from the fovea (nasal points 4–6 and temporal points 1–3), and at 2700-μm intervals from temporal point 3 (temporal points 4 and 5).

2.4. Statistical Analysis

All data analyses were performed with IBM SPSS Statistics for Windows (ver. 23.0; IBM Corp., Armonk, NY, USA). The paired t test was used to compare mean CT between the right and left eyes. Pearson's correlation coefficient (ρ), ICC, and CV values were obtained to determine the interocular symmetry of CT. The absolute differences in bilateral CT measurements were determined in all measurement areas. One-way analysis of variance (ANOVA) and Bonferroni correction were used to compare interocular CT differences among the nasal peripapillary, macular, and peripheral areas. Linear regression analysis was used to analyze the relationships of interocular CT differences in the nasal peripapillary, macular, and peripheral areas with various clinical factors. All interocular difference values (e.g., in SE, IOP, AL, and CT) were obtained by subtracting the left eye values from the right eye values. In all analyses, $p < 0.05$ was taken to indicate statistical significance.

3. Results

3.1. Demographics

Among a total of 154 healthy young adults without specific findings, 121 were excluded from the study due to high myopia, history of previous refractive surgery, subfoveal CT < 300 μm, unilateral uncomplicated pachychoroid, absence of pachyvessel and inner choroidal attenuation, etc. Thus, the final study population consisted of 33 subjects with bilateral uncomplicated pachychoroid (22 men and 11 women) and an average age of 27.55 ± 2.74 years. SE, IOP, and AL were not significantly different between the right and left eyes (all $p > 0.05$) (Table 1).

Table 1. Baseline characteristics of participants.

Characteristic		*p*-Value
Number of patients (no. of eyes)	33 (66)	N/A
Age (mean ± SD, years)	27.55 ± 2.74	N/A
Sex (male/female)	22/11	N/A
BCVA (mean ± SD, logMAR) *		0.670
Right	−0.02 ± 0.05	
Left	−0.03 ± 0.06	
Spherical equivalent (mean ± SD, diopters) *		0.988
Right	−2.43 ± 2.00	
Left	−2.42 ± 2.01	
Intraocular pressure (mean ± SD, mmHg) *		0.233
Right	15.52 ± 3.03	
Left	16.39 ± 2.89	
Axial length (mean ± SD, mm) *		0.927
Right	24.64 ± 1.05	
Left	24.61 ± 1.10	

* Comparison between right and left eyes using the paired *t* test. BCVA, best-corrected visual acuity; logMAR, logarithm of the minimum angle of resolution; SD, standard deviation.

3.2. Symmetry of Choroidal Thickness at Different Measurement Points

The CT measurements obtained by two different investigators (M.S.K. and Y.K.W.) showed excellent reproducibility (all ICCs > 0.9 and all CVs < 10%). The mean values of subfoveal CT were 384.14 ± 67.20 μm (minimum-maximum, 302.50–564.00 μm) in the right eye and 380.36 ± 71.23 μm (minimum-maximum, 305.50–595.00 μm) in the left eye. Table 2 summarizes the mean values of the bilateral CT measurements and interocular symmetry. The average CT measurements of the right and left eyes in the nasal peripapillary area (nasal points 1–3), macular area (nasal points 4–6, subfovea, temporal points 1–3), and peripheral area (temporal points 4 and 5) showed no statistically significant differences (all $p > 0.05$). In general, larger interocular correlation coefficients (ρ) were associated with larger ICC values and smaller CV values; the reverse relation was also observed. The interocular correlation coefficients of all points in the macular area (except nasal point 4 and temporal point 3; ρ = 0.577 and 0.667, respectively) were higher than those in the nasal peripapillary area. In addition, the interocular correlation coefficients of all points in the nasal peripapillary area were higher than those in the peripheral area (Figure 2).

Table 2. Comparison of choroidal thickness between the right and left eyes at 12 measurement points.

	Points	Choroidal Thickness (μm) (mean ± SD)		p-Value *	Measure of Symmetry		
		Right Eye	Left Eye		Interocular Correlation (ρ) (All, $p < 0.01$)	ICC (All, $p < 0.001$)	CV
Nasal peripapillary area	Nasal 1	277.64 ± 87.39	268.86 ± 77.63	0.446	0.685	0.815	13.52
	Nasal 2	268.89 ± 81.61	257.08 ± 78.36	0.232	0.766	0.862	12.95
	Nasal 3	232.56 ± 73.46	217.68 ± 68.22	0.130	0.701	0.699	15.34
Macular area	Nasal 4	218.63 ± 66.06	221.58 ± 61.92	0.769	0.577	0.752	14.75
	Nasal 5	294.79 ± 71.08	284.95 ± 70.26	0.199	0.850	0.898	8.93
	Nasal 6	346.77 ± 71.04	341.77 ± 72.15	0.473	0.909	0.917	6.43
	Subfovea	384.14 ± 67.20	380.36 ± 71.23	0.537	0.842	0.926	4.85
	Temporal 1	375.33 ± 70.22	380.36 ± 71.23	0.483	0.919	0.910	6.11
	Temporal 2	364.27 ± 62.61	377.90 ± 73.84	0.010	0.873	0.891	7.63
	Temporal 3	358.05 ± 78.09	371.26 ± 78.76	0.253	0.667	0.791	11.59
Peripheral area	Temporal 4	318.21 ± 73.61	320.58 ± 96.21	0.871	0.635	0.693	15.70
	Temporal 5	278.15 ± 86.25	263.14 ± 68.13	0.287	0.530	0.644	15.98

* Comparison of choroidal thickness between the right and left eyes by paired *t* test. CV, coefficient of variation; ICC, interclass correlation coefficient; ρ. Pearson's correlation coefficient; SD, standard deviation.

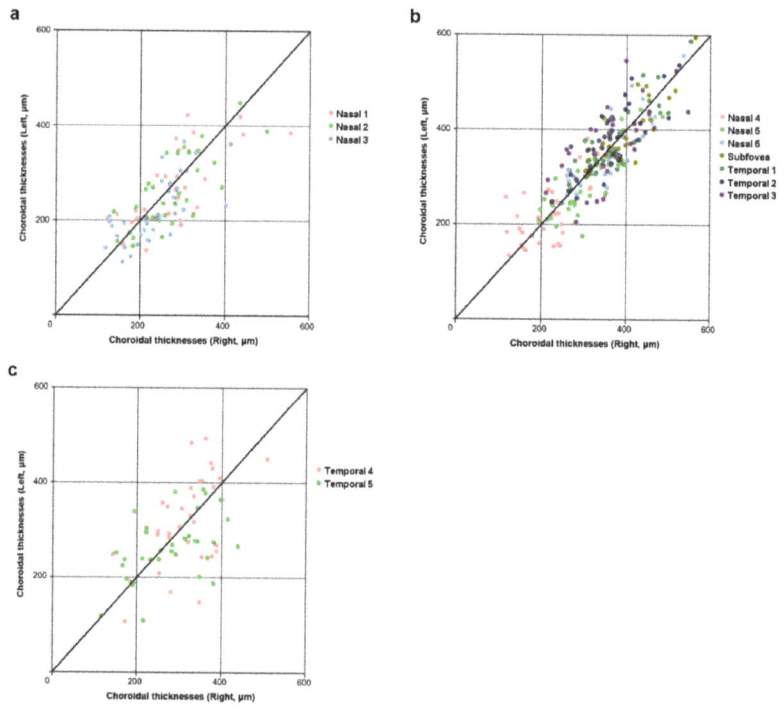

Figure 2. Scatter plots showing bilateral CT in uncomplicated pachychoroid subject in the nasal peripapillary (**a**), macular (**b**), and peripheral (**c**) areas. In the nasal peripapillary area (**a**), the scatter plot indicates weaker correlations than in the macular area (**b**), but stronger correlations than in the peripheral area (**c**) between right and left eye CT. CT, choroidal thickness.

3.3. Differences in CT Measurements by Points and Area

Table 3 shows the average absolute CT difference between the two eyes, measured at each of the 12 points. Similar to the symmetry results, the mean CT difference at all points in the macular area (except temporal point 3) was smaller than that at all points in the nasal peripapillary area. Furthermore, the mean CT difference was smaller at all points in the nasal peripapillary area than at any point in the peripheral area (Figure 3).

Table 3. Differences in absolute choroidal thickness between the right and left eyes at 12 measurement points.

Region		Difference in Choroidal Thickness (µm)	
		Mean ± SD	95% CI
Nasal peripapillary area	Nasal 1	51.29 ± 40.45	38.73–66.32
	Nasal 2	47.15 ± 30.87	37.42–59.07
	Nasal 3	46.06 ± 32.58	36.41–57.71
Macular area	Nasal 4	44.94 ± 34.36	33.14–56.45
	Nasal 5	35.62 ± 25.47	26.99–44.29
	Nasal 6	31.67 ± 23.62	23.49–40.12
	Subfovea	27.11 ± 23.28	19.77–35.01
	Temporal 1	33.15 ± 23.44	25.94–41.00
	Temporal 2	39.94 ± 25.70	31.03–48.69
	Temporal 3	56.52 ± 33.68	45.62–68.62
Peripheral area	Temporal 4	66.12 ± 48.07	49.81–84.60
	Temporal 5	60.59 ± 52.78	42.52–79.18

CI, confidence interval; SD, standard deviation.

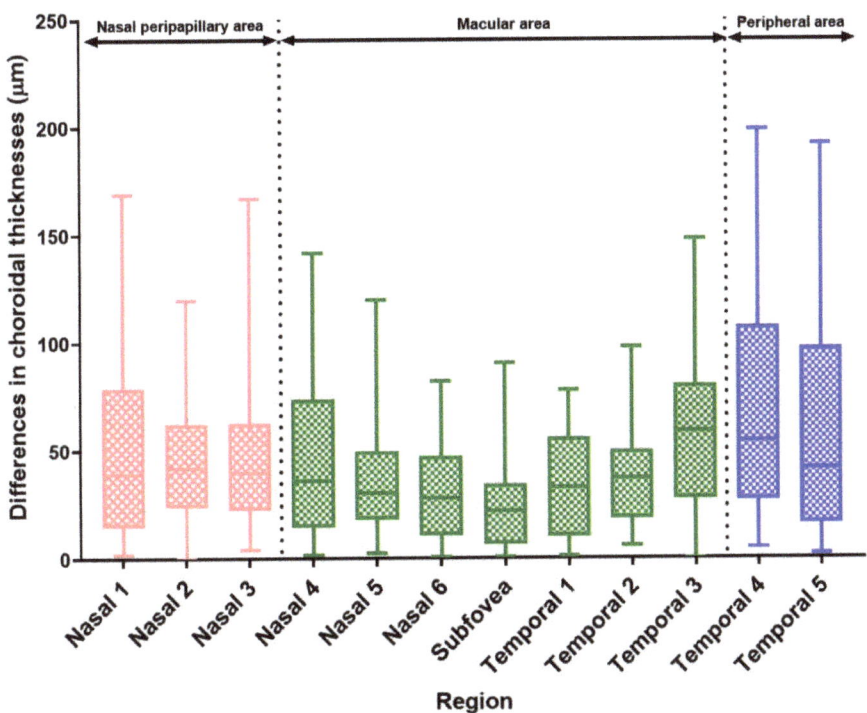

Figure 3. Box and whisker plots (2.5–97.5 percentile) of absolute interocular differences in CT according to region. CT differences were generally greater in the nasal peripapillary and peripheral areas than in the macular area. CT: choroidal thickness.

The mean absolute difference in CT increased gradually from the macular to the nasal peripapillary and peripheral areas (38.42 ± 28.59, 48.17 ± 34.60, and 63.36 ± 50.54 µm, respectively; $p < 0.001$, one-way ANOVA). In the Bonferroni post hoc test, the interocular absolute CT difference between the nasal peripapillary and peripheral areas was statistically significant ($p = 0.018$). The interocular absolute CT difference between macular and temporal areas was also statistically significant ($p < 0.001$). The absolute interocular CT difference between the nasal peripapillary and macular area showed a near significance ($p = 0.058$) (Table 4).

Table 4. Interocular difference in CT among the nasal peripapillary, macular, and peripheral areas.

		Region			Statistical Significance			
		Nasal Peripapillary Area	Macular Area	Peripheral Area	p *	p †	p ‡	p **
Difference in CT (μm)	Mean ± SD	48.17 ± 34.60	38.42 ± 28.59	63.36 ± 50.54	<0.001	0.058	0.018	<0.001
	95% CI	41.27–55.07	34.53–40.98	51.11–78.36				

CI, confidence interval; CT, choroidal thickness; SD, standard deviation. * Among the nasal peripapillary area, macular, peripheral areas (one-way analysis of variance). † Between the nasal peripapillary and macular areas (Bonferroni post hoc test). ‡ Between the nasal peripapillary and temporal areas (Bonferroni post hoc test). ** Between the macular and temporal areas (Bonferroni post hoc test).

3.4. Clinical Factors Associated with Differences in Interocular CT According to Area

Simple linear regression analysis was performed to analyze the relationships of interocular CT differences (right eye−left eye) in three different areas (nasal peripapillary, macular, and peripheral areas) with other clinical factors (e.g., age, sex, SE, IOP, and AL) (Table 5). In terms of macular area, the interocular CT difference showed a significant negative correlation with the interocular AL difference ($\beta = -6.226 \pm 3.025$, $p = 0.048$). In the nasal peripapillary and peripheral areas, the difference in CT was not significantly related to any clinical factor (all $p > 0.10$).

Table 5. Simple regression analysis of the relationships of clinical factors with the mean interocular difference in choroidal thickness by area.

	Simple Regression Analysis ($\beta \pm$ SD)					
Area	Nasal Peripapillary Area	p	Macular Area	p	Peripheral Area	p
Age	−5.058 ± 3.169	0.121	−0.185 ± 2.121	0.931	−5.235 ± 3.940	0.194
Sex (male = 0, female = 1)	9.538 ± 18.645	0.618	−1.792 ± 12.237	0.885	−18.966 ± 23.123	0.418
Interocular difference						
Intraocular pressure	−0.975 ± 1.908	0.613	−1.447 ± 1.205	0.239	−0.259 ± 2.354	0.913
Spherical equivalent	1.832 ± 2.816	0.520	3.069 ± 1.739	0.087	4.823 ± 3.374	0.163
Axial length	7.275 ± 4.839	0.143	−6.226 ± 3.025	0.048	−3.933 ± 6.118	0.525

Interocular differences were obtained by subtracting right eye values from left eye values. SD, standard deviation.

4. Discussion

In this study, we compared bilateral CT values among several points in the macular, nasal peripapillary, and peripheral areas using wide-field SS-OCT in subjects with uncomplicated pachychoroid. The degree of symmetry was generally high in the macular area (except nasal point 4 and temporal point 3) and low in the nasal peripapillary and peripheral areas. The interocular difference in CT increased gradually from the macular area to the nasal peripapillary and temporal areas ($p < 0.001$, one-way ANOVA), and the interocular difference in CT between the macular and nasal peripapillary area showed a near significance ($p = 0.058$) according to the post hoc Bonferroni test. This was assumed to be due to the low interocular symmetry of CT for nasal point 4 and temporal point 3 in the macular area.

According to a search of the PubMed database, no studies have analyzed interocular symmetry and differences in CT in uncomplicated pachychoroid patients. In particular, there have been no wide-field SS-OCT studies on the interocular symmetry of CT in the nasal peripapillary and peripheral areas. Most previous studies on the interocular symmetry of CT were mainly confined to foveal and parafoveal areas in healthy subjects rather than those with uncomplicated pachychoroid [2,24–27]. Therefore, this study is important in that it is the first to compare the interocular symmetry of CT among the nasal peripapillary, peripheral, and macular (foveal and parafoveal) areas using wide-field (16-mm) SS-OCT in subjects with uncomplicated pachychoroid.

Most of the studies mentioned above using Early Treatment Diabetic Retinopathy Study (ETDRS) maps or other methods reported that interocular CT in foveal and parafoveal areas showed high correlation coefficients and ICC values ($\rho > 0.8$, ICC > 0.9) [26–28]. Similarly, in the present study, CT measurements showed relatively high agreement ($\rho > 0.8$, ICC > 0.85) at the subfoveal, nasal 5, nasal 6, temporal 1, and temporal 2 points, which correspond to the center and inner ring (3-mm diameter area centered on the fovea) of the ETDRS map. However, CT measurements showed relatively low agreement at nasal point 4 and temporal point 3 ($\rho = 0.577$ and 0.667, respectively), corresponding to the outer ring of the ETDRS map. It is difficult to determine the reason for the low interocular symmetry of CT at these points. However, there have been several studies related to this issue. In the study by Chen et al. (mean (min, max) subfoveal CT = 334 (172, 568) μm in the right eye and 333 (133, 555) μm in the left eye) [26], the correlation coefficient for CT in the temporal area 3 mm from the fovea was 0.490, which was the lowest value among all areas measured in their study. In addition, other reports [29,30] posited that peripapillary CT variability could result from the presence of watershed zones, primarily near the optic disc [31]. The very low CT correlation coefficient for nasal point 4 compared to nasal point 5 in this study could be attributable to watershed zones.

To measure CT in the nasal peripapillary and peripheral areas in subjects with uncomplicated pachychoroid, wide-field imaging is required. Several studies measured peripheral choroidal CT using wide-field imaging [23,29,30,32,33]. However, to our knowledge, this is the first study to investigate interocular differences in CT in nasal peripapillary and peripheral areas in subjects with uncomplicated pachychoroid. In this study, the correlation coefficients of CT in the nasal peripapillary and peripheral areas were lower than in the macular area (except for nasal point 4 and temporal point 3), thus demonstrating that CT symmetry in the nasal peripapillary and peripheral areas is generally lower than in the macular area. However, the reason for these differences is not clear. In our previous study [23], CT measurements were compared between pachychoroid and "normochoroid eyes" using wide-field SS-OCT. Even in pachychoroid eyes, pachyvessels were sometimes absent from the nasal peripapillary and peripheral areas, leading to smaller than expected CT values. This may partly explain the greater interocular CT variation in nasal peripapillary and peripheral areas compared to the macular area.

CT is known to be affected by multiple factors. In this study, we also analyzed the relationships of interocular differences of CT with other clinical factors. In the macular area, interocular CT and AL differences had a significant negative correlation, i.e., the choroid in the macular area becomes thinner as the AL increases, and vice versa. However, in the nasal peripapillary and peripheral areas, no such correlations were seen. Thus, AL may have a greater effect on CT in the macular area than in the nasal peripapillary and peripheral areas, as suggested by previous studies [23,30]. Other factors, such as age, sex, IOP, and SE, also showed no relationships with interocular CT differences. However, only young adults were included in our study, and the age range was narrow (24–35 years; mean age = 27.55 years), which limited the generalizability of the findings. Age is known to be related to CT, but further research including detailed subgroup analyses is needed on this.

This study had some other limitations. CTs were measured manually, which can lead to measurement inaccuracy. However, the ICC and CV values showed good reproducibility, suggesting that any inaccuracy was minimal. Nevertheless, obtaining automatic CT measurements via software may be useful. We did not analyze other factors that may affect CT, such as mean arterial pressure or diurnal variation. Despite these limitations, this was the first study to compare CT among macular, nasal peripapillary, and peripheral areas in subjects with uncomplicated pachychoroid. In addition, the wide-field (16-mm) SS-OCT modality captured images without time lag, thus minimizing errors caused by time differences. Moreover, the image quality was higher, and the CT measurements were more precise in this study compared to other studies using SD-OCT or EDI-OCT. This study clearly demonstrated that interocular CT variation can occur in nasal peripapillary and peripheral areas.

In conclusion, interocular CT generally showed bilateral symmetry in our patients with uncomplicated pachychoroid, although this differed among areas. In addition, only interocular CT and AL differences were significantly correlated in the macular area; there were no significant associations for any other clinical factor. This suggests that the interocular CT difference in nasal peripapillary and peripheral areas is due to anatomical variation alone, rather than other clinical factors. Physicians should be aware of the possibility of interocular CT differences; when an uncomplicated pachychoroid patient exhibits an abnormal CT difference, it is important to perform detailed examinations to identify the factors, including other ophthalmic diseases, which may be responsible.

Author Contributions: Conceptualization: K.-Y.N. and J.-Y.K.; Data curation: M.-S.K., W.-H.L., and Y.-K.W.; Formal analysis and methodology: M.-S.K. and H.-B.L.; Visualization: H.-B.L. and Y.-K.W.; Writing—original draft: M.-S.K. and J.-Y.K.; Writing—review and editing: W.-H.L., K.-Y.N., and J.-Y.K. All authors have read and agreed to the published version of the manuscript.

Funding: This research received no external funding.

Institutional Review Board Statement: The study was conducted according to the guidelines of the Declaration of Helsinki and approved by the Institutional Review Board (or Ethics Committee) of Chungnam National University Hospital (Daejeon, Republic of Korea) (IRB File no: 2021-03-073-001; date of approval: 14 April 2021).

Informed Consent Statement: Informed consent was obtained from all subjects involved in the study.

Data Availability Statement: The data that support the findings of this study are available from the corresponding author upon reasonable request.

Conflicts of Interest: The authors declare no conflict of interest.

References

1. Fujimoto, J.; Swanson, E. The development, commercialization, and impact of optical coherence tomography. *Invest. Ophthalmol. Vis. Sci.* **2016**, *57*, OCT1–OCT13. [CrossRef]
2. Spaide, R.F.; Koizumi, H.; Pozonni, M.C. Enhanced depth imaging spectral-domain optical coherence tomography. *Am. J. Ophthalmol.* **2008**, *146*, 496–500. [CrossRef] [PubMed]
3. Potsaid, B.; Baumann, B.; Huang, D.; Barry, S.; Cable, A.E.; Schuman, J.S.; Duker, J.S.; Fujimoto, J.G. Ultrahigh speed 1050 nm swept source/Fourier domain OCT retinal and anterior segment imaging at 100,000 to 400,000 axial scans per second. *Opt. Express.* **2010**, *18*, 20029–20048. [CrossRef]
4. Waldstein, S.M.; Faatz, H.; Szimacsek, M.; Glodan, A.M.; Podkowinski, D.; Montuoro, A.; Simader, C.; Gerendas, B.S.; Schmidt-Erfurth, U. Comparison of penetration depth in choroidal imaging using swept source vs spectral domain optical coherence tomography. *Eye* **2015**, *29*, 409–415. [CrossRef]
5. Warrow, D.J.; Hoang, Q.V.; Freund, K.B. Pachychoroid pigment epitheliopathy. *Retina* **2013**, *33*, 1659–1672. [CrossRef] [PubMed]
6. Akkaya, S. Spectrum of pachychoroid diseases. *Int. Ophthalmol.* **2018**, *38*, 2239–2246. [CrossRef] [PubMed]
7. Cheung, C.M.G.; Lee, W.K.; Koizumi, H.; Dansingani, K.; Lai, T.Y.Y.; Freund, K.B. Pachychoroid disease. *Eye* **2019**, *33*, 14–33. [CrossRef]
8. Yanagi, Y. Pachychoroid disease: A new perspective on exudative maculopathy. *Jpn J. Ophthalmol.* **2020**, *64*, 323–337. [CrossRef]
9. Ersoz, M.G.; Karacorlu, M.; Arf, S.; Hocaoglu, M.; Sayman Muslubas, I. Pachychoroid pigment epitheliopathy in fellow eyes of patients with unilateral central serous chorioretinopathy. *Br. J. Ophthalmol.* **2018**, *102*, 473–478. [CrossRef] [PubMed]
10. Dansingani, K.K.; Balaratnasingam, C.; Naysan, J.; Freund, K.B. En face imaging of pachychoroid spectrum disorders with swept-source optical coherence tomography. *Retina* **2016**, *36*, 499–516. [CrossRef]
11. Kim, M.; Kim, S.S.; Koh, H.J.; Lee, S.C. Choroidal thickness, age, and refractive error in healthy Korean subjects. *Optom. Vis. Sci.* **2014**, *91*, 491–496. [CrossRef]
12. Xiong, S.; He, X.; Zhang, B.; Deng, J.; Wang, J.; Lv, M.; Zhu, J.; Zou, H.; Xu, X. Changes in choroidal thickness varied by age and refraction in children and adolescents: A one-year longitudinal study. *Am. J. Ophthalmol.* **2020**, *213*, 46–56. [CrossRef]
13. Li, X.Q.; Larsen, M.; Munch, I.C. Subfoveal choroidal thickness in relation to sex and axial length in 93 Danish university students. *Invest. Ophthalmol. Vis. Sci.* **2011**, *52*, 8438–8441. [CrossRef]

14. Flores-Moreno, I.; Lugo, F.; Duker, J.S.; Ruiz-Moreno, J.M. The relationship between axial length and choroidal thickness in eyes with high myopia. *Am. J. Ophthalmol.* **2013**, *155*, 314–319. [CrossRef]
15. Usui, S.; Ikuno, Y.; Uematsu, S.; Morimoto, Y.; Yasuno, Y.; Otori, Y. Changes in axial length and choroidal thickness after intraocular pressure reduction resulting from trabeculectomy. *Clin. Ophthalmol.* **2013**, *7*, 1155–1161. [CrossRef]
16. Akay, F.; Gundogan, F.C.; Yolcu, U.; Toyran, S.; Uzun, S. Choroidal thickness in systemic arterial hypertension. *Eur. J. Ophthalmol.* **2016**, *26*, 152–157. [CrossRef]
17. Baek, S.U.; Kim, J.S.; Kim, Y.K.; Jeoung, J.W.; Park, K.H. Diurnal variation of choroidal thickness in primary open-angle glaucoma. *J. Glaucoma.* **2018**, *27*, 1052–1060. [CrossRef] [PubMed]
18. Ersoz, M.G.; Karacorlu, M.; Arf, S.; Hocaoglu, M.; Sayman Muslubas, I. Outer nuclear layer thinning in pachychoroid pigment epitheliopathy. *Retina* **2018**, *38*, 957–961. [CrossRef] [PubMed]
19. Klein, T.; Huber, R. High-speed OCT light sources and systems. *Biomed. Opt Express.* **2017**, *8*, 828–859. [CrossRef] [PubMed]
20. Choudhry, N.; Golding, J.; Manry, M.W.; Rao, R.C. Ultra-widefield steering-based spectral-domain optical coherence tomography imaging of the retinal periphery. *Ophthalmology* **2016**, *123*, 1368–1374. [CrossRef]
21. Shinohara, K.; Shimada, N.; Moriyama, M.; Yoshida, T.; Jonas, J.B.; Yoshimura, N.; Ohno-Matsui, K. Posterior staphylomas in pathologic myopia imaged by widefield optical coherence tomography. *Invest. Ophthalmol. Vis. Sci.* **2017**, *58*, 3750–3758. [CrossRef]
22. Kakiuchi, N.; Terasaki, H.; Sonoda, S.; Shiihara, H.; Yamashita, T.; Tomita, M.; Shinohara, Y.; Sakoguchi, T.; Iwata, K.; Sakamoto, T. Regional differences of choroidal structure determined by wide-field optical coherence tomography. *Invest. Ophthalmol. Vis. Sci.* **2019**, *60*, 2614–2622. [CrossRef]
23. Lim, H.B.; Kim, K.; Won, Y.K.; Lee, W.H.; Lee, M.W.; Kim, J.Y. A comparison of choroidal thicknesses between pachychoroid and normochoroid eyes acquired from wide-field swept-source OCT. *Acta Ophthalmol.* **2021**, *99*, e117–e123. [CrossRef] [PubMed]
24. Akhtar, Z.; Rishi, P.; Srikanth, R.; Rishi, E.; Bhende, M.; Raman, R. Choroidal thickness in normal Indian subjects using swept source optical coherence tomography. *PLoS ONE* **2018**, *13*, e0197457. [CrossRef] [PubMed]
25. Al-Haddad, C.; El Chaar, L.; Antonios, R.; El-Dairi, M.; Noureddin, B. Interocular symmetry in macular choroidal thickness in children. *J. Ophthalmol.* **2014**, *2014*, 472391. [CrossRef] [PubMed]
26. Chen, F.K.; Yeoh, J.; Rahman, W.; Patel, P.J.; Tufail, A.; Da Cruz, L. Topographic variation and interocular symmetry of macular choroidal thickness using enhanced depth imaging optical coherence tomography. *Invest. Ophthalmol. Vis. Sci.* **2012**, *53*, 975–985. [CrossRef] [PubMed]
27. Orduna, E.; Sanchez-Cano, A.; Luesma, M.J.; Perez-Navarro, I.; Abecia, E.; Pinilla, I. Interocular symmetry of choroidal thickness and volume in healthy eyes on optical coherence tomography. *Ophthalmic Res.* **2018**, *59*, 81–87. [CrossRef]
28. Yang, M.; Wang, W.; Xu, Q.; Tan, S.; Wei, S. Interocular symmetry of the peripapillary choroidal thickness and retinal nerve fibre layer thickness in healthy adults with isometropia. *BMC Ophthalmol.* **2016**, *16*, 182. [CrossRef]
29. Rasheed, M.A.; Singh, S.R.; Invernizzi, A.; Cagini, C.; Goud, A.; Sahoo, N.K.; Cozzi, M.; Lupidi, M.; Chhablani, J. Wide-field choroidal thickness profile in healthy eyes. *Sci. Rep.* **2018**, *8*, 17166. [CrossRef]
30. Hoseini-Yazdi, H.; Vincent, S.J.; Collins, M.J.; Read, S.A.; Alonso-Caneiro, D. Wide-field choroidal thickness in myopes and emmetropes. *Sci. Rep.* **2019**, *9*, 3474. [CrossRef]
31. Hayreh, S.S. In vivo choroidal circulation and its watershed zones. *Eye* **1990**, *4*, 273–289. [CrossRef] [PubMed]
32. McNabb, R.P.; Grewal, D.S.; Mehta, R.; Schuman, S.G.; Izatt, J.A.; Mahmoud, T.H.; Jaffe, G.J.; Mruthyunjaya, P.; Kuo, A.N. Wide field of view of swept-source optical coherence tomography for peripheral retinal disease. *Br. J. Ophthalmol.* **2016**, *100*, 1377–1382. [CrossRef] [PubMed]
33. Mohler, K.J.; Draxinger, W.; Klein, T.; Kolb, J.P.; Wieser, W.; Haritoglou, C. Combined 60° wide-field choroidal thickness maps and high-definition en face vasculature visualization using swept-source megahertz OCT at 1050 nm. *Invest. Ophthalmol. Vis. Sci.* **2015**, *56*, 6284–6293. [CrossRef] [PubMed]

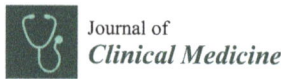

Article

An Artificial Intelligent Risk Classification Method of High Myopia Based on Fundus Images

Cheng Wan [1], Han Li [1], Guo-Fan Cao [2], Qin Jiang [2] and Wei-Hua Yang [2,*]

1. College of Electronic and Information Engineering, Nanjing University of Aeronautics and Astronautics, Nanjing 211100, China; wanch@nuaa.edu.cn (C.W.); lhlyx_mail@163.com (H.L.)
2. The Laboratory of Artificial Intelligence and Bigdata in Ophthalmology, The Affiliated Eye Hospital of Nanjing Medical University, Nanjing 210029, China; caoguofan587@163.com (G.-F.C.); jqin710@vip.sina.com (Q.J.)
* Correspondence: benben0606@139.com

Abstract: High myopia is a global ocular disease and one of the most common causes of blindness. Fundus images can be obtained in a noninvasive manner and can be used to monitor and follow up on many fundus diseases, such as high myopia. In this paper, we proposed a computer-aided diagnosis algorithm using deep convolutional neural networks (DCNNs) to grade the risk of high myopia. The input images were automatically classified into three categories: normal fundus images were labeled class 0, low-risk high-myopia images were labeled class 1, and high-risk high-myopia images were labeled class 2. We conducted model training on 758 clinical fundus images collected locally, and the average accuracy reached 98.15% according to the results of fivefold cross-validation. An additional 100 fundus images were used to evaluate the performance of DCNNs, with ophthalmologists performing external validation. The experimental results showed that DCNNs outperformed human experts with an area under the curve (AUC) of 0.9968 for the recognition of low-risk high myopia and 0.9964 for the recognition of high-risk high myopia. In this study, we were able to accurately and automatically perform high myopia classification solely using fundus images. This has great practical significance in terms of improving early diagnosis, prevention, and treatment in clinical practice.

Keywords: high myopia; fundus images; computer-aided diagnosis; risk classification

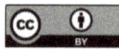

1. Introduction

High myopia is a global ocular disease. In recent years, its global incidence has increased significantly. The increasing number of people suffering from myopia and high myopia is not only a serious human health problem, but also a public management problem that affects social development. The cost of preventing and treating eye complications and vision loss in the nearly 1 billion people with high myopia is extremely high. Studies [1,2] have shown that, on a global scale, the loss of productivity due to uncorrected vision impairment is approximately USD 121.4 billion, while the cost of facilities and personnel required to establish refractive treatment services is as high as USD 20 billion [2]. The incidence of myopia in East Asia is significantly higher than that in Western countries, especially among young people in East Asia [1]. High-myopia fundus disease has become the second leading cause of blindness in China, and the trend tends towards a younger population [3]. Studies [1,2] have shown that in 2000, 2010, 2020, 2030, 2040, and 2050, the global prevalence of myopia for all age groups was/will be 22.9%, 28.3%, 34.0%, 39.9%, 45.2%, and 49.8%, respectively. Additionally, the prevalence of high myopia was/will be 2.7%, 4.0%, 5.2%, 6.1%, 7.7%, and 9.8%, respectively. It is estimated that by 2050, 4.758 billion people will suffer from myopia, and of these, 938 million will suffer from high myopia; this represents almost 50% and 10% of the world's total population, respectively [1]. According to the statistics, the overall incidence of myopia in children and adolescents in China is 53.6%, and the overall incidence of myopia in college students exceeds 90%. Among them, the prevalence of high myopia ranges from 6.69% to 38.4% [3]. Therefore, prevention and control of high myopia is a matter of great importance for society as a whole.

The difference between high myopia and low–medium myopia is that in high myopia, the refractive power in diopters is very high, usually characterized by a refractive error of ≤ -6.00 D. Moreover, it is mainly characterized by axial elongation. As myopia deepens and the axis of the eye grows longer, the visible retinal choroidal disease at the fundus becomes more severe, causing a range of serious complications, most of which lead to blindness. For this reason, high myopia-related fundus disease is a common cause of blindness worldwide and the second leading cause of blindness in China [3]. Although the terms "high myopia" and "pathological myopia" are often used interchangeably in daily life, they do not actually refer to the same disease. According to the consensus issued by the Optometry Group of the Ophthalmology Branch of the Chinese Medical Association in 2017 [3], high myopia can be divided into simple high myopia and pathological myopia. Although simple high myopia features high myopic diopters and has symptoms such as decreased vision, asthenopia, floaters, etc., it is not accompanied by serious fundus damage. However, the symptoms of pathological myopia include more serious impairment of visual function, such as occlusion, deformation, and visual ghosting, in addition to decreased vision, and the resulting fundus diseases are permanent and irreversible [3]. In addition, the degree of simple high myopia tends to be stable in adulthood, while the degree of pathological myopia deepens continuously as the course of disease progresses, accompanying the patient for life [4]. The potential risks of these two diseases are completely different. There is an urgent need for a standard risk-grading system with consistent nomenclature with which to classify different levels of risk for high myopia. This can then be used in different studies to assess the therapeutic utility. Therefore, we proposed an intelligent classification method for high myopia images according to the degree of potential risk. The specific classification rules are described in the Data Collection section below.

The traditional detection of high myopia mainly relies on artificial auxiliary methods such as diopter detection, eye axis measurement, and fundus color photography. However, manual testing and analysis rely on ophthalmologists, which is time-consuming and labor-intensive [4]. In addition, the shortage of ophthalmologists and medical equipment in areas with relatively poor medical resources leads to patients missing the optimal treatment period. For this reason, it is important to develop intelligent eye disease diagnostic methods based on fundus images. Clinically, for common fundus diseases such as diabetic retinopathy, macular degeneration, and glaucoma, fundus images have been widely used in disease diagnosis because they are noncontact, nondestructive, low-cost, easy to obtain, and easy to process.

In recent years, with the rapid development of the artificial intelligence technology and deep learning methods, many researchers have applied them to various image processing problems. New techniques and methods that analyze fundus images for high myopia have been continuously emerging [5–10]. These methods use computer-aided technologies to automatically analyze and diagnose lesions associated with high myopia in the absence of experienced ophthalmologists and professional optometry instruments. For example, Liu et al. [5] first proposed a system named PAMELA to detect pathological myopia. They used the support vector machine (SVM) approach in the machine learning technology to extract texture features in fundus images to diagnose pathological myopia. However, compared with the relatively simple SVM, deep learning methods can extract more abstract high-dimensional features, thus greatly improving recognition accuracy. Currently, most image classification methods are based on the convolutional neural network (CNN) model in deep learning. Varadarajan et al. [6], a research team from Google, introduced an attention mechanism into a CNN and trained a deep learning model to predict the refractive error. Through an attention heat map, it was shown that the fovea region of the retina has the largest contribution to the prediction. Dai et al. [7] designed a CNN model with two branches. One branch was used to distinguish between normal and abnormal fundus images, and the other branch was used to distinguish between simple high myopia and pathological myopia images. However, this model required two-step judgment, which has a lower prediction speed than the end-to-end direct classification method. The first task of the 2019 PALM Color Fundus Photographic Pathological Myopia Challenge [8] was the qualitative classification of pathological myopia. Participating teams used different CNN models [9–11] to predict the risk of pathological myopia using fundus images. However, these classifications only distinguished pathological myopia from nonpathological myopia, and certain fundus images classified as nonpathological myopia still have a certain high myopia risk (such as "simple high myopia" defined in [3]).

2. Materials and Methods

2.1. Data Collection

We referred to the rules of the International Photographic Classification and Grading System for Myopic Maculopathy [12]. Fundus images were classified into three categories according to the risk of disease: normal fundus, low-risk high myopia, and high-risk high myopia. Specifically, the label of normal fundus was class 0, and there are no significant lesions in this category. Low-risk high myopia was labeled class 1 based on the presence of tessellated fundus. High-risk high myopia was labeled class 2 due to the presence of more severe lesions in the fundus. These severe lesions include diffuse chorioretinal atrophy, patchy chorioretinal atrophy, and macular atrophy. Additional features such as lacquer cracks, choroidal neovascularization, and Fuchs spot were considered to be plus signs that did not fit into any particular category and could develop from or occur in any category.

The dataset used in this study was provided by the Affiliated Eye Hospital of Nanjing Medical University. All the images were obtained from multiple models of nonmydriatic fundus cameras, and the resolution of each image ranged from 512×512 to 2584×2000. There were no restrictions on the age or gender of the patients represented by the images. Our study followed the principles of the Declaration of Helsinki. The collected images were all anonymized, i.e., all the patient-related personal information was removed to avoid infringing on patient privacy; thus, there were no relevant patient statistics. The true label of each fundus image was decided upon by two ophthalmologists using the double-blind approach. Two identical diagnoses from the physicians formed the final result. When the two physicians provided different diagnoses, the judgment of an additional expert ophthalmologist was used as the final result.

The dataset used in this study included 858 color fundus images of patients of all ages. In order to exclude subjective factors, we used a random number seed to randomly divide all the fundus images into dataset A and dataset B. Dataset A was used to train the deep convolutional neural networks (DCNNs), and dataset B was the external validation dataset, which was used to compare the diagnostic performance of the intelligent model with that of the human expert. The intuitive distribution of data categories is shown in Table 1.

Table 1. Distribution information of datasets. Dataset A was used for training, and dataset B was used for external validation.

	Dataset A	Dataset B
Class 0	233	26
Class 1	339	53
Class 2	186	21
Total	758	100

2.2. Model Development

A total of 758 fundus images from dataset A were used to train the assisted diagnostic model. The trained DCNNs model can be used to efficiently obtain diagnostic results, i.e., for an input fundus image, the model automatically outputs the category to which the image belongs, namely the risk level of high myopia as predicted by the model. As the clinical data were collected from different camera instruments, the image resolution varied. Therefore, we first adjusted the size of all images to 224 × 224 for normalization, and carried out a series of preprocessing operations to enhance feature expression. These preprocessing operations mainly consisted of the following steps: quality assessment, contrast enhancement, image denoising, mean normalization, and variance normalization. Thereafter, we used the designed DCNNs for feature extraction and classification. The architecture of our proposed DCNNs is shown in Figure 1. Its basic network structure includes a convolution layer, a maximum/average pooling layer, a batch normalization layer, an activation layer, and a fully connected layer. Because the sample size of dataset A (which was used for training) was relatively small, there was a high risk of overfitting when the network model had too many parameters or too many layers. That is to say that when the accuracy of a network model on the training set is very high but the accuracy on a new dataset that has not been seen is very low, it does not have a powerful generalization ability. Therefore, the proposed DCNNs are mainly composed of a head convolution layer Conv1 and four continuous convolution modules named BasicBlocks. There are additional shortcut connections between the four convolution modules. Adding a shortcut connection is equivalent to adding all the information of the image of the previous layer in each block. To some extent, more original information is retained, and the possibility of a vanishing gradient problem in back propagation can be reduced. The final output of the fully connected layer was changed to three categories to accommodate the risk classification task of this study.

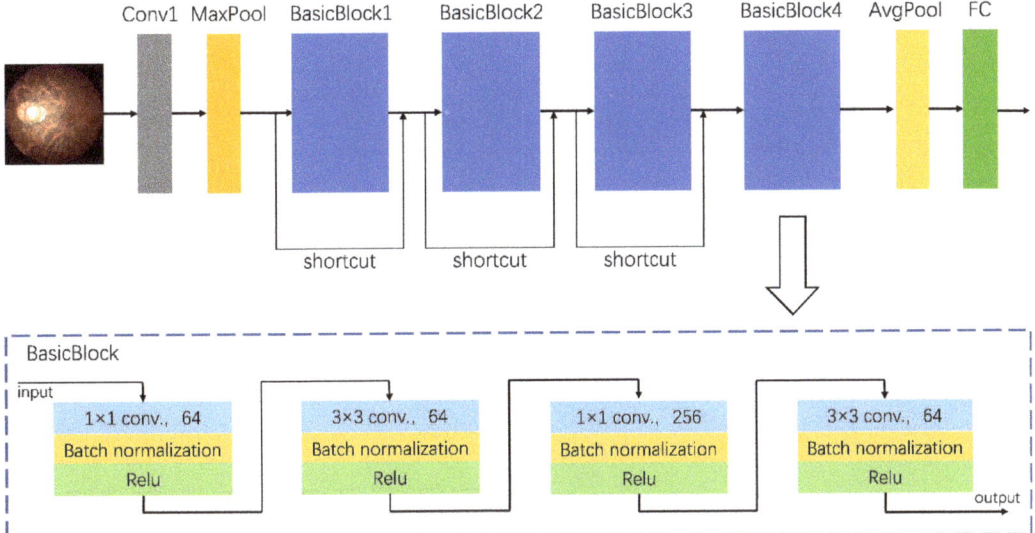

Figure 1. The architecture of the proposed deep convolutional neural networks. The grey block represents the input convolutional layer. The yellow blocks represent the maximum pooling layer or the average pooling layer. The blue blocks are four convolutional basic blocks whose detailed structure is shown at the bottom of the figure. The green block is the final full connected layer used for classification.

Experimental hardware: the CPU used was 3.60 GHz Intel(R) Core (TM) i7-7700 (Intel, Santa Clara, CA, USA); the GPU was NVIDIA GeForce RTX 2080-Ti (Micro-Star, Xinbei, China) with 16 GB of memory. Experimental software: the operating system used was Windows 7 × 64 (Windows 7, Microsoft, Redmond, WA, USA). The DCNNs model was built based on Pytorch (https://pytorch.org/, accessed on 17 July 2021) with Python

(Python 3.6.5, Python Software Foundation, Delaware, DE, USA). In the training process, the limited amount of training data increased the probability of an overfitting problem. In order to prevent overfitting and enhance the robustness of the model, we augmented the training data in many different ways, including random horizontal and vertical flips, rotating in random directions, and modifying the brightness, contrast, and saturation to cause color disturbances, etc. A total of 758 images from dataset A were augmented, and the number of samples after augmentation was five times the original, that is, a total of 3790 samples were utilized in the training process. The training process used fivefold cross-validation, with 80% of the samples used for training and 20% used for validation in each iteration. Furthermore, we adopted the label-smoothing regularization [13] and dropout [14] methods to further prevent overfitting. The total number of epochs in the training process was set to 100, and the initial learning rate was 0.000002. The learning rate was updated by adopting a strategy combining warm-up [13] and cosine annealing. The optimizer was RAdam [15], and the weight decay was set to 0.001.

2.3. Statistical Analysis

The collected data were randomly divided into two datasets: dataset A and dataset B. Model training was carried out on dataset A (a total of 758 images). Since the number of collected fundus images was relatively small, we needed to make full use of the data information to train DCNNs. Therefore, we adopted fivefold cross-validation in the training process. The specific steps were as described further. Dataset A was randomly divided into five parts. Each time, four parts were selected as the training set, and the remaining part was used as the test set. The cross-validation was repeated five times, and the average accuracy after the five cross-validations was taken as the final evaluation result of the DCNNs. The variance was reduced by averaging the results of the five different training groups. This way, the performance of the model was less sensitive to the division of data, and overfitting was reduced. On the other hand, cross-validation went through more iterations and thus avoided underfitting to some extent. The process of fivefold cross-validation is shown in Figure 2. This can effectively avoid the occurrence of overfitting and underfitting problems.

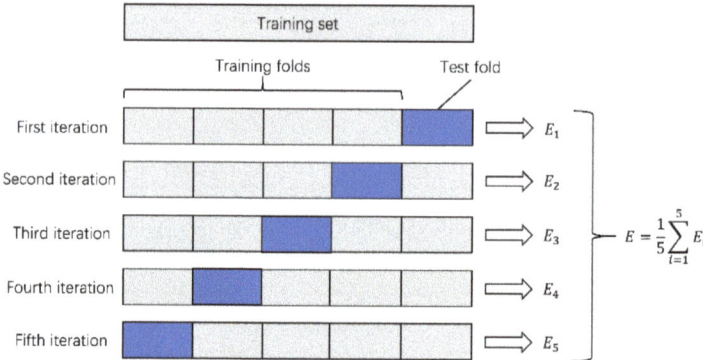

Figure 2. The process of fivefold cross-validation.

The 100 fundus images in dataset B were not used in the training process; instead, they were used as an additional test set for external validation. The 100 images were randomly selected by a computer program without any subjective bias, and the sample size of this study was calculated based on the sample size of previous studies. In order to evaluate the diagnostic level of our proposed algorithm in the real world, we compared the DCNNs model with another human expert. The human expert that participated in the external validation was a Chinese practicing physician who specialized in the clinical diagnosis and treatment of ophthalmic diseases. It should be noted that this human expert classified the cases independently and did not overlap with the group of ophthalmologists that annotated the dataset during the data collection process. To reduce the risk of prejudice caused by prior knowledge, the human expert was only allowed to observe the fundus lesions to determine the risk level of high myopia, without knowing the label information of the images or the patients' medical history. The label of each fundus image was judged as "normal" (class 0), "low-risk high myopia" (class 1), or "high-risk high myopia" (class 2), which was consistent with the classification standard of the DCNNs model. Finally, we recorded the diagnosis results of the human expert and compared them with the results of the DCNNs model.

We used a confusion matrix and receiver operating characteristic (ROC) curves to evaluate the classification performance. The confusion matrix placed the predicted labels and the true labels in the same table by category. In this table, we could clearly see the number of correct identifications and misidentifications in each category. Moreover, the area under the curve (AUC) value calculated using ROC curves could be used to evaluate the performance of a classifier. The closer the AUC is to 1.0, the better the classification effect. The number of true-positive (TP), true-negative (TN), false-positive (FP), and false-negative (FN) samples from each category was calculated using the confusion matrix, and accuracy, sensitivity, specificity, positive predicted value (PPV), and negative predicted value (NPV) could be easily calculated.

This was a multiclass (class 0, 1, 2) classification task. However, most of the aforementioned evaluation indicators are applicable to binary classification with only positive and negative classes. Therefore, we used two methods to evaluate the results of the multi-class classification task. One of the methods involved transforming the multiclassification problem into multiple separate binary classification problems, i.e., for the identification of low-risk high myopia, we only regarded the images labeled class 1 as positive samples; other images (class 0 and class 2) were regarded as negative samples. Similarly, for the identification of high-risk high myopia, only images labeled class 2 were treated as positive samples, while other images (class 0 and class 1) were treated as negative samples. Another method involved using multiclassification indicators directly defined by the kappa score and the Jaccard score to assess the overall performance. The calculation of the kappa score was based on the confusion matrix; its definition is as follows:

$$kappa = \frac{p_o - p_e}{1 - p_e} \qquad (1)$$

where p_o represents the total classification accuracy, and the representation of p_e is:

$$p_e = \frac{a_1 \times b_1 + a_2 \times b_2 + \ldots + a_c \times b_c}{n \times n} \qquad (2)$$

where a_i is the number of real samples of class i; a_i is the number of predicted samples of class i; and n is the total number of samples.

The Jaccard score measures the similarity between two sets of A and B as follows:

$$\text{Jaccard}(A, B) = \frac{|A \cap B|}{|A \cup B|} = \frac{|A \cap B|}{|A| + |B| - |A \cap B|} \qquad (3)$$

where the sets A and B represent the true label set and the predicted label set of all the samples, respectively.

2.4. Diagnosis Visualization

In order to more intuitively analyze the influence of each area in a fundus image on the classification results, analyze the causes of wrong classification, and reasonably explain certain seemingly unreasonable results output by the model, we used gradient weighted class activation mapping (Grad-CAM++) [16] to perform visual analysis of the DCNNs.

Class activation mapping (CAM) is a visual analysis method that expresses the importance of each pixel to the image classification in the form of a heat map by performing a weighted summation on the feature maps corresponding to the network weights. However, CAM needs to modify the network structure and retrain the model. Considering the simplicity of the practical application, we used Grad-CAM++ to conduct the visual analysis in this study. Grad-CAM++ does not need to modify the network structure, and the characteristics learned by the model can be intuitively displayed without reducing the classification accuracy, which makes the model more transparent and interpretable. Specifically, Grad-CAM++ removes the fully connected layer in DCNNs and uses the output of the second-to-last convolutional layer to complete the visualization. It can intuitively display the important areas that are helpful for classification. The more important areas are represented by the warmer colors in the heat map.

3. Results

The model training process was carried out on dataset A (which had 758 images, including 233 normal images, 339 low-risk high myopia images, and 168 high-risk high myopia images) The advantage of cross-validation is that the randomly generated subsamples are repeatedly used for training and validation at the same time, and the results are validated once each time. Thus, the accuracy of the algorithm can be estimated more accurately, and a more reliable and robust model can be obtained. The detailed quantitative results of our proposed DCNNs are shown in Table 2.

Table 2. Quantitative results of the proposed model on dataset A. Fold 0, fold 1, fold 2, fold 3, and fold 4 are the respective results in the fivefold cross-validation experiment.

	Training Loss	Training Accuracy	Valid Loss	Valid Accuracy
Fold 0	0.0026	100%	0.0369	98.68%
Fold 1	0.0026	100%	0.1295	96.69%
Fold 2	0.0044	100%	0.0560	98.01%
Fold 3	0.0042	100%	0.0423	98.68%
Fold 4	0.0017	100%	0.0401	98.00%
Average	0.0031	100%	0.0618	98.15%

In this study, 100 fundus images (26 normal images, 53 low-risk high myopia images, and 21 high-risk high myopia images) were randomly chosen for external validation. The vertical axis of the confusion matrix in Figure 3 is the true label, while the horizontal axis is the predicted label. In the confusion matrix in Figure 3, we can see that the number of correctly classified images located on the main diagonal in the confusion matrix of the DCNNs is significantly higher than that corresponding to the confusion matrix of the human expert. For the classification of the 26 normal fundus images, the results of the DCNNs were all correct, whereas the human expert only correctly classified 23 images and wrongly classified three images as low-risk high myopia. Using the confusion matrix, we were able to easily calculate the sensitivity, specificity, and other indicators. The performances of the DCNNs were compared with those of the human expert using descriptive statistics. All of the statistical tests in our study were two-sided, and a p-value less than 0.05 was considered significant. In terms of the overall classification accuracy, the correct and incorrect samples in the human expert diagnosis accounted for 93% and 7%, respectively. After using the DCNNs, the correct rate of diagnosis increased to 99% and the incorrect rate decreased to 1%. Seven samples that were incorrectly diagnosed by the human expert were correctly diagnosed using the DCNNs, and one sample that was correctly diagnosed by the human expert was incorrectly diagnosed after using DCNNs. McNemar's test showed that there was a statistically significant difference in the proportion of correct diagnoses before and after the DCNNs were used.

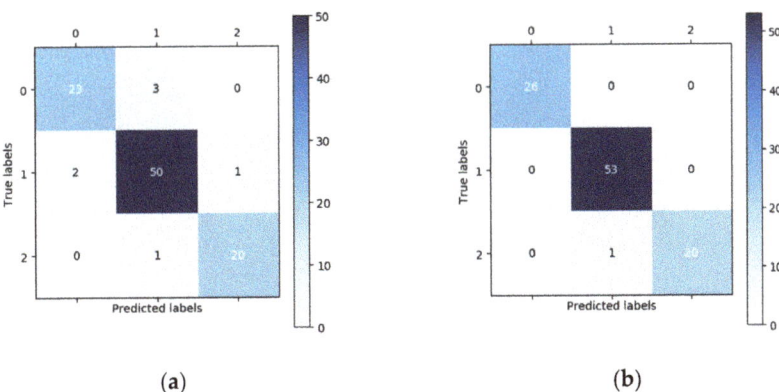

(a)　　　　　　　　　　　　　　(b)

Figure 3. Comparison of the classification performance of the DCNNs and the human expert in the external validation of dataset B. The results are shown as a confusion matrix in which the vertical axis represents the true labels and the horizontal axis represents the predicted labels. (**a**) The confusion matrix of the human expert. (**b**) The confusion matrix of the DCNNs.

Since the purpose of this study was to correctly identify high myopia images and decide upon risk classification, we only show the performance comparison between the DCNNs and the human expert as regards predicting low-risk high myopia (class 1) and high-risk high myopia (class 2). The specific results are shown in Tables 3 and 4. For the recognition of low-risk high myopia images (class 1), the DCNNs model had a superior performance in most indicators; the sensitivity and the NPV of the DCNNs were both 100%, while the sensitivity and the NPV of the human expert were 94.34% and 93.48%, respectively. For the recognition of high-risk high myopia images (class 2), the DCNNs model had a comparable sensitivity of 97.83% and an NPV of 98.75%, which is equivalent to those of the human expert. However, the DCNNs performed very well in specificity and PPV, both of which were 100%. It can also be seen from the ROC curves in Figure 4 that our proposed DCNNs had an AUC of 0.9968 for the recognition of low-risk high myopia and 0.9964 for the recognition of high-risk high myopia. Moreover, the sensitivity–specificity points corresponding to the human expert were all below the black curves corresponding to the DCNNs, which indicates that the DCNNs achieved a superior performance as compared to the human expert.

Table 3. Accuracy, sensitivity, specificity, PPV, and NPV of the recognition of low-risk high myopia (class 1).

	Accuracy	Sensitivity	Specificity	PPV	NPV
Human	93.00%	94.34%	91.48%	92.59%	93.48%
DCNNs	99.00%	100.00%	97.87%	98.14%	100.00%

Table 4. Accuracy, sensitivity, specificity, PPV, and NPV of the recognition of high-risk high myopia (class 2).

	Accuracy	Sensitivity	Specificity	PPV	NPV
Human	98.00%	95.24%	98.73%	95.23%	98.73%
DCNNs	99.00%	95.24%	100.00%	100.00%	98.75%

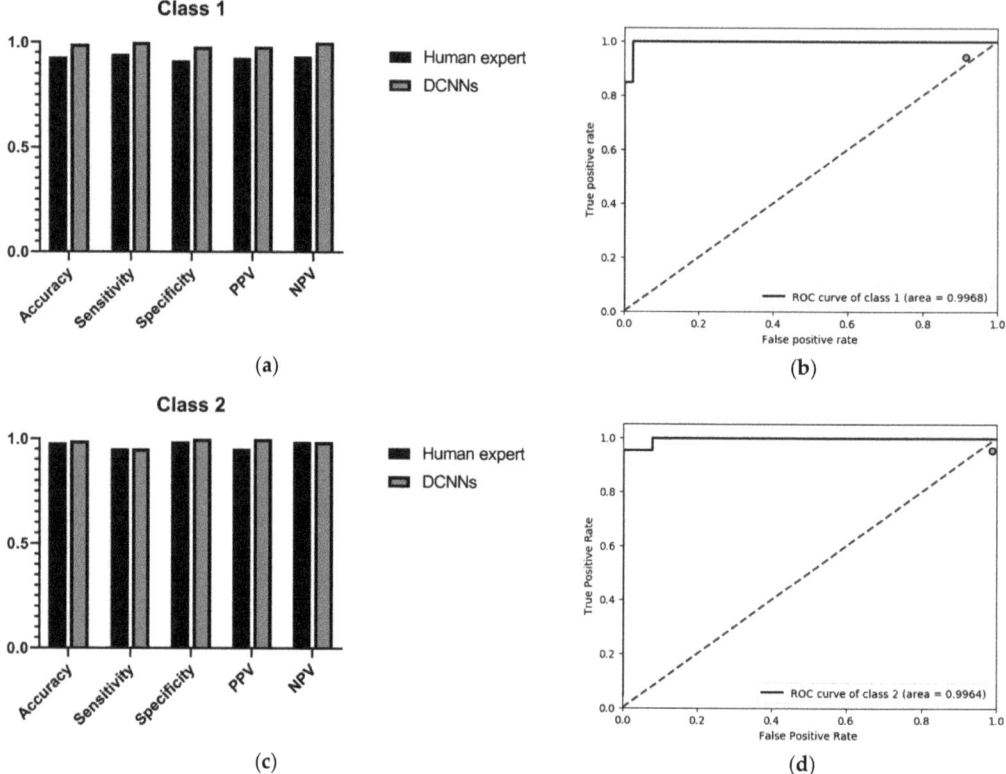

Figure 4. Evaluation results in the external validation dataset B. (**a**) Accuracy, sensitivity, specificity, PPV, NPV of the recognition of class 1; (**b**) ROC curves and AUC value of the recognition of class 1; (**c**) accuracy, sensitivity, specificity, PPV, NPV of the recognition of class 2; (**d**) ROC curves and AUC value of the recognition of Class 2.

In addition to transforming the multiclassification problem into several separate binary classification problems, we also directly introduced two multiclassification indicators to assess the overall performance: the kappa score and the Jaccard score. The kappa score is a method used in statistics to evaluate consistency. The higher the kappa value, the higher the classification accuracy of the algorithm. The Jaccard score is used to compare the similarities and differences between finite sample sets. In this study, we compared the similarities between the ground-truth set of the validation images and the corresponding prediction set. The larger the Jaccard score, the higher the sample similarity. We compared the performance of the DCNNs with that of the human expert in Table 5. The experimental results showed that both the kappa and Jaccard scores of the DCNNs were significantly better than those of the human expert.

Table 5. Overall performance of the multiclassification task.

	Kappa Score	Jaccard Score
Human	0.8842	0.8693
DCNNs	0.9834	0.9801

As shown in Figure 5, we used gradient activation heatmap Grad-CAM++ to analyze the fundus image area. From left to right, we can see the original fundus image, the corresponding heatmap, and the corresponding gradient activation heatmap (Grad-CAM++)

superimposed on the original image area. The warmer the color in the heatmap, the greater the influence on the classification prediction result. Figure 5a shows a high-risk high myopia fundus image with severe lesions, including diffuse chorioretinal atrophy, patchy chorioretinal atrophy, and macular atrophy. We can see that the DCNNs mainly focused on the macular area and the area of choroidal atrophy, rather than the background or other parts in the fundus.

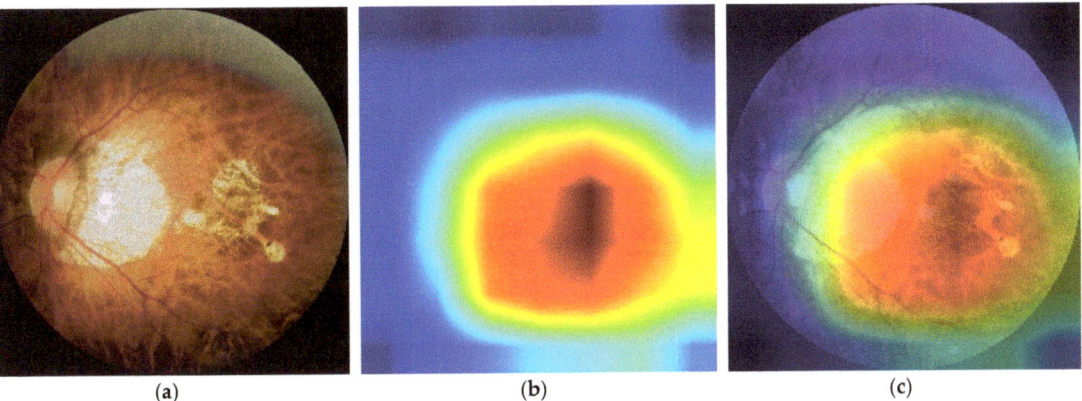

Figure 5. Visualization-based diagnosis by the DCNNs. (**a**) Original image. (**b**) Heatmap. (**c**) Grad-CAM++. Heatmaps and Grad-CAM++ showed that the DCNNs model focused on the macular area and the area of choroidal atrophy rather than the background.

4. Discussion

This study shows that the DCNNs model can be trained to detect high myopia and identify subtle lesion features in retinal fundus images in order to diagnose the risk of high myopia. Traditionally, myopia is diagnosed and classified through functional examinations (e.g., eye tests, optometry, microscopic field of vision tests, electrophysiological assessments) [17] or ocular coherence tomography (OCT), retinal autofluorescence (AF), fluorescein angiography (FA), or indocyanine green angiography (ICGA), which analyze the morphological changes of suspected pathological myopia [17]. Experimental results show that the DCNNs model is superior to or equivalent to a human expert in terms of accuracy, sensitivity, specificity, PPV, NPV, and other indicators. As compared with time-consuming and labor-intensive manual assisted examinations, the proposed method can reduce costs and improve diagnostic efficiency and accuracy. In addition, regarding the risk classification of high myopia, ophthalmologists are susceptible to subjective cognition and empirical impressions, which can lead to great differences in classification. The DCNNs model only performs feature extraction and prediction from the image level. It only needs to specify a standardized grading standard when labeling the training data, and the DCNNs model can give a prediction result that meets the grading standard.

As can be seen from Table 1, the fivefold training losses were very small, and the training accuracy remained at 100%, which indicates that the network model could adequately fit the training data. As a result of the relatively small size of the training dataset, we must pay attention to the possible overfitting problem. The average validation accuracy of the DCNNs was 98.15% according to the results of fivefold cross-validation, indicating that the model has good robustness. In the external validation set, we performed a classification performance comparison between the DCNNs and the human expert, which highlights the progress and practical significance of our method. In the randomly acquired external validation set, low-risk high myopia (class 1) accounted for more than half of the images. The unbalanced category distribution greatly increased the difficulty of classification. The confusion matrices in Figure 3 show that the human expert misdiagnosed three normal images as low-risk high myopia, missed two low-risk myopia cases and confused two images of low-risk and high-risk high myopia. The DCNNs correctly identified almost all the images, except for one that was considered to be a high-risk case image when in fact it was low-risk. On the one hand, when transforming the multiclassification problem into several separate binary classification problems, whether using the quantitative indicators such as accuracy, specificity, sensitivity, NPV, and PPV or the intuitive comparison of ROC curves, the DCNNs achieved a better or equal classification level as compared with the human expert. On the other hand, when directly using the kappa and Jaccard scores for the overall assessment of multiclassification problems, the scores of the DCNNs were both above 0.98, i.e., significantly better than those of the human expert. Since there are no clinical "gold standards" for the risk classification of high myopia, different ophthalmologists may have very different judgments due to the influence of subjective cognition and experience. As compared with ophthalmologists, DCNNs can always give prediction results that meet the given grading standards, which are not susceptible to other subjective factors and have higher generalization ability. The visualization results in Figure 5 show that the DCNNs model is hardly affected by the background when performing classification and mainly focuses on the macular area and the surrounding area of the optic disc in the fundus image. These areas are also the focus of the pathological characteristics of the fundus with high myopia, indicating that the classification of DCNNs is interpretable.

Most computer-aided algorithms for detecting high myopia are designed for binary classification. There are algorithms that only distinguish between normal and high myopia, or algorithms that only distinguish between normal and pathological myopia. However, it is also of great practical significance to classify the risk grade of high myopia. High myopia has obvious clinical manifestations, and physicians can easily judge whether there is high myopia based on the level of vision. However, assessing the severity of high myopia is a more challenging task. Even experienced ophthalmologists need to take great care in their observations in order to make a diagnosis. As compared with the model proposed by Dai [7] that judges the severity of high myopia according to two branches, our method achieves direct end-to-end classification and has significant advantages related to prediction speed. The real-world clinical value and utility of this study are as follows: the proposed intelligent classification model can be used in community hospitals and eye health institutions, such as physical examination institutions, and optician shops. When community doctors or staff at an institution collect fundus images, they will be able to predict the risk of high myopia and make recommendations to the patient, including certain recommendations regarding referrals.

Our study has several advantages. First, our DCNNs model can automatically determine the risk classification of high myopia. Using only retinal fundus images, it achieved a better diagnostic accuracy than a human expert. Moreover, it can automatically process data without manual assistance and with higher execution efficiency. Second, our model focuses on extracting morphological features from the image and making a prediction. This is not easily affected by subjective cognition and experience. No matter what grading standard is given, the prediction results of the network model are always consistent with the grading standard used to label the training data. Third, we applied the deep learning technology for the first time to classify the risk of high myopia. Not only did we automatically detect high myopia in the fundus images, but we also predicted its severity, which has a great clinical significance in real-life situations.

This study has several limitations. First, the distribution of sample categories was uneven. Low-risk high myopia images accounted for the largest proportion in the dataset, but normal fundus images would be the most common in real-life screening scenarios. In the confusion matrix, it can be seen that the diagnosis accuracy of the human expert for low-risk high myopia was lower than for high-risk high myopia. In future research, a larger sample size, a more balanced sample distribution, and more increased training data are required in order to improve the classification accuracy of our model. Second, the application of the DCNNs model needs to be evaluated using different ethnic groups in order to verify the robustness of our model in the risk classification of high myopia.

The research objects in this paper were all Asian, and, due to the limited dataset, no validation experiments on other races were conducted. Third, as a result of differences in the symptoms of high myopia in adolescents and elderly people, in the future, age, gender, family genetic history, and other factors should be considered when building intelligent models in order to improve the algorithm performance in the high myopia risk classification task.

5. Conclusions

Herein, we propose a method for risk classification of high myopia based on a DCNNs deep learning model which can automatically classify fundus images into three categories: normal, low-risk high myopia, and high-risk high myopia. The proposed method achieved a diagnosis accuracy superior to that of a human expert. Moreover, we applied the deep learning technology to the risk classification of high myopia for the first time. We believe that this method can be widely used in myopia screening and could be of great significance to clinical practice. This approach allows for the efficient and effective prediction of high myopia severity, which is conductive to assessing the potential risk and providing timely treatment.

Author Contributions: Conceptualization, G.-F.C., Q.J. and W.-H.Y.; methodology, C.W. and W.-H.Y.; software, H.L.; validation, H.L.; formal analysis, C.W. and W.-H.Y.; investigation, H.L.; resources, G.-F.C., Q.J. and W.-H.Y.; data curation, C.W. and W.-H.Y.; writing—original draft preparation, H.L.; writing—review and editing, C.W. and H.L.; visualization, H.L.; supervision, G.-F.C., Q.J. and W.-H.Y.; project administration, C.W. and W.-H.Y.; funding acquisition, C.W., G.-F.C., Q.J. and W.-H.Y. All authors have read and agreed to the published version of the manuscript.

Funding: This research was funded by the Chinese Postdoctoral Science Foundation, grant number 2019M661832; the Jiangsu Planned Projects for Postdoctoral Research Funds, grant number 2019K226; the Jiangsu Province Advantageous Subject Construction Project; the Nanjing Enterprise Expert Team Project.

Institutional Review Board Statement: Not applicable.

Informed Consent Statement: Informed consent was obtained from all the subjects involved in the study.

Data Availability Statement: The datasets analyzed during the current study are available from the corresponding author upon reasonable request.

Acknowledgments: The materials in this work were partly supported by the Affiliated Eye Hospital of Nanjing Medical University. The authors thank the data authors for providing valuable data.

Conflicts of Interest: The authors declare that there is no conflict of interest regarding the publication of this article.

References

1. Holden, B.A.; Fricke, T.R.; Wilson, D.A.; Jong, M.; Naidoo, K.S.; Sankaridurg, P.; Wong, T.Y.; Naduvilath, T.; Resnikoff, S. Global Prevalence of Myopia and High Myopia and Temporal Trends from 2000 through 2050. *Ophthalmology* **2016**, *123*, 1036–1042. [CrossRef] [PubMed]
2. Pan, C.W.; Dirani, M.; Cheng, C.Y.; Wong, T.Y.; Saw, S.M. The age-specific prevalence of myopia in Asia: A meta-analysis. *Optom. Vis. Sci.* **2015**, *92*, 258–266. [CrossRef]
3. Chinese Optometric Association. Expert consensus on the importance of prevention and control of high myopia. *Chin. J. Optom. Ophthalmol. Vis. Sci.* **2017**, *19*, 385–389. [CrossRef]
4. Ikuno, Y. Overview of The Complications of High Myopia. *Retina* **2017**, *37*, 2347–2351. [CrossRef]
5. Liu, J.; Wong, D.W.K.; Lim, J.H.; Tan, N.M.; Zhang, Z.; Li, H.; Yin, F.; Lee, B.; Saw, S.M.; Tong, L.; et al. Detection of Pathological Myopia by PAMELA with Texture-Based Features through an SVM Approach. *J. Healthc. Eng.* **2010**, *1*, 657574. [CrossRef]
6. Varadarajan, A.V.; Poplin, R.; Blumer, K.; Angermueller, C.; Ledsam, J.; Chopra, R.; Keane, P.A.; Corrado, G.S.; Peng, L.; Webster, D.R. Deep Learning for Predicting Refractive Error From Retinal Fundus Images. *Investig. Opthalmology Vis. Sci.* **2018**, *59*, 2861–2868. [CrossRef] [PubMed]
7. Dai, S.; Chen, L.; Lei, T.; Zhou, C.; Wen, Y. Automatic Detection Of Pathological Myopia And High Myopia On Fundus Images. In Proceedings of the 2020 IEEE International Conference on Multimedia and Expo (ICME), London, UK, 6–10 July 2020; pp. 1–6.

8. Huazhu, F.; Fei, L.; José, I.O. PALM: PAthoLogic Myopia Challenge. *Comput. Vis. Med. Imaging* **2019**. [CrossRef]
9. Freire, C.R.; Moura, J.C.C.; Barros, D.M.S. Automatic Lesion Segmentation and Pathological Myopia Classification in Fundus Images. *arXiv* **2020**, arXiv:2002.06382.
10. Hemelings, R.; Elen, B.; Blaschko, M.B.; Jacob, J.; Stalmans, I.; De Boever, P. Pathological myopia classification with simultaneous lesion segmentation using deep learning. *Comput. Methods Programs Biomed.* **2021**, *199*, 105920. [CrossRef] [PubMed]
11. Devda, J.; Eswari, R. Pathological Myopia Image Analysis Using Deep Learning. *Procedia Comput. Sci.* **2019**, *165*, 239–244. [CrossRef]
12. Ohno-Matsui, K.; Kawasaki, R.; Jonas, J.B.; Cheung, C.M.; Saw, S.M.; Verhoeven, V.J.; Klaver, C.C.; Moriyama, M.; Shinohara, K.; Kawasaki, Y.; et al. International Photographic Classification and Grading System for Myopic Maculopathy. *Am. J. Ophthalmol.* **2015**, *159*, 877–883. [CrossRef] [PubMed]
13. He, T.; Zhang, Z.; Zhang, H.; Zhang, Z.; Xie, J.; Li, M. Bag of Tricks for Image Classification with Convolutional Neural Networks. In Proceedings of the 2019 IEEE/CVF Conference on Computer Vision and Pattern Recognition (CVPR), Long Beach, CA, USA, 15–20 June 2019; pp. 558–567.
14. Srivastava, N.; Hinton, G.; Krizhevsky, A.; Sutskever, I.; Salakhutdinov, R. Dropout: A simple way to prevent neural networks from overfitting. *J. Mach. Learn. Res.* **2014**, *15*, 1929–1958.
15. Liu, L.; Jiang, H.; He, P. On the Variance of the Adaptive Learning Rate and Beyond. *arXiv* **2019**, arXiv:1908.03265.
16. Chattopadhay, A.; Sarkar, A.; Howlader, P.; Balasubramanian, V.N. Grad-cam++: Generalized gradient-based visual explanations for deep convolutional networks. In Proceedings of the IEEE Winter Conference on Applications of Computer Vision, Nevada, CA, USA, 12–14 March 2018; pp. 839–847.
17. Flitcroft, D.I.; He, M.; Jonas, J.B.; Jong, M.; Naidoo, K.; Ohno-Matsui, K.; Rahi, J.; Resnikoff, S.; Vitale, S.; Yannuzzi, L. IMI–Defining and classifying myopia: A proposed set of standards for clinical and epidemiologic studies. *Investig. Ophthalmol. Vis. Sci.* **2019**, *60*, M20–M30. [CrossRef] [PubMed]

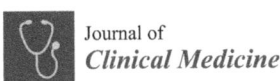

Review

Differences between *Mycobacterium chimaera* and *tuberculosis* Using Ocular Multimodal Imaging: A Systematic Review

Sandrine Anne Zweifel [1,2,*], Nastasia Foa [1], Maximilian Robert Justus Wiest [1,2], Adriano Carnevali [3], Katarzyna Zaluska-Ogryzek [4], Robert Rejdak [5,†] and Mario Damiano Toro [1,5,†]

1. Department of Ophthalmology, University Hospital Zurich, Frauenklinikstrasse 24, 8091 Zurich, Switzerland; foa.nastasia@gmail.com (N.F.); maximilian.wiest@usz.ch (M.R.J.W.); toro.mario@email.it (M.D.T.)
2. University of Zurich, 8091 Zurich, Switzerland
3. Department of Ophthalmology, University Magna Grecia of Catanzaro, 88100 Catanzaro, Italy; adrianocarnevali@unicz.it
4. Department of Pathophysiology, Medical University of Lublin, 20090 Lublin, Poland; katarzyna.zaluska-ogryzek@umlub.pl
5. Chair and Department of General and Pediatric Ophthalmology, Medical University of Lublin, 20079 Lublin, Poland; robertrejdak@yahoo.com
* Correspondence: sandrine.zweifel@usz.ch
† These authors equally contributed as last authors.

Abstract: Due to their non-specific diagnostic patterns of ocular infection, differential diagnosis between *Mycobacterium* (*M.*) *chimaera* and *tuberculosis* can be challenging. In both disorders, ocular manifestation can be the first sign of a systemic infection, and a delayed diagnosis might reduce the response to treatment leading to negative outcomes. Thus, it becomes imperative to distinguish chorioretinal lesions associated with *M. chimaera*, from lesions due to *M. tuberculosis* and other infectious disorders. To date, multimodal non-invasive imaging modalities that include ultra-wide field fundus photography, fluorescein and indocyanine green angiography, optical coherence tomography and optical coherence tomography angiography, facilitate in vivo examination of retinal and choroidal tissues, enabling early diagnosis, monitoring treatment response, and relapse detection. This approach is crucial to differentiate between active and inactive ocular disease, and guides clinicians in their decisional-tree during the patients' follow-up. In this review, we summarized and compared the available literature on multimodal imaging data of *M. chimaera* infection and tuberculosis, emphasizing similarities and differences in imaging patterns between these two entities and highlighting the relevance of multimodal imaging in the management of the infections.

Keywords: mycobacterium; multifocal choroiditis; fundus photography; biomicroscopy; multimodal imaging; fundus fluorescein angiography; indocyanine green angiography; fundus autofluorescence; optical coherence tomography angiography; optical coherence tomography

1. Introduction

Mycobacterium (M.) belongs to the genus of Actinobacteria, which consists of over 190 species, some of them causing serious health diseases in humans [1]. The most common pathogen is *M. tuberculosis*, which has a panoply of systemic manifestations, including ocular manifestations [1,2]. First discovered in 1882 by Robert Koch, *M. tuberculosis* is an intracellular slow-growing pathogen transmitted via the inhalation of aerosolized, bacteria-containing droplets. It is the etiologic agent of tuberculosis (TB), which remains a significant global public health burden [2–4].

In the last few years, *Mycobacterium chimaera*, a non-tuberculous mycobacterium (NTM), has gained awareness because of a worldwide hospital-acquired outbreak of disseminated infections following open-heart surgery [5–10]. *M. chimaera* is a non-tuberculous, slow-growing, mycobacterium that belongs to the Mycobacterium avium complex

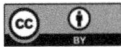

(MAC) [6,11,12]. Before its first identification, owing to ambiguous genetic features characterizing its strains, it had been wrongly identified as *M. avium*, *M. scrofulaceum*, or *M. intracellulare* by most of the clinical microbiology laboratories [5,11]. *M. chimaera* acts as an opportunistic pathogen. Before 2013, this mycobacterium was known to cause respiratory infections in immunocompromised individuals [5,6]. Since 2013, there has been an unprecedented increase in the incidence of *M. chimaera* infections, especially among individuals undergoing cardiopulmonary bypass surgery. It is primarily transmitted via thermoregulatory components of extracorporeal membrane oxygenation (ECMO) systems and water tanks of heater-cooler units (HCUs) [5,6]. With increased usage of ECMO systems and the ability to distinguish *M. chimaera* from other MAC bacteria, more attention has been given to this strain [5,11]. The first cases were observed in Switzerland in 2013. However, since then, *M. chimaera* affected cases have been reported in 11 other countries, including Canada, the USA, Europe, and Australia [11,12].

Both *M. chimaera* and *M. tuberculosis* cause disseminated infections, inducing granulomatous inflammation in multiple organs [6,13]. Tuberculosis (TB) generally affects the lungs, but can also affect other parts of the body. Only 10% of TB infections are symptomatic, manifested as a chronic cough along with fever and weight loss. If other organs are involved, a wide range of extra-pulmonary manifestations can also occur [4,13]. For example, ocular TB is a rare extrapulmonary manifestation of TB infection and a great imitator of other ocular pathologies [2]. The reported prevalence of tubercular uveitis varies widely, ranging from 0.2–2.7% in non-endemic regions to 5.6–10.5% in highly endemic regions [6,14,15]. If left untreated, progressive tuberculous infections kill about 50% of those affected [4]. Systemic symptoms and laboratory features of *M. chimaera* infections are also often non-specific and include unexplained low-grade fever, fatigue and sometimes also dyspnea [6]. Similarly, to a TB infection, if other organs are infected, additional organ-specific symptoms can occur [5,13,16,17]. In particular, it has been shown that the infection has a very strong proclivity for the eyes [7–10,18]. If not promptly diagnosed and treated, *M. chimaera* infections often become life-threatening [5,7,9].

While for TB infections, ocular and extraocular involvements have been described (including uveitis, retinal-choroidal lesions, optic neuropathy and endophthalmitis but also orbital, corneal, scleral, eyelid, conjunctival and lacrimal gland involvements) [2], for *M. chimaera* the most common ocular manifestation are chorioretinal lesions; mild anterior and intermediate uveitis and optic disc swelling. Secondary complications include macular and retinal neovascularization. Zweifel et al. [7,9] have demonstrated that choroidal manifestation lesions seem to reflect systemic disease activity and can be used as an early diagnostic biomarker for assessment of treatment efficacy [6–10].

To date, limited data exists about *M. chimaera* infections, a rare and often-lethal disease. Ophthalmologists should be aware of this recently described entity and its systemic and ocular findings. They may play a key role for differential diagnosis, for monitoring treatment response and detection of recurrences after discontinuation or adjustment of treatment due to adverse drug effect.

Differential diagnosis of ocular lesions can be often challenging, thus in this review we summarized and compared the available literature on ocular multimodal imaging data of *M. chimaera* and TB, emphasizing similarities and differences in imaging patterns between these two entities and highlighting the relevance of multimodal imaging in the management of the infections.

2. Materials and Methods

2.1. Search Methods for Identification of Studies

This systematic review was conducted and reported in accordance with the preferred reporting items for systematic reviews and meta-analyses guidelines [14]. The review protocol was not recorded at study design, and no registration number is available for consultation.

The methodology used for this comprehensive review consisted of a systematic search of all available articles exploring the current available diagnostic tools on M. *tuberculosis* and *chimaera*.

A comprehensive literature search of all original articles published up to August 2021 was performed in parallel by two authors (S.Z. and M.D.T.) using the PubMed, Cochrane library, Embase, and Scopus databases.

For the search strategy, we used the following keywords and Mesh terms: "M. *tuberculosis*", "M. *chimaera*", "Fundus photography", "Biomicroscopy", Fundus Fluorescein angiography", Indocyanine green angiography", "Fundus autofluorescence", "Ocular coherence tomography", and "Optical coherence tomography angiography". Furthermore, the reference lists of all identified articles were examined manually to identify any potential studies that were not captured by the electronic searches.

The search workflow was designed in adherence to the preferred reporting items for systematic reviews and meta-analyses (PRISMA) statement and according previous reports [14–17,19,20].

2.2. Eligibility Criteria

All studies available in the literature, reporting on original data on M. *tuberculosis* and *chimaera* infection with ocular involvement, were included, without restriction for study design, sample size, and intervention performed. Review articles or articles not written in English were excluded.

2.3. Data Collection

After preparation of the list of all electronic data captured, two reviewers (N.F. and M.R.J.W.) examined the titles and abstracts independently and identified relevant articles according to the eligibility criteria. Any disagreement was assessed by consensus and a third reviewer (A.C.) was consulted when necessary.

The reference lists of the analyzed articles were also considered as potential sources of information. For unpublished data, no effort was made to contact the corresponding authors.

3. Results

The results of the search strategy are summarized in Figure 1. From 510 articles extracted from the initial research, 425 abstracts were identified for screening and 41 of these met the inclusion/exclusion criteria for full-text review (Figure 1).

No data synthesis was possible for the heterogeneity of available data and the design of the available studies (i.e., case reports or case series). Thus, the current systematic review reports a qualitative analysis, detailed issue-by-issue below in narrative fashion.

3.1. Fundus Photography and Biomicroscopy

Using both fundus photography and biomicroscopy, chorioretinal lesions can be detected among patients infected by M. *chimaera*, but the extent of these lesions can vary widely [7,9,10]. Some patients have few inactive choroidal lesions, but others develop widespread lesions (progressive ocular disease). The lesions appear white/yellowish and usually have a round or ovoid shape. At the beginning they are usually small (50–300 mm diameter), but their size typically increases over 4 to 8 weeks in active disease. The lesions appear diffusely over both the posterior pole and the retinal periphery and have a particular uniform distribution [7,9,10]. In few patients, a stable period with clinically inactive lesions before progression to active ocular disease can occur. Indistinct borders on fundus photography represent a sign of activity, whereas inactive or quiescent patients have well-defined borders and appear as "punched-out" lesions. Active and inactive lesions, as well as atrophic lesions, can be observed close to each other in the same eye in patients with active ocular disease. Inactive lesions should be monitored as well, as many of them remain quiescent over time, however, after adaptation/stopping of antimycobacterial treatment, recurrence can be observed [9]. Nevertheless, the activity status of *M. chimaera* infection should not be determined only on the basis of biomicroscopy or color fundus photography findings. A comprehensive ophthalmological examination using multimodal imaging is required. Indeed, the diagnosis and monitoring of *M. chimaera* choroiditis require a detailed ophthalmic including wide-angle fundus photography, FA/ICG (if possible, using a wide-angle camera), EDI OCT, FAF and OCTA (if available) as proposed by Böni et al., should be performed [9].

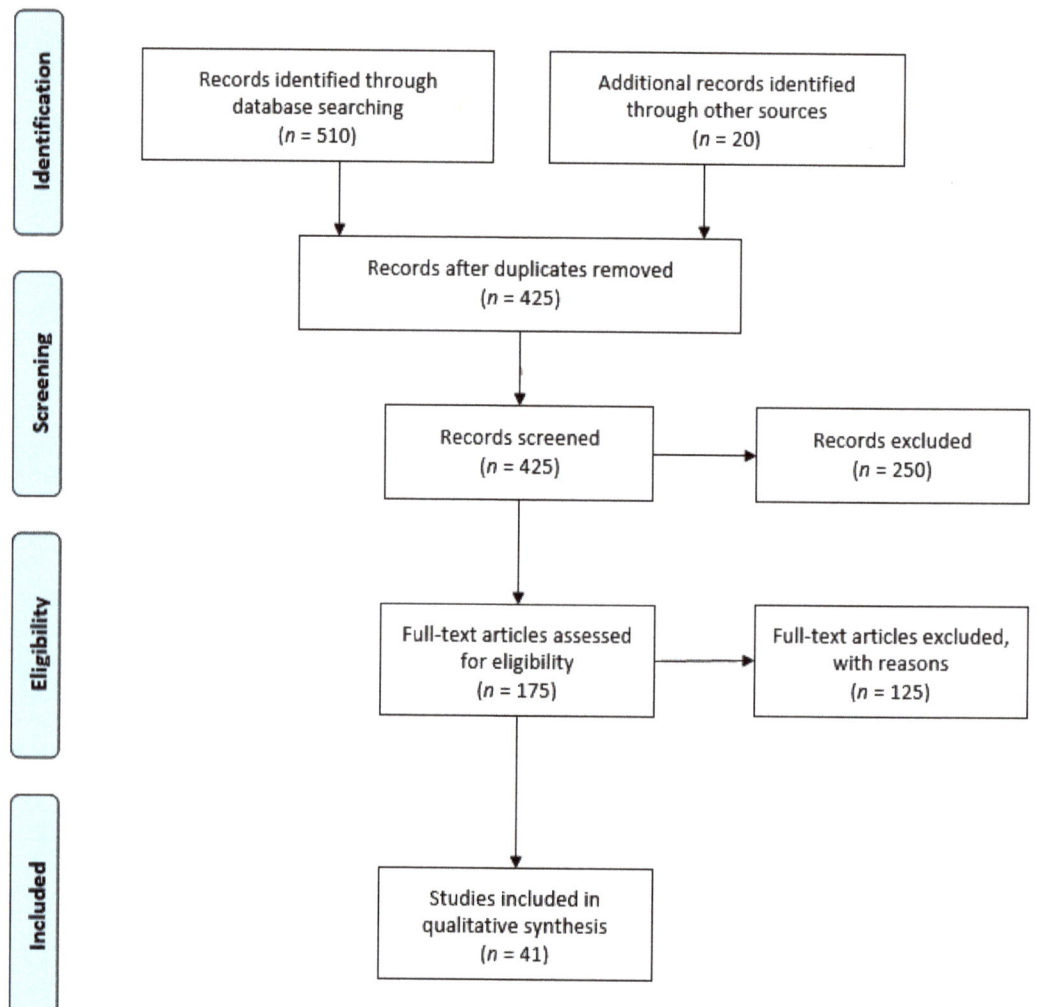

Figure 1. Preferred reporting items for systematic reviews and meta-analyses (PRISMA 2009) flowchart [14].

Biomicroscopy can be used to examine the anterior segment masses, single choroidal masses, or multifocal lesions, serpiginous-like choroiditis (SLC) and retinal vasculitis in intraocular TB patients [21,22]. Tubercle granulomas appear as ill-defined, yellowish, round-to-oval nodules that primarily involve the posterior pol. Furthermore, multiple, non-contiguous choroiditis might develop into a contiguous, diffused pattern called a serpiginous-like lesion, since it looks like serpiginous choroiditis. However, unlike serpiginous choroiditis, the serpiginous-like lesions tend to spare the fovea, are multifocal, and non-contiguous to the optic disc. In addition, unlike serpiginous choroiditis, the tuberculous serpiginous-like choroiditis (TB-SLC) cases exhibit an inflamed vitreous [2,23]. Usually, SLC develops in early to middle aged individuals. Choroidal granulomas are usually unilateral, large, solitary, elevated yellowish subretinal masses resembling a tumor. These granulomas are usually associated with an overlying exudative retinal detachment and located in the posterior fundus.

However, the diagnosis of ocular TB is still challenging, owing to the involvement of mixed tissues and heterogenous infections [24]. The emergence of more advanced TB diagnostic tools, such as IFN-γ release assays, radiodiagnostics, and molecular biology techniques has markedly improved the specificity of ocular TB diagnosis [25]. However, the sensitivity and specificity of current diagnostic tools is still suboptimal, which delays ocular TB diagnosis and treatment. The diagnosis of ocular TB is confirmed only when the causal bacteria are isolated from the ocular tissue. The status of presumed TB uveitis is determined if any of the following signs is observed: choroidal granuloma, retinal vasculitis with or without choroiditis, broad-based posterior synechiae, or serpiginous-like choroiditis (SLC) with a positive tuberculin skin test or QuantiFERON-TB Gold test, or any other relevant tests [26].

The ocular *M. chimaera* infection-induced chorioretinal lesions resemble ocular TB-induced multifocal choroiditis [27,28]. However, *M. chimaera* infection-induced lesions are uniformly distributed and rounded, whereas the TB-induced lesions are irregularly distributed and have variable shapes [9]. In addition, although ocular TB is manifested in several ways, none of the ocular *M. chimaera* cases exhibit any of these manifestations that are indicative of TB.

3.2. Fundus Fluorescein Angiography (FA)

FA shows potential in differentiating active from inactive disease, characterizing choroidal, optic disc, and retinal involvement, detecting complications, and monitoring treatment response [9,23].

The FA analysis of *M. chimaera*-infected cases shows the presence of active choroidal lesions that are hypofluorescent in early frames and stained in the later ones. However, early phase of FA usually shows hyperfluorescence of inactive lesions with hyperfluorescence in late phase according to a window defect. The fluorescent pattern for active and inactive lesions seems to be similar for both diseases. However, the shape and type of lesions, and also their distribution, differs between the two entities [9,22,24]. Contrary to the TB cases, the *M. chimaera*-infected cases do not present capillary nonperfusion, cystoid macular edema, or retinal vasculitis [7,9,10].

FA of choroidal granulomas and tubercles in ocular TB reveals active tubercles with hypofluorescence in early phases and hyperfluorescence in late phases, and inactive tubercles (healed) that exhibit transmission hyperfluorescence [23]. Large choroidal granulomas might exhibit hyperfluorescence in early phases and a dilated capillary bed, followed by a progressive increase in hyperfluorescence, and finally, pooling of dye in the subretinal space in the late phase. FA can also be used to diagnose retinal angiomatous proliferation (type 3 macular neovascularization) that develops alongside acute choroidal tubercle or granuloma and might require intravitreal antivascular endothelial growth factor (VEGF) therapy along with the usual therapy [23]. In SLC patients, FA reveals hypofluorescence in early phases and hyperfluorescence in the late phases. The lesions that are healed might exhibit either transmission hyperfluorescence or hypofluorescence in the early phase and staining in the late phase owing to late scleral staining through the thin choroid. During FA analysis, active lesions exhibit hypofluorescence in early phases with hyperfluorescence in late stages, while the inactive lesions exhibit hypofluorescence towards the center and hyperfluorescence towards the periphery [23]. Tuberculous retinal vasculitis is another manifestation of ocular TB. It primarily affects the veins and is occlusive in nature. Active vasculitis manifests in the form of severe perivenular cuffing with thick exudates, and is generally associated with focal choroiditis lesions, moderate vitritis, and retinal hemorrhages [16,24,27]. Occlusive retinal vasculitis might even lead to retinal neovascularization. Furthermore, this technique can also be used to diagnose cystoid macular edema, which is characterized by dye leakage and accumulation in cystic spaces around fovea, in a "petaloid" pattern, or to diagnose macular neovascularization that emerges at the border of an inactive choroidal lesion or optic disc neovascularization [22,24,25,27,28].

Clinically, tuberculous optic neuropathy is manifested as papillitis, retrobulbar optic neuropathy, and neuroretinitis. In cases with neuroretinitis or papillitis, FA reveals optic disc hyperfluorescence in early phases followed by leakage during the late phases [23].

The FA presentation of the chorioretinal lesions due to ocular *M. chimaera* is similar to multifocal choroiditis related to ocular TB. The fluorescent pattern for active and inactive lesions seem to be similar for both diseases. However, the shape and the type of lesions, and their distribution, differs between the two entities [9,22,24]. Additionally, retinal vasculitis was not observed in any of the patients with disseminated *M. chimaera* infection.

These aspects are summarized in Table 1, Figures 2 and 3.

Table 1. Classification and comparison of choroidal lesions due to *M. tuberculosis* and *M. chimaera* based on multimodal imaging.

	M. chimaera		*M. tuberculosis*	
	Active Lesion	Inactive Lesion/Lesion in Regression	Active Lesion	Inactive Lesion/Lesion in Regression
	Fundus Photography			
shape	ovoid to round	ovoid to round	ovoid to round	ovoid to round
border	Indistinct	well-demarcated	indistinct	well-demarcated
size	<1 optic disc diameter	<1 optic disc diameter	variable	variable
color	yellowish-white	whitish	grayish-white or yellowish	variable pigmentation
distribution	Uniform	uniform	SLC-like single or multifocal lesion	SLC-like single or multifocal lesion
FA				
early	Hypofluorescent	hyperfluorescent	hypofluorescent	hyperfluorescent
late	Hyperfluorescent	hyperfluorescent	hyperfluorescent	hyperfluorescent
ICGA	Hypocyanescent	hypocyanescent (in atrophic areas)/ isocyanescent	hypocyanescent	hypocyanescent
FAF	hypoautofluorescent	hypoautofluorescent (in atrophic areas)/ isoautofluorescent	hypoautofluorescent	hypoautofluorescent
EDI-OCT				
shape	full-thickness, round, well-defined borders	poorly defined margins	full-thickness, round, well defined borders	outer retinal, RPE irregularity similar to the choroid (complete resolution possible)
internal reflectivity	Hyporeflective	similar to the choroid	hyporeflective	
choroidal hypertransmission	Present	present	present	present
OCTA	CC flow reduction in the corresponding area of the lesions	CC flow reduction (in atrophic lesion)	CC flow reduction with few preserved islands in the center of the lesion	CC atrophy with visualization of medium-to-large choroidal vessels in the corresponding area

Abbreviations: M.: Mycobacterium; SLC: serpiginous like chorioiditis; FA: Fluoresceine angiography; ICGA: Indocyanine green angiography; FAF: Fundus autofluorescence; EDI-OCT: enhanced depth imaging optical coherence tomography angiography; RPE: retinal pigment epithelium; OCTA: optical coherence tomography angiography; CC: choriocapillaris.

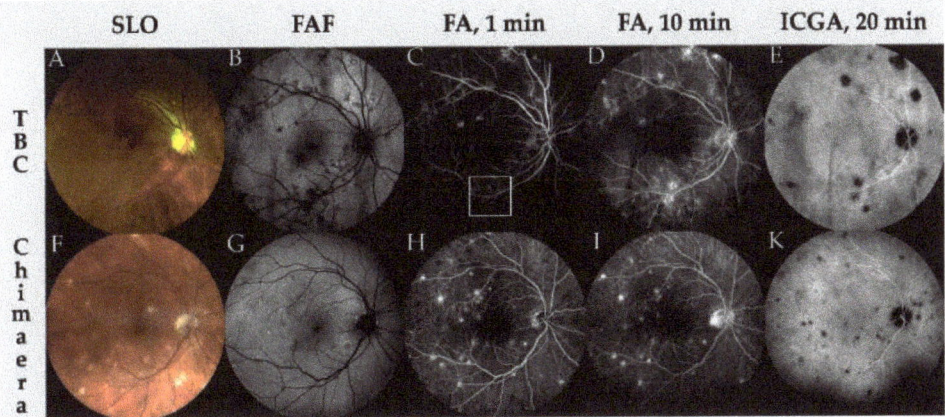

Figure 2. Multimodal imaging findings of patients suffering from multifocal choroiditis due to *M. tuberculosis* (TBC, **A–E**) and *M. chimaera* (**F–K**). In both scanning laser ophthalmoscopy images (SLO, **A,F**) choroidal granulomas can be observed. Note that panel A was acquired using an OPTOS device (OPTOS Inc., Marlborough, MA, USA) using a green and red laser, while panel F was acquired using a ZEISS Clarus device (Carl Zeiss Meditec, Inc., Dublin, CA, USA) with red, green and blue lasers, hence the difference in false color scheme. Fundus autofluorescence imaging (FAF, **B,G**) shows hypoautofluorescence at the location of choroidal granulomas, indicating loss of retinal pigment epithelium. In fluorescein angiography imaging at 1 min and 10 min (FA, **C,D,H,I**) early hypofluorescence in active lesions (panel C, inside white frame) and late-stage staining of choroidal granulomas can be appreciated. Note that in *M. chimaera*-associated multifocal choroiditis (MFC), hyperfluorescence seems to be more focused on the choroidal lesions while in *M. tuberculosis*-associated MFC the hyperfluorescences are more diffuse. In indocyanine green angiography imaging (ICGA, **E,K**), hypocyanescent lesions indicate the location of choroidal granulomas.

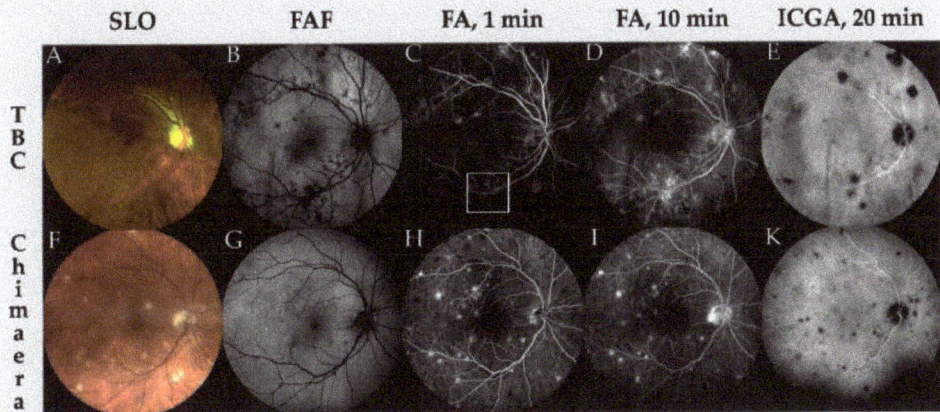

Figure 3. Typical imaging findings of ocular tuberculosis. Late stage fluoresceine angiography (FA; **A**) and optical coherence tomography (OCT; **B1**–near infrared fundus image; **B2**–OCT- B scan) of a 60-year-old female patient's left eye illustrating a hot disc and macular leakage in FA which corresponds to a cystoid macular edema with sub- and intraretinal fluid in the OCT images. OPTOS false-color scanning laser ophthalmoscopy (SLO; **C1,C3**) and FA (**C2,C4**) of a 46-year-old female patient. In the SLO color image of the right eye, optic disc edema, and multiple non-continuous choroidal granulomas are visible, the vitreous seems to be inflamed in the right eye. In the FA of the right eye (**C2**), a hot disc, vascular wall hyperfluorescence and staining of choroidal granulomas can be observed. However, there are no signs of vascular occlusion. The left eye shows no sign of infection (**C3,C4**).

3.3. Indocyanine Green Angiography (ICGA)

Because of its unique properties, ICGA lends itself to study the choroidal vasculature. In *M. chimaera*-infected eyes, multiple hypocyanescent lesions can be detected in ICGA in both early and late phases, many more compared to fundus photography or FA. ICG reveals the total lesion number and is, therefore, better suited to detect overall disease progression.

During the late phases of the ICGA examination, compared to inactive lesions, active lesions exhibit a stronger hypocyanescence for a longer duration. However, hypocyanescence of the lesions usually does not regress completely, even in clinically quiescent patients with clearly demarcated lesions on fundus photography. The persistence of hypocyanescence of these lesions is probably due to atrophy of the choriocapillaris/stromal choroid [9].

In TB posterior uveitis cases, ICGA reveals the presence of tubercular choroidal granulomas in choroidal stroma in the form of rounded hypocyanescent lesions during the dye transit and isocyanent lesions in the later phase [29,30]. In cases where the granuloma is present across the whole thickness of choroidal stroma, the lesions appear hypocyanescent throughout the course of the analysis. More than 90% of tuberculous granulomas are full thickness. Those granulomas have the same hypocyanescent behavior as *M. chimaera* lesions. As in multifocal choroiditis due to *M. chimaera*, most of the time, the tubercular granulomas visible on ICGA correspond to the hyporeflective lesions visible on EDI-OCT [23,31].

Compared to FA, ICGA is more efficient in examining the TB-SLC lesions. Even very subtle lesions can be identified on ICGA [22,29,30,32]. This is due to the involvement of the retinal pigment epithelium cells (RPE) that occurs later during the course of the disease. The SLC lesions are hypothesized to develop due to the occlusion of choriocapillaris that are visible in the form of irregularly-shaped hypocyanescent lesions during the early phase of the dye transit. They are still visible as hypocyanescent lesions during the late phases, because choriocapillaris are occluded and retain the dye. The healed stage is characterized on ICGA by better delineation of atrophic choroid [28,32].

3.4. Fundus Autofluorescence (FAF)

When using FAF in *M. chimaera*-infected eyes, active chorioretinal lesions appear as hyperautofluorescent areas in patients with progressive disease, whereas inactive lesions are usually hypoautofluorescent [7,9]. The hypoautofluorescence of the lesions is indicative of death of RPE and overlying photoreceptors. On the other hand, hyperautofluorescence of the lesions is indicative of loss of function. As in fundus photography, new active hyperautofluorescent lesions can often be observed close to atrophic hypoautofluorescent lesions. In the very late stages, lesions frequently show a confluent hypoautofluorescence, indicating a convergent loss of RPE [9].

Few studies have focused on the FAF patterns of TB granulomas. Gupta et al. [33] classified TB-SLC progression into four stages.

- Stage I: Acute lesions; poorly-demarcated amorphous hyperautofluorescence halo; lasts for 2 to 4 weeks
- Stage II: Lesions with a well-demarcated hypoautofluorescent border; lasts for 6 to 8 weeks
- Stage III: Lesions with mottled hypoautofluorescence and dispersed granular hyperautofluorescence
- Stage IV: Completely healed lesions with uniform hypoautofluorescence

The initial hyperautofluorescence has been attributed to the choroidal inflammation-induced fluorophore accumulation in the retina [34]. FAF has emerged as a powerful tool to monitor the TB serpiginoid lesion progression. It is advantageous over conventional angiography since the conventional technique is invasive and makes it difficult to interpret the results when the lesions comprise both active and inactive elements. FAF is also more efficient than ICGA, since ICGA cannot demarcate between healed and active lesions. Moreover, FAF can also provide the status of the RPE-photoreceptor complex [23].

3.5. Ocular Coherence Tomography (OCT)

In cases with progressive *M. chimaera* infection, enhanced depth imaging ocular coherence tomography (EDI-OCT) reveals rounded hyporeflective areas with significantly decreased choroidal vascularity. In EDI-OCT, the active lesions are generally well-demarcated and well correlated with hyporeflective regions, whereas inactive lesions are poorly demarcated and do not always correlate with hyporeflective regions. The thick lesions impact the adjoining RPE, making it irregularly shaped and attenuated. Choroidal hypertransmission can be observed in both inactive and active lesion. Choroidal lesions often underlie ellipsoid zones with altered integrity. In a previous case study, progressively large granuloma led to a Type 2 macular neovascularization with subretinal fluid development and concomitant visual decrease [9].

To date, no studies regarding the anterior segment OCT in patients with *M. chimaera* infection are available. In ocular TB, OCT of the anterior segment reveals a poorly-demarcated amorphous lesion, and synechiae and narrowing of anterior chamber exudates, corneal edema, and iridocorneal angle. The treatment of the condition usually leads to corneal edema regression and corneal thickness and exudate reduction [35].

In the case of intraretinal TB granuloma, OCT reveals a rounded, hyperreflective lesion in the neurosensory retina, which comprises a partially hyporeflective core underlying a hyperreflective area with surrounding neurosensory retinal detachment [36]. The presence of hyperreflective dots in the outer retina are attributed to proliferating RPE. Non-homogenous localized thickening is observed in the RPE/choriocapillaris complex under the retinal lesion devoid of any dome-shaped retinal elevation [23,36].

While describing the OCT characteristics of tuberculous choroidal granulomas, Salman et al. reported a local adhesion area (known as "contact sign") between the RPE–choriocapillaris layer and the overlying neurosensory retina [37]. Another study revealed the presence of nonhomogeneous lobulated patterns in tubercular choroidal granulomas [38]. This finding could be instrumental in the identification of smaller granulomas and in the differentiation between granulomas and normal large choroidal vessel lumens [39]. The proliferating RPE cells and granularity of outer photoreceptor layer reportedly contribute to the pathophysiology of choroidal granulomas [40,41].

In a previous study, EDI-OCT revealed choroidal infiltration with RPE elevation in lesion regions of TB-SLC patients [42]. In addition, SD-OCT can be used to reveal differences between active multifocal choroiditis and serpiginous choroiditis. In cases with serpiginous choroiditis, the structural alterations are limited to the outer retina. On the other hand, active multifocal choroiditis lesion is characterized by an increase in the reflectivity of inner retina [42]. Post-choroiditis treatment, the healed lesions exhibited increased reflectivity of only the outer retina region.

In the active choroiditis phase, there is either no change or a slight increase in the thickness of the retina; however, its thickness decreases mildly after the lesion has healed, which might be attributed to retinal atrophy [41]. With an increase in the thickness of the choroid, its reflectivity increases (also known as "waterfall effect"), which is attributed to inflammatory cell infiltration [43]. In a previous study, Bansal et al. [44] described the SD-OCT changes in the outer retina of an SLC patient. Their findings showed a correlation between the OCT and FAF findings. For instance, the spread of hyperreflectivity into the outer retina on OCT corresponded to the alterations in the photoreceptor outer segment tips, the RPE layers, and photoreceptor ellipsoid and myoid junction. They also reported a thickening of RPE/Bruch's membrane complex in the areas with lesions [44].

Furthermore, OCT can be used for the diagnosis and monitoring of uveitic macular edema too. Individuals with presumed ocular TB exhibit varied patterns of macular edema, such as serous retinal detachment, diffuse macular edema, and cystoid macular edema. The central macular thicknesses observed on OCT can be used as an indicator of treatment response [45].

3.6. Optical Coherence Tomography Angiography (OCTA)

Before the emergence of OCTA, ICGA was the only imaging modality available for the assessment of choroidal circulation. OCTA proved to be highly efficient non-invasive imaging technique that could be used to attain high resolution in vivo images. With disease progression, a reduction in the flow could be observed in the choriocapillaris/inner choroid image obtained using OCTA for the regions containing lesions observed in the images from ICGA. Similar to ICGA, OCTA could detect a higher number of lesions compared to that detected using other conventional techniques, such as FA and fundus photography. Böni et al. [9] reported that OCTA was able to reveal neovascular flow overlying a large chorioretinal lesion in their case study. The OCTA image corroborated the presence of neovascular flow in the area of subretinal hyperreflective material (SHRM), as detected using the structural OCT. The OCTA image of the neovascular lesion revealed the presence of small- and medium-caliber vessels with branched tiny vessels and arcades at vessel termini. Intravitreal anti–vascular endothelial growth factor (anti-VEGF) treatment was administered, which led to significant amelioration of the neovascular membrane. Follow-up assessment revealed a reduction in retinal thickness, SHRM, and area and density of the neovascular membrane [9].

Intraocular TB induces an inflammatory choriocapillopathy [37,40]. As in *M. chimaera* eyes, OCTA reveals a choriocapillaris flow reduction in the corresponding area of the ICGA-detected lesions in TB-SLC patients. These regions appear as well-delineated hyporeflective regions dispersed with few choriocapillaris spots towards the center of the lesion. The affected regions could be more precisely determined using OCTA than ICGA. During lesion healing, some patients may develop choriocapillaris atrophy [46,47].

In addition, OCTA facilitates vascular abnormality detection among these patients [48]. Previously, OCTA was used for the detection of macular neovascularization in a TB-SLC patient [49]. In this study, OCTA could efficiently differentiate between the neovascular membrane and the various retinochoroidal layers of the abnormal vascular network [49]. OCTA has also been deemed to be useful to monitor TB-SLC progression and its worsening post-therapy (unpublished data). Taken together, OCTA holds great potential in the diagnosis and management of posterior uveitic entities. Future studies with large sample sizes using OCTA could further elucidate the pathophysiology of this disease [23,49].

4. Conclusions

M. chimaera and *M. tuberculosis* infections can be very aggressive and can lead to death. A timely diagnosis of those infections is not always easy. Multimodal imaging of ocular findings can lead to an early diagnosis and a prompt initiation of anti-tuberculosis therapy, preventing poor patient outcomes. Furthermore, it gives the possibility to differentiate active and inactive ocular lesion and, because of the likely association with systemic disease activity, it plays a critical role for monitoring patients under treatment and for evaluation in the follow-up after discontinuation of treatment or treatment adjustment due to adverse drug effect.

Author Contributions: Conceptualization, S.A.Z., A.C. and M.D.T.; methodology, S.A.Z. and M.D.T.; software, S.A.Z. and M.D.T.; validation, A.C., M.D.T. and R.R.; formal analysis, S.A.Z. and M.D.T.; investigation, N.F., M.R.J.W. and K.Z.-O.; visualization and supervision, R.R. and M.D.T.; Writing—original draft, S.A.Z., N.F. and M.D.T.; Writing—review and editing, all coauthors; project administration, M.D.T. and R.R.; funding acquisition, S.A.Z. All authors have read and agreed to the published version of the manuscript.

Funding: This research received no external funding.

Institutional Review Board Statement: Not applicable.

Informed Consent Statement: All patients gave informed consent to publish their clinical data.

Data Availability Statement: Data are available on reasonable request to the corresponding author.

Conflicts of Interest: The authors declare no conflict of interest.

References

1. Waman, V.P.; Vedithi, S.C.; Thomas, S.E.; Bannerman, B.P.; Munir, A.; Skwark, M.J.; Malhotra, S.; Blundell, T.L. Mycobacterial genomics and structural bioinformatics: Opportunities and challenges in drug discovery. *Emerg. Microbes Infect.* **2019**, *8*, 109–118. [CrossRef] [PubMed]
2. Neuhouser, A.J.; Sallam, A. Ocular Tuberculosis. In *StatPearls*; StatPearls Publishing LLC.: Treasure Island, FL, USA, 2021.
3. Furin, J.; Cox, H.; Pai, M. Tuberculosis. *Lancet* **2019**, *393*, 1642–1656. [CrossRef]
4. Talip, B.A.; Sleator, R.D.; Lowery, C.J.; Dooley, J.S.; Snelling, W.J. An Update on Global Tuberculosis (TB). *Infect. Dis. Res. Treat.* **2013**, *6*, 39–50. [CrossRef]
5. Riccardi, N.; Monticelli, J.; Antonello, R.M.; Luzzati, R.; Gabrielli, M.; Ferrarese, M.; Codecasa, L.; Di Bella, S.; Giacobbe, D.R. Mycobacterium chimaera infections: An update. *J. Infect. Chemother. Off. J. Jpn. Soc. Chemother.* **2020**, *26*, 199–205. [CrossRef] [PubMed]
6. Hasse, B.; Hannan, M.M.; Keller, P.M.; Maurer, F.P.; Sommerstein, R.; Mertz, D.; Wagner, D.; Fernández-Hidalgo, N.; Nomura, J.; Manfrin, V.; et al. International Society of Cardiovascular Infectious Diseases Guidelines for the Diagnosis, Treatment and Prevention of Disseminated Mycobacterium chimaera Infection Following Cardiac Surgery with Cardiopulmonary Bypass. *J. Hosp. Infect.* **2020**, *104*, 214–235. [CrossRef] [PubMed]
7. Zweifel, S.A.; Mihic-Probst, D.; Curcio, C.A.; Barthelmes, D.; Thielken, A.; Keller, P.M.; Hasse, B.; Böni, C. Clinical and Histopathologic Ocular Findings in Disseminated Mycobacterium chimaera Infection after Cardiothoracic Surgery. *Ophthalmology* **2017**, *124*, 178–188. [CrossRef] [PubMed]
8. Deaner, J.D.; Lowder, C.Y.; Pichi, F.; Gordon, S.; Shrestha, N.; Emami-Naeini, P.; Sharma, S.; Srivastava, S.K. Clinical and Multimodal Imaging Findings in Disseminated Mycobacterium Chimaera. *Ophthalmol. Retin.* **2021**, *5*, 184–194. [CrossRef] [PubMed]
9. Böni, C.; Al-Sheikh, M.; Hasse, B.; Eberhard, R.; Kohler, P.; Hasler, P.; Erb, S.; Hoffmann, M.; Barthelmes, D.; Zweifel, S.A. Multimodal imaging of choroidal lesions in disseminated mycobacterium chimera infection after cardiothoracic surgery. *Retina* **2019**, *39*, 452–464. [CrossRef]
10. Ma, J.; Ruzicki, J.L.; Carrell, N.W.; Baker, C.F. Ocular manifestations of disseminated Mycobacterium chimaera infection after cardiothoracic surgery. *Can. J. Ophthalmol.* **2021**. [CrossRef]
11. Ortiz-Martínez, Y.; Galindo-Regino, C.; González-Hurtado, M.R.; Vanegas-Pastrana, J.J.; Valdes-Villegas, F. State of the art on Mycobacterium chimaera research: A bibliometric analysis. *J. Hosp. Infect.* **2018**, *100*, e159–e160. [CrossRef]
12. Achermann, Y.; Rössle, M.; Hoffmann, M.; Deggim, V.; Kuster, S.; Zimmermann, D.R.; Bloemberg, G.; Hombach, M.; Hasse, B. Prosthetic valve endocarditis and bloodstream infection due to *Mycobacterium chimaera*. *J. Clin. Microbiol.* **2013**, *51*, 1769–1773. [CrossRef]
13. Sia, J.K.; Rengarajan, J. Immunology of Mycobacterium tuberculosis Infections. *Microbiol. Spectr.* **2019**, *7*. [CrossRef] [PubMed]
14. Moher, D.; Liberati, A.; Tetzlaff, J.; Altman, D.G. Preferred reporting items for systematic reviews and meta-analyses: The PRISMA statement. *PLoS Med.* **2009**, *6*, e1000097. [CrossRef] [PubMed]
15. Tognetto, D.; Giglio, R.; Vinciguerra, A.L.; Milan, S.; Rejdak, R.; Rejdak, M.; Zaluska-Ogryzek, K.; Zweifel, S.; Toro, M.D. Artificial Intelligence Applications and Cataract Management: A Systematic Review. *Surv. Ophthalmol.* **2021**, *9*, 004. [CrossRef]
16. Posarelli, C.; Sartini, F.; Casini, G.; Passani, A.; Toro, M.D.; Vella, G.; Figus, M. What Is the Impact of Intraoperative Microscope-Integrated OCT in Ophthalmic Surgery? Relevant Applications and Outcomes. A Systematic Review. *J. Clin. Med.* **2020**, *9*, 1682. [CrossRef]
17. Plyukhova, A.A.; Budzinskaya, M.V.; Starostin, K.M.; Rejdak, R.; Bucolo, C.; Reibaldi, M.; Toro, M.D. Comparative Safety of Bevacizumab, Ranibizumab, and Aflibercept for Treatment of Neovascular Age-Related Macular Degeneration (AMD): A Systematic Review and Network Meta-Analysis of Direct Comparative Studies. *J. Clin. Med.* **2020**, *9*, 1522. [CrossRef]
18. Kongwattananon, W.; Brod, R.D.; Kodati, S. Mycobacterium Chimaera Choroiditis. *Ophthalmol. Retina* **2021**, *5*, 542. [CrossRef] [PubMed]
19. Toro, M.D.; Nowomiejska, K.; Avitabile, T.; Rejdak, R.; Tripodi, S.; Porta, A.; Reibaldi, M.; Figus, M.; Posarelli, C.; Fiedorowicz, M. Effect of Resveratrol on In Vitro and In Vivo Models of Diabetic Retinopathy: A Systematic Review. *Int. J. Mol. Sci.* **2019**, *20*, 3503. [CrossRef]
20. Toro, M.D.; Gozzo, L.; Tracia, L.; Cicciù, M.; Drago, F.; Bucolo, C.; Avitabile, T.; Rejdak, R.; Nowomiejska, K.; Zweifel, S.; et al. New Therapeutic Perspectives in the Treatment of Uveal Melanoma: A Systematic Review. *Biomedicines* **2021**, *9*, 1311. [CrossRef]
21. Scriven, J.E.; Scobie, A.; Verlander, N.Q.; Houston, A.; Collyns, T.; Cajic, V.; Kon, O.M.; Mitchell, T.; Rahama, O.; Robinson, A.; et al. Mycobacterium chimaera infection following cardiac surgery in the United Kingdom: Clinical features and outcome of the first 30 cases. *Clin. Microbiol. Infect.* **2018**, *24*, 1164–1170. [CrossRef]
22. Kohler, P.; Kuster, S.P.; Bloemberg, G.; Schulthess, B.; Frank, M.; Tanner, F.C.; Rössle, M.; Böni, C.; Falk, V.; Wilhelm, M.J.; et al. Healthcare-associated prosthetic heart valve, aortic vascular graft, and disseminated Mycobacterium chimaera infections subsequent to open heart surgery. *Eur. Heart J.* **2015**, *36*, 2745–2753. [CrossRef]
23. Agarwal, A.; Mahajan, S.; Khairallah, M.; Mahendradas, P.; Gupta, A.; Gupta, V. Multimodal Imaging in Ocular Tuberculosis. *Ocul. Immunol. Inflamm.* **2017**, *25*, 134–145. [CrossRef] [PubMed]
24. Testi, I.; Agrawal, R.; Mehta, S.; Basu, S.; Nguyen, Q.; Pavesio, C.; Gupta, V. Ocular tuberculosis: Where are we today? *Indian J. Ophthalmol.* **2020**, *68*, 1808–1817. [CrossRef]

25. Vasconcelos-Santos, D.V.; Zierhut, M.; Rao, N.A. Strengths and weaknesses of diagnostic tools for tuberculous uveitis. *Ocul. Immunol. Inflamm.* **2009**, *17*, 351–355. [CrossRef]
26. Brunner, D.R.; Zweifel, S.A.; Barthelmes, D.; Meier, F.; Böni, C. Review of people with retinal vasculitis and positive QuantiFERON(®)-TB Gold test in an area nonendemic for tuberculosis. *Int. Ophthalmol.* **2018**, *38*, 2389–2395. [CrossRef] [PubMed]
27. Gupta, V.; Shoughy, S.S.; Mahajan, S.; Khairallah, M.; Rosenbaum, J.T.; Curi, A.; Tabbara, K.F. Clinics of ocular tuberculosis. *Ocul. Immunol. Inflamm.* **2015**, *23*, 14–24. [CrossRef]
28. Agrawal, R.; Gupta, B.F.; González-López, J.J.M.P.; Cardoso, J.M.; Triantafullopoulou, I.M.; Grant, R.M.; Addison, P.K.F.; Westcott, M.F.; Pavesio, C.E.F. Spectrum of Choroidal Involvement in Presumed Ocular Tuberculosis: Report from a Population with Low Endemic Setting for Tuberculosis. *Ocul. Immunol. Inflamm.* **2017**, *25*, 97–104. [CrossRef]
29. Milea, D.; Fardeau, C.; Lumbroso, L.; Similowski, T.; Lehoang, P. Indocyanine green angiography in choroidal tuberculomas. *Br. J. Ophthalmol.* **1999**, *83*, 753. [CrossRef] [PubMed]
30. Wolfensberger, T.J.; Piguet, B.; Herbort, C.P. Indocyanine green angiographic features in tuberculous chorioretinitis. *Am. J. Ophthalmol.* **1999**, *127*, 350–353. [CrossRef]
31. Agarwal, R.; Iezhitsa, L.; Agarwal, P. Pathogenetic role of magnesium deficiency in ophthalmic diseases. *Biometals* **2013**, *27*, 5–18. [CrossRef]
32. Herbort, C.P.; LeHoang, P.; Guex-Crosier, Y. Schematic interpretation of indocyanine green angiography in posterior uveitis using a standard angiographic protocol. *Ophthalmology* **1998**, *105*, 432–440. [CrossRef]
33. Gupta, A.; Bansal, R.; Gupta, V.; Sharma, A. Fundus autofluorescence in serpiginouslike choroiditis. *Retina* **2012**, *32*, 814–825. [CrossRef]
34. Feeney, L. Lipofuscin and melanin of human retinal pigment epithelium. Fluorescence, enzyme cytochemical, and ultrastructural studies. *Invest. Ophthalmol. Vis. Sci.* **1978**, *17*, 583–600. Available online: https://iovs.arvojournals.org/article.aspx?articleid=2175722 (accessed on 11 August 2021). [PubMed]
35. Hashida, N.; Terubayashi, A.; Ohguro, N. Anterior segment optical coherence tomography findings of presumed intraocular tuberculosis. *Cutan. Ocul. Toxicol.* **2011**, *30*, 75–77. [CrossRef] [PubMed]
36. Pirraglia, M.P.; Tortorella, P.; Abbouda, A.; Toccaceli, F.; La Cava, M. Spectral domain optical coherence tomography imaging of tubercular chorioretinitis and intraretinal granuloma. Intraretinal tuberculosis: A case report. *Int. Ophthalmol.* **2015**, *35*, 445–450. [CrossRef]
37. Salman, A.; Parmar, P.; Rajamohan, M.; Vanila, C.G.; Thomas, P.A.; Jesudasan, C.A. Optical coherence tomography in choroidal tuberculosis. *Am. J. Ophthalmol.* **2006**, *142*, 170–172. [CrossRef] [PubMed]
38. Invernizzi, A.; Mapelli, C.; Viola, F.; Cigada, M.; Cimino, L.; Ratiglia, R.; Staurenghi, G.; Gupta, A. Choroidal granulomas visualized by enhanced depth imaging optical coherence tomography. *Retina* **2015**, *35*, 525–531. [CrossRef]
39. Parchand, S.M.; Sharma, K.; Sharma, A.; Singh, R. Unusual choroidal mass. *Case Rep.* **2013**, *2013*, bcr2013200286. [CrossRef]
40. Saxena, S.; Singhal, V.; Akduman, L. Three-dimensional spectral domain optical coherence tomography imaging of the retina in choroidal tuberculoma. *Case Rep.* **2013**, *2013*, bcr2012008156. [CrossRef]
41. Mahendradas, P.; Madhu, S.; Kawali, A.; Govindaraj, I.; Gowda, P.B.; Vinekar, A.; Shetty, N.; Shetty, R.; Shetty, B.K. Combined depth imaging of choroid in uveitis. *J. Ophthalmic. Inflamm. Infect.* **2014**, *4*, 18. [CrossRef]
42. van Velthoven, M.E.; Ongkosuwito, J.V.; Verbraak, F.D.; Schlingemann, R.O.; de Smet, M.D. Combined en-face optical coherence tomography and confocal ophthalmoscopy findings in active multifocal and serpiginous chorioretinitis. *Am. J. Ophthalmol.* **2006**, *141*, 972–975. [CrossRef] [PubMed]
43. Gallagher, M.J.; Yilmaz, T.; Cervantes-Castañeda, R.A.; Foster, C.S. The characteristic features of optical coherence tomography in posterior uveitis. *Br. J. Ophthalmol.* **2007**, *91*, 1680–1685. [CrossRef]
44. Bansal, R.; Kulkarni, P.; Gupta, A.; Gupta, V.; Dogra, M.R. High-resolution spectral domain optical coherence tomography and fundus autofluorescence correlation in tubercular serpiginouslike choroiditis. *J. Ophthalmic. Inflamm. Infect.* **2011**, *1*, 157–163. [CrossRef]
45. Al-Mezaine, H.S.; Al-Muammar, A.; Kangave, D.; Abu El-Asrar, A.M. Clinical and optical coherence tomographic findings and outcome of treatment in patients with presumed tuberculous uveitis. *Int. Ophthalmol.* **2008**, *28*, 413–423. [CrossRef] [PubMed]
46. De Luigi, G.; Mantovani, A.; Papadia, M.; Herbort, C.P. Tuberculosis-related choriocapillaritis (multifocal-serpiginous choroiditis): Follow-up and precise monitoring of therapy by indocyanine green angiography. *Int. Ophthalmol.* **2012**, *32*, 55–60. [CrossRef]
47. Knecht, P.B.; Papadia, M.; Herbort, C.P. Secondary choriocapillaritis in infectious chorioretinitis. *Acta Ophthalmol.* **2013**, *91*, e550–e555. [CrossRef] [PubMed]
48. Agrawal, R.; Xin, W.; Keane, P.A.; Chhablani, J.; Agarwal, A. Optical coherence tomography angiography: A non-invasive tool to image end-arterial system. *Expert Rev. Med. Devices* **2016**, *13*, 519–521. [CrossRef]
49. Yee, H.Y.; Keane, P.A.; Ho, S.L.; Agrawal, R. Optical Coherence Tomography Angiography of Choroidal Neovascularization Associated with Tuberculous Serpiginous-like Choroiditis. *Ocul. Immunol. Inflamm.* **2016**, *24*, 699–701. [CrossRef]

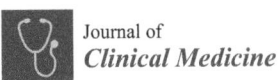

Journal of
Clinical Medicine

Article

Anterior-Segment Swept-Source Ocular Coherence Tomography and Scheimpflug Imaging Agreement for Keratometry and Pupil Measurements in Healthy Eyes

Francisco Pérez-Bartolomé [1,2], Carlos Rocha-De-Lossada [3,4,5], José-María Sánchez-González [6,*], Silvia Feu-Basilio [2], Josep Torras-Sanvicens [2] and Jorge Peraza-Nieves [2]

1. Department of Ophthalmology, Hospital Universitario Puerta de Hierro, 28222 Majadahonda, Spain; franciscoperezbartolome@gmail.com
2. Department of Ophthalmology, Clinic Institute of Ophthalmology, Hospital Clinic of Barcelona, University of Barcelona, 08036 Barcelona, Spain; silviafeub@gmail.com (S.F.-B.); jts29206@gmail.com (J.T.-S.); jorge.peraza.nieves@gmail.com (J.P.-N.)
3. Department of Ophthalmology (Qvision), Vithas Virgen del Mar Hospital, 04120 Almería, Spain; carlosrochadelossada5@gmail.com
4. Department of Ophthalmology, Hospital Virgen de Las Nieves, 18014 Granada, Spain
5. Department of Ophthalmology, Ceuta Medical Center, 51001 Ceuta, Spain
6. Department of Physics of Condensed Matter, Optics Area, Vision Science Research Group (CIVIUS), Pharmacy Faculty, University of Seville, 41012 Sevilla, Spain
* Correspondence: jsanchez80@us.es; Tel.: +34-955-42-08-61

Abstract: This study examines agreement between the devices Anterion® and Pentacam HR® used for corneal and pupil measurements in healthy eyes. The parameters compared between the two devices were: anterior Km (D), anterior K2 (D), anterior K1 (D), anterior K1 axis (°), anterior astigmatism (D), anterior K max (D), posterior Km (D), posterior K2 (D), posterior K1 (D), posterior K1 axis (°), posterior astigmatism (D), CCT (μm), thinnest point thickness (μm), thinnest point X-coordinate (mm), thinnest point Y-coordinate (mm), pupil diameter (mm), pupil center-corneal vertex distance (mm) (angle kappa), pupil centroid angle (°), pupil centroid X-coordinate (mm), and pupil centroid Y-coordinate (mm). The Student's t test for independent samples identified significant differences ($p < 0.005$) between devices for the measurements anterior and posterior flat K axis, posterior flat K, steep K, and mean K. For these last three measurements, although significant, none of the differences were clinically relevant. Corneal power and thickness measurements except Kf axis showed excellent agreement between Anterion and Pentacam. In a clinical setting we would not recommend the interchangeable use of Pentacam and Anterion for measurement of pupil parameters.

Keywords: anterior-segment swept-source; ocular coherence tomography; Scheimpflug imaging; agreement analysis; pupil measurements

1. Introduction

Precise measurement of both corneal power and pupil diameter has progressively gained importance in parallel with the development of cataract and refractive surgery procedures [1]. Central corneal thickness (CCT), and mean (Km), flat (Kf) and steep (Ks) keratometry, along with pupil diameter (PD), are main determining factors for excimer laser ablation and/or multifocal intraocular lens (MIOL) implantation [2,3]. One of the devices most used in clinical practice for these measurements is the Pentacam® HR (OCULUS Optikgeräte GmbH), a rotating Scheimpflug camera system designed to visualize the anterior segment that is able to measure corneal topography, elevation of the anterior and posterior corneal surface, corneal thickness, and anterior chamber angle [1,4].

Based on a completely different technology, the Anterion® (Heidelberg Engineering, Heidelberg, Germany) is a multimodal imaging device introduced in 2019 [5]. Through anterior segment swept-source optical coherence tomography (OCT), it can be used to measures axial length for ocular biometry and can also be used to image the anterior segment. The cornea display of the device offers a wide range of anterior segment parameters such as anterior and posterior keratometry, central corneal thickness, elevation measures, and pupil size.

For anterior segment measurements, studies have shown variable repeatability and reproducibility between Pentacam® HR and Anterion, and between Anterion and other OCT-based devices, such as CASIA (Tomey Corporation, Nagoya, Japan) [6–10]. With regard to the latest research, Brunner et al. [11] investigated repeatability coefficients and limits of agreement comparing Pentacam HR, Orbscan IIz, and Tomey Casia SS-1000 measurements. However, to the best of our knowledge, no investigation has compared pupil measurements provided by Anterion and Pentacam HR. The aim of the present study was to determine agreement between these two devices for both keratometry and pupil measurements in healthy individuals.

2. Materials and Methods

This was a prospective cross-sectional study. The study protocol was approved by the Ethics committee of the Hospital Clinic de Barcelona (HCB/2021/0388) and adhered to the principles of the Declaration of Helsinki. Informed consent was obtained from each participant at the time of enrollment.

2.1. Study Population

Participants were 56 healthy volunteers recruited among hospital staff and their relatives. While examinations were performed in both eyes, only data for one eye were analyzed. Inclusion criteria were age ≥ 18 years, no history of ocular surgery or contact lens use, and no corneal disease, ocular trauma, or systemic collagen disease.

2.2. Devices

The Anterion device uses swept-source AS-OCT technology with a 1300 nm wavelength light source, and speed of 50,000 A-scans/second. This device images the anterior segment of the eye at an axial depth of 14 mm, lateral width of 16.5 mm, in-tissue axial resolution less than 10 μm and lateral resolution 30–45 mm [12]. All measurements are assisted by eye-tracking technology centered on the corneal vertex [12].

The Pentacam HR uses a rotating Scheimpflug camera which takes 100 images of 500 measurement points on the anterior and posterior corneal surfaces over 180 degrees of rotation [13]. Elevation data from all these images are combined to form a three-dimensional reconstruction of corneal shape within the same diameter optic zones as Anterion.

2.3. Examination Protocol

All patients underwent a complete ophthalmic examination, including distance-corrected visual acuity measurement, anterior segment bio-microscopy and fundus examination. After three minutes of dark adaptation, the same experienced ophthalmologist performed a single scan of both eyes, first using the cornea mode of Anterion and then the Pentacam HR in standard light conditions.

Subjects were instructed to maintain the imaged eye on the central fixation target built into each device. Only scans of optimal quality indicated as over 95% by the Pentacam HR and as "green" by the Anterion were included in the analysis. Subjects with eye conditions that could affect fixation and the quality of data acquisition such as corneal disease, cataract or any maculopathy were excluded. Scans obtained in subjects with suspected or confirmed keratoconus (Kmax index >48 D, irregular astigmatism, infero-temporal displacement of the thinnest corneal point or an abnormal Belin-Ambrosio Pentacam analysis) or another corneal ectasia were also discarded.

Data from the Anterion wavefront analysis were exported to an excel sheet. From each device, 20 parameters were automatically exported: 11 related to both anterior and posterior corneal surface measurements: Kf, Km, Ks, Kf axis and astigmatism; four related to corneal thickness: CCT, thinnest point and its location; five related to pupil measurements: PD, center from visual axis (angle kappa), pupil center angle (between pupil center plane and corneal surface) and position with vectors X and Y. The same parameters of the Pentacam were manually entered in the same excel sheet used for the Anterion data. Both eyes were examined, but only right eye data were included. If right eye was not suitable for inclusion, left eye data was included.

2.4. Statistical Analysis

All data were analyzed using SPSS (version 22.0, IBM Corp., Armonk, NY, USA) and Excel software (2016, Microsoft Corp., Redmond, WA, USA). Results are expressed as the mean ± standard deviation (SD). Significance was set at $p < 0.05$. The Shapiro-Wilk test was used to confirm the normal distribution of data ($p > 0.05$). Initially, the Student's t test for independent samples was used to identify differences between devices.

Inter-device agreement for each corneal aberration parameter was assessed through mean differences, paired t-test for mean differences, and 95% confidence intervals and limits of agreement (LoA). Bland-Altman plots were also constructed using the LoAs to compare both devices. Sample size calculation was based on recent studies that have analyzed agreement between AS-OCT and Scheimpflug devices [6,7]. For a 2-sided level of significance (α) at 0.05 and power (β) of 80%, the sample-size calculation indicated that a minimum of 50 participants was required to detect a difference of 0.1 µm in all measurements.

3. Results

The 56 subjects recruited were 32 women (57.14%) and 24 men (42.85%) of mean age 52.35 years ± 20.2 SD (21–78). Table 1 provides a descriptive analysis of the study sample. The Student's t test for independent samples identified significant differences ($p < 0.05$) between devices for the measurements of anterior and posterior flat K axis, posterior flat K, steep K, and mean K. For these last three measurements, although significant, none of the differences were clinically relevant.

Table 1. Descriptive analysis. Comparison of corneal parameters between the Anterion and Pentacam HR devices.

Parameter	Anterion	Pentacam HR	*p* Value
Anterior Km (D)	43.52 ± 1.54 (40.50–47.25)	42.93 ± 1.52 (40.00–46.20)	0.43
Anterior K2 (D)	44.01 ± 1.64 (40.65–47.81)	43.92 ± 1.59 (41.00–47.70)	0.80
Anterior K1 (D)	43.07 ± 1.56 (40.21–46.71)	42.93 ± 1.52 (40.00–46.20)	0.68
Anterior K1 axis (°)	109.93 ± 62.71 (1.00–180)	76.61 ± 69.64 (0.30–179.90)	0.01 *
Anterior astigmatism (D)	0.93 ± 0.81 (0.05–4.70)	0.98 ± 0.66 (0.00–3.40)	0.77
Anterior K max (D)	44.51 ± 1.72 (40.98–47.56)	44.59 ± 1.76 (41.30–47.40)	0.83
Posterior Km (D)	−6.14 ± 0.27 (−6.94–−5.55)	−6.30 ± 0.28 (−7.00–−5.70)	<0.01 *
Posterior K2 (D)	−6.29 ± 0.30 (−7.38–−5.66)	−6.57 ± 0.86 (−12.00–−5.80)	0.04 *
Posterior K1 (D)	−5.99 ± 0.25 (−6.54–−5.44)	−6.14 ± 0.27 (−6.80–−5.60)	<0.01 *
Posterior K1 axis (°)	124.56 ± 71.69 (0.00–180)	75.87 ± 76.74 (1.10–179.30)	<0.01 *
Posterior astigmatism (D)	−0.30 ± 0.13 (−0.84–−0.04)	0.32 ± 0.13 (0.00–0.60)	0.61
CCT (µm)	546.41 ± 32 (474–615)	552.17 ± 38.05 (479–702)	0.43
TPT (µm)	541.52 ± 31.91 (472–613)	547.06 ± 36.49 (477–674)	0.44

Table 1. Cont.

Parameter	Anterion	Pentacam HR	p Value
TPP X (mm)	−0.49 ± 0.63 (−1.64–1.04)	−0.38 ± 0.49 (−1.06–0.95)	0.37
TPP Y (mm)	−0.37 ± 0.35 (−1.43–0.44)	−0.33 ± 0.28 (−1.31–0.37)	0.47
Pupil diameter (mm)	5.74 ± 1.34 (2.90–7.80)	3.82 ± 1.60 (1.66–7.06)	<0.01 *
PCP (mm) angle kappa	0.37 ± 0.18 (0.07–1.05)	0.26 ± 0.14 (0.05–0.71)	0.003 *
PCA (°, degrees)	162.89 ± 69.38 (3.00–347)	194.99 ± 78.87 (18.90–359)	0.04 *
PCP X (mm)	−0.22 ± 0.28 (−0.89–0.57)	−0.13 ± 0.23 (−0.63–0.46)	0.12
PCP Y (mm)	0.04 ± 0.20 (−0.55–0.48)	−0.01 ± −0.14 (−0.33–0.29)	0.10

Data were presented as mean ± standard deviation (range) * Statistically significant differences with Student's t test for independent samples. Km = mean keratometry, K1: flat keratometry, K2: steep keratometry, CCT: central corneal thickness, D: diopters TPT: thinnest point thickness, TPP: thinnest point posterior, PCD: pupil center distance, PCA: pupil center angle, PCP: pupil center posterior, μm: microns, mm: millimeters.

Overall, mean differences were small, with narrow limits of agreement (LOA) (Table 2, Figures 1 and 2). Although the paired t-test revealed significant differences for all the parameters studied (except posterior steep K, $p = 0.051$), differences in absolute values were generally close to 0. Thus, overall, good agreement was found between the Anterion and Pentacam measures. Nonetheless, we found some exceptions. Both anterior and posterior Kf axis showed poor agreement between devices (large mean difference with wide LOA) (Table 2 and Figure 1). For pupil measurements, positions in the X and Y axis were highly concordant, but PD, pupil center from visual axis (angle kappa) and pupil center angle were not (Table 2 and Figure 3).

Table 2. Inter-device measurement agreement between Anterion and Pentacam HR.

Parameter	Difference	95% LoA	p Value	CI (95%)
Anterior Km (D)	0.09 ± 0.26	−0.41–0.60	<0.01 *	0.67–0.90
Anterior K2 (D)	0.08 ± 0.41	−0.72–0.89	<0.01 *	0.97–0.99
Anterior K1 (D)	0.13 ± 0.27	−0.39–0.66	<0.01 *	0.98–0.99
Anterior K1 axis (°)	33.32 ± 65.57	−95.19–161.83	<0.01 *	0.41–0.82
Anterior astig. (D)	−0.04 ± 0.45	−0.92–0.84	<0.01 *	0.81–0.94
Anterior K max (D)	−0.07 ± 0.53	−1.13–0.97	<0.01 *	0.95–0.98
Posterior Km (D)	0.16 ± 0.10	−0.03–0.36	<0.01 *	0.93–0.98
Posterior K2 (D)	0.28 ± 0.80	−1.29–1.85	0.051	−0.10–0.66
Posterior K1 (D)	0.15 ± 0.08	−0.01–0.32	<0.01 *	0.94–0.98
Posterior K1 axis (°)	48.69 ± 88.68	−125.12–222.50	0.02 *	−0.00–0.69
Posterior astig. (D)	0.014 ± 0.10	−0.18–0.21	<0.01 *	0.67–0.90
CCT (μm)	−5.76 ± 18.22	−41.47–29.95	<0.01 *	0.87–0.96
TPT (μm)	−5.54 ± 18.08	−40.99–29.91	<0.01 *	0.86–0.95
TPP X (mm)	−0.10 ± 0.35	−0.79–0.58	<0.01 *	0.80–0.94
TPP Y (mm)	−0.04 ± 0.20	−0.44–0.34	<0.01 *	0.80–0.93
Pupil diameter (mm)	1.92 ± 1.16	−0.35–4.20	<0.01 *	0.67–0.90
PCP (mm) angle kappa	0.10 ± 0.15	−0.19–0.40	<0.01 *	0.46–0.83
PCA (°, degrees)	−32.10 ± 115.72	−261.20–197.02	<0.01 *	0.46–0.78
PCP X (mm)	−0.08 ± 0.14	−0.36–0.19	<0.01 *	0.85–0.95
PCP Y (mm)	0.05 ± 0.16	−0.27–0.39	<0.01 *	0.43–0.82

Data were presented as mean ± standard deviation * Statistically significant differences with Student's t test for paired samples. CI: confidence interval, LoA: limits of agreement, Km: mean keratometry, K1: flat keratometry, K2: steep keratometry, CCT: central corneal thickness. TPT: thinnest point thickness, TPP: thinnest point posterior, PCD: pupil center distance, PCA: pupil center angle, PCP: pupil center posterior, D: diopters, μm: microns, mm: millimeters.

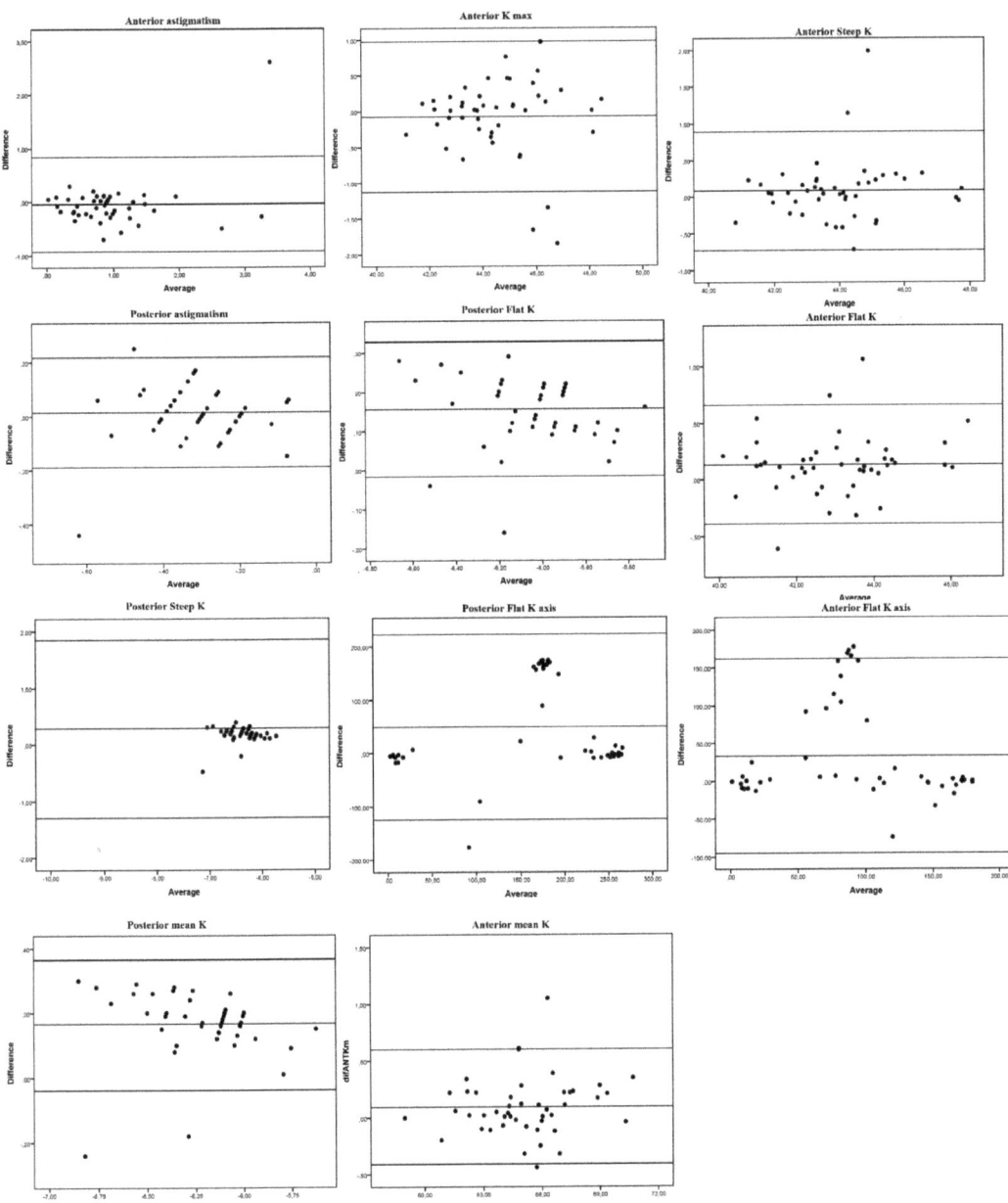

Figure 1. Bland-Altman plots of mean differences against averages of anterior and posterior corneal surface keratometry readings. Mean, lower and upper limits of agreement (±1.96 SD, standard deviation). Left: anterior vertical coma. Right: total vertical coma.

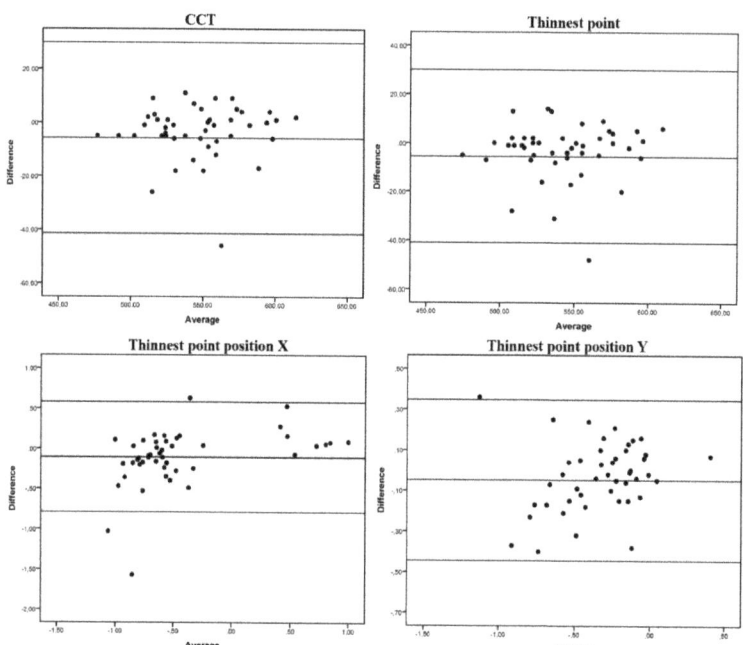

Figure 2. Bland-Altman plots of mean differences against averages of pachy-metric measurements. Mean, lower and upper limits of agreement (±1.96 SD, standard deviation).

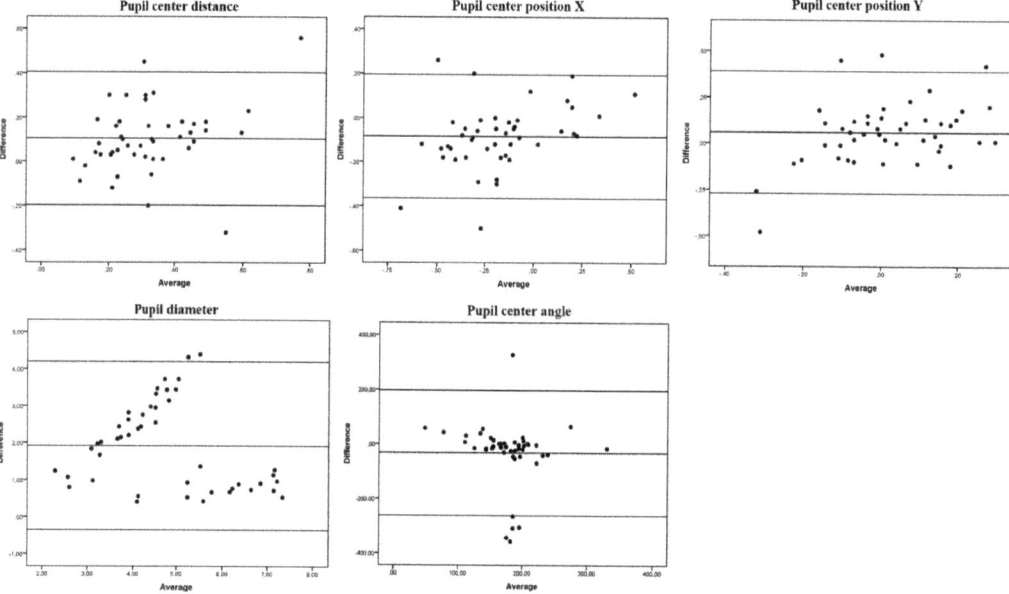

Figure 3. Bland-Altman plots of mean differences against averages of pupil measurements. Mean, lower and upper limits of agreement (±1.96 SD, standard deviation).

4. Discussion

Anterior segment measurements are used as cut-offs for patient and ocular surgical method selection. In this study, excellent agreement was observed between both devices for kerato-metric and pachy-metric measurements, while pupil parameter measurements usually differed significantly. PD has been described as a main factor in indicating refractive surgery [2,3]. In addition, scotopic larger pupils can overlap ablation optic zones and optic diameters of MIOL resulting in poor night vision and halos [14]. PD is influenced by the light of the media and undergoes size reduction with accommodation [4]. Therefore, it is not clear whether the Pentacam is able to provide clinically useful information prior to refractive surgery as it uses a 450-nm visible blue light-emitting diode which can induce miosis. In effect, here we recorded a smaller PD with the Pentacam (3.82 ± 1.6 vs. 5.74 ± 1.34) (Table 1). Being based on OCT technology, Anterion does not induce such intense miosis and could theoretically be a better method to measure mesopic PD. Güçlü et al. [15] reported that IOL-Master 700, another OCT-based biometer, is a useful device that is interchangeable with Pentacam for keratometry values and axis, but not for white-to-white distance (WTW), anterior chamber depth (ACD), and CCT. In their study, mean PD determined in healthy eyes was 6.4 ± 1.4 mm with IOL-Master 700 and 4.5 ± 1.3 mm with Pentacam [15]. In our study, slightly smaller PDs were recorded but with the same trend, probably because we included older subjects. Our Bland-Altman plots indicated great disparity with wide LOAs (-0.35–4.2) for our PD measurements (Figure 3). Therefore, we would not recommend the interchangeable use of Pentacam and Anterion for PD measurements.

Recently, besides PD, much attention has been paid to other causes of disturbing ocular symptoms after MIOL implantation, such as glare and halos. Studies so far have shown that any large deviation between the optical center or visual axis and the pupillary axis of the MIOL can lead to higher-order aberrations postoperatively, compromising visual quality [16–19]. Both Pentacam and Anterior are able to determine the position of the pupil center through two vectors (X and Y), the angle kappa (radial distance between visual axis and the center of the pupil) and the pupil center angle (angle between the pupil center plane and corneal surface). Above all, angle kappa has emerged as a useful parameter to consider when planning MIOL implantation. Berdahl and Waring suggested that a MIOL should not be implanted if the preoperative angle kappa is larger than one half the diameter of the central optical region of the multifocal IOL [20]. Fu et al. analyzed 57 eyes of 29 patients undergoing MIOL implantation and concluded that an angle kappa distance greater than 0.5 mm could influence objective visual quality (optical scattering) [21].

In our study sample, mean angle Kappa measurements were 0.37 ± 0.18 mm with the Anterion and 0.26 ± 0.14 mm ($p < 0.005$) with Pentacam, and Bland Altman plots revealed slight dispersion and a small mean difference (0.1 mm ± 0.15). Both devices could be useful in measuring this parameter in clinical practice, but again they should not be considered interchangeable. Likewise, significant differences were found for pupil center angle (Table 1), with a large mean difference ($-32.1° \pm 115.72$) and wide LOAs (-261.2–197.02). On the contrary, pupil center positions X and Y showed excellent agreement and a low mean difference between devices.

Overall excellent agreement was observed for both kerato-metric and pachy-metric measurements. Posterior Kf, Ks and Km differed significantly between devices, but mean differences were small and clinically irrelevant. Several studies have compared the performance of Anterion and other devices [6–10], but only one has provided agreement for posterior corneal surface readings [8]. Overall, for biometric measures, Anterion seems to be more interchangeable with other OCT devices such as CASIA or IOL-Master 700. Tañá-Rivero et al. detected significant differences in WTW measurements taken with the Anterion, IOLMaster 700 (Carl Zeiss Meditec AG, Carl Zeiss Meditec, Jena, Germany) and Pentacam HR, yet concluded that, in clinical terms, Anterion could be considered interchangeable with both these devices [6]. Recently, this group obtained comparable values of keratometry, J0 and J45 vectors, lens thickness, and axial length using the same three devices, but, again, significant differences emerged for anterior chamber depth and central corneal thickness data [7]. Showing the same trend as our results, average posterior corneal power (PCP) and PCP astigmatism were highly repeatable, and agreement was good between the four devices.

Our study has some limitations. While a repeatability analysis was beyond the scope of this study, we only accepted optimal quality images, and all were taken by an experienced ophthalmologist in similar conditions of darkness. While a larger sample would have allowed us to detect more subtle differences, we believe that our sample was sufficiently large to detect clinically meaningful variations. Future research should include an inter-observer analysis in order to improve anterior segment pathologies specificity without reducing the sensitivity [11].

5. Conclusions

In summary, corneal power and thickness measurements, except Kf axis, showed excellent agreement between Anterion and Pentacam. Agreement for pupillary position in X and Y vectors x and y components of the pupil-glint vectors was good, but pupil center distance (angle Kappa), PD and pupil center angle showed poor agreement and, overall, differed significantly between both devices.

By way of overall conclusion, in a clinical setting we would not recommend the interchangeable use of Pentacam and Anterion for measurement of pupil parameters; we would only recommend the interchangeable use of Pentacam and Anterion for corneal measurements.

Author Contributions: Conceptualization, F.P.-B., C.R.-D.-L., J.-M.S.-G., S.F.-B., J.P.-N. and J.T.-S.; methodology, F.P.-B., C.R.-D.-L., J.-M.S.-G., S.F.-B., J.P.-N. and J.T.-S.; validation, F.P.-B., C.R.-D.-L., J.-M.S.-G., S.F.-B., J.P.-N. and J.T.-S.; formal analysis, F.P.-B., C.R.-D.-L., J.-M.S.-G., S.F.-B., J.P.-N. and J.T.-S.; investigation, F.P.-B., C.R.-D.-L., J.-M.S.-G., S.F.-B., J.P.-N. and J.T.-S.; resources, F.P.-B., C.R.-D.-L., J.-M.S.-G., S.F.-B., J.P.-N. and J.T.-S.; data curation, F.P.-B., C.R.-D.-L., J.-M.S.-G., S.F.-B., J.P.-N. and J.T.-S.; writing—original draft preparation, F.P.-B., C.R.-D.-L., J.-M.S.-G., S.F.-B., J.P.-N. and J.T.-S.; writing—review and editing, F.P.-B., C.R.-D.-L., J.-M.S.-G., S.F.-B., J.P.-N. and J.T.-S.; visualization, F.P.-B., C.R.-D.-L., J.-M.S.-G., S.F.-B., J.P.-N. and J.T.-S.; supervision, F.P.-B., C.R.-D.-L., J.-M.S.-G., S.F.-B., J.P.-N. and J.T.-S. All authors have read and agreed to the published version of the manuscript.

Funding: This research received no external funding.

Institutional Review Board Statement: The study was conducted according to the guidelines of the Declaration of Helsinki and approved by the Ethics Committee of Hospital Clinic of Barcelona (protocol code HCB/2021/0388).

Informed Consent Statement: Informed consent was obtained from all subjects involved in the study.

Data Availability Statement: The data presented in this study are available on request from the corresponding author. The data are not publicly available due to the data is part of a research project.

Conflicts of Interest: The authors declare no conflict of interest.

References

1. Beggs, S.; Short, J.; Rengifo-Pardo, M.; Ehrlich, A. Applications of the Excimer Laser: A Review. *Dermatol. Surg.* **2015**, *41*, 1201–1211. [CrossRef] [PubMed]
2. Myung, D.; Schallhorn, S.; Manche, E.E. Pupil size and LASIK: A review. *J. Refract. Surg.* **2013**, *29*, 734–741. [CrossRef]
3. Hjortdal, J.; Møller-Pedersen, T.; Ivarsen, A.; Ehlers, N. Corneal power, thickness, and stiffness: Results of a prospective randomized controlled trial of PRK and LASIK for myopia. *J. Cataract Refract. Surg.* **2005**, *31*, 21–29. [CrossRef] [PubMed]
4. Yazici, A.T.; Bozkurt, E.; Alagoz, C.; Alagoz, N.; Pekel, G.; Kaya, V.; Yilmaz, O.F. Central corneal thickness, anterior chamber depth, and pupil diameter measurements using visante OCT, orbscan, and pentacam. *J. Refract. Surg.* **2010**, *26*, 127–133. [CrossRef]
5. Schiano-Lomoriello, D.; Hoffer, K.J.; Abicca, I.; Savini, G. Repeatability of automated measurements by a new anterior segment optical coherence tomographer and biometer and agreement with standard devices. *Sci. Rep.* **2021**, *11*, 983. [CrossRef] [PubMed]
6. Tañá-Rivero, P.; Aguilar-Córcoles, S.; Rodríguez-Prats, J.L.; Montés-Micó, R.; Ruiz-Mesa, R. Agreement of white-to-white measurements with swept-source OCT, Scheimpflug and color LED devices. *Int. Ophthalmol.* **2021**, *41*, 57–65. [CrossRef]

7. Tañá-Rivero, P.; Aguilar-Córcoles, S.; Tello-Elordi, C.; Pastor-Pascual, F.; Montés-Micó, R. Agreement between 2 swept-source OCT biometers and a Scheimpflug partial coherence interferometer. *J. Cataract Refract. Surg.* **2021**, *47*, 488–495. [CrossRef] [PubMed]
8. Gjerdrum, B.; Gundersen, K.G.; Lundmark, P.O.; Aakre, B.M. Repeatability of OCT-based versus scheimpflug-and reflection-based keratometry in patients with hyperosmolar and normal tear film. *Clin. Ophthalmol.* **2020**, *14*, 3991–4003. [CrossRef]
9. Chan, P.P.-M.; Lai, G.; Chiu, V.; Chong, A.; Yu, M.; Leung, C.K.-S. Anterior chamber angle imaging with swept-source optical coherence tomography: Comparison between CASIAII and ANTERION. *Sci. Rep.* **2020**, *10*, 18771. [CrossRef]
10. Pardeshi, A.A.; Song, A.E.; Lazkani, N.; Xie, X.; Huang, A.; Xu, B.Y. Intradevice repeatability and interdevice agreement of ocular biometric measurements: A comparison of two swept-source anterior segment oct devices. *Transl. Vis. Sci. Technol.* **2020**, *9*, 1–9. [CrossRef]
11. Brunner, M.; Czanner, G.; Vinciguerra, R.; Romano, V.; Ahmad, S.; Batterbury, M.; Britten, C.; Willoughby, C.E.; Kaye, S.B. Improving precision for detecting change in the shape of the cornea in patients with keratoconus. *Sci. Rep.* **2018**, *8*, 12345. [CrossRef]
12. Applegate, R.A.; Sarver, E.J.; Khemsara, V. Are all aberrations equal? *J. Refract. Surg.* **2002**, *18*, S556–S562. [CrossRef]
13. Cicchetti, D.V. Guidelines, Criteria, and Rules of Thumb for Evaluating Normed and Standardized Assessment Instruments in Psychology. *Psychol. Assess.* **1994**, *6*, 284–290. [CrossRef]
14. Muñoz, G.; Albarrán-Diego, C.; Ferrer-Blasco, T.; Sakla, H.F.; García-Lázaro, S. Visual function after bilateral implantation of a new zonal refractive aspheric multifocal intraocular lens. *J. Cataract Refract. Surg.* **2011**, *37*, 2043–2052. [CrossRef]
15. Güçlü, H.; Akaray, İ.; Kaya, S.; Sattarpanah, S.; Çınar, A.C.; Sakallıoğlu, K.; Korkmaz, S.; Gürlü, V. Agreement of Anterior Segment Parameters Between Scheimpflug Topography and Swept-Source Optical Coherence Based Optic Biometry in Keratoconus and Healthy Subjects. *Eye Contact Lens* **2021**, *47*, 539–545. [CrossRef] [PubMed]
16. Harrer, A.; Hirnschall, N.; Tabernero, J.; Artal, P.; Draschl, P.; Maedel, S.; Findl, O. Variability in angle κ and its influence on higher-order aberrations in pseudophakic eyes. *J. Cataract Refract. Surg.* **2017**, *43*, 1015–1019. [CrossRef] [PubMed]
17. Shimizu, K.; Ito, M. Dissatisfaction after Bilateral Multifocal Intraocular Lens Implantation: An Electrophysiology Study. *J. Refract. Surg.* **2011**, *27*, 309–312. [CrossRef] [PubMed]
18. Karhanová, M.; Pluháček, F.; Mlčák, P.; Vláčil, O.; Šín, M.; Marešová, K. The importance of angle kappa evaluation for implantation of diffractive multifocal intra-ocular lenses using pseudophakic eye model. *Acta Ophthalmol.* **2015**, *93*, e123–e128. [CrossRef]
19. Tchah, H.; Nam, K.; Yoo, A. Predictive factors for photic phenomena after refractive, rotationally asymmetric, multifocal intraocular lens implantation. *Int. J. Ophthalmol.* **2017**, *10*, 241–245. [CrossRef]
20. Moshirfar, M.; Hoggan, R.; Muthappan, V. Angle Kappa and its importance in refractive surgery. *Oman J. Ophthalmol.* **2013**, *6*, 151–158. [CrossRef]
21. Fu, Y.; Kou, J.; Chen, D.; Wang, D.; Zhao, Y.; Hu, M.; Lin, X.; Dai, Q.; Li, J.; Zhao, Y.E. Influence of angle kappa and angle alpha on visual quality after implantation of multifocal intraocular lenses. *J. Cataract Refract. Surg.* **2019**, *45*, 1258–1264. [CrossRef] [PubMed]

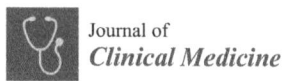

Article

Changes in Peripapillary and Macular Vessel Densities and Their Relationship with Visual Field Progression after Trabeculectomy

Jooyoung Yoon, Kyung Rim Sung * and Joong Won Shin

Department of Ophthalmology, College of Medicine, University of Ulsan, Asan Medical Center, Seoul 05505, Korea; cec1204@naver.com (J.Y.); sideral@hanmail.net (J.W.S.)
* Correspondence: sungeye@gmail.com; Tel.: +82-2-3010-3680; Fax: +82-2-470-6440

Abstract: The aim of this study was to determine the factors associated with visual field (VF) deterioration after trabeculectomy, including the peripapillary vessel density (pVD) and macular vessel density (mVD) changes assessed by optical coherence tomography angiography (OCT-A). Primary open-angle glaucoma patients with more than two years of follow-up after trabeculectomy were included. pVD was calculated in a region defined as a 750 µm-wide elliptical annulus extending from the optic disc boundary. mVD was calculated in the parafoveal (1–3 mm) and perifoveal (3–6 mm) regions. VF deterioration was defined as the rate of mean deviation (MD) worse than −1.5 dB/year. The change rates of pVD and mVD were compared between the deteriorated VF and non-deteriorated VF groups. The factors associated with the rate of MD were determined by linear regression analyses. VF deterioration was noted in 14 (21.5%) of the 65 eyes that underwent trabeculectomy. The pVD (−2.26 ± 2.67 vs. −0.02 ± 1.74%/year, $p \leq 0.001$) reduction rate was significantly greater in the deteriorated VF group than in the non-deteriorated VF group, while that of parafoveal ($p = 0.267$) and perifoveal ($p = 0.350$) VD did not show a significant difference. The linear regression analysis showed that the postoperative MD reduction rate was significantly associated with the rate of pVD reduction ($p = 0.016$), while other clinical parameters and preoperative vascular parameters did not show any association. Eyes with greater loss of peripapillary retinal circulation after trabeculectomy tended to exhibit VF deterioration. The assessment of peripapillary vascular status can be an adjunctive strategy to predict visual function after trabeculectomy.

Keywords: primary open-angle glaucoma; optical coherence tomography angiography; vessel density; visual field; progression

Citation: Yoon, J.; Sung, K.R.; Shin, J.W. Changes in Peripapillary and Macular Vessel Densities and Their Relationship with Visual Field Progression after Trabeculectomy. *J. Clin. Med.* **2021**, *10*, 5862. https://doi.org/10.3390/jcm10245862

Academic Editors: Vito Romano, Yalin Zheng and Mariantonia Ferrara

Received: 8 November 2021
Accepted: 13 December 2021
Published: 14 December 2021

Publisher's Note: MDPI stays neutral with regard to jurisdictional claims in published maps and institutional affiliations.

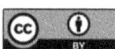

Copyright: © 2021 by the authors. Licensee MDPI, Basel, Switzerland. This article is an open access article distributed under the terms and conditions of the Creative Commons Attribution (CC BY) license (https://creativecommons.org/licenses/by/4.0/).

1. Introduction

Glaucoma causes progressive structural abnormalities in the optic nerve head (ONH) and the loss of visual function [1]. The mainstay of glaucoma treatment is slowing down the disease progression by preventing further ONH damage. The lowering of intraocular pressure (IOP) is the only proven way to slow down the disease progression [2,3]. Elevated IOP is a well-known risk factor for glaucoma [4–7]; however, several vascular factors also play a role in the pathophysiology of glaucoma development and progression [8]. Previous studies have evaluated the changes of the ocular hemodynamic in the ophthalmic artery, ONH, and retinal vasculature [9,10] after medical or surgical IOP reduction.

OCT angiography (OCT-A) is a non-invasive technique that can provide quantitative and reproducible vascular information of the ONH and retina [11]. OCT-A allows the precise visualization of the retinal capillary network [12] layer by layer, and a reduction of the vessel density (VD) assessed by OCT-A showed a correlation with the structural and functional parameters in glaucoma patients [13–15].

Increased or stable microcirculation after the surgical lowering of IOP has been reported [16–20]. However, research outcomes evaluating the clinical implication of postoperative microvascular changes in association with the visual prognosis are limited. Hence, we aimed to evaluate the longitudinal peripapillary and macular microcirculation changes after the surgical IOP reduction and their association with the postoperative visual field (VF) changes.

2. Materials and Methods

In this retrospective observational study, we recruited primary open-angle glaucoma (POAG) patients who underwent trabeculectomy by a single surgeon (KRS) at the glaucoma clinic of Asan Medical Center (Seoul, Korea) between November 2016 and January 2019. All the study procedures were performed in accordance with the principles of the Declaration of Helsinki. The Institutional Review Board of Asan Medical Center approved this study. The requirement for written informed consent was waived due to the retrospective design.

2.1. Participants

At the baseline examination, all the participants underwent complete ophthalmologic examinations; best-corrected visual acuity (BCVA), refractometry, slit-lamp biomicroscopy, Goldmann applanation tonometry, gonioscopy, stereoscopic optic disc/retinal nerve fiber layer (RNFL) photography, ultrasound pachymetry, standard automated perimetry (Humphrey Field analyzer with Swedish Interactive Threshold Algorithm standard 24-2 test; Carl Zeiss Meditec, Dublin, CA, USA), and OCT-A (AngioVue, Optovue Inc., Fremont, CA, USA).

The inclusion criteria of this study were as follows: patients diagnosed with POAG, with BCVA of logMAR +0.30 (Snellen 20/40) or better, a spherical refraction of −8.0 to +3.0 diopters (D), a cylinder correction within ±3 D, and clear ocular media. POAG was defined as having an open angle on gonioscopy, RNFL defects, or glaucomatous optic disc changes (neuroretinal rim thinning, disc excavation, or disc hemorrhage), and corresponding VF defects. Participants with any ophthalmic or neurological disease other than glaucoma that can affect ONH were excluded. If both eyes met the inclusion criteria, one eye was selected at random. The participants were followed-up for ≥2 years after the trabeculectomy.

Trabeculectomy was performed in patients with progressive glaucomatous changes that could not be controlled with maximum tolerated medical therapy (MTMT) and in those with an elevated IOP that could cause additional ONH damage. A single experienced glaucoma specialist (KRS) performed all surgical interventions. All glaucoma medications were continued up to the time of the surgery. Eyes with persistent hypotony maculopathy after trabeculectomy or eyes with other macular abnormalities, such as an epiretinal membrane or age-related macular degeneration, were excluded from the study. Patients who received other intraocular surgery during the 2-year follow-up period were also excluded from the study.

2.2. Trabeculectomy

Trabeculectomy was performed by a single surgeon (KRS). A 6- to 7-mm horizontal incision was made in the superior area, and the conjunctiva and Tenon's capsule were carefully dissected for preparation of the fornix-based conjunctival flap. A limbus-based half-thickness scleral flap (2.5 × 2 mm) was then prepared. 0.2% mitomycin C-soaked sponge was applied under the sub-Tenon space for 2 min and copious irrigation with balanced salt solution (BSS) was performed in order to wash out the mitomycin C. The sclerectomy was made with the Kelly Descemet punch under the partial scleral flap, and the peripheral iridectomy was performed through the sclerectomy site. The scleral flap was closed with a single 9-0 nylon suture. The conjunctiva and Tenon's capsule are secured with a 8-0 vicryl interrupted suture followed by running sutures. Bleb elevation and integrity of the conjunctival closure were checked. Topical corticosteroid (1.0% prednisolone), cycloplegics, and an antibiotic (0.5% moxifloxacin) were prescribed for approximately 1 month postoperatively, depending on the eye condition.

2.3. VF Assessment

Only the reliable VF test results were included in the analysis. A reliable VF test result was defined by the presence of false-positive errors < 15%, false-negative errors < 15%, and fixation loss < 20%. A glaucomatous VF defect was defined as the presence of a cluster of three or more non-edge contiguous points on a pattern deviation plot with a p-value < 5% (one of which had a p-value < 1%), confirmed by at least two consecutive examinations; pattern standard deviation with a p-value < 5%; or glaucoma hemifield test result outside normal limits. The VF was assessed before the surgery, and 6 months, 1 year, 1.5 years, and 2 years postoperatively. VF progression was defined as the rate of mean deviation (MD) worse than -1.5 dB annually [21]. At least five qualified VF examinations were required to be included.

2.4. OCT-A Imaging

The AngioVue OCT-A imaging system enables non-invasive visualization of the ophthalmic microvasculature. The dynamic motion of the moving particles, such as red blood cells, was captured using this system, with a split-spectrum amplitude-decorrelation angiography algorithm used to identify the perfused vessels. In this study, the peripapillary vasculature was measured in a 4.5×4.5 mm region centered on the optic disc, and within a slab from the internal limiting membrane to the posterior border of the RNFL. The peripapillary VD (pVD) was calculated in a region defined as a 750 μm-wide elliptical annulus extending from the optic disc boundary. The macular vasculature was measured in a 6.0×6.0 mm region centered on the fovea, and within a slab from the internal limiting membrane to the posterior border of the inner plexiform layer. The macular VD was calculated in the parafoveal and perifoveal regions, defined as concentric circular areas with an inner and outer diameter of 1 mm and 3 mm, and 3 mm and 6 mm, respectively. All the scans were evaluated for quality. The reasons for exclusion were poor image quality, defined as the signal strength index < 48; poor clarity; localized weak signals caused by artifacts, such as floaters; residual motion artifacts visible as irregular vessel patterns or disc boundaries on the en face angiogram; or segmentation failure. At least five qualified OCT-A examinations were required to be included. The circumpapillary retinal nerve fiber layer (RNFL) thickness and ganglion cell complex (GCC) thickness were also assessed using the same device.

2.5. Statistical Analysis

The normality was tested using the Kolmogorov-Smirnov test for all continuous variables. The baseline clinical characteristics were compared between the eyes with relatively stable VF and those with deteriorated VF after trabeculectomy using either an independent t-test or Mann-Whitney test as appropriate. A linear mixed model was performed to determine the postoperative change rate of IOP, and the OCT-A driven vascular and structural parameters. Repeated measures ANOVA was used to compare the postoperative changes of each parameter. Univariate and multivariate linear regression analyses, including the OCT-A driven vascular parameters, were used to determine the factors associated with the VF MD change rate after the trabeculectomy. A p-value < 0.1 in the univariate analysis was included in the multivariate analysis. The statistical analysis was performed using the SPSS software, version 20 (IBM Corp., Armonk, NY, USA). p-value ≤ 0.05 was considered statistically significant.

3. Results

Of the 81 eyes of 81 patients initially enrolled, 16 eyes were excluded due to the poor quality, poor clarity, and segmentation failure of the OCT-A image. Sixty-five eyes of 65 patients (38 male, 27 female) with successful trabeculectomy and qualified visual field tests were included in the final analysis. The baseline characteristics are described in Table 1. Postoperative VF deterioration was observed in 14 eyes (21.5%) when assessed for two years postoperatively. The preoperative clinical characteristics, including age, VF

MD, and IOP did not differ between the two groups. VD parameters, RNFL, and GCC thickness, which were assessed before surgery, also did not differ between the groups. No significant postoperative complications, such as prolonged hypotony and inadequate IOP control, were observed in both groups. Topical medications were prescribed based on the patients' postoperative condition. 1.59 ± 1.03 topical medications were used in the total population after the surgery, while 1.57 ± 1.02 in the progression group, and 1.59 ± 1.04 in the non-progression group were used, respectively. The difference in the number of postoperative topical medications between the progression and non-progression groups was not statistically significant ($p = 0.957$).

Table 1. Baseline demographics and the clinical characteristics of the VF progression and non-progression group.

Variables	Total ($n = 65$)	Progression ($n = 14$)	Non-Progression ($n = 51$)	p-Value *
Age (years)	54.8 ± 13.3	55.7 ± 13.5	54.6 ± 13.4	0.778
Sex, male/female	38/27	8/6	30/21	0.911
Topical medications, n	2.8 ± 0.6	2.6 ± 0.5	2.8 ± 0.6	0.322
Self-reported history of HTN, n (%)	20 (30.8%)	4 (28.6%)	16 (31.4%)	0.842
Self-reported history of DM, n (%)	8 (12.3%)	2 (14.3%)	6 (11.8%)	0.801
VF MD (dB)	-16.6 ± 7.9	-13.8 ± 6.7	-17.4 ± 8.1	0.137
IOP (mmHg)	19.9 ± 8.4	20.5 ± 7.9	20.0 ± 9.2	0.860
SE (D)	-2.3 ± 3.1	-3.0 ± 3.6	-2.1 ± 2.9	0.301
Axial length (mm)	24.9 ± 1.8	25.1 ± 1.8	24.9 ± 1.7	0.675
Central corneal thickness (μm)	530.1 ± 45.5	513.1 ± 51.5	533.8 ± 43.8	0.195
Peripapillary VD (%)	34.75 ± 5.85	34.25 ± 5.55	34.86 ± 5.98	0.780
Foveal VD (%)	15.99 ± 6.46	15.45 ± 5.37	16.14 ± 6.77	0.728
Parafoveal VD (%)	41.73 ± 4.99	39.77 ± 4.78	42.27 ± 4.96	0.098
Perifoveal VD (%)	37.75 ± 3.80	36.25 ± 3.53	38.16 ± 3.80	0.096
RNFL thickness (μm)	65.92 ± 8.83	66.23 ± 6.35	65.84 ± 9.41	0.889
GCC thickness (μm)	69.59 ± 7.48	67.54 ± 5.22	70.12 ± 7.92	0.271

Independent t-test for numerical variables; Mann-Whitney test for non-numerical variables. * $p \leq 0.05$ was considered statistically significant. Abbreviations: HTN, Hypertension; DM, Diabetes mellitus; VF MD, Visual field mean deviation; SE, Spherical equivalence; VD, vessel density; RNFL, Retinal nerve fiber layer; GCC, Ganglion cell complex.

The postoperative change rate of clinical parameters is described in Tables 2 and 3, and Figure 1. The VF MD rate of the deteriorated VF group was -2.46 ± 0.77 dB/year, while that of the non-progression VF group was 0.06 ± 0.89 dB/year ($p < 0.001$). The rate of pVD ($p \leq 0.001$) and RNFL thickness ($p = 0.039$) differed between the two groups, while foveal VD ($p = 0.054$) showed marginal difference. The parafoveal VD ($p = 0.267$) and perifoveal VD ($p = 0.350$) did not show significant difference. The rate of IOP ($p = 0.672$) and other structural parameters, such as GCC ($p = 0.198$) thickness, did not differ between the groups.

The baseline clinical characteristics and postoperative change rates of each OCT-A parameter were analyzed using univariate and multivariate linear regression analyses to determine the factors associated with the VF MD change rate after trabeculectomy (Table 4). None of the preoperative parameters showed an association with the postoperative VF MD rate. However, the rate of pVD ($p = 0.006$) and foveal VD ($p = 0.057$) in the univariate analysis showed a possible association with the postoperative VF MD rate; additionally, the multivariate analysis revealed that only the postoperative reduction rate of pVD showed a correlation ($p = 0.016$).

A representative case example is shown in Figure 2. A 43-year-old woman with POAG exhibited a gradual loss of peripapillary microcirculation after trabeculectomy along with progressive glaucomatous VF progression (a). A 25-year-old woman with POAG showed stable peripapillary retinal microcirculation and VF after trabeculectomy when assessed for two years with a similar level of preoperative VF MD and IOP reduction after trabeculectomy (b).

Table 2. Comparison of the postoperative change rate of the parameters between the VF progression and non-progression group.

Variables, Mean ± SD [95% CI]	Total (n = 65)	Progression (n = 14)	Non-Progression (n = 51)	p-Value *
VF MD change rate (dB/year)	−0.49 ± 1.35 (−0.82, −0.15)	−2.46 ± 0.77 (−2.91, −2.01)	0.06 ± 0.89 (−0.19, 0.30)	<0.001 *
IOP reduction rate (mmHg/year)	−3.43 ± 4.56 (−4.56, −2.30)	−3.89 ± 4.13 (−6.28, −1.51)	−3.30 ± 4.70 (−4.63, −1.98)	0.672
Peripapillary VD change rate (%/year)	−0.50 ± 2.17 (−1.04, 0.04)	−2.26 ± 2.67 (−3.81, −0.72)	−0.02 ± 1.74 (−0.51, 0.47)	<0.001 *
Foveal VD change rate (%/year)	−0.28 ± 3.55 (−1.16, 0.60)	−1.62 ± 2.52 (−3.08, −0.17)	0.09 ± 3.73 (−0.96, 1.13)	0.054
Parafoveal VD change rate (%/year)	−0.80 ± 2.97 (−1.54, −0.07)	−1.59 ± 2.71 (−3.15, −0.02)	−0.59 ± 3.03 (−1.43, 0.26)	0.267
Perifoveal VD change rate (%/year)	−0.72 ± 1.97 (−1.21, −0.23)	−1.16 ± 1.55 (−2.06, −0.27)	−0.60 ± 2.06 (−1.18, −0.02)	0.350
RNFL thickness change rate (μm/year)	−0.70 ± 3.82 (−1.66, 0.26)	−2.64 ± 3.80 (−4.93, −0.34)	−0.20 ± 3.70 (−1.25, 0.85)	0.039 *
GCC thickness change rate (μm/year)	0.59 ± 3.51 (−0.31, 1.47)	1.72 ± 3.52 (−0.41, 3.85)	0.31 ± 3.49 (−0.67, 1.29)	0.198

Independent t-test. * $p \leq 0.05$ was considered statistically significant. Abbreviations: VF MD, Visual field mean deviation; IOP, intraocular pressure; VD, vessel density; RNFL, Retinal nerve fiber layer; GCC, Ganglion cell complex.

Table 3. Comparison of the postoperative changes of VF MD, IOP and peripapillary VD between the VF progression and non-progression group.

Variables, Mean ± SD		Total (n = 65)	Progression (n = 14)	Non-Progression (n = 51)	p-Value *
VF MD (dB)	Pre-op	−16.62 ± 7.92	−15.32 ± 5.91	−17.19 ± 8.01	<0.001 *
	Post-op 0.5yr	−16.88 ± 8.01	−17.49 ± 7.23	−16.47 ± 8.27	
	Post-op 1yr	−17.01 ± 7.81	−18.88 ± 5.88	−16.39 ± 8.06	
	Post-op 1.5yr	−16.98 ± 7.80	−19.43 ± 6.75	−16.44 ± 8.05	
	Post-op 2yr	−17.36 ± 8.16	−20.07 ± 6.55	−16.65 ± 8.10	
IOP (mmHg)	Pre-op	19.85 ± 8.42	20.50 ± 7.92	19.67 ± 8.62	0.789
	Post-op 0.5yr	11.55 ± 2.92	11.57 ± 2.53	11.55 ± 3.04	
	Post-op 1yr	12.42 ± 2.97	12.71 ± 2.89	12.33 ± 3.01	
	Post-op 1.5yr	12.78 ± 2.92	12.57 ± 2.82	12.84 ± 2.98	
	Post-op 2yr	12.98 ± 2.87	12.71 ± 2.52	13.06 ± 2.98	
Peripapillary VD (%)	Pre-op	34.75 ± 5.85	34.36 ± 5.55	34.86 ± 5.98	0.001 *
	Post-op 0.5yr	33.92 ± 6.33	31.13 ± 4.93	34.62 ± 6.51	
	Post-op 1yr	35.79 ± 6.18	30.42 ± 3.89	36.24 ± 6.50	
	Post-op 1.5yr	34.54 ± 6.62	31.18 ± 3.20	35.45 ± 6.96	
	Post-op 2yr	32.27 ± 4.22	30.28 ± 3.01	32.47 ± 4.35	

Repeated measures ANOVA * $p \leq 0.05$ was considered statistically significant. Abbreviations: VF MD, Visual field mean deviation; IOP, intraocular pressure; VD, vessel density.

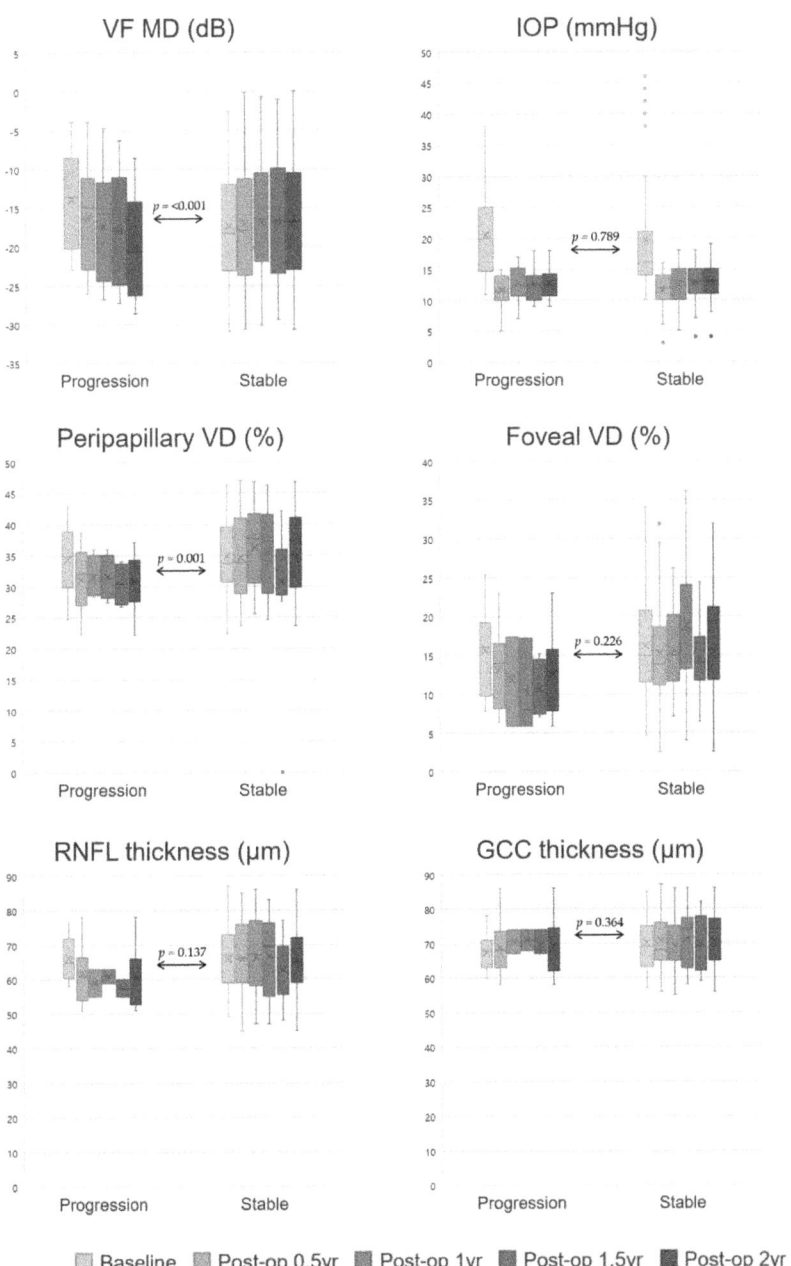

Figure 1. Comparison of postoperative parameter changes between the VF progression and non-progression group. Repeated measures ANOVA was used to compare the post-operative changes of each parameter, and the *p*-values of repeated measures ANOVA were presented. X: average value, horizontal line: median value, dots: outliers. Abbreviations: GCC, ganglion cell complex; IOP, intraocular pressure; RNFL, retinal nerve fiber layer; VD, vessel density; VF MD, visual field mean deviation.

Table 4. Univariable and multivariable linear regression analyses to determine the factors associated with the visual field change rate after trabeculectomy.

Variables	Univariable		Multivariable ($p < 0.1$ in Univariable)	
	B ± SD	p-Value *	B ± SD	p-Value *
Age (years)	0.003 ± 0.013	0.814		
SE (D)	0.018 ± 0.055	0.739		
Central corneal thickness (μm)	0.005 ± 0.004	0.135		
Baseline IOP (mmHg)	−0.001 ± 0.019	0.961		
Baseline VF MD (dB)	−0.034 ± 0.021	0.112		
Baseline peripapillary VD (%)	−0.013 ± 0.029	0.648		
Baseline foveal VD (%)	−0.024 ± 0.026	0.369		
Baseline parafoveal VD (%)	0.009 ± 0.034	0.800		
Baseline perifoveal VD (%)	0.024 ± 0.045	0.586		
Baseline RNFL thickness (μm)	−0.013 ± 0.019	0.499		
Baseline GCC thickness (μm)	0.022 ± 0.023	0.341		
Postoperative IOP reduction rate (mmHg/year)	0.011 ± 0.037	0.771		
Postoperative peripapillary VD change rate (%/year)	0.209 ± 0.074	0.006	0.186 ± 0.075	0.016
Postoperative foveal VD change rate (%/year)	0.090 ± 0.046	0.057	0.065 ± 0.046	0.160
Postoperative parafoveal VD change rate (%/year)	0.078 ± 0.056	0.175		
Postoperative perifoveal VD change rate (%/year)	0.059 ± 0.086	0.496		
RNFL thickness change rate (μm/year)	0.075 ± 0.044	0.098		
GCC thickness change rate (μm/year)	−0.047 ± 0.048	0.335		

* $p \leq 0.05$ was considered statistically significant. Abbreviations: SD, standard deviation; VF MD, visual field mean deviation; IOP, intraocular pressure; SE, spherical equivalence; VD, vessel density; RNFL, retinal nerve fiber layer; GCC, ganglion cell complex.

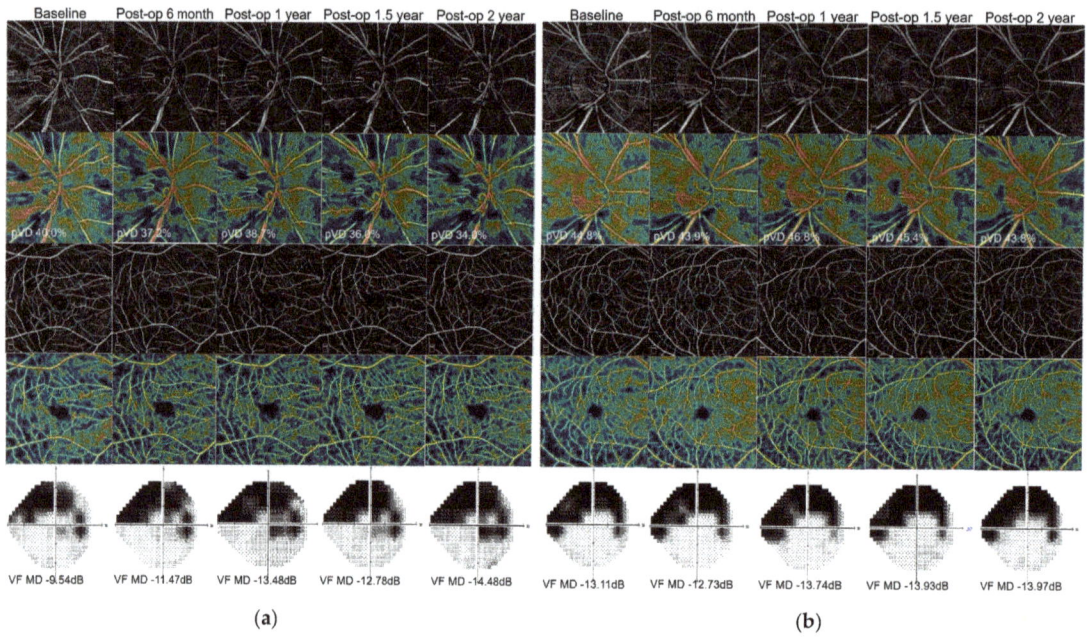

Figure 2. (**a**) A 43-year-old woman with POAG exhibited a gradual loss of peripapillary microcirculation after trabeculectomy along with progressive glaucomatous VF progression. (**b**) A 25-year-old woman with POAG showed stable peripapillary retinal microcirculation and VF after trabeculectomy when assessed for 2 years with a similar level of preoperative VF MD and IOP reduction after trabeculectomy. Abbreviations: POAG, primary open angle glaucoma; VF, visual field; IOP, intraocular pressure.

4. Discussion

Our study demonstrated a two-year VF change after trabeculectomy in POAG eyes and the factors associated with the postoperative VF deterioration. The deteriorated VF group showed a faster rate of pVD than the non-deteriorated VF group. Furthermore, the rate of pVD was the only factor associated with that of VF MD. The baseline clinical characteristics or the change rates of other structural parameters, or macular area VD were not relevant to postoperative VF changes.

Trabeculectomy is the most commonly performed glaucoma surgery in patients with inadequate IOP control or progression of glaucoma despite MTMT. Trabeculectomy can slow the rate of glaucomatous deterioration; however, it does not completely stop the disease progression in the long term, and some studies reported the continuous deterioration of VF despite successful IOP control after trabeculectomy [22–24]. Hence, factors other than IOP should be sought and considered for the care of glaucoma patients who have undergone trabeculectomy. This study demonstrated the association between the postoperative pVD change and VF MD rates, which indicates that peripapillary retinal circulation change could provide insight into postoperative VF change in glaucoma patients.

Studies [16–20,25] have evaluated the change of peripapillary and retinal microvasculature following a large amount of IOP reduction in glaucoma patients. Some studies [17,18,20] reported limited or no significant VD change, while others [16,19,25] have documented microvascular improvement after IOP reduction. Zeboulon et al. [20] reported a limited change in the whole peripapillary VD change and increased focal peripapillary vascular loss 1 month after deep nonpenetrating sclerotomy. Lommatzsch et al. [18] reported that no significant changes were detectable in the papillary or macular VD, RNFL, or macular ganglion cell layer thickness after trabeculectomy in open-angle glaucoma patients. Kim et al. [17] showed no significant change in the microcirculation of the peripapillary retina and choroid 3 months postoperatively after trabeculectomy in POAG patients. Contrarily, Shin et al. [19] showed that 19 (61.3%) of 31 eyes exhibited peripapillary microvascular improvement in the circumpapillary capillary dropout area three months after the trabeculectomy. Hollo et al. [16] also observed pVD improvement after large IOP reduction by topical medication in young patients with high untreated IOP. Liu et al. [25] reported the increase of vessel densities in the optic nerve head and the peripapillary area after applying prostaglandin analog for more than three weeks in the treatment-naïve eyes.

These studies demonstrated peripapillary and macular VD changes after trabeculectomy or large IOP reduction during a relatively short follow-up period (three to six months). However, in this study, we followed up with the patients who underwent trabeculectomy for two years and investigated the correlation between VD change and VF deterioration. To the best of our knowledge, this is the first study describing the association of VD with VF outcome after trabeculectomy. The diagnostic potential of macular and peripapillary OCT-A-determined VD loss in early glaucoma has been reported [11,15,26]. Along with these studies, our study showed that the assessment of peripapillary retinal circulation can be used as a predictor of visual function after IOP lowering surgery. GCC thickness change rate and the change rates of other vascular parameters did not show any difference between the deteriorated and the non-deteriorated VF groups and were not related to the postoperative VF MD change rate. Considering that most glaucoma patients who have undergone trabeculectomy already have a substantial loss of VF, a biomarker reflecting visual function change is important in the care of advanced glaucoma patients.

It is unclear why some eyes showed a decrease of peripapillary VD despite successful IOP reduction. A significant IOP decrease after trabeculectomy is known to reduce the depth of the lamina cribrosa [27–29]. Additionally, this level of LC depth reduction has shown an association with microvascular improvement after trabeculectomy [17,19]. However, in another study on the long-term shape and depth of LC after trabeculectomy, although most eyes showed long-term flattening and shallowing of the LC, some eyes showed a deepened LC from the baseline. Therefore, the authors concluded that a reduction of IOP plays an important role in the early phase of LC change; however, LC remodeling may play a crucial role in a stable IOP in the later phase [30]. Hence, such remodeling of LC may lead to VD reduction and glaucomatous VF deterioration.

This study has some limitations. First, we excluded 16 eyes due to the poor image quality, poor clarity, and segmentation failure of OCT-A. This could be a limitation of the current OCT-A technology. Second, the study population was of a single ethnicity; thus, the results may not be directly applied to other ethnic groups. Third, the sample size was relatively small, suggesting the need for further study with a larger population. Lastly, the follow-up period was two years postoperatively, which may be relatively short considering that glaucoma is a progressive degenerative disease. A study with a longer duration may confirm our findings.

5. Conclusions

This study demonstrated that a greater loss of peripapillary microvasculature after trabeculectomy is associated with visual function deterioration up to two years after surgery. This is the first study showing the relationship between the retinal microvasculature and visual function change after trabeculectomy. POAG patients with greater peripapillary capillary decrease after the IOP lowering surgery may experience VF deterioration; therefore, careful monitoring is warranted in these patients. Additionally, our results suggest the potential use of OCT-A measured peripapillary VD as a biomarker for predicting the visual function after trabeculectomy.

Author Contributions: Conceptualization, J.Y., K.R.S. and J.W.S.; methodology, J.Y., K.R.S. and J.W.S.; formal analysis, J.Y., K.R.S. and J.W.S.; investigation, J.Y., K.R.S. and J.W.S.; resources, J.Y., K.R.S. and J.W.S.; writing—original draft preparation, J.Y.; writing—review and editing, K.R.S. and J.W.S.; supervision, K.R.S. All authors have read and agreed to the published version of the manuscript.

Funding: This research received no external funding.

Institutional Review Board Statement: The study was conducted according to the guidelines of the Declaration of Helsinki, and approved by the Institutional Review Board of Asan Medical Center (IRB no. 2021-1284, date of approval: 19 August 2021).

Informed Consent Statement: Patient consent was waived due to the retrospective nature of this study, and due to the subjects' anonymity and minimal risk to patients.

Data Availability Statement: The data used to support the findings of this study are included in the article, and are available on request from the corresponding author.

Conflicts of Interest: The authors declare no conflict of interest.

References

1. Weinreb, R.N.; Khaw, P.T. Primary open-angle glaucoma. *Lancet* **2004**, *363*, 1711–1720. [CrossRef]
2. Collaborative Normal-Tension Glaucoma Study Group. Comparison of glaucomatous progression between untreated patients with normal-tension glaucoma and patients with therapeutically reduced intraocular pressures. *Am. J. Ophthalmol.* **1998**, *126*, 487–497.
3. Heijl, A.; Leske, M.C.; Bengtsson, B.; Hyman, L.; Bengtsson, B.; Hussein, M. Reduction of intraocular pressure and glaucoma progression: Results from the Early Manifest Glaucoma Trial. *Arch. Ophthalmol.* **2002**, *120*, 1268–1279. [CrossRef] [PubMed]
4. Gordon, M.O.; Beiser, J.A.; Brandt, J.D.; Heuer, D.K.; Higginbotham, E.J.; Johnson, C.A.; Keltner, J.L.; Miller, J.P.; Parrish, R.K.; Wilson, M.R. The Ocular Hypertension Treatment Study: Baseline factors that predict the onset of primary open-angle glaucoma. *Arch. Ophthalmol.* **2002**, *120*, 714–720. [CrossRef]
5. Investigators, A. The Advanced Glaucoma Intervention Study (AGIS): 7. The relationship between control of intraocular pressure and visual field deterioration. *Am. J. Ophthalmol.* **2000**, *130*, 429–440.
6. Kass, M.A.; Heuer, D.K.; Higginbotham, E.J.; Johnson, C.A.; Keltner, J.L.; Miller, J.P.; Parrish, R.K.; Wilson, M.R.; Gordon, M.O. The Ocular Hypertension Treatment Study: A randomized trial determines that topical ocular hypotensive medication delays or prevents the onset of primary open-angle glaucoma. *Arch. Ophthalmol.* **2002**, *120*, 701–713. [CrossRef]
7. Leske, M.C.; Heijl, A.; Hussein, M.; Bengtsson, B.; Hyman, L.; Komaroff, E. Factors for glaucoma progression and the effect of treatment: The early manifest glaucoma trial. *Arch. Ophthalmol.* **2003**, *121*, 48–56. [CrossRef]
8. Yanagi, M.; Kawasaki, R.; Wang, J.J.; Wong, T.Y.; Crowston, J.; Kiuchi, Y. Vascular risk factors in glaucoma: A review. *Clin. Exp. Ophthalmol.* **2011**, *39*, 252–258. [CrossRef]

9. Deokule, S.; Vizzeri, G.; Boehm, A.; Bowd, C.; Weinreb, R.N. Association of visual field severity and parapapillary retinal blood flow in open-angle glaucoma. *J. Glaucoma* **2010**, *19*, 293–298. [CrossRef]
10. Logan, J.; Rankin, S.; Jackson, A. Retinal blood flow measurements and neuroretinal rim damage in glaucoma. *Br. J. Ophthalmol.* **2004**, *88*, 1049–1054. [CrossRef]
11. Jia, Y.; Wei, E.; Wang, X.; Zhang, X.; Morrison, J.C.; Parikh, M.; Lombardi, L.H.; Gattey, D.M.; Armour, R.L.; Edmunds, B. Optical coherence tomography angiography of optic disc perfusion in glaucoma. *Ophthalmology* **2014**, *121*, 1322–1332. [CrossRef]
12. Spaide, R.F.; Klancnik, J.M.; Cooney, M.J. Retinal vascular layers imaged by fluorescein angiography and optical coherence tomography angiography. *JAMA Ophthalmol.* **2015**, *133*, 45–50. [CrossRef]
13. Akagi, T.; Iida, Y.; Nakanishi, H.; Terada, N.; Morooka, S.; Yamada, H.; Hasegawa, T.; Yokota, S.; Yoshikawa, M.; Yoshimura, N. Microvascular density in glaucomatous eyes with hemifield visual field defects: An optical coherence tomography angiography study. *Am. J. Ophthalmol.* **2016**, *168*, 237–249. [CrossRef]
14. Holló, G. Vessel density calculated from OCT angiography in 3 peripapillary sectors in normal, ocular hypertensive, and glaucoma eyes. *Eur. J. Ophthalmol.* **2016**, *26*, e42–e45. [CrossRef]
15. Liu, L.; Jia, Y.; Takusagawa, H.L.; Pechauer, A.D.; Edmunds, B.; Lombardi, L.; Davis, E.; Morrison, J.C.; Huang, D. Optical coherence tomography angiography of the peripapillary retina in glaucoma. *JAMA Ophthalmol.* **2015**, *133*, 1045–1052. [CrossRef]
16. Holló, G. Influence of large intraocular pressure reduction on peripapillary OCT vessel density in ocular hypertensive and glaucoma eyes. *J. Glaucoma* **2017**, *26*, e7–e10. [CrossRef]
17. Kim, J.-A.; Kim, T.-W.; Lee, E.J.; Girard, M.J.; Mari, J.M. Microvascular changes in peripapillary and optic nerve head tissues after trabeculectomy in primary open-angle glaucoma. *Investig. Ophthalmol. Vis. Sci.* **2018**, *59*, 4614–4621. [CrossRef]
18. Lommatzsch, C.; Rothaus, K.; Koch, J.; Heinz, C.; Grisanti, S. Retinal perfusion 6 months after trabeculectomy as measured by optical coherence tomography angiography. *Int. Ophthalmol.* **2019**, *39*, 2583–2594. [CrossRef]
19. Shin, J.W.; Sung, K.R.; Uhm, K.B.; Jo, J.; Moon, Y.; Song, M.K.; Song, J.Y. Peripapillary microvascular improvement and lamina cribrosa depth reduction after trabeculectomy in primary open-angle glaucoma. *Investig. Ophthalmol. Vis. Sci.* **2017**, *58*, 5993–5999. [CrossRef]
20. Zéboulon, P.; Lévêque, P.-M.; Brasnu, E.; Aragno, V.; Hamard, P.; Baudouin, C.; Labbé, A. Effect of surgical intraocular pressure lowering on peripapillary and macular vessel density in glaucoma patients: An optical coherence tomography angiography study. *J. Glaucoma* **2017**, *26*, 466–472. [CrossRef]
21. Verma, S.; Nongpiur, M.E.; Atalay, E.; Wei, X.; Husain, R.; Goh, D.; Perera, S.A.; Aung, T. Visual Field Progression in Patients with Primary Angle-Closure Glaucoma Using Pointwise Linear Regression Analysis. *Ophthalmology* **2017**, *124*, 1065–1071. [CrossRef]
22. Ehrnrooth, P.; Puska, P.; Lehto, I.; Laatikainen, L. Progression of visual field defects and visual loss in trabeculectomized eyes. *Graefe's Arch. Clin. Exp. Ophthalmol.* **2005**, *243*, 741–747. [CrossRef]
23. Kotecha, A.; Spratt, A.; Bunce, C.; Garway-Heath, D.F.; Khaw, P.T.; Viswanathan, A. Optic disc and visual field changes after trabeculectomy. *Investig. Ophthalmol. Vis. Sci.* **2009**, *50*, 4693–4699. [CrossRef]
24. Shigeeda, T.; Tomidokoro, A.; Araie, M.; Koseki, N.; Yamamoto, S. Long-term follow-up of visual field progression after trabeculectomy in progressive normal-tension glaucoma. *Ophthalmology* **2002**, *109*, 766–770. [CrossRef]
25. Liu, C.; Umapathi, R.M.; Atalay, E.; Schmetterer, L.; Husain, R.; Boey, P.Y.; Aung, T.; Nongpiur, M.E. The Effect of Medical Lowering of Intraocular Pressure on Peripapillary and Macular Blood Flow as Measured by Optical Coherence Tomography Angiography in Treatment-naive Eyes. *J. Glaucoma* **2021**, *30*, 465–472. [CrossRef]
26. Rao, H.L.; Pradhan, Z.S.; Weinreb, R.N.; Reddy, H.B.; Riyazuddin, M.; Dasari, S.; Palakurthy, M.; Puttaiah, N.K.; Rao, D.A.; Webers, C.A. Regional comparisons of optical coherence tomography angiography vessel density in primary open-angle glaucoma. *Am. J. Ophthalmol.* **2016**, *171*, 75–83. [CrossRef]
27. Lee, E.J.; Kim, T.-W. Lamina cribrosa reversal after trabeculectomy and the rate of progressive retinal nerve fiber layer thinning. *Ophthalmology* **2015**, *122*, 2234–2242. [CrossRef]
28. Lee, E.J.; Kim, T.-W.; Weinreb, R.N.; Kim, H. Reversal of lamina cribrosa displacement after intraocular pressure reduction in open-angle glaucoma. *Ophthalmology* **2013**, *120*, 553–559. [CrossRef]
29. Quigley, H.; Arora, K.; Idrees, S.; Solano, F.; Bedrood, S.; Lee, C.; Jefferys, J.; Nguyen, T.D. Biomechanical responses of lamina cribrosa to intraocular pressure change assessed by optical coherence tomography in glaucoma eyes. *Investig. Ophthalmol. Vis. Sci.* **2017**, *58*, 2566–2577. [CrossRef]
30. Kadziauskienė, A.; Jašinskienė, E.; Ašoklis, R.; Lesinskas, E.; Rekašius, T.; Chua, J.; Cheng, C.-Y.; Mari, J.M.; Girard, M.J.; Schmetterer, L. Long-term shape, curvature, and depth changes of the lamina cribrosa after trabeculectomy. *Ophthalmology* **2018**, *125*, 1729–1740. [CrossRef]

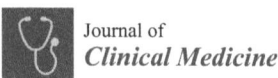

Review

In Vivo Confocal Microscopy Evaluation in Patients with Keratoconus

Alvin Wei Jun Teo [1], Hassan Mansoor [2], Nigel Sim [3], Molly Tzu-Yu Lin [4] and Yu-Chi Liu [1,4,5,6,*]

[1] Department of Cornea and External Eye Disease, Singapore National Eye Centre, Singapore 168751, Singapore; alvin.teo@mohh.com.sg
[2] Al Shifa Trust Eye Hospital, Jhelum Road, Rawalpindi 46000, Pakistan; hassan-mansoor@hotmail.com
[3] Yong Loo Lin School of Medicine, National University of Singapore, Singapore 168751, Singapore; sim.nigel@u.nus.edu
[4] Tissue Engineering and Cell Therapy Group, Singapore Eye Research Institute, Singapore 169856, Singapore; molly.lin.t.y@seri.com.sg
[5] Cornea and Refractive Surgery Group, Singapore Eye Research Institute, Singapore 169856, Singapore
[6] Ophthalmology and Visual Sciences Academic Clinical Program, Duke-NUS Medical School, Singapore 169857, Singapore
* Correspondence: liuchiy@gmail.com

Abstract: Keratoconus is the most common primary corneal ectasia characterized by progressive focal thinning. Patients experience increased irregular astigmatism, decreased visual acuity and corneal sensitivity. Corneal collagen crosslinking (CXL), a minimally invasive procedure, is effective in halting disease progression. Historically, keratoconus research was confined to ex vivo settings. In vivo confocal microscopy (IVCM) has been used to examine the corneal microstructure clinically. In this review, we discuss keratoconus cellular changes evaluated by IVCM before and after CXL. Cellular changes before CXL include decreased keratocyte and nerve densities, disorganized subbasal nerves with thickening, increased nerve tortuosity and shortened nerve fibre length. Repopulation of keratocytes occurs up to 1 year post procedure. IVCM also correlates corneal nerve status to functional corneal sensitivity. Immediately after CXL, there is reduced nerve density and keratocyte absence due to mechanical removal of the epithelium and CXL effect. Nerve regeneration begins after 1 month, with nerve fibre densities recovering to pre-operative levels between 6 months to 1 year and remains stable up to 5 years. Nerves remain tortuous and nerve densities are reduced. Corneal sensitivity is reduced immediately postoperatively but recovers with nerve regeneration. Our article provides comprehensive review on the use of IVCM imaging in keratoconus patients.

Keywords: keratoconus; corneal nerves; in-vivo confocal microscopy (IVCM); cornea cross-linking (CXL); corneal sensitivity

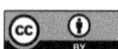

1. Introduction

Keratoconus is an ectatic condition of the cornea that is characterised by progressive thinning and steepening, causing significant visual morbidity. Reported prevalence ranges from 0.3 to 3300 per 100,000, depending on diagnostic criteria and geographic location [1]. The pathophysiology of keratoconus is multifactorial. Environmental (microtrauma), genetics, and biochemical factors play a role in disease [1]. Eye rubbing is one of the important environmental factors of keratoconus. Repetitive, prolonged and greater force of eye rubbing is associated with its progression [2]. Patient factors include atopy such as asthma and hay fever [3], and usage of contact lens wear [4,5]. As for genetic factors, alterations in Lysyl oxidase (LOX), Collagen Type V Alpha 1 Chain (COL5A1), and Forkhead box protein O1 (FOXO1) gene have been correlated to keratoconus pathogenesis [6–8]. Other studies have also shown that relatives of patients with keratoconus have a high prevalence of undiagnosed keratoconus [9,10]. In addition, biochemical factors such as increased protease activity cause collagen cross-linkages in the stroma to be broken down [11].

There has been much interest in corneal nerve structure, function and their role in corneal health and disease [12]. Corneal nerves beside their sensory function also secrete neuromediators that are vital to the development and maintenance of the cornea. It is hence important to understand the function and morphology of corneal nerves in diseased states. In keratoconus, attempts to understand corneal nerves were previously confined to ex vivo studies or cornea buttons with severe disease with staining techniques [13]. Most recently, the use of confocal microscopy in analysing keratoconic corneas have been instrumental in understanding the microstructural changes in vivo.

In vivo confocal microscopy (IVCM) is a non-invasive imaging modality that has been used to examine and quantify the cellular structure of the cornea in vivo [14,15]. It attains images by optical sectioning, where a light is focused via a small aperture onto the tissue, and in focus light is processed while light from out of focus planes are attenuated. The term "confocal" means that there is a common focal point between the illumination and collection systems. An en face image can be processed once the scan proceeds serially through the cornea depth. This allows microstructures such as corneal epithelium, and stromal keratocytes to be imaged at a cellular level [16,17]. Although the field of view of a single image is small (typically 0.16 mm^2), multiple IVCM images can be constructed into a mosaic image using automatic tissue classification algorithms for large-area visualisation and analysis [18]. The laser scanning confocal microscope is the most advanced of these and is the only design that is commercially available currently. It achieves 800 times magnification, lateral resolution of 1 μm, and axial resolution of 4 μm [14]. IVCM has thus emerged as a promising tool to study ocular and systemic diseases causing corneal neuropathies [19]. With the advancement of analytic tools, it allows for reliable longitudinal assessment on corneal nerve changes with good measurement repeatability and reproducibility [20–22].

The introduction of crosslinking in 2003 provided a minimally invasive treatment option for patients with keratoconus to halt disease progression [23]. This procedure has also shown good long-term results, effectively halting the progression of corneal ectasia, with stabilization of refractive status and topographical changes [24–26]. In conventional protocols, the epithelium is removed for better riboflavin and UV-A absorption. Other variations such as transepithelial CXL in which the corneal epithelium is left intact, have also been suggested to reduce the risk of infection, improve postoperative patient comfort and aid visual recovery.

Many studies have now depicted corneal nerve changes in the keratoconic cornea before and after crosslinking using in vivo confocal microscopy images. With increasing recognition of the important role corneal nerves play in maintaining structure and function of the cornea, we aim to summarize the literature regarding the use of in vivo confocal microscopy in the keratoconic cornea before and after CXL in this review. Aspects related to corneal nerve morphology, corneal sensation, and protocols in CXL are presented.

2. Systematic Review Methodology

Four international databases (Web of Science, PubMed, Scopus, and Google Scholar) were searched for relevant articles. All cross-sectional and longitudinal studies discussing keratoconus, cross linking and corneal sensitivity in the body, figures, or tables of the article were accepted without any restrictions.

2.1. Search Strategy

Key words such as "keratoconus", "corneal sensitivity", "cross-sectional studies", "longitudinal studies", "in vivo confocal microscopy" "cornea collagen cross-linking", and "corneal nerves" were used to search the databases of Web of Science, PubMed, Google Scholar, and Scopus from inception to December 2021. Relevant articles had their reference lists reviewed for articles of interest as well.

2.2. Inclusion Criteria

All stages of the study followed the PRISMA guidelines. Observational epidemiological studies including cross-sectional, case–control, and cohort studies that had a population-based design were included in the study. If several studies were conducted in a certain population, the higher quality study was included in the analysis. Studies from 2010 were preferably chosen to ensure the review is updated. Studies which did not meet one or more inclusion criteria were excluded from the study. The outcome of the study was the function and morphology of corneal nerves, in vivo confocal microscopy, collagen crosslinking and corneal sensitivity.

Two reviewers (A.W.J.T. and Y.C.L.) screened all retrieved articles by title and abstract initially. Only original research articles written in English were included. Analysis reviews, editorials, opinions were excluded. The articles retrieved were then curated manually to assess relevance to the study's objective. Additionally, the reference lists of remaining studies were checked to identify further relevant articles that may have been overlooked during the initial process. All the eligible articles were obtained and fully read.

We excluded articles where IVCM findings were not mentioned in the results of the full text article. Studies where recovery of full text was not possible, even after searching the available medical databases and/or contacting the corresponding authors, were excluded. Disagreements were settled through discussion with an expert for arbitration.

2.3. Data Extraction and Quality Evaluation of the Studies

The initial database search with the above keywords identified 265 papers. After excluding articles where full text was not available (21), 244 articles were left. After going through title and screening through the abstract and applying our inclusion/exclusion criteria (26 were reviews) 218 studies were left. After full text-retrieval and further curation, 84 studies remained.

3. Corneal Nerve Function and Anatomy

The cornea is a highly innervated structure. Corneal nerves originate from the ophthalmic branch of the trigeminal nerve [27]. The main stromal nerve bundles enter the human cornea radially at the corneoscleral limbus at a distance of 293 ± 106 μm from the ocular surface and are distributed uniformly throughout the corneal circumference [28]. Soon after entering the cornea, each stromal nerve bundle gives rise through repetitive branching to varying numbers of progressively smaller and smaller stromal nerves that anastomose frequently, often at highly acute branch points, to form a moderately dense midstromal plexus. Most midstromal nerve fibres turn abruptly 90 degrees and continued into the narrow band of anterior stroma located immediately beneath bowman's membrane, and gives rise to a dense, roughly two-dimensional, subepithelial plexus [29]. The subepithelial plexus has a characteristic plexiform appearance due to the anastomosis of tortuous nerve fibres, with it being denser in the peripheral and intermediate cornea than the central region. Straight fibres from the subepithelial plexus generally penetrate Bowman's membrane and continued into the corneal epithelium, with other nerves becoming subbasal nerves that course parallel to the ocular surface near the interface of Bowman's membrane and the basal epithelium (Figure 1). Subbasal nerves form a gentle spiral-like clockwise assemblage of long, curvilinear nerve fibres that converge on an imaginary center, or vortex, located inferior and slightly nasal to the corneal apex. This assembly is believed to be influenced by the electromagnetic fields of the eye [30]. They then form intraepithelial terminals that are distributed abundantly throughout the epithelium.

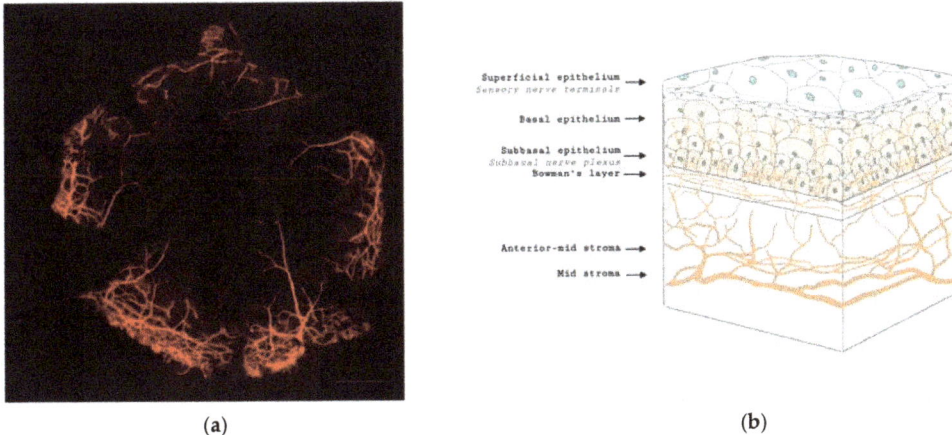

Figure 1. Anatomy of corneal nerves. (**a**) Whole mount staining with anti-class β III tubulin of mice cornea showing the distributions of corneal nerve. Scale bar: 500 μm. (**b**) Cross section of corneal nerves. (**b**) is created by Biorender.

Corneal nerves have afferent and efferent function, conveying touch and pain, as well as producing neuromediators such as neurotrophins and neuropeptides that is thought to play a role in its pathophysiology. These serve as trophic factors in ocular homeostasis and maintaining corneal microstructure. Corneal epithelial, stromal cells and endothelial cells also contribute to the diversity of neuromediators in the cornea by producing neurotrophins [31]. Neurotrophins, such as nerve growth factor (NGF), regulate neuronal development, survival, death and plasticity [12]. In keratoconus, the high affinity receptor of NGF, tyrosine kinase receptor A, was found in high levels and is thought to be due to heterologous upregulation for maintenance of unmyelinated corneal nerves [32]. Another neurotrophin, ciliary neurotrophic factor (CNTF) which is important for protection of the cornea from oxidative radical damage, had a higher expression of its mRNA in keratoconus as compared to normal eyes [32].

Neuropeptides are released slowly, act over an extended period, involved in neurotransmission and have a paracrine function. Calcitonin gene-related peptide (CGRP) plays an important role in the nociceptive pathway in the cornea, by activating factors such as bradykinin and stimulating the release of nitrous oxide [33]. These effects help produce a favorable neurochemical environment that enhances neural activity. Vasoactive intestinal peptide (VIP) is another important neuropeptide, playing a role in corneal wound healing [34] by exerting anti-inflammatory effects in a signaling pathway dependent manner [12,35]. Work by Sacchetti and colleagues analysed 12 keratoconic corneas obtained post keratoplasty and found that keratoconic corneas showed significantly higher CGRP and VIP levels as compared to controls. This increase is thought to be due to an attempt by sensory nerves to counteract degenerative changes in keratoconus [36].

4. Cellular and Corneal Nerve Morphological Changes in Keratoconus

4.1. Microstructural Changes

A lack of animal models for keratoconus renders investigation into the cellular changes difficult, and excised corneas usually represent severe disease. In ex-vivo studies, Brookes et al., found an increase in enzymatic activity in stromal keratocytes with immunohistochemical staining, and this change leads to destruction of the cornea [13]. In a study analysing corneal buttons with severe keratoconus using the acetylcholinesterase technique, stromal nerves were thickened, increasingly tortuous and disorganised with looping and coiling. Subbasal nerves showed loss of their radial, clockwise whorl configuration with tortuosity and localized thickening [37]. These staining techniques, however, can only be applied to in-vitro or ex-vivo corneas but not study corneas in vivo [38].

Several changes of the corneal cell and nerve microstructure in patients with keratoconus have been observed on IVCM images (Figure 2). Corneal stromal keratocytes (CSKs) are a population of quiescent mesenchymal-derived cells residing between collagen lamellae [39]. The cell density is the highest in the anterior 10% of the stroma and decreases posteriorly. CSKs possess dendritic processes to connect with neighboring cells, forming a highly organized syncytium throughout the stroma [40]. Some keratocytes are located in the vicinity of stromal nerves and occasionally enwrap nerve fibres with cytoplasmic extensions, suggesting an interdependence of the two [29]. Studies comparing keratoconic corneas and healthy controls found that there was generally lower stromal keratocyte density (Figure 2e,f) [41,42], with pronounced reflectivity and irregular arrangement of the stromal keratocytes [41,43]. There is loss of corneal stromal thickness over time, postulated to be due to a release of degradative enzymes [44]. These changes in cell densities may also be secondary to other factors such as contact lens wear [42,45,46].

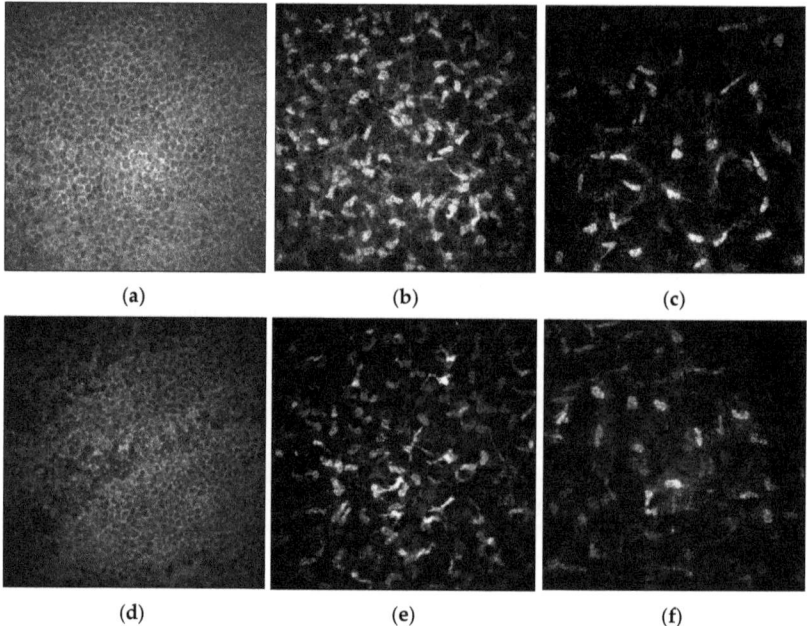

Figure 2. In-vivo confocal microscopy (IVCM) imaging of the corneal epithelium, anterior stromal keratocytes and posterior stromal keratocytes in healthy (a–c, respectively) and keratoconic eyes (d–f, respectively). Cell densities of the corneal epithelium, anterior stromal keratocytes and posterior stromal keratocytes are reduced in keratoconic eyes relative to healthy subjects. Scale bar: 100 µm.

IVCM images of the corneal nerve plexus in keratoconic eyes showed that nerve fibre bundles were tortuous and formed closed loops within the apex of the cone. In severe keratoconus, there was abrupt termination of the nerve fibres in the region of the cone. The subbasal nerve architecture was also abnormal, with predominantly oblique and horizontal orientation of subbasal nerve fibres at the apex, and the curvilinear orientation at the base of the cone differed markedly from the normal inferocentral whorl-like region seen in the normal cornea. Mean densities were also reduced at $10{,}478 \pm 2188$ µm/mm^2 as compared to normal corneas ($21{,}668 \pm 1411$ µm/mm^2) [47]. An increase in nerve fibre tortuosity and diameter were observed [42,46]. The mean diameter of stromal nerve fibres was reported to be significantly greater in subjects with keratoconus compared to control subjects (10.2 ± 4.6 µm versus 5.5 ± 1.9 µm) [46]. These findings were supported in a larger study of 145 patients in which participants were stratified into the manifest keratoconus group, the subclinical keratoconus group, the relatives of keratoconus group and the control group. They found that there was no significant difference between the subbasal nerve diameter amongst all groups, but the mean stromal nerve diameter in all three keratoconus groups (8.0 ± 3.5 µm to 8.8 ± 3.5 µm) was significantly higher than the control group (5.4 ± 2.1 µm; $p < 0.001$) [48]. Enlargement of nerves were thought to be related to impairment of nerve function, while increased nerve tortuosity was a morphologic marker of nerve regeneration [49]. A comparison of corneal nerve morphology between healthy and keratoconic corneas is demonstrated in Figure 3.

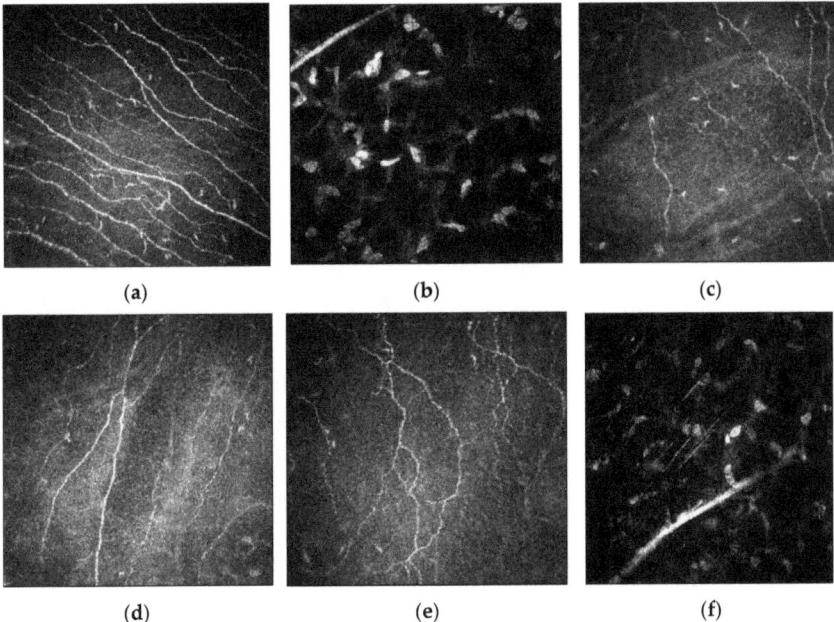

Figure 3. Morphology of corneal nerves evaluated by IVCM imaging in healthy and keratoconic corneas. (**a**) Subbasal nerve plexus with almost parallel nerve fibre bundles as observed in healthy corneas. (**b**) Normal stromal nerves in healthy corneas. (**c–e**) IVCM images demonstrate decreased nerve fibre density, thickened subbasal nerves and tortuous nerve paths in keratoconic corneas, respectively. (**f**) Thickened stromal nerves in keratoconic corneas. Scale bar: 100 µm.

Changes to the corneal nerve fibre length and subbasal nerve plexus were also noted in patients with keratoconus. The nerve fibre length was reduced significantly (16.4 ± 1.9 mm/mm^2) compared to healthy corneas (23.8 ± 3.3 mm/mm^2), and the subbasal nerve plexus was significantly more tortuous [50].

There is an increased risk in the first 6 years for young, unilateral keratoconus patients with a normal eye developing keratoconus in that eye subsequently [51,52]. However, our current imaging tools have not yielded any methods used to screen for keratoconus efficiently. IVCM analysis so far does not show any predictive factors. Studies analysing the fellow normal eye of a patient with keratoconus in one eye compared with normal controls showed that there were no significant differences between corneal nerve fibre densities, length, and branch densities [53]. Another study showed that there was a significant difference in the stromal keratocyte densities of subclinical keratoconus and controls, but there were no significant differences in subbasal nerve densities and diameters [48].

The corneal cellular and nerve changes in keratoconus are summarized in Table 1.

Table 1. Results of main studies investigating cellular and corneal nerve changes in keratoconus.

Author	Assessment	Number of Eyes	Findings
Brookes et al. [13] 2003	Excised corneas	10 KCN, 3 controls	• Using immunohistochemistry, localised nerve thickenings and anterior keratocyte nuclei were seen wrapping around corneal nerves—postulated to play a role in disease pathology.
Aqaba et al. [37] 2011	Excised corneas	14 KCN, 6 controls	• Using acetylcholinesterase staining technique, 71% of keratoconic corneas demonstrated central stromal nerve changes such as thickening, tortuosity, nerve spouting and overgrowth.
Mocan et al. [42] 2008	IVCM assessment	68 KCN, 22 controls	• Lower anterior stromal, mid-stromal and posterior stromal keratocyte density, lower endothelial cell density, subbasal long nerve density and thicker corneal nerves were found in keratoconus.
Patel et al. [47] 2006	IVCM assessment	4 KCN	• Abnormal subbasal nerves with a tortuous network of nerve fibre bundles were present at the apex. • Central subbasal nerve density was significantly lower in keratoconus corneas.
Flockerzi et al. [50] 2020	IVCM assessment	23 KCN	• Subbasal nerves are shorter and are more tortuous in the keratoconus cornea.
Mannion et al. [46] 2007	IVCM assessment	1 KCN	• Thicker nerve fibre bundles in the stroma and reduced nerve fibre density were found in the subepithelial plexus of the keratoconus cornea.
Mannion et al. [54] 2005	IVCM assessment	13 KCN, 13 controls	• Mean diameter of nerve fibres in stroma was found to be greater in subjects with keratoconus compared to controls. • There was altered orientation of the nerve fibres in keratoconus.
Ozgurhan et al. [48] 2013	IVCM assessment	30 KCN, 32 subclinical KCN, 53 KCN relatives, 30 controls	• Stromal keratocyte densities were significantly lower in all KCN groups as compared to controls. • Significantly higher mean stromal nerve diameter was noted in all KCN groups as compared to controls.
Patel et al. [55] 2009	IVCM assessment	27 KCN, 31 controls	• Subbasal nerve density and basal epithelial density were significantly lower than controls in all keratoconic eyes.

Table 1. Cont.

Author	Assessment	Number of Eyes	Findings
Pahuja et al. [53] 2016	IVCM assessment	33 normal eyes of KCN, 30 controls	• Significant difference in corneal nerve fibre densities and length between keratoconus eyes and control eyes. • No significant difference between unaffected eye of keratoconus patient and controls

KCN, keratoconus; IVCM, in-vivo confocal microscopy.

4.2. Relationship between Corneal Nerves and Corneal Sensitivity in Keratoconus

Evaluation of corneal sensitivity in diseased states is important as it serves as a functional measure of corneal nerves, which have important role in maintaining normal cellular structure and function as described earlier. However, it is known that clinical function and nerve alterations may not always correlate. Clinical symptoms can be present in the absence of visible nerve pathology and vice-versa [12].

Despite substantial nerve remodeling, the effect on corneal sensitivity is equivocal. Early studies using the Cochet–Bonnet aesthesiometer suggested that corneal sensitivity in keratoconus patients decreased in proportion to worsening disease severity [56,57]. However, the contact aesthesiometer is relatively crude and has certain limitations such as a limited stimulus range and an inability to distinguish subtle changes in corneal sensitivity [58,59]. A newer way of measuring corneal sensation such as the Belmonte non-contact gas aesthesiometer was developed to overcome these limitations. Using gas aesthesiometry, corneal sensation was found to be significantly reduced in keratoconus patients with mechanical, chemical and thermal stimulation, independent of severity of disease [60]. Hence, results in the literature may vary with the use of different aesthesiometers. Moreover, the use of rigid contact lens, a common management for keratoconus, is a confounding factor. The contact lens is known to reduce corneal sensitivity in normal and keratoconus corneas [61,62]. This has given rise to varying results, with some studies showing reduced corneal sensation in keratoconus patients [57,60,62], while some showed no difference between keratoconus patients and controls after adjusting for contact lens wear [54,55].

5. Corneal Nerve and Cellular Changes, and Corneal Sensitivity after Crosslinking

5.1. Corneal Nerve and Cellular Changes

A number of studies showed initial nerve degeneration that occurred immediately after CXL but nerves regenerated over time [63–65]. In a rabbit study, Xia et al., showed an initial absence of subepithelial nerve plexus with nerve fibre debris and nerve degeneration within 7 days of undergoing epithelium-off CXL. Fine nerve fibres were then found to be sprouting from neighboring non-injured nerve fibres in the deeper corneal stroma 7 days after CXL. The regenerating nerves made a tortuous progression toward the centre of the cornea to penetrate the denervated areas. They were found in excess throughout the anterior stroma, with the corneal nerve fibre density returning to normal levels by 180 days. Although there was a reduction in corneal sensitivity in the first 7 days after CXL, significant corneal nerve regeneration resulted in restoration of corneal sensitivity 90 days after the procedure. Rabbit corneas that underwent transepithelial CXL had no changes to the corneal nerves [63].

Clinical studies subsequently analysed IVCM images of keratoconus patients who underwent CXL at intervals of 1, 3, 6-months and 1-year post procedure. At one month after CXL, there is rarefaction of keratocytes associated with honeycomb-like stromal edema in the anterior 300 µm of the cornea (Figure 4). Hyper-reflective microparticles, representing keratocyte apoptotic bodies, are also visible (Figure 4d) [64]. After 3 months, there is keratocyte repopulation with increased density of the extracellular matrix and resolution in stromal haze after 3 months. There is also collagen compaction by new structured fibres in the anterior-mid stroma [64–66]. The subepithelial nerve fibres regenerated more rapidly than the stromal nerve fibres from the surrounding non-irradiated area between the second and third postoperative months. At 6 months postoperatively, there is a dense keratocyte population with increased extracellular matrix density. Subepithelial nerve regeneration is almost complete with restored corneal sensitivity [65,67]. However, not all eyes follow the same timeframe, with a study finding a slight delay in the regeneration of the subepithelial plexus in 68.8% of eyes at 6 months after CXL [68]. In another study, disconnected neural fibres were observed under the Bowman's lamina 6 months post-CXL [64]. However, the number of fibres increased progressively, and interconnections began to resemble the preoperative sub-epithelial plexus structure 12 months after CXL. The nerve fibre regeneration process is characterized by the presence of native subepithelial nerve flocks simulating Langerhans cells in a "pseudodendritic pattern". Langerhans cells were detectable between the second and third month after CXL, suggesting transient postoperative inflammation or an initial reinnervation process characterized by sprouting nerve fibres (Figure 5) [64]. At 12 months, the subepithelial nerve plexus and densities recover to preoperative values with repopulation of keratocytes [69,70].

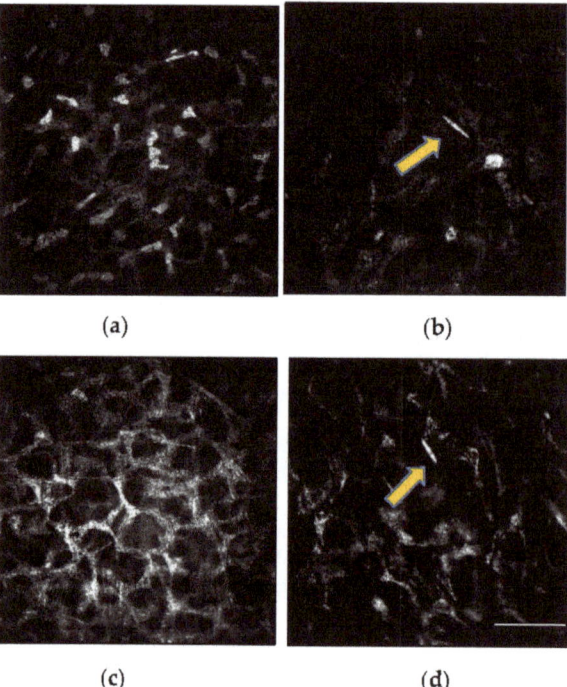

Figure 4. IVCM images of the anterior corneal stroma after CXL. (**a**) Rarefaction of keratocytes and elongated nuclei (masked necrotic keratocytes) are observed. (**b**) Reduction in keratocyte density with the presence of a fine needle-like opacity (yellow arrow), suggestive of apoptosis of keratocytes. (**c**) Anterior stromal honeycomb similar to edema, comprising of hyper-reflective cytoplasm and extracellular lacunae are evident (**d**). Repopulation of the cross-linked area with activated keratocytes. A needle-like opacity (yellow arrow) is also detectable, indicating apoptotic keratocytes. Scale bar: 100 μm.

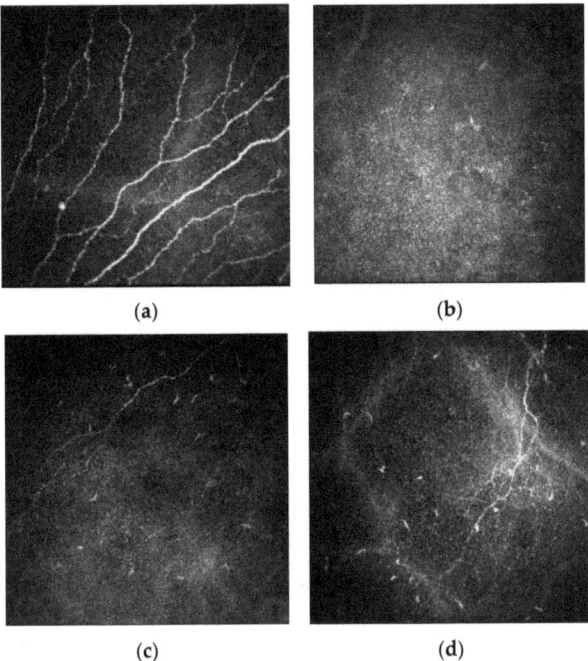

Figure 5. IVCM images demonstrating corneal nerve architecture before and after CXL. (**a**) Thickened subbasal nerves as noticed in a keratoconic cornea before CXL. (**b**) There is decreased nerve fibre density 1-month post-CXL. (**c**) At 4-months after CXL, there is an initial re-innervation process characterized by sprouting nerve fibres. Langerhans cells are also detectable, suggestive of transient post-CXL inflammation. (**d**) Increased nerve fibre density and tortuosity 1-year after CXL. Scale bar: 100 μm.

In a 5-year prospective study, patients with early-stage keratoconus who underwent conventional CXL had similar changes in the first year as described earlier. After 1 year, there was a continual increase in the median nerve fibre density with nerves adopting configurations of increasing loops, crossings and tortuosity. They also adopted radial, circumferential, or mixed orientations as they regenerated. Final nerve densities matched preoperative nerve densities but remained reduced relative to healthy corneas [71] (Figure 5).

In corneas thinner than 400 μm, it was traditionally thought to be a contraindication due to the potential for endothelium toxicity. Various methods utilizing contact lens [72], Hypotonic riboflavin solution [73,74], and epithelial island cross linking techniques [75] have been used to overcome this limitation. The effect on corneal nerves were found to be similar as compared to conventional CXL protocols. There was an absence of the subbasal nerve plexus and significant keratocyte apoptosis in the first postoperative month. By six months, near total recovery of the subepithelial nerve plexus had occurred [72,73]. Anterior stromal keratocyte density were reduced with corneas showing significant keratocyte apoptosis [73,75]. There was gradual recovery of keratocytes but this did not reach pre op levels (572 vs. 368, $p < 0.007$) at the end of 6 months [73]. Endothelial cell density were similar pre- and post-operatively in contact lens assisted CXL and epithelial island CXL [72,75] but there was a decrease in protocol utilizing hypotonic riboflavin from 2895 to 2660 ($p < 0.005$) [73]. Endothelial cell morphology remained the same, with no corneal edema [73]. While these results are promising, they are limited by their small study population and relatively short study follow up, with long term studies needed to prove their safety and efficacy.

The effect on corneal nerves following accelerated CXL or transepithelial CXL has also been studied. The subbasal nerve densities of 153 eyes undergoing accelerated and conventional epithelium-off CXL were investigated using IVCM images. There was a significant decrease in subbasal nerve density of the conventional CXL group than the accelerated CXL throughout the study period except on the final visit of 15 months postoperatively. This difference was thought to be due to the longer time of ultraviolet light exposure in the conventional protocol [76].

Studies evaluating the effect of transepithelial CXL on corneal nerves show less consistent results. Studies found that unlike the conventional epithelium-off treatment, subepithelial and anterior midstromal nerve fibres in transepithelial CXL remained present [77,78]. On follow-up visits within 6 months with IVCM, the nerves showed increased reflectivity with a granular appearance, and had irregular paths with branch anomalies. However, other studies report a significant decrease in the number of nerve fibres at one month after transepithelial CXL, with recovery to pre operative densities at 6 months [79–81]. This suggests that mechanical removal of the epithelium in CXL is not the only explanation for the reduction in corneal nerve densities. CXL itself may have a role in altering the cornea nerve plexus. Subsequent studies used iontophoresis, a technique used to drive negatively charged riboflavin across the intact epithelium, in transepithelial crosslinking protocols [79,82]. With regards to the corneal stroma, lacunar edema, apoptotic keratocytes and activated keratocytes with elongated membrane processes are seen 3 months postoperatively. The effect of newer variations on corneal nerves such as pulsed transepithelial CXL [83] or the usage of supplemental oxygen is yet to be investigated [84]. Table 2 summarises the main studies investigating corneal nerve and cellular changes after CXL in keratoconus.

Table 2. Results of main studies investigating corneal cell and nerve alternations after CXL in keratoconus.

Author	Study and CXL Protocol	N. of Eyes	Follow Up	Findings
Xia et al. [63] 2011	Longitudinal study, transepithelial or epithelium-off conventional CXL	108 rabbit eyes	180 days	• Immediate reduction of corneal sensitivity and decrease in nerve density after conventional CXL. • Gradual recovery to normal levels occurred at 90 days and 180 days respectively. • Rabbits that underwent transepithelial CXL showed no significant difference in cornea sensitivity.
Mazzotta et al. [64] 2015	Longitudinal study; epithelium-off CXL	84 eyes	12 months	• Regeneration of subepithelial and stromal nerves was complete with fully restored corneal sensitivity 12 months after CXL.
Mazzotta et al. [65] 2008	Longitudinal study; epithelium-off CXL	44 eyes	3 years	• Immediate disappearance of subepithelial plexus and anterior-mid stromal nerve fibres after CXL, with restoration of nerve plexus and full corneal sensitivity at one year after CXL.
Parissi et al. [71] 2016	Longitudinal study; epithelium-off CXL	19 eyes	5 years	• Nerves continued to regenerate 5 years after CXL but remained reduced relative to normal corneas. • More nerve loops, crossings and greater crossing angles were observed.

Table 2. Cont.

Author	Study and CXL Protocol	N. of Eyes	Follow Up	Findings
Al-aqaba et al. [78] 2012	Cross-sectional study; transepithelial or epithelium-off CXL	8 eyes	N/A	• Absence of subbasal nerves in the epithelium-off CXL group was attributed to mechanical removal of epithelium. • Subbasal nerves were detected immediately after transepithelial CXL. • Stromal nerves had localised swellings with disruption of axonal membrane and loss of axonal continuity within the treatment zone.
Zare et al. [68] 2016	Longitudinal study; epithelium-off CXL	32 eyes	6 months	• At 1 month, subepithelial nerve plexus was absent in 25 eyes (78.1%) and was reduced in 7 eyes (21.9%). The plexus was absent in 22 eyes (68.8%) and reduced in 10 eyes (31.3%) at 6 months.
Jordan et al. [70] 2014	Longitudinal study; epithelium-off CXL	38 eyes	12 months	• Mean subbasal nerve density decreased significantly at 1, 3, and 6 months, with a return to preoperative values at 12 months postoperatively.
Mazzotta et al. [72] 2016	Longitudinal study; contact lens assisted epithelium-off CXL	10 eyes	6 months	• Corneal reinnervation was fully restored at 6 months. • Keratocyte apoptosis occurred after the procedure but this recovered at 6 months. • No changes to endothelial cell count.
Sufi et al. [73] 2021	Longitudinal study; epithelium-off CXL with hypotonic riboflavin	10 eyes	6 months	• Absence of the subbasal nerve plexus at the first postoperative month. There was nearly total regeneration of subepithelial nerve plexus at end of 6 months. • Anterior stromal keratocyte densities were reduced even at the end of 6 months. • Endothelial cell densities decreased from 2895 to 2660 cells/mm^2.
Mazzotta et al. [75] 2014	Longitudinal study; epithelial island CXL	10 eyes	12 months	• Keratocyte apoptosis and nerve fibre loss under the epithelial island and de-epithelialized ring at 1 month postoperatively. • No change in endothelial cell densities after the procedure.
Kymionis et al. [69] 2009	Longitudinal study; epithelium-off CXL	5 eyes	12 months	• The subepithelial nerve plexus was absent within the CXL treatment zone at the first postoperative month. • There was reinnervation at 3 months, with keratocyte repopulation at 6 months.

Table 2. Cont.

Author	Study and CXL Protocol	N. of Eyes	Follow Up	Findings
Hashemian et al. [76] 2014	Longitudinal study; epithelium-off or AXL	153 eyes	15 months	• Anterior stromal keratocyte density and subbasal nerve density decreased significantly in AXL and CXL groups 1 month postoperatively. • Both nerve parameters were significantly decreased in the conventional CXL group for 1 year but were comparable with AXL at 15 months.
Caporossi et al. [77] 2012	Longitudinal study; transepithelial CXL	10 eyes	6 months	• Subepithelial and stromal nerve fibres were present immediately post procedure. There was limited apoptosis of keratocytes.
Bouheraoua et al. [81] 2014	Longitudinal study; transepithelial CXL, epithelium-off CXL or AXL	45 eyes	6 months	• Compared to preoperative values, the mean corneal subbasal nerve and anterior stromal keratocyte densities were significantly lower at 6 months in the epithelium-off CXL and AXL groups. • Postoperative values of subbasal nerve and anterior stromal keratocyte densities were comparable to the preoperative values in the transepithelial group.
Filippello et al. [80] 2012	Longitudinal study; transepithelial CXL	20 eyes	18 months	• Stromal Keratocytes and nerve fibres decreased in number (approximately 25%) after transepithelial CXL. They returned to pretreatment levels about 6 months after the procedure.
Jouve et al. [79]. 2017	Longitudinal study; transepithelial CXL using iontophoresis or Epithelium-off CXL	80 eyes	24 months	• Mean corneal subbasal nerve and anterior stromal keratocyte densities were significantly lower than preoperative values in both groups, but there was faster recovery to preoperative levels in the transepithelial group (6 months vs. 12 months).
Ozgurhan et al. [85] 2015	Longitudinal study epithelium-off AXL	30 eyes	12 months	• Corneal sensitivity significantly decreased at 3 months but increased to preoperative ranges after 6 months. • There was still a significant decrease in mean subbasal nerve fibre density at 6 months postoperative but restored to preoperative values at 12 months.
Unlu et al. [86] 2017	Longitudinal study; epithelium-off CXL	30 eyes	6 months	• Mean corneal sensation decreased in the first month and recovered to preoperative levels at 6 months. Subbasal nerve plexus gradually regenerated to almost preoperative levels at 6 months.

CXL, corneal crosslinking; AXL, accelerated crosslinking.

5.2. Changes in Corneal Sensitivity in Relation to Corneal Nerve Status after CXL

Besides evaluating corneal nerve metrics, ocular surface sensitivity and integrity are functional measures of corneal nerve status. Wasilewski and colleagues analysed corneal tactile sensitivity using the Cochet–Bonnet aesthesiometer in patients after CXL. The median sensitivity was 53.0 ± 8.7 mm preoperatively, 20.0 ± 16.2 mm at 7 days, 33.0 ± 16.4 mm at 30 days, 40 ± 12.6 mm at 90 days and 45 ± 9.2 mm at 180 days [87]. Decreased sensation was thought to be due to removal of the epithelium, and recovery of sensation was thought to correlate to nerve regeneration as described earlier in this review. In another study reporting the time course of ocular surface sensitivity changes using the Cochet–Bonnet aesthesiometer, the mean sensitivity was 59.0 ± 3.0 mm before CXL, decreased to 52.0 ± 13.0 mm at 3 months, and recovered to preoperative levels at 6 months with no further change at 12 months and at 5 years [71].

With regards to accelerated CXL, a study showed that the mean corneal sensation, measured by the Cochet–Bonnet aesthesiometer, decreased from 56.0 ± 5.4 mm before surgery, to 11.0 ± 4.5 mm and 33.0 ± 10.3 mm, in the first and third month after CXL, but recovered to preoperative values at 6 months. The mean subbasal nerve densities were significantly decreased up to 6 months postoperatively and recovered to preoperative levels only 12 months after procedure. This suggested that the recovery of corneal sensitivity preceded recovery of subbasal nerve densities to preoperative levels [85], implying that clinical function and nerve morphology may not always correlate.

Tolerance to RGP lenses after CXL has also been investigated by comparing corneal sensation, corneal nerve changes and lens wearing times. The mean corneal sensation, assessed by the Cochet–Bonnet aesthesiometer, decreased from 0.44 ± 0.05 g/mm^2 to 1.19 ± 0.72 g/mm^2 at 1 month, but improved to 0.48 ± 0.06 g/mm^2 and 0.44 ± 0.05 g/mm^2 at 3 to 6 months postoperatively. No subepithelial plexus could be visualised at one month but there was gradual restoration of corneal innervation with comparable preoperative levels at 6 months. Patients were more tolerant of RGP lenses with increased wearing times at the end of the 6-month study. Contribution of the flattening effect of CXL and a potential decrease in corneal sensitivity was thought to improve wearing of contact lenses [86].

6. Future Applications of IVCM in Keratoconus

IVCM images have been thought to be usable as a screening tool in patients with diabetic corneal neuropathy. Corneal nerve length and thickness have been reported to be early markers of eye involvement in patients with type 2 diabetes [88]. With the incorporation of deep learning techniques, artificial intelligence-based algorithm could provide rapid and good localisation performance for the quantification of corneal nerve biomarkers [89]. At this time of writing, there has not been any articles utilizing artificial intelligence techniques to analyse IVCM images in keratoconus. Although the prevalence of keratoconus is less than diabetes, we believe it could play a supplemental role to the armament of methods used to screen keratoconus.

The evaluation of subclinical or forme fruste keratoconus currently does not have any consensus. Although advances in corneal tomography and biomechanical assessments have made keratoconus diagnosis easier in the early stages, evaluation of these cases remain challenging [90]. Current evidence in the literature using IVCM images of corneal nerves taken from eyes with forme fruste keratoconus is limited. Larger study populations with well-defined inclusion criteria would possibly allow us to better understand nerve changes occurring in this subset of patients with very early keratoconus and possibly provide an opportunity for screening.

As described earlier, neuromediators secreted by corneal nerves play an important role in corneal health. There have been attempts to correlate neuromediator profiles with the severity of keratoconus [91]. We postulate that analysis of IVCM images along with neuromediator profiles and proteomic or metabolomic studies may uncover new insights into the pathophysiology of keratoconus.

7. Conclusions

Keratoconus presents with cornea ectasia that causes significant visual disability from a young age. Recent research has shown the possible role of corneal nerves in the pathophysiology of the disease. Aside from clinical examination, keratometric, topographical and biomechanical assessments that demonstrate clinical severity, IVCM has allowed accurate and reliable in-vivo evaluation of keratoconus at a cellular level, replacing the need for pathologic studies to understand the cellular and tissue changes. On IVCM evaluation, keratoconic corneas showed lower stromal keratocyte densities, thicker corneal nerves, reduced nerve fibre length, increased nerve tortuosity and irregular orientation, leading to decreased corneal sensitivity. However, the decreased sensitivity may not be positively correlated with the severity of the disease. Immediately after CXL, the subbasal nerve plexus, anterior and mid-stromal nerve densities were significantly reduced in the first six months, but these recovered gradually with restoration to preoperative levels by 12 months. The continued study of keratoconus with IVCM will allow us to further investigate the role that corneal nerves play in its pathophysiology, as well as the corneal nerve changes secondary to keratoconus. This has potential to allow further treatments on modulating corneal neuropathic changes to be developed in the future.

Author Contributions: A.W.J.T. and Y.-C.L. were responsible for conceptualization, data curation, writing the manuscript, editing and project administration. H.M. was responsible for visualization and authoring parts of the manuscript. N.S. and M.T.-Y.L. contributed to writing the manuscript. Y.-C.L. provided supervision. All authors have read and agreed to the published version of the manuscript.

Funding: This research received no external funding.

Data Availability Statement: Not applicable.

Conflicts of Interest: The authors declare no conflict of interest.

References

1. Ferrari, G.; Rama, P. The keratoconus enigma: A review with emphasis on pathogenesis. *Ocul. Surf.* **2020**, *18*, 363–373. [CrossRef]
2. Sahebjada, S.; Al-Mahrouqi, H.H.; Moshegov, S.; Panchatcharam, S.M.; Chan, E.; Daniell, M.; Baird, P.N. Eye rubbing in the aetiology of keratoconus: A systematic review and meta-analysis. *Graefes Arch. Clin. Exp. Ophthalmol.* **2021**, *259*, 2057–2067. [CrossRef] [PubMed]
3. Sugar, J.; Macsai, M.S. What causes keratoconus? *Cornea* **2012**, *31*, 716–719. [CrossRef]
4. Macsai, M.S.; Varley, G.A.; Krachmer, J.H. Development of keratoconus after contact lens wear. Patient characteristics. *Arch. Ophthalmol.* **1990**, *108*, 534–538. [CrossRef]
5. Nauheim, J.S.; Perry, H.D. A clinicopathologic study of contact-lens-related keratoconus. *Am. J. Ophthalmol.* **1985**, *100*, 543–546. [CrossRef]
6. Ates, K.M.; Estes, A.J.; Liu, Y. Potential underlying genetic associations between keratoconus and diabetes mellitus. *Adv. Ophthalmol. Pract. Res.* **2021**, *1*, 100005. [CrossRef]
7. Dudakova, L.; Liskova, P.; Trojek, T.; Palos, M.; Kalasova, S.; Jirsova, K. Changes in lysyl oxidase (LOX) distribution and its decreased activity in keratoconus corneas. *Exp. Eye Res.* **2012**, *104*, 74–81. [CrossRef] [PubMed]
8. Lu, Y.; Vitart, V.; Burdon, K.P.; Khor, C.C.; Bykhovskaya, Y.; Mirshahi, A.; Hewitt, A.W.; Koehn, D.; Hysi, P.G.; Ramdas, W.D.; et al. Genome-wide association analyses identify multiple loci associated with central corneal thickness and keratoconus. *Nat. Genet.* **2013**, *45*, 155–163. [CrossRef]
9. Karimian, F.; Aramesh, S.; Rabei, H.M.; Javadi, M.A.; Rafati, N. Topographic evaluation of relatives of patients with keratoconus. *Cornea* **2008**, *27*, 874–878. [CrossRef]
10. Kaya, V.; Utine, C.A.; Altunsoy, M.; Oral, D.; Yilmaz, O.F. Evaluation of corneal topography with Orbscan II in first-degree relatives of patients with keratoconus. *Cornea* **2008**, *27*, 531–534. [CrossRef]
11. Mackiewicz, Z.; Määttä, M.; Stenman, M.; Konttinen, L.; Tervo, T.; Konttinen, Y.T. Collagenolytic proteinases in keratoconus. *Cornea* **2006**, *25*, 603–610. [CrossRef] [PubMed]
12. Al-Aqaba, M.A.; Dhillon, V.K.; Mohammed, I.; Said, D.G.; Dua, H.S. Corneal nerves in health and disease. *Prog. Retin. Eye Res.* **2019**, *73*, 100762. [CrossRef] [PubMed]
13. Brookes, N.H.; Loh, I.P.; Clover, G.M.; Poole, C.A.; Sherwin, T. Involvement of corneal nerves in the progression of keratoconus. *Exp. Eye Res.* **2003**, *77*, 515–524. [CrossRef]
14. Erie, J.C.; McLaren, J.W.; Patel, S.V. Confocal microscopy in ophthalmology. *Am. J. Ophthalmol.* **2009**, *148*, 639–646. [CrossRef]

15. Guthoff, R.F.; Zhivov, A.; Stachs, O. In vivo confocal microscopy, an inner vision of the cornea—A major review. *Clin. Exp. Ophthalmol.* **2009**, *37*, 100–117. [CrossRef]
16. Tavakoli, M.; Hossain, P.; Malik, R.A. Clinical applications of corneal confocal microscopy. *Clin. Ophthalmol.* **2008**, *2*, 435–445. [CrossRef]
17. Stewart, S.; Liu, Y.C.; Lin, M.T.; Mehta, J.S. Clinical Applications of In Vivo Confocal Microscopy in Keratorefractive Surgery. *J. Refract. Surg.* **2021**, *37*, 493–503. [CrossRef]
18. Allgeier, S.; Bartschat, A.; Bohn, S.; Peschel, S.; Reichert, K.M.; Sperlich, K.; Walckling, M.; Hagenmeyer, V.; Mikut, R.; Stachs, O.; et al. 3D confocal laser-scanning microscopy for large-area imaging of the corneal subbasal nerve plexus. *Sci. Rep.* **2018**, *8*, 7468. [CrossRef]
19. So, W.Z.; Wong, S.Q.; Tan, H.C.; Mehta, J.S.; Liu, Y.C. Diabetic cornea neuropathy as the surrogate marker for diabetic peripheral neuropathy. *Neural Regen Res.* **2021**, *9*, 3956. [CrossRef]
20. Mansoor, H.; Tan, H.C.; Lin, M.T.; Mehta, J.S.; Liu, Y.C. Diabetic Corneal Neuropathy. *J. Clin. Med.* **2020**, *9*, 3956. [CrossRef]
21. Chin, J.Y.; Yang, L.W.Y.; Ji, A.J.S.; Nubile, M.; Mastropasqua, L.; Allen, J.C.; Mehta, J.S.; Liu, Y.C. Validation of the Use of Automated and Manual Quantitative Analysis of Corneal Nerve Plexus Following Refractive Surgery. *Diagnostics* **2020**, *10*, 493. [CrossRef] [PubMed]
22. Liu, Y.C.; Jung, A.S.J.; Chin, J.Y.; Yang, L.W.Y.; Mehta, J.S. Cross-sectional Study on Corneal Denervation in Contralateral Eyes Following SMILE Versus LASIK. *J. Refract. Surg.* **2020**, *36*, 653–660. [CrossRef] [PubMed]
23. Wollensak, G.; Spoerl, E.; Seiler, T. Riboflavin/ultraviolet-a-induced collagen crosslinking for the treatment of keratoconus. *Am. J. Ophthalmol.* **2003**, *135*, 620–627. [CrossRef]
24. Marafon, S.B.; Kwitko, S.; Marinho, D.R. Long-term results of accelerated and conventional corneal cross-linking. *Int. Ophthalmol.* **2020**, *40*, 2751–2761. [CrossRef]
25. Meiri, Z.; Keren, S.; Rosenblatt, A.; Sarig, T.; Shenhav, L.; Varssano, D. Efficacy of Corneal Collagen Cross-Linking for the Treatment of Keratoconus: A Systematic Review and Meta-Analysis. *Cornea* **2016**, *35*, 417–428. [CrossRef]
26. Raiskup-Wolf, F.; Hoyer, A.; Spoerl, E.; Pillunat, L.E. Collagen crosslinking with riboflavin and ultraviolet-A light in keratoconus: Long-term results. *J. Cataract Refract. Surg.* **2008**, *34*, 796–801. [CrossRef] [PubMed]
27. Al-Aqaba, M.A.; Fares, U.; Suleman, H.; Lowe, J.; Dua, H.S. Architecture and distribution of human corneal nerves. *Br. J. Ophthalmol.* **2010**, *94*, 784–789. [CrossRef] [PubMed]
28. Marfurt, C.F.; Cox, J.; Deek, S.; Dvorscak, L. Anatomy of the human corneal innervation. *Exp. Eye Res.* **2010**, *90*, 478–492. [CrossRef]
29. Müller, L.J.; Marfurt, C.F.; Kruse, F.; Tervo, T.M. Corneal nerves: Structure, contents and function. *Exp. Eye Res.* **2003**, *76*, 521–542. [CrossRef]
30. Dua, H.S.; Gomes, J.A. Clinical course of hurricane keratopathy. *Br. J. Ophthalmol.* **2000**, *84*, 285–288. [CrossRef]
31. Lambiase, A.; Manni, L.; Bonini, S.; Rama, P.; Micera, A.; Aloe, L. Nerve growth factor promotes corneal healing: Structural, biochemical, and molecular analyses of rat and human corneas. *Investig. Ophthalmol. Vis. Sci.* **2000**, *41*, 1063–1069.
32. Chung, E.S.; Lee, K.H.; Kim, M.; Chang, E.J.; Chung, T.Y.; Kim, E.K.; Lee, H.K. Expression of neurotrophic factors and their receptors in keratoconic cornea. *Curr. Eye Res.* **2013**, *38*, 743–750. [CrossRef]
33. Ceruti, S.; Villa, G.; Fumagalli, M.; Colombo, L.; Magni, G.; Zanardelli, M.; Fabbretti, E.; Verderio, C.; van den Maagdenberg, A.M.; Nistri, A.; et al. Calcitonin gene-related peptide-mediated enhancement of purinergic neuron/glia communication by the algogenic factor bradykinin in mouse trigeminal ganglia from wild-type and R192Q Cav2.1 Knock-in mice: Implications for basic mechanisms of migraine pain. *J. Neurosci.* **2011**, *31*, 3638–3649. [CrossRef] [PubMed]
34. Liu, Y.-C.; Hin-FaiYam, G.; Tzu-YuLin, M.; EriciaTeo; Koh, S.-K.; LuDeng; LeiZhou; LouisTong; Mehta, J.S. Comparison of tear proteomic and neuromediator profiles changes between small incision lenticule extraction (SMILE) and femtosecond laser-assisted in-situ keratomileusis (LASIK). *J. Adv. Res.* **2021**, *29*, 67–81. [CrossRef]
35. Yang LW, Y.; Mehta, J.S.; Liu, Y.C. Corneal neuromediator profiles following laser refractive surgery. *Neural Regen. Res.* **2021**, *16*, 2177. [CrossRef] [PubMed]
36. Sacchetti, M.; Scorcia, V.; Lambiase, A.; Bonini, S. Preliminary evidence of neuropeptides involvement in keratoconus. *Acta Ophthalmol.* **2015**, *93*, e315–e316. [CrossRef] [PubMed]
37. Al-Aqaba, M.A.; Faraj, L.; Fares, U.; Otri, A.M.; Dua, H.S. The morphologic characteristics of corneal nerves in advanced keratoconus as evaluated by acetylcholinesterase technique. *Am. J. Ophthalmol.* **2011**, *152*, 364–376.e361. [CrossRef] [PubMed]
38. Liu, Y.C.; Lin, M.T.; Mehta, J.S. Analysis of corneal nerve plexus in corneal confocal microscopy images. *Neural Regen. Res.* **2021**, *16*, 690–691. [CrossRef] [PubMed]
39. West-Mays, J.A.; Dwivedi, D.J. The keratocyte: Corneal stromal cell with variable repair phenotypes. *Int. J. Biochem. Cell Biol.* **2006**, *38*, 1625–1631. [CrossRef] [PubMed]
40. Yam, G.H.; Fuest, M.; Zhou, L.; Liu, Y.C.; Deng, L.; Chan, A.S.; Ong, H.S.; Khor, W.B.; Ang, M.; Mehta, J.S. Differential epithelial and stromal protein profiles in cone and non-cone regions of keratoconus corneas. *Sci. Rep.* **2019**, *9*, 2965. [CrossRef]
41. Hollingsworth, J.G.; Efron, N.; Tullo, A.B. In vivo corneal confocal microscopy in keratoconus. *Ophthalmic Physiol. Opt.* **2005**, *25*, 254–260. [CrossRef]
42. Mocan, M.C.; Yilmaz, P.T.; Irkec, M.; Orhan, M. In vivo confocal microscopy for the evaluation of corneal microstructure in keratoconus. *Curr. Eye Res.* **2008**, *33*, 933–939. [CrossRef]

43. Uçakhan, O.O.; Kanpolat, A.; Ylmaz, N.; Ozkan, M. In vivo confocal microscopy findings in keratoconus. *Eye Contact Lens* **2006**, *32*, 183–191. [CrossRef] [PubMed]
44. Kim, W.J.; Rabinowitz, Y.S.; Meisler, D.M.; Wilson, S.E. Keratocyte apoptosis associated with keratoconus. *Exp. Eye Res.* **1999**, *69*, 475–481. [CrossRef] [PubMed]
45. Bitirgen, G.; Ozkagnici, A.; Malik, R.A.; Oltulu, R. Evaluation of contact lens-induced changes in keratoconic corneas using in vivo confocal microscopy. *Investig. Ophthalmol. Vis. Sci.* **2013**, *54*, 5385–5391. [CrossRef] [PubMed]
46. Mannion, L.S.; Tromans, C.; O'Donnell, C. Corneal nerve structure and function in keratoconus: A case report. *Eye Contact Lens* **2007**, *33*, 106–108. [CrossRef]
47. Patel, D.V.; McGhee, C.N. Mapping the corneal sub-basal nerve plexus in keratoconus by in vivo laser scanning confocal microscopy. *Investig. Ophthalmol. Vis. Sci.* **2006**, *47*, 1348–1351. [CrossRef]
48. Ozgurhan, E.B.; Kara, N.; Yildirim, A.; Bozkurt, E.; Uslu, H.; Demirok, A. Evaluation of corneal microstructure in keratoconus: A confocal microscopy study. *Am. J. Ophthalmol.* **2013**, *156*, 885–893.e882. [CrossRef]
49. Kawabuchi, M.; Chongjian, Z.; Islam, A.T.; Hirata, K.; Nada, O. The effect of aging on the morphological nerve changes during muscle reinnervation after nerve crush. *Restor. Neurol. Neurosci.* **1998**, *13*, 117–127.
50. Flockerzi, E.; Daas, L.; Seitz, B. Structural changes in the corneal subbasal nerve plexus in keratoconus. *Acta Ophthalmol.* **2020**, *98*, e928–e932. [CrossRef]
51. Koh, S.; Inoue, R.; Maeda, N.; Kabata, D.; Shintani, A.; Jhanji, V.; Klyce, S.D.; Maruyama, K.; Nishida, K. Long-term Chronological Changes in Very Asymmetric Keratoconus. *Cornea* **2019**, *38*, 605–611. [CrossRef]
52. Li, X.; Yang, H.; Rabinowitz, Y.S. Longitudinal study of keratoconus progression. *Exp. Eye Res.* **2007**, *85*, 502–507. [CrossRef]
53. Pahuja, N.K.; Shetty, R.; Nuijts, R.M.; Agrawal, A.; Ghosh, A.; Jayadev, C.; Nagaraja, H. An In Vivo Confocal Microscopic Study of Corneal Nerve Morphology in Unilateral Keratoconus. *Biomed. Res. Int.* **2016**, *2016*, 5067853. [CrossRef]
54. Simo Mannion, L.; Tromans, C.; O'Donnell, C. An evaluation of corneal nerve morphology and function in moderate keratoconus. *Cont. Lens Anterior Eye* **2005**, *28*, 185–192. [CrossRef]
55. Patel, D.V.; Ku, J.Y.; Johnson, R.; McGhee, C.N. Laser scanning in vivo confocal microscopy and quantitative aesthesiometry reveal decreased corneal innervation and sensation in keratoconus. *Eye* **2009**, *23*, 586–592. [CrossRef]
56. Millodot, M.; Owens, H. Sensitivity and fragility in keratoconus. *Acta Ophthalmol.* **1983**, *61*, 908–917. [CrossRef] [PubMed]
57. Dogru, M.; Karakaya, H.; Ozçetin, H.; Ertürk, H.; Yücel, A.; Ozmen, A.; Baykara, M.; Tsubota, K. Tear function and ocular surface changes in keratoconus. *Ophthalmology* **2003**, *110*, 1110–1118. [CrossRef]
58. Lum, E.; Murphy, P.J. Effects of ambient humidity on the Cochet-Bonnet aesthesiometer. *Eye* **2018**, *32*, 1644–1651. [CrossRef] [PubMed]
59. Golebiowski, B.; Papas, E.; Stapleton, F. Assessing the sensory function of the ocular surface: Implications of use of a non-contact air jet aesthesiometer versus the Cochet-Bonnet aesthesiometer. *Exp. Eye Res.* **2011**, *92*, 408–413. [CrossRef]
60. Dienes, L.; Kiss, H.J.; Perényi, K.; Nagy, Z.Z.; Acosta, M.C.; Gallar, J.; Kovács, I. Corneal Sensitivity and Dry Eye Symptoms in Patients with Keratoconus. *PLoS ONE* **2015**, *10*, e0141621. [CrossRef]
61. Murphy, P.J.; Patel, S.; Marshall, J. The effect of long-term, daily contact lens wear on corneal sensitivity. *Cornea* **2001**, *20*, 264–269. [CrossRef]
62. Mandathara, P.S.; Stapleton, F.J.; Kokkinakis, J.; Willcox, M.D. Pilot Study of Corneal Sensitivity and Its Association in Keratoconus. *Cornea* **2017**, *36*, 163–168. [CrossRef]
63. Xia, Y.; Chai, X.; Zhou, C.; Ren, Q. Corneal nerve morphology and sensitivity changes after ultraviolet A/riboflavin treatment. *Exp. Eye Res.* **2011**, *93*, 541–547. [CrossRef] [PubMed]
64. Mazzotta, C.; Hafezi, F.; Kymionis, G.; Caragiuli, S.; Jacob, S.; Traversi, C.; Barabino, S.; Randleman, J.B. In Vivo Confocal Microscopy after Corneal Collagen Crosslinking. *Ocul. Surf.* **2015**, *13*, 298–314. [CrossRef] [PubMed]
65. Mazzotta, C.; Traversi, C.; Baiocchi, S.; Caporossi, O.; Bovone, C.; Sparano, M.C.; Balestrazzi, A.; Caporossi, A. Corneal healing after riboflavin ultraviolet-A collagen cross-linking determined by confocal laser scanning microscopy in vivo: Early and late modifications. *Am. J. Ophthalmol.* **2008**, *146*, 527–533. [CrossRef]
66. Mazzotta, C.; Caporossi, T.; Denaro, R.; Bovone, C.; Sparano, C.; Paradiso, A.; Baiocchi, S.; Caporossi, A. Morphological and functional correlations in riboflavin UV A corneal collagen cross-linking for keratoconus. *Acta Ophthalmol.* **2012**, *90*, 259–265. [CrossRef]
67. Mazzotta, C.; Balestrazzi, A.; Traversi, C.; Baiocchi, S.; Caporossi, T.; Tommasi, C.; Caporossi, A. Treatment of progressive keratoconus by riboflavin-UVA-induced cross-linking of corneal collagen: Ultrastructural analysis by Heidelberg Retinal Tomograph II in vivo confocal microscopy in humans. *Cornea* **2007**, *26*, 390–397. [CrossRef]
68. Zare, M.A.; Mazloumi, M.; Farajipour, H.; Hoseini, B.; Fallah, M.R.; Mahrjerdi, H.Z.; Abtahi, M.A.; Abtahi, S.H. Effects of Corneal Collagen Crosslinking on Confocal Microscopic Findings and Tear Indices in Patients with Progressive Keratoconus. *Int. J. Prev. Med.* **2016**, *7*, 132. [CrossRef]
69. Kymionis, G.D.; Diakonis, V.F.; Kalyvianaki, M.; Portaliou, D.; Siganos, C.; Kozobolis, V.P.; Pallikaris, A.I. One-year follow-up of corneal confocal microscopy after corneal cross-linking in patients with post laser in situ keratosmileusis ectasia and keratoconus. *Am. J. Ophthalmol.* **2009**, *147*, 774–778.e771. [CrossRef]
70. Jordan, C.; Patel, D.V.; Abeysekera, N.; McGhee, C.N. In vivo confocal microscopy analyses of corneal microstructural changes in a prospective study of collagen cross-linking in keratoconus. *Ophthalmology* **2014**, *121*, 469–474. [CrossRef]

71. Parissi, M.; Randjelovic, S.; Poletti, E.; Guimarães, P.; Ruggeri, A.; Fragkiskou, S.; Wihlmark, T.B.; Utheim, T.P.; Lagali, N. Corneal Nerve Regeneration After Collagen Cross-Linking Treatment of Keratoconus: A 5-Year Longitudinal Study. *JAMA Ophthalmol.* **2016**, *134*, 70–78. [CrossRef]
72. Mazzotta, C.; Jacob, S.; Agarwal, A.; Kumar, D.A. In Vivo Confocal Microscopy After Contact Lens-Assisted Corneal Collagen Cross-linking for Thin Keratoconic Corneas. *J. Refract. Surg.* **2016**, *32*, 326–331. [CrossRef] [PubMed]
73. Sufi, A.R.; Soundaram, M.; Gohil, N.; Keenan, J.D.; Prajna, N.V. Structural Changes in Thin Keratoconic Corneas Following Crosslinking with Hypotonic Riboflavin: Findings on In Vivo Confocal Microscopy. *J. Ophthalmic Vis. Res.* **2021**, *16*, 325–337. [CrossRef]
74. Raiskup, F.; Spoerl, E. Corneal cross-linking with hypo-osmolar riboflavin solution in thin keratoconic corneas. *Am. J. Ophthalmol.* **2011**, *152*, 28–32.e21. [CrossRef] [PubMed]
75. Mazzotta, C.; Ramovecchi, V. Customized epithelial debridement for thin ectatic corneas undergoing corneal cross-linking: Epithelial island cross-linking technique. *Clin. Ophthalmol.* **2014**, *8*, 1337–1343. [CrossRef] [PubMed]
76. Hashemian, H.; Jabbarvand, M.; Khodaparast, M.; Ameli, K. Evaluation of corneal changes after conventional versus accelerated corneal cross-linking: A randomized controlled trial. *J. Refract. Surg.* **2014**, *30*, 837–842. [CrossRef]
77. Caporossi, A.; Mazzotta, C.; Baiocchi, S.; Caporossi, T.; Paradiso, A.L. Transepithelial corneal collagen crosslinking for keratoconus: Qualitative investigation by in vivo HRT II confocal analysis. *Eur. J. Ophthalmol.* **2012**, *22* (Suppl. S7), S81–S88. [CrossRef]
78. Al-Aqaba, M.; Calienno, R.; Fares, U.; Otri, A.M.; Mastropasqua, L.; Nubile, M.; Dua, H.S. The effect of standard and transepithelial ultraviolet collagen cross-linking on human corneal nerves: An ex vivo study. *Am. J. Ophthalmol.* **2012**, *153*, 258–266.e252. [CrossRef]
79. Jouve, L.; Borderie, V.; Sandali, O.; Temstet, C.; Basli, E.; Laroche, L.; Bouheraoua, N. Conventional and Iontophoresis Corneal Cross-Linking for Keratoconus: Efficacy and Assessment by Optical Coherence Tomography and Confocal Microscopy. *Cornea* **2017**, *36*, 153–162. [CrossRef]
80. Filippello, M.; Stagni, E.; Buccoliero, D.; Bonfiglio, V.; Avitabile, T. Transepithelial cross-linking in keratoconus patients: Confocal analysis. *Optom. Vis. Sci.* **2012**, *89*, e1–e7. [CrossRef]
81. Bouheraoua, N.; Jouve, L.; El Sanharawi, M.; Sandali, O.; Temstet, C.; Loriaut, P.; Basli, E.; Borderie, V.; Laroche, L. Optical coherence tomography and confocal microscopy following three different protocols of corneal collagen-crosslinking in keratoconus. *Investig. Ophthalmol. Vis. Sci.* **2014**, *55*, 7601–7609. [CrossRef] [PubMed]
82. Lombardo, M.; Serrao, S.; Rosati, M.; Ducoli, P.; Lombardo, G. Biomechanical changes in the human cornea after transepithelial corneal crosslinking using iontophoresis. *J. Cataract Refract. Surg.* **2014**, *40*, 1706–1715. [CrossRef]
83. Ziaei, M.; Vellara, H.; Gokul, A.; Patel, D.; McGhee, C.N.J. Prospective 2-year study of accelerated pulsed transepithelial corneal crosslinking outcomes for Keratoconus. *Eye* **2019**, *33*, 1897–1903. [CrossRef] [PubMed]
84. Mazzotta, C.; Sgheri, A.; Bagaglia, S.A.; Rechichi, M.; Di Maggio, A. Customized corneal crosslinking for treatment of progressive keratoconus: Clinical and OCT outcomes using a transepithelial approach with supplemental oxygen. *J. Cataract Refract. Surg.* **2020**, *46*, 1582–1587. [CrossRef] [PubMed]
85. Ozgurhan, E.B.; Celik, U.; Bozkurt, E.; Demirok, A. Evaluation of subbasal nerve morphology and corneal sensation after accelerated corneal collagen cross-linking treatment on keratoconus. *Curr. Eye Res.* **2015**, *40*, 484–489. [CrossRef] [PubMed]
86. Ünlü, M.; Yüksel, E.; Bilgihan, K. Effect of corneal cross-linking on contact lens tolerance in keratoconus. *Clin. Exp. Optom.* **2017**, *100*, 369–374. [CrossRef]
87. Wasilewski, D.; Mello, G.H.; Moreira, H. Impact of collagen crosslinking on corneal sensitivity in keratoconus patients. *Cornea* **2013**, *32*, 899–902. [CrossRef]
88. dell'Omo, R.; Cifariello, F.; De Turris, S.; Romano, V.; Di Renzo, F.; Di Taranto, D.; Coclite, G.; Agnifili, L.; Mastropasqua, L.; Costagliola, C. Confocal microscopy of corneal nerve plexus as an early marker of eye involvement in patients with type 2 diabetes. *Diabetes Res. Clin. Pract.* **2018**, *142*, 393–400. [CrossRef]
89. Williams, B.M.; Borroni, D.; Liu, R.; Zhao, Y.; Zhang, J.; Lim, J.; Ma, B.; Romano, V.; Qi, H.; Ferdousi, M.; et al. An artificial intelligence-based deep learning algorithm for the diagnosis of diabetic neuropathy using corneal confocal microscopy: A development and validation study. *Diabetologia* **2020**, *63*, 419–430. [CrossRef]
90. Henriquez, M.A.; Hadid, M.; Izquierdo, L., Jr. A Systematic Review of Subclinical Keratoconus and Forme Fruste Keratoconus. *J. Refract. Surg.* **2020**, *36*, 270–279. [CrossRef]
91. Kolozsvári, B.L.; Petrovski, G.; Gogolák, P.; Rajnavölgyi, É.; Tóth, F.; Berta, A.; Fodor, M. Association between mediators in the tear fluid and the severity of keratoconus. *Ophthalmic Res.* **2014**, *51*, 46–51. [CrossRef] [PubMed]

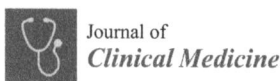

Article

Association of Neuroretinal Thinning and Microvascular Changes with Hypertension in an Older Population in Southern Italy

Alfredo Niro [1,†], Giancarlo Sborgia [2,*,†], Luisa Lampignano [3], Gianluigi Giuliani [2], Fabio Castellana [3], Roberta Zupo [3], Ilaria Bortone [3], Pasquale Puzo [2], Angelo Pascale [2], Valentina Pastore [2], Rosa Buonamassa [2], Roberta Galati [2], Marco Bordinone [2], Flavio Cassano [2], Chiara Griseta [3], Sarah Tirelli [3], Madia Lozupone [2], Vitoantonio Bevilacqua [4], Francesco Panza [2], Rodolfo Sardone [3], Giovanni Alessio [2] and Francesco Boscia [2]

1. Eye Clinic, Hospital "SS. Annunziata", ASL Taranto, 74100 Taranto, Italy; alfred.nir@tiscali.it
2. Department of Basic Medical Sciences, Neuroscience and Sense Organs, University of Bari "Aldo Moro", 70124 Bari, Italy; giuliani_gianluigi@hotmail.it (G.G.); puzopasquale@gmail.com (P.P.); pascaleangelo@gmail.com (A.P.); valentinapastore@hotmail.it (V.P.); rosabuona@hotmail.it (R.B.); robertaga@hotmail.it (R.G.); marcoab313@hotmail.it (M.B.); f.cassano@hotmail.it (F.C.); madia.lozupone@gmail.com (M.L.); f_panza@hotmail.com (F.P.); giovanni.alessio@uniba.it (G.A.); francesco.boscia@uniba.it (F.B.)
3. Unit of Research Methodology and Data Sciences for Population Health, "Salus in Apulia Study", National Institute of Gastroenterology "Saverio de Bellis", Research Hospital, 70013 Castellana Grotte, Italy; luisa.lampignano@irccsdebellis.it (L.L.); fabio.castellana@irccsdebellis.it (F.C.); roberta.zupo@irccsdebellis.it (R.Z.); ilaria.bortone@gmail.com (I.B.); chiaragriseta@gmail.com (C.G.); sarahtirelli93@gmail.com (S.T.); rodolfo.sardone@irccsdebellis.it (R.S.)
4. Department of Electrical and Information Engineering, Polytechnic University of Bari, 70126 Bari, Italy; vitoantonio.bevilacqua@poliba.it
* Correspondence: gcsborgia@hotmail.it; Tel.: +39-0805478916
† They contributed equally as co-first authors.

Abstract: Background: Retinal microvasculature assessment at capillary level may potentially aid the evaluation of early microvascular changes due to hypertension. We aimed to investigate associations between the measures obtained using optical coherence tomography (OCT) and OCT-angiography (OCT-A) and hypertension, in a southern Italian older population. Methods: We performed a cross-sectional analysis from a population-based study on 731 participants aged 65 years+ subdivided into two groups according to the presence or absence of blood hypertension without hypertensive retinopathy. The average thickness of the ganglion cell complex (GCC) and the retinal nerve fiber layer (RNFL) were measured. The foveal avascular zone area, vascular density (VD) at the macular site and of the optic nerve head (ONH) and radial peripapillary capillary (RPC) plexi were evaluated. Logistic regression was applied to assess the association of ocular measurements with hypertension. Results: GCC thickness was inversely associated with hypertension (odds ratio (OR): 0.98, 95% confidence interval (CI): 0.97–1). A rarefaction of VD of the ONH plexus at the inferior temporal sector (OR: 0.95, 95% CI: 0.91–0.99) and, conversely, a higher VD of the ONH and RPC plexi inside optic disc (OR: 1.07, 95% CI: 1.04–1.10; OR: 1.04, 95% CI: 1.02–1.06, respectively) were significantly associated with hypertension. Conclusion: A neuroretinal thinning involving GCC and a change in capillary density at the peripapillary network were related to the hypertension in older patients without hypertensive retinopathy. Assessing peripapillary retinal microvasculature using OCT-A may be a useful non-invasive approach to detect early microvascular changes due to hypertension.

Keywords: hypertension; older adults; optical coherence tomography; optical coherence tomography angiography; ganglion cell complex; optic nerve head; radial peripapillary capillary

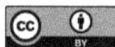

1. Introduction

Hypertension, a major risk factor for cardiovascular deaths globally, is expected to affect 1.56 billion adults worldwide by 2025 [1]. It can cause end-organ damage, in the form of cardiovascular disease and nephropathy, resulting in 9.4 million deaths per year around the world [2]. Moreover, many studies have indicated a link between obesity and hypertension, particularly in older people [3]. The prevalence of hypertension rises with age, but it is an easily treatable risk factor for the most prevalent causes of multimorbidity and death in older adults. In particular, hypertension also causes microvascular damage in both the cerebral and retinal circulations [4]. Because the retinal and cerebral vessels share embryological and anatomical characteristics, they may show similar patterns of damage attributable to hypertension.

The value of retinal imaging as a tool to evaluate the ocular effect of hypertension and its importance in making an early prediction of patients' risk of developing cerebrovascular disease has previously been described [5]. In recent years, hypertensive subjects without hypertensive retinopathy have been shown through optical coherence tomography (OCT) to have a lower thickness of ganglion cell complex (GCC) [6,7] and retinal nerve fiber layer (RNFL) [6–8]. Moreover, OCT-angiography (OCT-A) revealed a reduced macular capillary density in hypertensive subjects without related retinopathy [8–10]. Previous OCT-A studies have also reported a decreased macular perfusion, along with GCC thinning, in subjects with essential hypertension [9,11]. Those studies were only focused on macular vascular plexi. However, the optic nerve head (ONH) and radial peripapillary capillary (RPC) plexi at the peripapillary site have a key role in the vascular supply of inner neuroretinal layers, including the ganglion cell layer (GCL) and RNFL [12,13]. In recent OCT-A studies, RPC plexus impairment was more evident in older subjects [14], diabetic patients with and without diabetic retinopathy [15], and hypertensive patients with and without retinopathy [8,10].

The aim of the present study was to investigate linear relationships between the retinal features obtained on both OCT and OCT-A scans and blood hypertension, in an older population (aged 65+ years), without related retinopathy, of a cross-sectional study in southern Italy.

2. Materials and Methods

2.1. Study Population and Design

Data used in the present study were drawn from the population based GreatAGE Study conducted on subjects aged over 65 years, residents of Castellana Grotte, Bari (Puglia Region, southern Italy) participating in the Salus in Apulia Study. The general sampling population was the 19,675 residents listed in the health registry office on 31 December 2014, of whom 4021 subjects were aged 65 years or older. The study design and data collection methods have been described in detail elsewhere [16].

This study presents data from a subpopulation of the study that underwent ophthalmological assessment including OCT and OCT-A (n = 731) and were without diabetes mellitus, demyelinating disorders, cardiac diseases. All participants signed informed consent, and the study was approved in 2014 and again in 2019 by the IRB of the National Institute of Gastroenterology "S. De Bellis", where all the examinations described in this study were performed. The present study adhered to the "Standards for Reporting Diagnostic Accuracy Studies" (STARD) guidelines (http://www.stard-statement.org/, accessed on 1 December 2021, the "Strengthening the Reporting of Observational Studies in Epidemiology" (STROBE) guidelines (https://www.strobe-statement.org/, accessed on 1 December 2021) and is in accordance with the Helsinki Declaration of 1975.

2.2. Clinical and Anthropometric Assessment

Height was measured to the nearest 0.5 cm using a wall-mounted stadiometer (Seca 711; Seca, Hamburg, Germany). Body weight was determined to the nearest 0.1 kg using a calibrated balance beam scale (Seca 711; Seca, Hamburg, Germany). BMI was calculated by dividing body weight (kg) by the square of height (m^2). Waist circumference (WC) was measured at the narrowest part of the abdomen, or area between the tenth rib and the iliac crest (minimum circumference). Office blood pressure measurement was performed four times at 3-h intervals, from 8 am to 5 pm on a single day, following the Hypertension Clinical Practice Guideline [17]. The mean values of the systolic (SBP) and diastolic (DBP) blood pressure for each patient were used in this study. Hypertension was defined as present in participants with elevated BP at the time of examination (SPB $\geq$ 130 mm Hg or DBP $\geq$ 80 mm Hg) according to American Heart Association criteria [17]. Education was defined by years of schooling. Smoking was assessed with the single categorized question "Are you a current smoker?". All participants underwent standardized neuropsychological tests as detailed elsewhere [18] and the Mini-Mental State Examination (MMSE) to assess global cognition [18]. The diagnosis of mild cognitive impairment (MCI) was made according to the Diagnostic and Statistical Manual of Mental Disorders, Fifth Edition (DSM-5) criteria, as detailed elsewhere [18], A blood sample was collected in the morning after overnight fasting to measure fasting blood glucose (FBG), glycated hemoglobin (HbA1c), total cholesterol, high-density lipoprotein (HDL) cholesterol, and low-density lipoprotein (LDL) cholesterol and triglycerides.

2.3. Ophthalmological Assessment

Each participant underwent a complete ophthalmic examination including best-corrected visual acuity (BCVA) measurement, slit-lamp biomicroscopy, intraocular pressure (IOP) measurement, and funduscopy. BCVA was recorded as Snellen visual acuity and converted to the logarithm of minimal angle of resolution (LogMar) units for statistical analysis. Then, we performed OCT and OCT-A using Optovue RTVue XR 100 AVANTI, Optovue, Inc. (Fremont, CA, USA). OCT-A analyzes retinal vasculature after identification and segmentation of multiple retinal layers using the AngioVue module with Optovue RTVue AVANTI software (version 2015.100.0.35, Optovue, Inc., Fremont, CA, USA). The Angio Retina mode (3×3 mm^2) and the Angio Disc (4.5×4.5 mm^2) mode were employed. RTvue software includes the Optovue's Motion Correction Technology (MCT™, Optovue, Inc., Fremont, CA, USA) and 3D Projection Artifact Technology. Furthermore, the software provided the signal strength index (SSI), which represents the scan's reflectance signal strength, and a quality index (Q-score), representing the overall quality of the image, taking into account factors like SSI and motion artefacts [19]. In the present study, we only included images with a Q-score of 6 or above, SSI above 60, and without motion or shadow artefacts. The examinations were performed blinded by trained ophthalmologists. The vessel density (VD, %), defined as the percentage area occupied by the vessels in the corresponding region, was automatically measured by the built-in OCT device software. VD measurement was undertaken in the optic disc area, in the total peripapillary area, and in each of the six peripapillary sectors in two different layers, the ONH layer (Figure 1A,E) and the RPC layer (Figure 1B,F). Each layer corresponds with an en-face structural image. The software defines the peripapillary area as a 1.0 mm wide round annulus extending from the optic disc boundary and the inside optic disc area as a 2.0 mm diameter circle involving the optic disc. The peripapillary and the inside optic disc areas together composed the whole peripapillary area (4.0 mm-diameter round whole image). The peripapillary area, in turn, was divided into six peripapillary sectors. (Figure 1A,B,E,F). The software-provided peripapillary sectors are based on the Garway–Heath map [20]. The OCT angiograms centered on the fovea were automatically segmented to define the superficial plexus from 3 µm below the internal limiting membrane to 15 µm below the inner plexiform layer and the deep plexus from 15 to 70 µm below the inner plexiform layer. The VD at each macular plexus, superficial VD (SVD) and deep VD (DVD), was calculated for the whole 3 mm circle area centered on the fovea (whole retina), for the area between the outer 3 mm circle and the inner 1 mm circle (parafoveal quadrant), and for the area inside the central 1 mm circle (foveal quadrant) (Figure 1C,D,G,H).

The measurement of the foveal avascular zone (FAZ, mm^2) at the deep capillary plexus (Figure S1) was performed as described in detail elsewhere [21]. The thickness (µm) of the GCC, composed of the thickness of RNFL, GCL and inner plexiform layer (IPL), at the macular area, and, separately, of the RNFL, were measured at the same time using the same OCT (Figure S2).

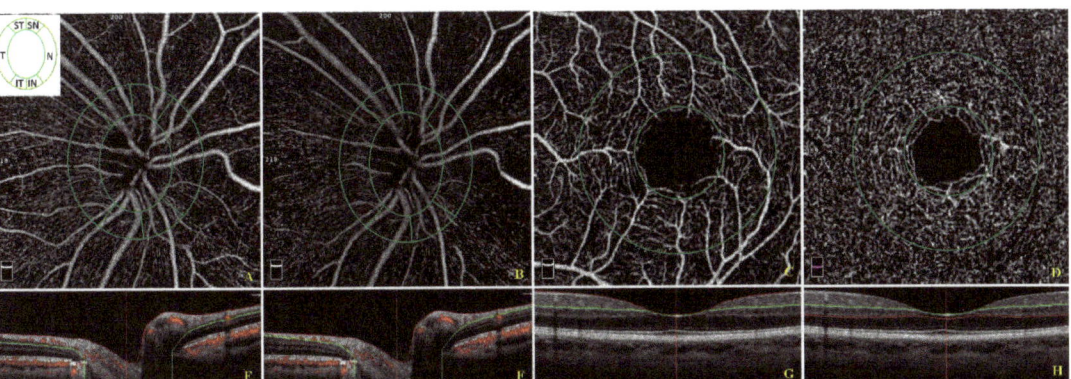

Figure 1. Optical coherence tomographic (OCT) angiographic images of the papillary region and macular region and corresponding structural OCT scans. The papillary vessel density measurement included measurements of the optic nerve head (ONH) (**A**) and radial peripapillary capillary (RPC) (**B**) plexi in an area of $4.5 \times 4.5\,\text{mm}^2$. The papillary area was subdivided into an optic disc area (inside optic disc, surrounded by the inner green circle) and six peripapillary regions (nasal, inferior nasal, inferior temporal, temporal, superior temporal, superior nasal) between the two green rings (**A**,**B**). The macular vessel density measurement included measurements of the superficial (**C**) and deep vascular (**D**) plexi in an area of $3 \times 3\,\text{mm}^2$. The macular area was divided into a foveal and parafoveal area between two concentric circles with a 1 mm diameter and 3 mm diameter, respectively (**C**,**D**). The colored lines (red and green) in horizontal OCT B-scans show segmentation lines defining the different depths in the retinal tissue. The ONH plexus is segmented from the inner limiting membrane to 150 µm below the inner limiting membrane (**E**). The RPC plexus is segmented from the upper boundary of the inner limiting membrane to the lower boundary of the nerve fiber layer (**F**). The superficial capillary plexus is segmented from approximately 3 µm below the inner limiting membrane to 15 µm below the inner plexiform layer (**G**). The deep capillary plexus is segmented from 15 µm below the inner plexiform layer to 70 µm below the inner plexiform layer (**H**).

Exclusion criteria for all study participants were IOP > 22 mmHg, history of glaucoma, optic neuropathies, retinal diseases including any fundus findings suggesting hypertensive retinopathy (Grade 1–2 (Mild), 3 (Moderate), 4 (severe), according to the Keith–Wagener–Barker or Mitchell–Wong classification system) [22], a recent history of intraocular surgery, ocular trauma, and an obvious media opacity that could interfere with the OCT analysis.

2.4. Statistical Analyses

Continuous variables were expressed as mean ± standard deviation (SD) and categorical variables as proportion (%). Statistical significance was set with a *p*-value lesser than or equal to 0.05, with 95% confidence intervals (CI).

The whole sample was subdivided into two groups according to the presence or absence of hypertension. Due to the diffuse non-normal distribution of all variables (using the Shapiro distribution test), Wilcoxon rank sum test was performed to assess differences between the groups for continuous variables and Chi squared test for categorical variables. Logistic regression models were applied to assess associations between the unitary increases of OCT-A parameters that showed significant differences among the groups, as independent variables, and a hypertensive status as outcome. We built two hierarchical nested models: an unadjusted model and a fully adjusted model, adjusted for age, sex, BMI, MMSE, and IOP.

To reduce selection bias and simplify the reading of results we used a complete randomization algorithm for the eye selection assigning the corresponding value (left or right eye) to the new variable thus created. Moreover, we performed the Bonferroni corrected *p*-value in every model for every single OCT covariate.

Statistical analysis was performed with RStudio software, Version 1.4.1106 using additional packages: idyverse, randomizeR, rstatistix, Epi, kable.

3. Results

3.1. Descriptive Analysis

From 2016 to 2019, 892 of the 1929 participants in the Salus in Apulia Study underwent ophthalmological examinations. In addition, 124 subjects were excluded due to lack of data about hypertension, 20 due to glaucoma, 12 to hypertensive retinopathy, and 5 to erroneous scans including scans with segmentation failure. Overall, 731 participants were eligible for the final analysis presented in this study.

The average age of the participants was 73.4 ± 6.1 years, with a higher percentage of females (n = 434, 59.4%). The main sociodemographic and clinical characteristics of the whole sample, subdivided according to the presence/absence of hypertension, are shown in Table 1.

Table 1. Sociodemographic and clinical variables in subjects with and without hypertension. The Salus in Apulia Study (n = 731).

	Without Hypertension		With Hypertension		p *
	Mean ± SD/ Sample Size	Median (Min to Max)	Mean ± SD/ Sample Size	Median (Min to Max)	
Sociodemographic Assessment					
Subjects (%)	114 (15.6)		617 (84.4)		
Age (years)	73.2 ± 5.8	71.5 (65 to 89)	73.4 ± 6.1	72 (65 to 95)	0.93
Sex					0.23$^{\chi^2}$
Males (%)	52 (45.6)	–	245 (39.7)	–	
Females (%)	62 (54.4)	–	372 (60.3)	–	
Male/Female (%)	83.9		65.9		
Smokers	9 (7.9)	–	36 (5.8)	–	0.40$^{\chi^2}$
Waist circumference (cm)	99.7 ± 11.9	98 (70 to 127)	103.8 ± 10.2	104 (70 to 139)	<0.01
BMI (kg/m^2)	27.3 ± 4.6	27.3 (18.4 to 43)	28.3 ± 4.7	27.9 (18.5 to 47.7)	0.04
MMSE	26.1 ± 3.9	27 (13 to 30)	26.5 ± 4.1	28 (1 to 30)	0.33
MCI	9 (7.9)	–	117 (19)	–	<0.01
Metabolic Assessments					
SBP (mmHg)	115.3 ± 6.4	120 (100 to 125)	136.1 ± 13	140 (100 to 180)	<0.01
DBP (mmHg)	68.2 ± 4.6	70 (50 to 75)	79.6 ± 6.7	80 (40 to 100)	<0.01
HbA1c (mmol/mol) HbA1c (%)	39.7 ± 9.5 5.8	39 (18 to 92) 5.7 (3.8 to 10.6)	39.6 ± 9.2 5.8	38 (19 to 128) 5.6 (3.9 to 13.9)	0.77
Total cholesterol (mg/dL)	178.4 ± 34.7	178 (85 to 270)	186.6 ± 37.2	186 (79 to 386)	0.04
Triglycerides (mg/dL)	93 ± 47.8	84.4 (17 to 292)	104.7 ± 55.6	92 (30 to 520)	0.02
RBC (10^6 cells/mm^3)	4.7 ± 0.5	4.6 (3.2 to 6.8)	4.8 ± 1.5	4.8 (2.9 to 40.8)	<0.01
Hemoglobin (g/dL)	13.4 ± 1.3	13.4 (9.5 to 16.9)	13.9 ± 1.5	13.9 (9 to 18.5)	<0.01

BMI: body mass index; MMSE: Mini Mental State Examination; MCI: mild cognitive impairment; SBP: systolic blood pressure; DBP diastolic blood pressure; HbA1c: glycated hemoglobin; RBC: Red Blood Cell. All data are shown as mean ± standard deviation (SD)/sample size, median (min to max) for continuous variables and as (%) for proportions. * Wilcoxon sum rank test; $^{\chi^2}$ Chi squared test.

Older people with hypertension (higher SBP and DBP; p < 0.01, respectively) had a significantly greater waist circumference (p < 0.01) and BMI (p = 0.04). Moreover, the MCI prevalence was higher in subjects with hypertension ($p < 0.01$). Regarding blood tests, older people with hypertension had higher serum total cholesterol ($p = 0.04$), triglycerides levels ($p = 0.02$), Red Blood Cell count ($p < 0.01$), and hemoglobin ($p < 0.01$). Other sociodemographic characteristics of the whole population study, subdivided according to the presence/absence of hypertensive condition, not significantly different among the groups, are shown in the Table S1.

3.2. Analysis of Ophthalmological Parameters

Table 2 shows the ophthalmological parameters in older subjects with and without hypertension. BCVA and IOP were not significantly different between the groups.

Table 2. Ophthalmological variables in subjects with and without hypertension. The Salus in Apulia Study ($n = 731$).

	Without Hypertension		With Hypertension		
	Mean ± SD	Median (Min to Max)	Mean ± SD	Median (Min to Max)	p Value *
BCVA (LogMar)	0.13 ± 0.3	0.03 (0 to 1.6)	0.11 ± 0.2	0.03 (0 to 1.8)	0.70
IOP (mmHg)	14.9 ± 3.4	14.4 (10 to 22)	14.7 ± 3.1	14.5 (9 to 21)	0.14
GCC thickness (μm)	99.2 ± 18	96.5 (65 to 237.8)	95.4 ± 12.6	94.5 (44.7 to 180.1)	0.04
RNFL thickness (μm)	97.6 ± 10.7	98 (62 to 128)	95.5 ± 11	96 (57 to 127)	0.06
ONH peripapillary inferior temporal VD (%)	63.7 ± 4.8	64.5 (46.2 to 71.9)	62.2 ± 5.8	62.8 (38.9 to 72.3)	0.02
ONH inside Optic Disc VD (%)	58.6 ± 8.2	59.4 (28.7 to 72.6)	60.8 ± 6.4	62.1 (35.7 to 72.9)	<0.01
RPC inside Optic Disc VD (%)	38.7 ± 10.6	37.8 (13.3 to 67.2)	42.9 ± 10.8	43 (13.3 to 67.2)	<0.01
SSI	61.3 ± 10.4	62 (34 to 87.6)	62.6 ± 11.1	63.7 (2.1 to 87.6)	0.20

BCVA: best-corrected visual acuity; IOP: intraocular pressure; GCC: ganglion cell complex; RNFL: retinal nerve fiber layer; ONH: optic nerve head; VD: vascular density; RPC: radial peripapillary capillary; SSI, signal strength index; * Wilcoxon sum rank test.

The mean GCC thickness was slightly lower in patients with hypertension ($p = 0.04$). Mean RNFL thickness was slightly lower in the hypertension group than in subjects without hypertension with a significance rather close to the value 0.05 ($p = 0.06$). VD of ONH plexus at the inferior temporal sector was significantly lower in subjects with than without hypertension ($p = 0.02$). Conversely, VD of the ONH and RPC inside the optic disc was significantly higher in subjects with than without hypertension ($p < 0.01$). No significant difference was found between the groups regarding VD of ONH and RPC networks at the other sectors analyzed, FAZ area, and SVD and DVD at the foveal and parafoveal sites. However, all measurements of VD at the macular site revealed slightly higher values in hypertensive patients (Table S2).

3.3. Regression Models

The increase of GCC thickness was inversely associated with hypertension (OR: 0.98; 95% CI: 0.97–1). Also, the unitary increase of VD of the ONH plexus at the inferior temporal sector of the peripapillary area (OR:0.95, 95% CI: 0.91–0.99) was inversely associated with hypertensive condition. Conversely, the increase of VD of the ONH (OR:1.07, 95% CI: 1.04–1.10) and RPC inside Optic Disc (OR:1.04, 95% CI: 1.02–1.06) were directly associated with hypertension (Table 3).

Table 3. Logistic regression models on hypertension status (Yes/No) as dependent variable and regressors. N: 731.

	Raw Model			Adjusted Model				
	OR	CI 95%	Stand. Err.	OR	CI 95%	Stand. Err.	p	Adj. p
GCC Thickness (µm)	0.98	0.97 to 0.99	0.01	0.98	0.97 to 0.99	0.01	0.01	0.04
Age (years)				1	0.97 to 1.04	0.01	0.58	0.99
Sex (Female)				1.26	0.83 to 1.82	0.21	0.42	0.99
BMI (Kg/m^2)				1.04	1.00 to 1.09	0.02	0.06	0.36
IOP				1.07	0.96 to 1.19	0.05	0.21	0.99
MMSE				1.03	0.98 to 1.09	0.02	0.22	0.99
ONH peripapillary Inferior Temporal VD (%)	0.95	0.91 to 0.99	0.02	0.95	0.91 to 0.99	0.02	0.01	0.05
Age (years)				1.01	0.97 to 1.05	0.01	0.61	0.99
Sex (Female)				1.17	0.77 to 1.79	0.21	0.45	0.99
BMI (Kg/m^2)				1.04	1.00 to 1.09	0.02	0.07	0.49
IOP				1.07	0.96 to 1.19	0.05	0.20	0.99
MMSE				1.04	0.98 to 1.09	0.02	0.18	0.99
ONH Inside Optic Disc VD (%)	1.06	1.03 to 1.10	0.01	1.07	1.04 to 1.10	0.06	<0.01	<0.01
Age (years)				1.02	0.98 to 1.06	0.02	0.27	0.99
Sex (Female)				1.22	0.80 to 1.88	0.20	0.34	0.99
BMI (Kg/m^2)				1.04	0.99 to 1.09	0.04	0.06	0.42
Mean IOP				1.07	0.96 to 1.19	0.07	0.18	0.99
MMSE				1.02	0.97 to 1.08	0.02	0.32	0.99
RPC Inside Optic Disc VD (%)	1.04	1.02 to 1.05	0.01	1.04	1.02 to 1.06	0.01	<0.01	<0.01
Age (years)				1.03	0.99 to 1.07	0.01	0.18	0.99
Sex (Female)				1.11	0.72 to 1.71	0.21	0.63	0.99
BMI (Kg/m^2)				1.04	0.99 to 1.09	0.02	0.08	0.56
IOP				1.09	0.98 to 1.21	0.05	0.10	0.70
MMSE				1.04	0.98 to 1.09	0.02	0.17	0.99

GCC: ganglion cell complex; BMI: Body Mass Index; IOP: intraocular pressure; MMSE: Mini Mental State Evaluation; ONH: optic nerve head; VD: vascular density; RPC: radial peripapillary capillary.

All other OCT-A parameters not associated with hypertension in the models are reported in Table S3.

4. Discussion

In the present study conducted in an older population-based sample, on OCT, thinner GCC was observed in hypertensive subjects. On OCT-A, a capillary rarefaction at the inferior temporal sector of the ONH peripapillary plexus and, conversely, a higher density of the ONH and RPC network inside optic disc were significantly associated with hypertensive condition.

In our population-based sample, older people with hypertension had a higher BMI and waist circumference, suggesting the relationship between obesity and blood hypertension in older adults, as recently reported [23]. The MCI prevalence was also higher in hypertensive subjects, confirming the potential role of hypertension as risk factor for MCI (reduced function in memory, thinking, and other cognitive domains, but not affecting everyday functioning), as previously reported [24].

In the present study, the lowest average value for GCC and RNFL, was observed in older individuals with blood hypertension as compared to the control group. These findings were consistent with previous studies [6,10,11]. The reduced thickness of the inner neuroretinal layers observed, suggesting neural damage, was hypothesized to be related to microvascular abnormalities in patients with blood hypertension [10], similar to the proposed mechanism underlying the reduction of RNFL in diabetic patients without retinopathy [25]. An association with the hypertensive condition was mainly observed for GCC thickness, and this could be explained by the early damage of the GCL-IPL, containing ganglion cells bodies and dendrites, that precedes the damage of the axons in RNFL [26], as well as by the exclusion from the present study of patients with hypertensive retinopathy. On OCT-A, the larger difference in the average VD of the peripapillary networks between hypertensive patients and control subjects was reported at the inferior temporal sector of the ONH network and inside the optic disc of the RPC plexus. The vessels of ONH and RPC vascular networks have a relatively constant caliber and few anastomoses, paralleling the RNFL in the peripapillary area, which display a characteristic linear morphological pattern [27]. In healthy subjects, these networks are more prominent in the peripheral arcuate nerve fiber layer region, as well as in the temporal sectors, where the thinnest RNFL was located [27,28]. This opposite distribution could be due to the activity-vascular related mechanism by which denser temporal RPC exists to fulfill the highly metabolic requirements of photoreceptors, ganglion cells, and retinal pigment epithelial cells within the macular area [28], despite the reported association between RNFL thickness and peripapillary VD [29] supports the idea that the perfusion of RPC may be proportional to the quantity of RNFL supplied [12]. The peripapillary plexus is considered to be crucial for the homeostasis and function of the ganglion cells and their axons in the RNFL [30], and a reduced VD has been observed in early glaucoma [31] and non-arteritic ischemic optic neuropathy [32], associated with a reduced RNFL and GCC thickness [33]. Therefore, we may hypothesize that in the hypertensive condition the reduced thickness of GCC and RNFL could be related to the vascular rarefaction in a peripapillary sector with a high metabolic requirement. An increased vascular density inside the optic disc was recently observed in hypertensive subjects without related retinopathy [8,34], consistent with our finding. This is probably due to the increased reflux venous resistance related to hypertension vascular damage and the poor regulatory capacity of papillary ONH and RPC networks causing blood flow restriction and consequent vessels dilatation interpreted as an increased capillary density by OCT-A [8,34]. In contrast with previous results [8,11,34], we found a slightly lower vascular density of the macular superficial and deep vascular plexi and a slight enlargement of deep FAZ in normotensive individuals, with no significant difference as compared to hypertensive patients. Although these differences between the groups fall in the range of normal variation of macular vessel density measurements, as previously reported [35], they deserve some consideration. The mechanism underlying the association between blood hypertension and macular capillary density remains unclear. Previous studies have indicated a reduced retinal VD in hypertension as a possible effect of vascular narrowing due to an increased vascular resistance [4,11,36,37], which may impair blood flow. However, first of all, we should consider some technical limits of OCT-A whereby a slow blood flow above a minimum threshold detected by the machine may be wrongly reflected as a vascular rarefaction or even an area of non-perfusion on OCT-A images [37], and some optical parameters, such as the axial length of the eye, and in particular myopic condition, that could induce noise in the image, making the vascular network appear artificially denser because of the larger area being scanned under smaller magnification [38]. Furthermore, the results of 11 studies on macular vessels rarefaction reported in a recent meta-analysis [39] should be analyzed considering the Asiatic ethnicity of most of the study populations (9 out of 11 studies considered Asiatic populations) [8,10,11,34,40–44], and the inclusion of patients with hypertensive retinopathy in the study groups [10,44].

In the present study, the differences in VD between older subjects with and without hypertension showed a different trend at peripapillary and macular sites. Peripapillary vessels originate from two systems, the central retinal artery and the short posterior ciliary arteries, whereas macular vessels originate only from the central retinal artery [45]. The posterior ciliary arteries might suffer more severe damage than the retinal vascular system in glaucoma [46], diabetic retinopathy [15], and obstructive sleep apnea syndrome [45], because they are probably more prone to structural alterations due to high intraocular pressure, microangiopathy and hypercapnia, respectively. Therefore, the different origins and sizes of the vessels between the peripapillary and parafoveal areas might explain our findings, suggesting different damage to the vessels in different vascular systems attributable to hypertension.

The strengths of the present study included: a standardized measurement of daytime blood pressure in office setting, which might better reflect the hemodynamic load over the 24 h period than one single blood pressure measurement and could be more correlated with end-organ damage of arteries and heart [47,48]; OCT scanning combined with an ophthalmological clinical examination to avoid optical interferences due to ocular media abnormalities. Furthermore, we considered randomly the measurements of one eye for each subject as a good practice for statistical analysis [49] although, in all age groups, a moderate degree of interocular asymmetry in retinal layer thickness, including GCC and RNFL [50,51], and retinal vascular features [52], in both normotension and hypertension [53], was previously reported. However, some limitations and questions need to be considered. ONH parameters (rim, cup, etc.) were not analyzed in this study. We did not measure the ocular perfusion pressure as the net pressure gradient causing blood to flow to the eye, because of its limitations in reflecting the true perfusion pressure at the ONH, influenced by several variables as diurnal variations in the blood pressure and IOP [54], diurnal-to-nocturnal decreases in retinal and ONH blood flow in older patients [55], and intracranial pressure [56]. Moreover, the RPC plexus contains multilayered capillaries that are overlapping on en-face OCT images, complicating the ability to detect small capillary losses [31]. The macular deep vascular plexus is notoriously affected by projection artefacts which may lead to erroneous findings; one of these measures is the axial length, that was lacking in this study setting. Nor did we analyze in OCT-A the choriocapillaris, which appears as a mesh-like homogeneous tissue whose single vessels are usually not discernible. Measurement of the choriocapillaris network could be less precise than that of the intraretinal vascular networks [57]. A limit in methodology of the present study include the definition of the hypertensive status that was not based on previous clinical diagnosis as well as the presence of hypertensive medication, and the cross-sectional nature of the data, preventing assessment of the direction of the association, with a high risk of reverse causality bias.

In conclusion, the present findings confirmed a thinner GCC and microvascular changes at the peripapillary area in older hypertensive individuals than in age-matched healthy subjects. This conclusion and the higher MCI prevalence in hypertensive subjects suggests a link between central and peripheric neural damage with systemic vascular disregulation. Assessment of the peripapillary retinal microvasculature using OCT-A may be a useful non-invasive technique to detect early microvascular changes due to hypertension. Further larger studies, particularly with longitudinal cohort or randomized clinical trial designs, are needed to test the effectiveness of retinal capillary density as a novel biomarker in predicting the incidence and progression of hypertension-related microvascular complications, also at the population level.

Supplementary Materials: The following supporting information can be downloaded at: https://www.mdpi.com/article/10.3390/jcm11041098/s1, Table S1. Sociodemographic and clinical variables in subjects with and without hypertension. The Salus in Apulia Study ($n = 731$). Table S2. Ophthalmological variables in subjects with and without hypertension. The Salus in Apulia Study

(n = 731). Table S3. Logistic regression models on Hypertension status (Yes/No) as dependent variable and regressors. N:731. Figure S1. Optical coherence tomographic angiographic (OCT-A) image of the foveal avascular zone (FAZ) areas at the deep vascular plexus. The FAZ area border (inner yellow line) was outlined automatically, and the surface area was then measured in square millimeters using built-in software under the flow option of the instrument in the deep vascular plexus (A) The colored lines (red and green) in horizontal OCT B-scans show segmentation lines defining the depths in the retinal tissue (B). Figure S2. Optical coherence tomographic images of the ganglion cell complex (GCC) and retinal nerve fiber layer (RNFL) thickness. The device measures GCC and RNFL thickness within an automatically rendered 7 mm^2 area, centered 1 mm temporally to the fovea. The system produces a color-coded thickness map for interpretation. (A,C) Thicker regions of GCC and RNFL are displayed as yellow and orange, whereas thinner regions are displayed as blue and green. Acquired thicknesses are compared with values from a normative database and displayed as a significance map. The color-coded map shows the corresponding probabilities of deviation from the normal range based on comparison with an age-matched control group of healthy subjects. (B,D) Cross-sectional B-scan displays the segmentation used for GCC and RNFL analysis. (B) The traced boundaries for the GCC scan (white lines) include the inner limiting membrane and the outer IPL. (D) The traced boundaries for the RNFL scan (colored lines) include the inner limiting membrane and the outer IPL.

Author Contributions: Conceptualization: R.S., L.L. and A.N.; Methodology, R.S., F.P. and G.A.; Formal Analysis, F.C. (Fabio Castellana) and S.T.; Investigation: L.L., A.N., G.G., I.B., R.Z., P.P., A.P., V.P., C.G., R.B., R.G., M.B. and F.C. (Flavio Cassano); Data Curation, F.C. (Fabio Castellana) and V.B.; Writing—Original Draft Preparation, L.L. and A.N.; Writing—Review and Editing, R.S., F.P. and M.L.; Supervision: G.S., F.B. and G.A.; Project Administration, R.S. Funding Acquisition, R.S. All authors have read and agreed to the published version of the manuscript.

Funding: This study was funded by the Italian Ministry of Health with "Italian Network on aging 2019" Grant.

Institutional Review Board Statement: The study was conducted in accordance with the Declaration of Helsinki, and approved by the Institutional Review Board (or Ethics Committee) of the National Institute of Gastroenterology "S. De Bellis" (Approval Code: 68/CE De Bellis; Approval Date: 9 April 2019).

Informed Consent Statement: Informed consent was obtained from all subjects involved in the study.

Data Availability Statement: The data that support the findings of the present study are available from the corresponding author (GS) upon reasonable request.

Acknowledgments: We thank the "Salus in Apulia" Research Team. This manuscript is the result of the research work on frailty undertaken by the "Research Network on Aging" team, supported by the resources of the Italian Ministry of Health—Research Networks of National Health Institutes. We thank M.V. Pragnell, B.A., for her precious help as native English supervisor. We thank the General Practitioners of Castellana Grotte, for their fundamental role in the recruitment of participants to these studies: Cecilia Olga Maria Campanella, Annamaria Daddabbo, Giosuè Dell'aera, Rosalia Francesca Giustiniano, Massimo Guzzoni Iudice, Savino Lomuscio, Rocco Lucarelli, Antonio Mazzarisi, Mariana Palumbo, Maria Teresa Persio, Rosa Vincenza Pesce, Gabriella Puzzovivo, Pasqua Maria Romano, Cinzia Sgobba, Francesco Simeone, Paola Tartaglia, and Nicola Tauro.

Conflicts of Interest: The authors declare no conflict of interest.

References

1. Kearney, P.M.; Whelton, M.; Reynolds, K.; Muntner, P.; Whelton, P.K.; He, J. Global burden of hypertension: Analysis of worldwide data. *Lancet* **2005**, *365*, 217–223. [CrossRef]
2. Lim, S.S.; Vos, T.; Flaxman, A.D.; Danaei, G.; Shibuya, K.; Adair-Rohani, H.; AlMazroa, M.A.; Amann, M.; Anderson, H.R.; Andrews, K.G.; et al. A comparative risk assessment of burden of disease and injury attributable to 67 risk factors and risk factor clusters in 21 regions, 1990–2010: A systematic analysis for the Global Burden of Disease Study 2010. *Lancet* **2012**, *380*, 2224–2260. [CrossRef]
3. Fields, L.E.; Burt, V.L.; Cutler, J.A.; Hughes, J.; Roccella, E.J.; Sorlie, P. The burden of adult hypertension in the United States 1999 to 2000: A rising tide. *Hypertension* **2004**, *44*, 398–404. [CrossRef] [PubMed]
4. Wong, T.Y.; Mitchell, P. The eye in hypertension. *Lancet* **2007**, *369*, 425–435. [CrossRef]

5. MacGillivray, T.J.; Trucco, E.; Cameron, J.R.; Dhillon, B.; Houston, J.G.; Van Beek, E.J. Retinal imaging as a source of biomarkers for diagnosis, characterization and prognosis of chronic illness or long-term conditions. *Br. J. Radiol.* **2014**, *87*, 20130832. [CrossRef]
6. Akay, F.; Gündoğan, F.C.; Yolcu, U.; Toyran, S.; Tunç, E.; Uzun, S. Retinal structural changes in systemic arterial hypertension: An OCT study. *Eur. J. Ophthalmol.* **2016**, *26*, 436–441. [CrossRef]
7. Lee, M.W.; Lee, W.H.; Park, G.S.; Lim, H.-B.; Kim, J.-Y. Longitudinal Changes in the Peripapillary Retinal Nerve Fiber Layer Thickness in Hypertension: 4-Year Prospective Observational Study. *Investig. Ophthalmol. Vis. Sci.* **2019**, *60*, 3914–3919. [CrossRef]
8. Hua, D.; Xu, Y.; Zeng, X.; Yang, N.; Jiang, M.; Zhang, X.; Yang, J.; He, T.; Xing, Y. Use of optical coherence tomography angiography for assessment of microvascular changes in the macula and optic nerve head in hypertensive patients without hypertensive retinopathy. *Microvasc. Res.* **2020**, *129*, 103969. [CrossRef]
9. Pascual-Prieto, J.; Burgos-Blasco, B.; Avila Sanchez-Torija, M.; Fernández-Vigo, J.I.; Arriola-Villalobos, P.; Barbero Pedraz, M.A.; García-Feijoo, J.; Martínez-de-la-Casa, J.M. Utility of optical coherence tomography angiography in detecting vascular retinal damage caused by arterial hypertension. *Eur. J. Ophthalmol.* **2020**, *30*, 579–585. [CrossRef]
10. Peng, Q.; Hu, Y.; Huang, M.; Wu, Y.; Zhong, P.; Dong, X.; Wu, Q.; Liu, B.; Li, C.; Xie, J.; et al. Retinal Neurovascular Impairment in Patients with Essential Hypertension: An Optical Coherence Tomography Angiography Study. *Investig. Ophthalmol. Vis. Sci.* **2020**, *61*, 42. [CrossRef]
11. Lim, H.B.; Lee, M.W.; Park, J.H.; Kim, K.; Jo, Y.J.; Kim, J.Y. Changes in Ganglion Cell-Inner Plexiform Layer Thickness and Retinal Microvasculature in Hypertension: An Optical Coherence Tomography Angiography Study. *Am. J. Ophthalmol.* **2019**, *199*, 167–176. [CrossRef] [PubMed]
12. Yu, P.K.; Cringle, S.J.; Yu, D.Y. Correlation between the radial peripapillary capillaries and the retinal nerve fibre layer in the normal human retina. *Exp. Eye Res.* **2014**, *129*, 83–92. [CrossRef] [PubMed]
13. Chandrasekera, E.; An, D.; McAllister, I.L.; Yu, D.Y.; Balaratnasingam, C. Three-Dimensional Microscopy Demonstrates Series and Parallel Organization of Human Peripapillary Capillary Plexuses. *Investig. Ophthalmol. Vis. Sci.* **2018**, *59*, 4327–4344. [CrossRef] [PubMed]
14. Chang, R.; Nelson, A.J.; LeTran, V.; Vu, B.; Burkemper, B.; Chu, Z.; Fard, A.; Kashani, A.H.; Xu, B.Y.; Wang, R.K.; et al. Systemic Determinants of Peripapillary Vessel Density in Healthy African Americans: The African American Eye Disease Study. *Am. J. Ophthalmol.* **2019**, *207*, 240–247. [CrossRef]
15. Huang, J.; Zheng, B.; Lu, Y.; Gu, X.; Dai, H.; Chen, T. Quantification of Microvascular Density of the Optic Nerve Head in Diabetic Retinopathy Using Optical Coherence Tomographic Angiography. *J. Ophthalmol.* **2020**, *2020*, 5014035. [CrossRef]
16. Castellana, F.; Lampignano, L.; Bortone, I.; Zupo, R.; Lozupone, M.; Griseta, C.; Daniele, A.; De Pergola, G.; Giannelli, G.; Sardone, R.; et al. Physical Frailty, Multimorbidity, and All-Cause Mortality in an Older Population From Southern Italy: Results from the Salus in Apulia Study. *J. Am. Med. Dir. Assoc.* **2021**, *22*, 598–605. [CrossRef]
17. Whelton, P.K.; Carey, R.M.; Aronow, W.S.; Casey, D.E.; Collins, K.J.; Dennison Himmelfarb, C.; DePalma, S.M.; Gidding, S.; Jamerson, K.A.; Jones, D.W.; et al. 2017 ACC/AHA/AAPA/ABC/ACPM/AGS/APhA/ASH/ASPC/NMA/PCNA Guideline for the Prevention, Detection, Evaluation, and Management of High Blood Pressure in Adults: A Report of the American College of Cardiology/American Heart Association Task Force on Clinical Practice Guidelines. *Hypertension* **2018**, *71*, e13–e115.
18. Sardone, R.; Battista, P.; Donghia, R.; Lozupone, M.; Tortelli, R.; Guerra, V.; Grasso, A.; Griseta, C.; Castellana, F.; Zupo, R.; et al. Age-Related Central Auditory Processing Disorder, MCI, and Dementia in an Older Population of Southern Italy. *Otolaryngol.—Head Neck Surg.* **2020**, *163*, 348–355. [CrossRef]
19. Czakó, C.; István, L.; Ecsedy, M.; Récsán, Z.; Sándor, G.; Benyó, F.; Horváth, H.; Papp, A.; Resch, M.; Borbándy, Á.; et al. The effect of image quality on the reliability of OCT angiography measurements in patients with diabetes. *Int. J. Retina Vitreous* **2019**, *5*, 46. [CrossRef]
20. Garway-Heath, D.F.; Poinoosawmy, D.; Fitzke, F.W.; Hitchings, R.A. Mapping the visual field to the optic disc in normal tension glaucoma eyes. *Ophthalmology* **2000**, *107*, 1809–1815. [CrossRef]
21. Shahlaee, A.; Pefkianaki, M.; Hsu, J.; Ho, J.C. Measurement of Foveal Avascular Zone Dimensions and its Reliability in Healthy Eyes Using Optical Coherence Tomography Angiography. *Am. J. Ophthalmol.* **2016**, *161*, 50–55.e1. [CrossRef] [PubMed]
22. Downie, L.E.; Hodgson, L.A.; DSylva, C.; McIntosh, R.L.; Rogers, S.L.; Connell, P.; Wong, T.Y. Hypertensive retinopathy: Comparing the Keith-Wagener-Barker to a simplified classification. *J. Hypertens.* **2013**, *31*, 960–965. [CrossRef] [PubMed]
23. Zhang, W.; He, K.; Zhao, H.; Hu, X.; Yin, C.; Zhao, X.; Shi, S. Association of body mass index and waist circumference with high blood pressure in older adults. *BMC Geriatr.* **2021**, *21*, 260. [CrossRef] [PubMed]
24. Luck, T.; Luppa, M.; Briel, S.; Riedel-Heller, S.G. Incidence of mild cognitive impairment: A systematic review. *Dement. Geriatr. Cogn. Disord.* **2010**, *29*, 164–175. [CrossRef]
25. Jeon, S.J.; Kwon, J.W.; La, T.Y.; Park, C.K.; Choi, J.A. Characteristics of Retinal Nerve Fiber Layer Defect in Nonglaucomatous Eyes with Type II Diabetes. *Investig. Ophthalmol. Vis. Sci.* **2016**, *57*, 4008–4015. [CrossRef]
26. Scuderi, G.; Fragiotta, S.; Scuderi, L.; Iodice, C.M.; Perdicchi, A. Ganglion Cell Complex Analysis in Glaucoma Patients: What Can It Tell Us? *Eye Brain.* **2020**, *12*, 33–44. [CrossRef]
27. Mase, T.; Ishibazawa, A.; Nagaoka, T.; Yokota, H.; Yoshida, A. Radial Peripapillary Capillary Network Visualized Using Wide-Field Montage Optical Coherence Tomography Angiography. *Investig. Ophthalmol. Vis. Sci.* **2016**, *57*, OCT504–OCT510. [CrossRef]

28. Liu, G.; Wang, Y.; Gao, P. Distributions of Radial Peripapillary Capillary Density and Correlations with Retinal Nerve Fiber Layer Thickness in Normal Subjects. *Med. Sci. Monit.* **2021**, *27*, e933601. [CrossRef]
29. She, X.; Guo, J.; Liu, X.; Zhu, H.; Li, T.; Zhou, M.; Wang, F.; Sun, X. Reliability of Vessel Density Measurements in the Peripapillary Retina and Correlation with Retinal Nerve Fiber Layer Thickness in Healthy Subjects Using Optical Coherence Tomography Angiography. *Ophthalmologica* **2018**, *240*, 183–190. [CrossRef]
30. Yu, D.Y.; Cringle, S.J.; Balaratnasingam, C.; Morgan, W.H.; Paula, K.Y.; Su, E.N. Retinal ganglion cells: Energetics, compartmentation, axonal transport, cytoskeletons and vulnerability. *Prog. Retin. Eye Res.* **2013**, *36*, 217–246. [CrossRef]
31. Mansoori, T.; Sivaswamy, J.; Gamalapati, J.S.; Balakrishna, N. Radial Peripapillary Capillary Density Measurement Using Optical Coherence Tomography Angiography in Early Glaucoma. *J. Glaucoma* **2017**, *26*, 438–443. [CrossRef] [PubMed]
32. Cerdà-Ibáñez, M.; Duch-Samper, A.; Clemente-Tomás, R.; Torrecillas-Picazo, R.; Ruiz del Río, N.; Manfreda-Dominguez, L. Correlation Between Ischemic Retinal Accidents and Radial Peripapillary Capillaries in the Optic Nerve Using Optical Coherence Tomographic Angiography: Observations in 6 Patients. *Ophthalmol. Eye Dis.* **2017**, *9*, 1179172117702889. [CrossRef] [PubMed]
33. Augstburger, E.; Zéboulon, P.; Keilani, C.; Baudouin, C.; Labbé, A. Retinal and Choroidal Microvasculature in Nonarteritic Anterior Ischemic Optic Neuropathy: An Optical Coherence Tomography Angiography Study. *Investig. Ophthalmol. Vis. Sci.* **2018**, *59*, 870–877. [CrossRef] [PubMed]
34. Hua, D.; Xu, Y.; Zhang, X.; He, T.; Chen, C.; Chen, Z.; Xing, Y. Retinal microvascular changes in hypertensive patients with different levels of blood pressure control and without hypertensive retinopathy. *Curr. Eye Res.* **2021**, *46*, 107–114. [CrossRef] [PubMed]
35. You, Q.S.; Chan, J.C.; Ng, A.L.; Choy, B.K.; Shih, K.C.; Cheung, J.J.; Wong, J.K.; Shum, J.W.; Ni, M.Y.; Lai, J.S.; et al. Macular Vessel Density Measured with Optical Coherence Tomography Angiography and Its Associations in a Large Population-Based Study. *Investig. Ophthalmol. Vis. Sci.* **2019**, *60*, 4830–4837. [CrossRef] [PubMed]
36. Bosch, A.J.; Harazny, J.M.; Kistner, I.; Friedrich, S.; Wojtkiewicz, J.; Schmieder, R.E. Retinal capillary rarefaction in patients with untreated mild-moderate hypertension. *BMC Cardiovasc. Disord.* **2017**, *17*, 300. [CrossRef] [PubMed]
37. Kannenkeril, D.; Harazny, J.M.; Bosch, A.; Ott, C.; Michelson, G.; Schmieder, R.E.; Friedrich, S. Retinal vascular resistance in arterial hypertension. *Blood Press.* **2018**, *27*, 82–87. [CrossRef]
38. Yang, Y.; Wang, J.; Jiang, H.; Yang, X.; Feng, L.; Hu, L.; Wang, L.; Lü, F.; Shen, M. Retinal Microvasculature Alteration in High Myopia. *Investig. Ophthalmol. Vis. Sci.* **2016**, *57*, 6020–6030. [CrossRef]
39. Tan, W.; Yao, X.; Le, T.-T.; Tan, A.C.S.; Cheung, C.Y.; Chin, C.W.L.; Schmetterer, L.; Chua, J. The Application of Optical Coherence Tomography Angiography in Systemic Hypertension: A Meta-Analysis. *Front. Med.* **2021**, *8*, 778330. [CrossRef]
40. Xu, Q.; Sun, H.; Huang, X.; Qu, Y. Retinal microvascular metrics in untreated essential hypertensives using optical coherence tomography angiography. *Graefe's Arch. Clin. Exp. Ophthalmol.* **2021**, *259*, 395–403. [CrossRef]
41. Chua, J.; Le, T.T.; Tan, B.; Ke, M.; Li, C.; Wong, D.W.; Tan, A.; Lamoureux, E.; Wong, T.Y.; Chin, C.W.; et al. Choriocapillaris microvasculature dysfunction in systemic hypertension. *Sci. Rep.* **2021**, *11*, 4603. [CrossRef] [PubMed]
42. Sun, C.; Ladores, C.; Hong, J.; Nguyen, D.Q.; Chua, J.; Ting, D.; Schmetterer, L.; Wong, T.Y.; Cheng, C.Y.; Tan, A. Systemic hypertension associated retinal microvascular changes can be detected with optical coherence tomography angiography. *Sci. Rep.* **2020**, *10*, 9580. [CrossRef] [PubMed]
43. Shin, Y.I.; Nam, K.Y.; Lee, W.H.; Ryu, C.K.; Lim, H.B.; Jo, Y.J.; Kim, J.Y. Peripapillary microvascular changes in patients with systemic hypertension: An optical coherence tomography angiography study. *Sci. Rep.* **2020**, *10*, 6541. [CrossRef] [PubMed]
44. Lee, W.H.; Park, J.H.; Won, Y.; Lee, M.W.; Shin, Y.I.; Jo, Y.J.; Kim, J.Y. Retinal microvascular change in hypertension as measured by optical coherence tomography angiography. *Sci. Rep.* **2019**, *9*, 156. [CrossRef]
45. Yu, J.; Xiao, K.; Huang, J.; Sun, X.; Jiang, C. Reduced Retinal Vessel Density in Obstructive Sleep Apnea Syndrome Patients: An Optical Coherence Tomography Angiography Study. *Investig. Ophthalmol. Vis. Sci.* **2017**, *58*, 3506–3512. [CrossRef]
46. Hosking, S.L.; Harris, A.; Chung, H.S.; Jonescu-Cuypers, C.P.; Kagemann, L.; Hilton, E.J.R.; Garzozi, H. Ocular haemodynamic responses to induced hypercapnia and hyperoxia in glaucoma. *Br. J. Ophthalmol.* **2004**, *88*, 406–411. [CrossRef]
47. Dell'Oro, R.; Lonati, L.; Mineo, M.; Buzzi, S.; Seravalle, G.; Facchetti, R.; Parati, G.; Mancia, G.; Grassi, G. Relationship between 24-h ambulatory blood pressure and retinal vascular abnormal-ities in hypertension. *J. Hypertens.* **2010**, *28*, e41. [CrossRef]
48. Grassi, G.; Schmieder, R.E. The renaissance of the retinal microvascular network assessment in hypertension: New challeng-es. *J. Hypertens.* **2011**, *29*, 1289–1291. [CrossRef]
49. Armstrong, R.A. Statistical guidelines for the analysis of data obtained from one or both eyes. *Ophthalmic Physiol. Opt.* **2013**, *33*, 7–14. [CrossRef]
50. Yang, M.; Wang, W.; Xu, Q.; Tan, S.; Wei, S. Interocular symmetry of the peripapillary choroidal thickness and retinal nerve fibre layer thickness in healthy adults with isometropia. *BMC Ophthalmol.* **2016**, *16*, 182. [CrossRef]
51. Lee, S.Y.; Jeoung, J.W.; Park, K.H.; Kim, D.M. Macular ganglion cell imaging study: Interocular symmetry of ganglion cell-inner plex-iform layer thickness in normal healthy eyes. *Am. J. Ophthalmol.* **2015**, *159*, 315–323.e2. [CrossRef] [PubMed]
52. Cameron, J.R.; Megaw, R.D.; Tatham, A.J.; McGrory, S.; MacGillivray, T.J.; Doubal, F.N.; Wardlaw, J.M.; Trucco, E.; Chandran, S.; Dhillon, B. Lateral thinking—Interocular symmetry and asymmetry in neurovascular patterning, in health and disease. *Prog. Retin. Eye Res.* **2017**, *59*, 131–157. [CrossRef] [PubMed]

53. Robertson, G.; Fleming, A.; Williams, M.C.; Trucco, E.; Quinn, N.; Hogg, R.; McKay, G.J.; Kee, F.; Young, I.; Pellegrini, E.; et al. Association between hypertension and retinal vascular features in ultra-widefield fundus imaging. *Open Heart* **2020**, *7*, e001124. [CrossRef]
54. Baek, S.U.; Kim, Y.K.; Ha, A.; Kim, Y.W.; Lee, J.; Kim, J.-S.; Jeoung, J.W.; Park, K.H. Diurnal change of retinal vessel density and mean ocular perfusion pressure in patients with open-angle glaucoma. *PLoS ONE* **2019**, *14*, e0215684. [CrossRef] [PubMed]
55. Kida, T.; Liu, J.H.; Weinreb, R.N. Effect of aging on nocturnal blood flow in the optic nerve head and macula in healthy hu-man eyes. *J. Glaucoma* **2008**, *17*, 366–371. [CrossRef] [PubMed]
56. Berdahl, J.P.; Fautsch, M.P.; Stinnett, S.S.; Allingham, R.R. Intracranial pressure in primary open angle glaucoma, normal tension glauco-ma, and ocular hypertension: A case-control study. *Investig. Ophthalmol. Vis. Sci.* **2008**, *49*, 5412–5418. [CrossRef]
57. Wang, Q.; Chan, S.; Yang, J.Y.; You, B.; Wang, Y.X.; Jonas, J.B.; Wei, W.B. Vascular Density in Retina and Choriocapillaris as Measured by Optical Coherence To-mography Angiography. *Am. J. Ophthalmol.* **2016**, *168*, 95–109. [CrossRef]

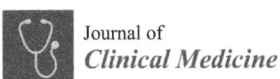

Article

Topographic Outcomes in Keratoconus Surgery: Epi-on versus Epi-off Iontophoresis Corneal Collagen Cross-Linking

Pasquale Napolitano [1], Fausto Tranfa [2], Luca D'Andrea [2,3,*], Ciro Caruso [4], Michele Rinaldi [5], Alberto Mazzucco [2], Nicola Ciampa [2], Antonietta Melenzane [2] and Ciro Costagliola [2]

[1] Department of Medicine and Health Sciences "Vincenzo Tiberio", University of Molise, 86100 Campobasso, Italy; napolitano.pasquale1989@gmail.com
[2] Department of Neurosciences, Reproductive Sciences and Dentistry, Eye Clinic, University of Naples "Federico II", 80138 Naples, Italy; fausto.tranfa@unina.it (F.T.); mazzucco.alberto@libero.it (A.M.); nicolaciampa3@gmail.com (N.C.); antonietta.melenzane@unina.it (A.M.); ciro.costagliola@unina.it (C.C.)
[3] Public Health Department, Università degli Studi di Napoli "Federico II", 80138 Naples, Italy
[4] Corneal Transplant Center, Pellegrini Hospital, Via Portamedina alla Pignasecca, 41, 80127 Napoli, Italy; cirocarusoeye@gmail.com
[5] Department of Ophthalmology, University Della Campania Luigi Vanvitelli, 80138 Naples, Italy; michrinaldi@libero.it
* Correspondence: dandrea.luca91@gmail.com; Tel.: +39-33-3637-0527

Abstract: Background: Corneal collagen cross-linking (CXL) has become the gold standard for mild and moderate stages to stop the progression of keratoconus. We analyzed some corneal topography indices to compare iontophoresis epi-on and iontophoresis epi-off techniques throughout a two-year follow-up. Methods: A total of 64 eyes of 49 patients who underwent CXL were recruited. In 30 eyes the epi-off technique was performed, whereas the remaining 34 eyes were treated with the epi-on technique. All patients underwent a complete ophthalmologic examination that included CDVA, central and thinnest corneal thickness, Schirmer test I, TBUT test, and the Ocular Surface Disease Index. Results: In both groups, a significant improvement in visual function was recorded. No statistically significant differences between Kmax, Mean K, Flat K, Steep K values were found. Statistically significant differences ($p < 0.05$) between the epi-on and epi-off groups' pachymetry before and after 24 months follow-up as well as between the epi-on and epi-off groups' topographically thinnest point in the immediate post-surgery and 24 months after surgery were recorded. Conclusion: Our study highlighted that both techniques are valid in mid-term corneal stabilization. The advantage of the new iontophoresis epi-off cross-linking technique could be found in a faster imbibing time of the cornea, therefore reducing surgical times, with a lower risk of complications.

Keywords: corneal collagen cross-linking; keratoconus; epi-on technique; epi-off technique; iontophoresis; cornea; pachymetry; thinnest point; CXL; OSDI

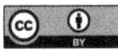

1. Introduction

Keratoconus (KC) is a corneal ectasia and diverse genetic, environmental, and biochemical factors have been associated with it. Increased systemic levels of pro-inflammatory factors, including interleukin-6, tumor necrosis factor-α, and matrix metalloproteinase-9 were found, suggesting that KC may have an inflammatory component [1]. Nevertheless, the etiopathological mechanisms are still not completely elucidated [2]. Keratoconus is characterized by the thinning of the corneal stroma, which leads to the cornea taking a conical shape, generating irregular astigmatism, and increasing the level of higher-order aberrations, with the consequent progressive deterioration of vision [2]. The typical onset of KC is puberty [3,4], with pediatric patients showing the highest rate and speed of progression [5]. In this light, prompt surgical intervention has been suggested in children and adolescents [6,7]. Corneal collagen cross-linking (CXL) has become the gold standard for mild and moderate stages to stop the progression of ectasia [6,8]. This technique aims to strengthen the stromal collagen by induction of collagen bonds activated by ultraviolet light. Thanks to the use of riboflavin-soaked cornea [9], the cross-links between corneal lamellae can increase the biomechanical strength and stability of the cornea or slow the progression of keratoconus. The standard Dresden cross-linking protocol has been shown to lead to keratoconus stabilization over a mid-term and long-term follow-up [10,11]. The standard corneal cross-linking procedure includes the removal of corneal epithelium to achieve adequate penetration of riboflavin into the stroma. Unfortunately, epithelial removal may be responsible for crosslinking-related complications, i.e., vision impairment, risk of infection, and postoperative pain [12]. In the attempt to avoid the side effects induced by epithelial debridement, a trans-epithelial cross-linking technique has been recently introduced [13–15].

For both techniques, the first step is represented by a corneal soak. This step is realized with or without epithelial debridement and requires about 30 min. Iontophoresis guarantees a faster delivery (5 min) of charged molecules into corneal stroma through a small electric current. The second step consists of the activation of penetrated riboflavin with ultraviolet A (UVA) light for about 9 min; the intensity of the UVA light source is 10 mW/cm^2. The last step is the same for both techniques [10,15,16].

This study has aimed to analyze some corneal topography indices comparing, after corneal collagen crosslinking, iontophoresis epi-on (without epithelial debridement) and iontophoresis epi-off (with epithelial debridement) techniques throughout the two-year follow-up period.

2. Materials and Methods

A prospective interventional study, approved by the institution's review board and in accordance with the Declaration of Helsinki, was conducted on patients affected by keratoconus, referred to the Unit of Ophthalmology of the University of Naples "Federico II" from January 2018 to December 2020. We included patients affected by KC and listed for CXL surgery according to the following criteria: (1) patients with progressive keratoconus (1 diopter increase in the steepest meridian during a 6-month observation period); (2) Stage 2 or 3 of keratoconus (Amsler–Krumeich classification); (3) Corrected distance visual acuity (CDVA) < 0.4 logMAR; and (4) central clear cornea and minimum corneal thickness of at least 450 μm.

We divided patients into two groups through the block randomization method of treatment depending on the treatment performed: CXL by iontophoresis with or without epithelium removal.

2.1. Surgical Procedure

Corneal cross-linking was performed by instilling dextran-free hypo-osmolar riboflavin containing benzalkonium chloride (Ricrolin+, SOOFT, Montegiorgio, Italy) on the cornea by iontophoresis to increase the permeability of the epithelium for 5 min.

A return electrode was placed on the skin of the frontal region; meanwhile, the corneal iontophoresis electrode was attached to the cornea through a vacuum adsorption device. The corneal electrode was filled with approximately 0.5 mL Ricrolin+ to fully immerse the stainless-steel mesh. To follow, the device was connected to a current generator (I-ON XL, SOOFT, Montegiorgio, Italy) with 1 mA current.

At the end of iontophoresis, a UVA light was then focused on the apex of the cornea, 10 mW/cm^2 (UV-X 2000; IROC Innocross AG, Zug, Switzerland) for 9 min. During irradiation, drops of balanced solution were applied to the cornea every 1 min to keep moisture to avoid complications.

When the epi-off CXL technique was performed, the corneal epithelium was mechanically removed with a blunt spatula immediately before the application of Riboflavin. Subsequently, the CXL throughout iontophoresis was performed as an epi-on technique as explained before, and a contact lens was placed onto the ocular surface and removed after one week [17].

Postoperatively, an ophthalmic gel of 0.15% sodium hyaluronate, 1% xanthan gum, and 0.3% netilmicin (Xanternet Gel, SIFI, Catania, Italy) was prescribed 6 times a day until complete epithelial regrowth (epithelial integrity was assessed with fluorescein staining). In patients who underwent epi-on iontophoresis CXL, in whom a contact lens was not used, dexamethasone 21-phosphate 0.15% drops were prescribed 4 times a day for 10 days and 0.15% sodium hyaluronate, Riboflavin, L-Leucin, L-Prolin, L-Glycin, and L-ysin drops (Ribolisin free, Sooft) 6 times daily for 45 days. In patients who underwent epi-off iontophoresis CXL, after contact lens removal, dexamethasone 21-phosphate 0.15% drops were prescribed 4 times a day for 10 days and 0.15% sodium hyaluronate, Riboflavin, L-Leucin, L-Prolin, L-Glycin, and L-Lysin drops (Ribolisin free, Sooft) 6 times daily for 45 days. In addition, all patients received oral amino acid supplements (Aminoftal; Sooft) for the first 7 postoperative days in effort to promote epithelial healing.

2.2. Ophthalmic Examination

Each patient underwent clinical preoperative examination, including manifest refraction, Slit Lamp Examination, and corneal topography (Pentacam, Oculus, Wetzlar, Germany), recorded at 1 month, 3 months, 6 months, 12 months, and 24 months after surgery. Several topographic parameters were analyzed including Kmax; Mean K; Steep K; Flat K; True Net Power; Mean Corneal Thickness; and Thinnest corneal point. Corneal Tomography was also focused on the presence/absence of inflammatory cells and the activation of corneal keratocytes which is related to the development of fibrosis [18–20]. The considered Pentacam parameters provide information about corneal refractive power, calculated thanks to the Sheimpflug principles. The Scheimpflug system consists of a rotational slit camera producing a three-dimensional model of the anterior segment of the eye from 138,000 elevation points. Studying this model, the operator is able to measure the dioptric corneal power in each point and axis of the anterior segment (Kmax, Mean K, Steep K, Flat K) and measure corneal power in total (true Net Power) by computing the power of the anterior and posterior corneal surface without taking in consideration corneal thickness. The study of Corneal Thickness profile enables one to collocate the reduction in corneal depth in the corneal profile, allowing one to correlate them with the highest and steepest points of the cornea.

Symptoms evaluation was performed before and one month after surgery using the Ocular Surface Index (OSDI) questionnaire.

2.3. Statistical Analysis

The statistical analysis was carried out using IBM SPSS 25 for Mac (SPSS Inc., Chicago, IL, USA). The averages were compared by an ANOVA test unchanged according to Bonferroni. In all the statistical tests, 5% was used as a significant value.

3. Results

A total of 64 eyes of 49 patients underwent CXL, 30 using the epi-off technique, and 34 eyes the epi-on (Table 1). The mean age of patients was 26 ± 4.2. In the epi-off group, CDVA converted in logMAR were at baseline 0.3 ± 0.1 and improved to 0.22 ± 0.14 at 2 years follow-up clinical examination. In the epi-on group, the visual acuity values converted in logMAR improved from 0.22 ± 0.1 at baseline to 0.09 ± 0 at the last follow-up. We found no statistically significant differences between the two groups ($p = 0.9$).

The statistical analysis performed (Table 2) showed no statistically significant difference between Kmax, Mean K, Flat K, Steep K values before and 24 months after surgery in both groups.

The mean K at baseline was 47.20 ± 2.90 D and 48.00 ± 2.50 D in the epi-off and epi-on groups, respectively. After two years of follow-up, these two values remained unchanged, 47.16 ± 3.15 D in the epi-off group and 48.82 ± 4.06 D in the epi-on group, with no statistically significant differences between the groups ($p = 0.57$).

Table 1. Patients' Demographics.

		Frequency	Percentage
Gender			
	Male	32	65.30%
	Female	17	34.69%
Age			
	Mean age of all patients	26 ± 4.2	
	Mean age of Epi-on group	25 ± 5.6	
	Mean age of Epi-off group	27 ± 6.3	
Eyes			
	Treated	64	65%
	Untreated	34	34.70%
Technique			
	Epi-on	34	53%
	Epi-off	30	47%

Table 2. Postoperative Outcomes.

	T0	T3	T6	T12	T24	ANOVA
Differences with Respect to Preoperative CDVA (Logmar)						
Epi-on		0.22 ± 0.1	0.15 ± 0.2	0.09 ± 0	0.09 ± 0	0.9
Epi-off		0.3 ± 0.1	0.3 ± 0.1	0.22 ± 0.14	0.22 ± 0.14	
Kmax (D)						
Epi-on	53.6 ± 1.4	54.2 ± 0.8	53.2 ± 3.5	55.6 ± 0.7	55.9 ± 0.7	0.96
Epi-off	58.1 ± 9.2	58.8 ± 1.76	58.8 ± 7	55.9 ± 1.8	56.2 ± 1.8	
Mean K (D)						
Epi-on	48.00 ± 2.50	47.96 ± 3.25	48.2 ± 1.75	48.96 ± 2.80	48.82 ± 4.06	0.57
Epi-off	47.20 ± 2.90	46.89 ± 4.15	47.1 ± 1.75	47.00 ± 2.40	47.16 ± 3.15	
Steep K (D)						
Epi-on	46.75 ± 3.87	46.55 ± 2.97	46.15 ± 4.07	45.75 ± 4.17	47.05 ± 2.82	0.69
Epi-off	47.75 ± 3.20	47.45 ± 2.79	47.15 ± 3.00	47.62 ± 4.20	47.55 ± 3.12	
Flat K (D)						
Epi-on	45.62 ± 2.09	44.92 ± 2.09	45.23 ± 3.12	45.11 ± 2.65	45.42 ± 1.83	0.44
Epi-off	44.62 ± 2.63	44.99 ± 2.74	45.10 ± 3.00	44.92 ± 1.68	45.02 ± 2.03	
True net power (d)						
Epi-on	2.8 ± 1.7	3.2 ± 1.2	2.5 ± 0.1	3.2 ± 0.1	3.4 ± 0.4	0.67
Epi-off	4.5 ± 2.8	5 ± 0.6	3.7 ± 0.07	5.6 ± 0.7	5.7 ± 1.2	
Mean corneal thickness (μm)						
Epi-on	491.5 ± 11.3	484.8 ± 24	495.9 ± 19	489.5 ± 13.4	490.5 ± 13.4	0.7
Epi-off	500.5 ± 22.6	481 ± 24.5	499.7 ± 63.6	513 ± 3.1	515 ± 4	
Thinnest point (μm)						
Epi-on	466.2 ± 15.5	463 ± 26.1	473.2 ± 4.2	463 ± 22.6	467 ± 19	0.72
Epi-off	475.8 ± 21.9	452.1 ± 19	463.2 ± 31.8	491 ± 12	497 ± 27	
OSDI score						
Epi-on	4.89 ± 1.32	5.78 ± 1.2	6.89 ± 0.1	9.87 ± 2.5	11.62 ± 2.12	0.98
Epi-off	4.58 ± 1.18	8.01 ± 0.6	9.12 ± 0.23	12.45 ± 1.32	13.65 ± 2.15	

T0 = baseline; T3 = 3 months postoperatively; T6 = 6 months postoperatively; T12 = 12 months postoperatively; T24 = 24 months postoperatively; ANOVA= p value of the difference between groups; CDVA = corrected distance visual acuity; CXL = corneal cross-linking; I-CXL =transepithelial iontophoresis; I-SCXL = iontophoresis with epithelial debridement.

Steep K and flat K at baseline were 47.75 ± 3.20 D and 44.62 ± 2.63 D, respectively, in the epi-off group. After two years of follow-up, these values remained unchanged at 47.55 ± 3.12 D and 45.02 ± 2.03 D with no statistically significant differences between the two groups ($p = 0.69$). In the epi-on group, Steep K and flat K at baseline were 46.75 ± 3.87 D and 45.62 ± 2.09 D, respectively. After two years of follow-up, these values remained unchanged at 47.05 ± 2.82 D and 45.42 ± 1.83 D with no statistically significative differences between the two groups ($p = 0.44$).

On the contrary, the Kmax mean values were 53.6 ± 1.4 D for the epi-on technique and 58.1 ± 9.2 D in the epi-off group at baseline and of 55.9 ± 0.7 D and 56.2 ± 1.8 D, respectively, with a statistically significant difference ($p < 0.05$) between the epi-on and epi-off groups' pachymetry before and after 24 months follow up.

After 2 years, the mean corneal thickness was not significantly changed in both groups, from 491.5 ± 1.3 μm to 467.41 ± 19 μm for the epi-on group ($p = 0.7$) and from 475.41 ± 21.9 μm to 497 ± 27 μm for the epi-off group ($p = 0.7$).

Contrarily, a statistically significant difference ($p < 0.05$) of the topographically thinnest point immediately post-surgery and 24 months after surgery emerged. Thickness average values were higher in patients who underwent epi-off surgery; indeed, the mean pre-surgery thinnest point was 478 μm, and after 24 months of follow-up, it was 518 μm (Figure 1). Particularly, no significant changes in both groups, from 466.2 ± 15.5 μm to 467.41 ± 19 μm for the epi-on group ($p = 0.7$) and from 475.41 ± 21.9 μm to 497 ± 27 μm ($p = 0.7$) in the epi-off group, occurred after 2 years of follow-up.

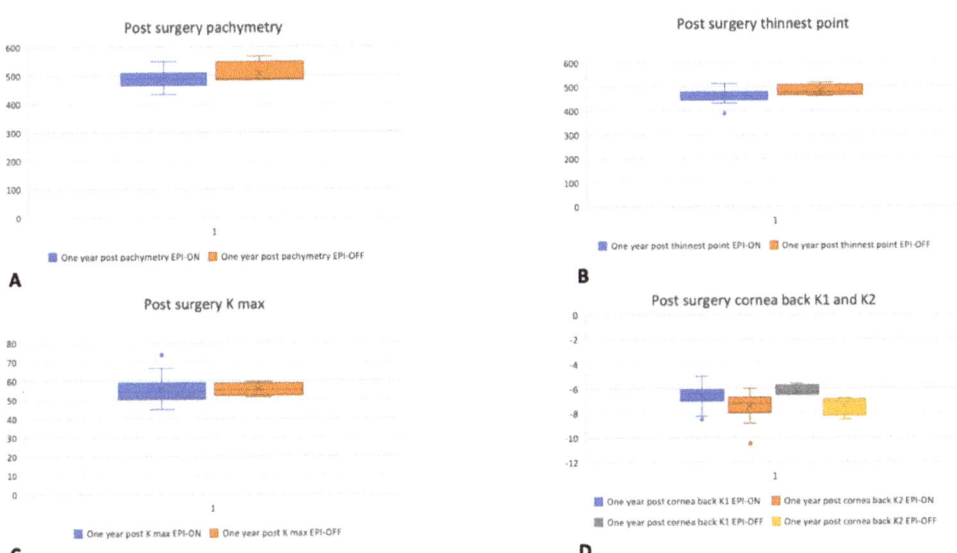

Figure 1. Kmax (**A**), Pachymetry (**B**), thinnest point (**C**), and cornea back (**D**) topographic outcomes before surgery and after one year of follow-up in the epi-on and epi-off groups.

The ANOVA Univariate analysis highlighted no statistically significant differences in the Average Pachymetry and the Topographically Thinnest Point between groups during the follow-up period; this is best displayed in Figure 1. Moreover, statistically significant differences between Kmax values before surgery and after 1 month ($p < 0.008$), 3 months ($p > 0.001$), and 6 months of the follow-up period ($p > 0.002$) were identified. On the one hand, during the follow-up period, Kmax values were on average higher than time zero. On the opposite side, the Kmax values came back to the before surgery values at the last follow-up after 24 months.

Lastly, the data collected from the OSDI© questionnaire highlighted at the baseline a score of 4.58 ± 1.18 and 4.89 ± 1.32, respectively, in the epi-off and epi-on groups. After 2 years of follow up, the score increased to 13.65 ± 2.15 in epi-off group ($p < 0.01$) and 11.62 ± 2.12 in epi-on ($p < 0.04$). We also found a statistically significant difference between the two groups ($p < 0.02$).

4. Discussion

Corneal collagen cross-linking stops the progression of keratoconus through new covalent bonds between collagen fibers, which increase the strengthens and the rigidity of the cornea by more than 300% [21], with a parallel improvement in both the refractive and topographic features of treated corneas [22,23]. Wollensak et al. [15], in a non-randomized pilot study conducted on 22 patients, described a clinical technique to halt the KC progression in all treated eyes. The study highlighted a halt in the progression of all treated eyes. Thereafter, several studies confirmed the Wollensak results, demonstrating the efficacy of corneal cross-linking in halting the progression of keratoconus. One of the largest trials including 241 eyes was conducted by Raiskup-Wolf et al. [10], who emphasized that the treatment was able to decrease the steepness of the cone, improving subjective visual symptoms, and, consequently, uncorrected (UDVA) and corrected (CDVA) distance visual acuities [16].

Most of the complications related to standard CXL are associated with epithelial removal, i.e., postoperative pain, stromal haze, infection, and corneal melting [24,25]. Other alternatives, avoiding total removal of the epithelium, have been suggested in order to improve safety, including partial de-epithelialization, epithelial disruption, the creation of an epithelial flap (Epi-Flap CXL), and several trans-epithelial CXL techniques. The potential advantages of trans-epithelial techniques are reduced treatment time, prevention of slow visual recovery, and less risk of serious side effects and complications (postoperative pain, infection) while maintaining the same efficacy of the standard epi-off procedure [26–31]. Shalchi et al. [32] compared the results of standard epi-off CXL with a metanalysis of 45 papers referred on transepithelial CXL with a total of 5 papers in the management of progressive keratoconus. The majority of studies on standard CXL have shown a reduction in the maximum simulated keratometry, whereas transepithelial corneal CXL did not halt keratoconus progression in about 75% of cases within 1 year [33]. Moreover, the shortening riboflavin delivery time from 30 to 5 min is not negligible. Our study supports the concept that CXL with Iontophoresis is effective in halting the progression of keratoconus without the side effects of epithelial removal, encountered the performing standard epi-off CXL procedure. In addition, the comparison between epi-on and epi-off techniques, both with the iontophoretic corneal soak in our series, confirmed their efficacy in halting keratoconus progression. With the epi-off iontophoretic approach, we guaranteed a deep penetration of riboflavin with a shorter time of delivery. Moreover, epithelial debridement and repair can determine a better quality of vision with a reduction in higher-order aberration thanks to a better distribution of the epithelium from the base to the apex of the cone [34] Furthermore, unlike standard treatment, we found a great recovery of the corneal shape and thickness in patients who underwent epithelium removal before iontophoresis CXL. These outcomes could be related to the epithelium reparative process that regularizes the corneal surface [35].

In addition, keratocyte repopulation is related to stromal growing factors influencing the correct orientation of stromal lamellae and nerve regeneration. In fact, survived keratocytes were stimulated by stromal fibroblast through neurotrophic and inflammatory factors [18–20,36]. This regenerative process requires new structural and enzymatic protein to be available. The obtainability of amino acids becomes essential for the correct stromal and nerve regeneration. As a result, the topical and oral supplementation of essential amino acids may contribute to a better and faster corneal restoration [37].

Standard Dresden protocol CXL (S-CXL) is used as a treatment of progressive keratoconus in pediatric and adult patients, and its efficacy is widely reported in numerous studies [38–41]. Nevertheless, this technique presents two disadvantages: It is time-consuming (about 60 min for each surgery) and requires epithelial debridement. With the introduction of transepithelial CXL and subsequently of Iontophoretic cross-linking (I-CXL), the same outcomes were achieved with shorter surgery time and no corneal manipulation. Cantemir et al. [42], with a 3-year follow-up study, showed that I-CXL is not inferior to S-CXL for stopping the progression of keratoconus with faster recovery of visual acuity. Jouve et al. [43] reported that I-CXL halted the progression of keratoconus more efficiently compared to S-CXL with regard to the flattening effect. The introduction of I-CXL with epithelial debridement (SI-CXL) was designed as an improvement in S-CXL. The main outcome of the study underscored the non-statistically significant difference between the protocols about visual acuity, topographic indices, keratometry, and OSDI after 2 years of follow-up. SI-CXL induced less corneal thinning and a significantly higher reduction in higher-order aberrations and coma with a better visual outcome. In 2019, Vinciguerra et al. [35] compared S-CXL, I-CXL, and SI-CXL focusing on refractive, topographic, tomographic, and aberrometric outcomes demonstrating that SI-CXL was not inferior compared to the other techniques. Cifariello et al. [44] were the first to analyze OSDI© (Ocular Surface Disease Index) differences in patients who underwent CXL. According to their previous study, we evaluated the degree of ocular discomfort in patients treated with I-CXL and SI-CXL. The results showed an increase in OSDI score to 13.65 ± 2.15 in the epi-off group ($p < 0.01$) and 11.62 ± 2.12 in the epi-on group ($p < 0.04$) at 2 years of follow-up. A statistically significant difference between the two groups ($p < 0.02$) was found.

5. Conclusions

In conclusion, we brought to light that both techniques are valid in long-term corneal stabilization. Moreover, the mechanical removal of the corneal epithelium would still seem the most valid method to obtain a better saturation of corneal stroma with the photosensitizer and better postoperative results. The advantage of the new iontophoresis epi-off cross-linking technique could be the faster corneal imbibing related to the iontophoretic soak and the better visual acuity with a reduction in higher-order aberration linked to epithelium debridement.

Author Contributions: Data curation, A.M. (Alberto Mazzucco); investigation, A.M. (Antonietta Melenzane) and N.C.; project administration, C.C. (Ciro Costagliola); supervision, F.T.; validation, C.C. (Ciro Caruso) and M.R.; writing—review and editing, P.N. and L.D. All authors have read and agreed to the published version of the manuscript.

Funding: This research received no external funding.

Institutional Review Board Statement: The clinical study was conducted according to the ethical standards of the Declaration of Helsinki. Patients were informed about the nature and purpose of the trial, and they provided informed consent. The approval of the institutional review/ethics committee (IRB) of the Corneal Transplant Center Pellegrini Hospital, Napoli, Italy, was obtained (authorization 1269/2017).

Informed Consent Statement: Informed consent was obtained from all subjects involved in the study.

Data Availability Statement: The data presented in this study are available on request from the corresponding author.

Conflicts of Interest: The authors declare no conflict of interest.

References

1. McKay, T.B.; Serjersen, H.; Hjortdal, J.; Zieske, J.D.; Karamichos, D. Characterization of Tear Immunoglobulins in a Small-Cohort of Keratoconus Patients. *Sci. Rep.* **2020**, *10*, 9426. [CrossRef] [PubMed]
2. Santodomingo-Rubido, J.; Carracedo, G.; Suzaki, A.; Villa-Collar, C.; Vincent, S.J.; Wolffsohn, J.S. Keratoconus: An updated review. *Contact Lens Anterior Eye* **2022**, 101559. [CrossRef] [PubMed]
3. Olivo-Payne, A.; Abdala-Figuerola, A.; Hernandez-Bogantes, E.; Pedro-Aguilar, L.; Chan, E.; Godefrooij, D. Optimal management of pediatric keratoconus: Challenges and solutions. *Clin. Ophthalmol.* **2019**, *13*, 1183–1191. [CrossRef]

4. Choi, J.A.; Kim, M.S. Progression of keratoconus by longitudinal assessment with corneal topography. *Investig. Ophthalmol. Vis. Sci.* **2012**, *53*, 927–935. [CrossRef] [PubMed]
5. Padmanabhan, P.; Rachapalle Reddi, S.; Rajagopal, R.; Natarajan, R.; Iyer, G.; Srinivasan, B.; Narayanan, N.; Lakshmipathy, M.; Agarwal, S. Corneal Collagen Cross-Linking for Keratoconus in Pediatric Patients-Long-Term Results. *Cornea* **2017**, *36*, 138–143. [CrossRef]
6. Chatzis, N.; Hafezi, F. Progression of keratoconus and efficacy of pediatric [corrected] corneal collagen cross-linking in children and adolescents. *J. Refract. Surg.* **2012**, *28*, 753–758. [CrossRef]
7. Miller, C.; Castro, H.M.; Ali, S.F. Collagen Crosslinking for Keratoconus Management in the Pediatric Population. *Int. Ophthalmol. Clin.* **2022**, *62*, 33–44. [CrossRef]
8. Chan, C. Corneal Cross-Linking for Keratoconus: Current Knowledge and Practice and Future Trends. *Asia-Pac. J. Ophthalmol.* **2020**, *9*, 557–564. [CrossRef]
9. Wollensak, G.; Spoerl, E.; Seiler, T. Stress-strain measurements of human and porcine corneas after riboflavin-ultraviolet-A-induced cross-linking. *J. Cataract Refract. Surg.* **2003**, *29*, 1780–1785. [CrossRef]
10. Raiskup-Wolf, F.; Hoyer, A.; Spoerl, E.; Pillunat, L.E. Collagen crosslinking with riboflavin and ultraviolet-A light in keratoconus: Long-term results. *J. Cataract Refract. Surg.* **2008**, *34*, 796–801. [CrossRef]
11. Salman, A.; Ali, A.; Rafea, S.; Omran, R.; Kubaisi, B.; Ghabra, M.; Darwish, T. Long-term visual, anterior and posterior corneal changes after crosslinking for progressive keratoconus. *Eur. J. Ophthalmol.* **2022**, *32*, 50–58. [CrossRef] [PubMed]
12. Lombardo, M.; Serrao, S.; Raffa, P.; Rosati, M.; Lombardo, G. Novel Technique of Transepithelial Corneal Cross-Linking Using Iontophoresis in Progressive Keratoconus. *J. Ophthalmol.* **2016**, *2016*, 7472542. [CrossRef] [PubMed]
13. Bikbova, G.; Bikbov, M. Transepithelial corneal collagen cross-linking by iontophoresis of riboflavin. *Acta Ophthalmol.* **2014**, *92*, e30–e34. [CrossRef] [PubMed]
14. Mastropasqua, L.; Nubile, M.; Calienno, R.; Mattei, P.A.; Pedrotti, E.; Salgari, N.; Mastropasqua, R.; Lanzini, M. Corneal cross-linking: Intrastromal riboflavin concentration in iontophoresis-assisted imbibition versus traditional and transepithelial techniques. *Am. J. Ophthalmol.* **2014**, *157*, 623–630.e1. [CrossRef]
15. Wollensak, G.; Spoerl, E.; Seiler, T. Riboflavin/ultraviolet-a-induced collagen crosslinking for the treatment of keratoconus. *Am. J. Ophthalmol.* **2003**, *135*, 620–627. [CrossRef]
16. De Bernardo, M.; Capasso, L.; Tortori, A.; Lanza, M.; Caliendo, L.; Rosa, N. Trans epithelial corneal collagen crosslinking for progressive keratoconus: 6 months follow up. *Contact Lens Anterior Eye* **2014**, *37*, 438–441. [CrossRef]
17. Vinciguerra, P.; Romano, V.; Rosetta, P.; Legrottaglie, E.F.; Kubrak-Kisza, M.; Azzolini, C.; Vinciguerra, R. Iontophoresis-Assisted Corneal Collagen Cross-Linking with Epithelial Debridement: Preliminary Results. *Biomed. Res. Int.* **2016**, *2016*, 3720517. [CrossRef]
18. Pei, Y.; Sherry, D.M.; McDermott, A.M. Thy-1 distinguishes human corneal fibroblasts and myofibroblasts from keratocytes. *Exp. Eye Res.* **2004**, *79*, 705–712. [CrossRef]
19. Jester, J.V.; Budge, A.; Fisher, S.; Huang, J. Corneal keratocytes: Phenotypic and species differences in abundant protein expression and in vitro light-scattering. *Investig. Ophthalmol. Vis. Sci.* **2005**, *46*, 2369–2378. [CrossRef]
20. West-Mays, J.A.; Dwivedi, D.J. The keratocyte: Corneal stromal cell with variable repair phenotypes. *Int. J. Biochem. Cell Biol.* **2006**, *38*, 1625–1631. [CrossRef]
21. Spörl, E.; Huhle, M.; Kasper, M.; Seiler, T. Artificial stiffening of the cornea by induction of intrastromal cross-links. *Der Ophthalmol.* **1997**, *94*, 902–906. [CrossRef] [PubMed]
22. Caporossi, A.; Baiocchi, S.; Mazzotta, C.; Traversi, C.; Caporossi, T. Parasurgical therapy for keratoconus by riboflavin-ultraviolet type A rays induced cross-linking of corneal collagen: Preliminary refractive results in an Italian study. *J. Cataract Refract. Surg.* **2006**, *32*, 837–845. [CrossRef] [PubMed]
23. Grewal, D.S.; Brar, G.S.; Jain, R.; Sood, V.; Singla, M.; Grewal, S.P. Corneal collagen crosslinking using riboflavin and ultraviolet-A light for keratoconus: One-year analysis using Scheimpflug imaging. *J. Cataract Refract. Surg.* **2009**, *35*, 425–432. [CrossRef]
24. Mazzotta, C.; Balestrazzi, A.; Baiocchi, S.; Traversi, C.; Caporossi, A. Stromal haze after combined riboflavin-UVA corneal collagen cross-linking in keratoconus: In vivo confocal microscopic evaluation. *Clin. Exp. Ophthalmol.* **2007**, *35*, 580–582. [CrossRef]
25. Eberwein, P.; Auw-Hädrich, C.; Birnbaum, F.; Maier, P.C.; Reinhard, T. Hornhauteinschmelzung nach Cross-Linking und tiefer lamellärer Keratoplastik ("DALK") bei Keratokonus [Corneal melting after cross-linking and deep lamellar keratoplasty in a keratoconus patient]. *Klin Monbl Augenheilkd* **2008**, *225*, 96–98. [CrossRef] [PubMed]
26. Zaheryani, S.M.S.; Movahedan, H.; Salouti, R.; Mohaghegh, S.; Javadpour, S.; Shirvani, M.; Kasraei, F.; Bamdad, S. Corneal Collagen Cross-Linking Using Epithelium Disruptor Instrument in Progressive Keratoconus. *J. Curr. Ophthalmol.* **2020**, *32*, 256–262. [CrossRef] [PubMed]
27. Hashemi, H.; Miraftab, M.; Hafezi, F.; Asgari, S. Matched comparison study of total and partial epithelium removal in corneal cross-linking. *J. Refract. Surg.* **2015**, *31*, 110–115. [CrossRef]
28. Galvis, V.; Tello, A.; Carreño, N.I.; Ortiz, A.I.; Barrera, R.; Rodriguez, C.J.; Ochoa, M.E. Corneal Cross-Linking (with a Partial Deepithelization) in Keratoconus with Five Years of Follow-Up. *Ophthalmol. Eye Dis.* **2016**, *8*, 17–21. [CrossRef]
29. Borroni, D.; Bonzano, C.; Hristova, R.; Rachwani-Anil, R.; Sánchez-González, J.M.; de Lossada, C.R. Epithelial Flap Corneal Cross-linking. *J. Refract. Surg.* **2021**, *37*, 741–745. [CrossRef]

30. Hersh, P.S.; Lai, M.J.; Gelles, J.D.; Lesniak, S.P. Transepithelial corneal crosslinking for keratoconus. *J. Cataract Refract. Surg.* **2018**, *44*, 313–322. [CrossRef]
31. Vinciguerra, P.; Romano, V.; Rosetta, P.; Legrottaglie, E.F.; Piscopo, R.; Fabiani, C.; Azzolini, C.; Vinciguerra, R. Transepithelial Iontophoresis Versus Standard Corneal Collagen Cross-linking: 1-Year Results of a Prospective Clinical Study. *J. Refract. Surg.* **2016**, *32*, 672–678. [CrossRef] [PubMed]
32. Shalchi, Z.; Wang, X.; Nanavaty, M.A. Safety and efficacy of epithelium removal and transepithelial corneal collagen crosslinking for keratoconus. *Eye* **2015**, *29*, 15–29. [CrossRef] [PubMed]
33. Bottós, K.M.; Schor, P.; Dreyfuss, J.L.; Nader, H.B.; Chamon, W. Effect of corneal epithelium on ultraviolet-A and riboflavin absorption. *Arq. Bras. De Oftalmol.* **2011**, *74*, 348–351. [CrossRef] [PubMed]
34. Kobashi, H.; Rong, S.S.; Ciolino, J.B. Transepithelial versus epithelium-off corneal crosslinking for corneal ectasia. *J. Cataract Refract. Surg.* **2018**, *44*, 1507–1516. [CrossRef]
35. Vinciguerra, P.; Rosetta, P.; Legrottaglie, E.F.; Morenghi, E.; Mazzotta, C.; Kaye, S.B.; Vinciguerra, R. Iontophoresis CXL With and Without Epithelial Debridement Versus Standard CXL: 2-Year Clinical Results of a Prospective Clinical Study. *J. Refract Surg.* **2019**, *35*, 184–190. [CrossRef]
36. Yam, G.H.; Williams, G.P.; Setiawan, M.; Yusoff, N.Z.; Lee, X.W.; Htoon, H.M.; Zhou, L.; Fuest, M.; Mehta, J.S. Nerve regeneration by human corneal stromal keratocytes and stromal fibroblasts. *Sci. Rep.* **2017**, *7*, 45396. [CrossRef]
37. Roszkowska, A.M.; Rusciano, D.; Inferrera, L.; Severo, A.A.; Aragona, P. Oral Aminoacids Supplementation Improves Corneal Reinnervation after Photorefractive Keratectomy: A Confocal-Based Investigation. *Front. Pharmacol.* **2021**, *12*, 680734. [CrossRef]
38. Caporossi, A.; Mazzotta, C.; Baiocchi, S.; Caporossi, T. Long-term results of riboflavin ultraviolet a corneal collagen cross-linking for keratoconus in Italy: The Siena eye cross study. *Am. J. Ophthalmol.* **2010**, *149*, 585–593. [CrossRef]
39. Vinciguerra, R.; Romano, M.R.; Camesasca, F.I.; Azzolini, C.; Trazza, S.; Morenghi, E.; Vinciguerra, P. Corneal cross-linking as a treatment for keratoconus: Four-year morphologic and clinical outcomes with respect to patient age. *Ophthalmology* **2013**, *120*, 908–916. [CrossRef]
40. Theuring, A.; Spoerl, E.; Pillunat, L.E.; Raiskup, F. Hornhautkollagenvernetzung mit Riboflavin und UVA-Licht bei Patienten mit progressivem Keratokonus: 10-Jahres-Ergebnisse [Corneal collagen cross-linking with riboflavin and ultraviolet-A light in progressive keratoconus. Results after 10-year follow-up]. *Ophthalmologe* **2015**, *112*, 140–147. [CrossRef]
41. Wittig-Silva, C.; Chan, E.; Islam, F.M.; Wu, T.; Whiting, M.; Snibson, G.R. A randomized, controlled trial of corneal collagen cross-linking in progressive keratoconus: Three-year results. *Ophthalmology* **2014**, *121*, 812–821. [CrossRef] [PubMed]
42. Cantemir, A.; Alexa, A.I.; Galan, B.G.; Anton, N.; Ciuntu, R.E.; Danielescu, C.; Chiselita, D.; Costin, D. Iontophoretic collagen cross-linking versus epithelium-off collagen cross-linking for early stage of progressive keratoconus—3 years follow-up study. *Acta Ophthalmol.* **2017**, *95*, e649–e655. [CrossRef] [PubMed]
43. Jouve, L.; Borderie, V.; Sandali, O.; Temstet, C.; Basli, E.; Laroche, L.; Bouheraoua, N. Conventional and Iontophoresis Corneal Cross-Linking for Keratoconus: Efficacy and Assessment by Optical Coherence Tomography and Confocal Microscopy. *Cornea* **2017**, *36*, 153–162. [CrossRef] [PubMed]
44. Cifariello, F.; Minicucci, M.; Di Renzo, F.; Di Taranto, D.; Coclite, G.; Zaccaria, S.; De Turris, S.; Costagliola, C. Epi-Off versus Epi-On Corneal Collagen Cross-Linking in Keratoconus Patients: A Comparative Study through 2-Year Follow-Up. *J. Ophthalmol.* **2018**, *2018*, 4947983. [CrossRef] [PubMed]

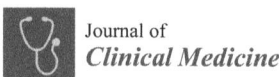

Article

Improvement in Dacryoendoscopic Visibility after Image Processing Using Comb-Removal and Image-Sharpening Algorithms

Sujin Hoshi [1,*], Kuniharu Tasaki [1], Kazushi Maruo [2], Yuta Ueno [1], Haruhiro Mori [1], Shohei Morikawa [1], Yuki Moriya [1], Shoko Takahashi [1], Takahiro Hiraoka [1] and Tetsuro Oshika [1]

1. Department of Ophthalmology, Faculty of Medicine, University of Tsukuba, 1-1-1 Tennoudai, Tsukuba 305-8575, Japan; k.tasaki1986@gmail.com (K.T.); yu_ueno71@yahoo.co.jp (Y.U.); moririn21@gmail.com (H.M.); s0711715@yahoo.co.jp (S.M.); yuki.morika.429@gmail.com (Y.M.); shoko.takahashi.05@gmail.com (S.T.); thiraoka@md.tsukuba.ac.jp (T.H.); oshika@eye.ac (T.O.)
2. Department of Biostatistics, Faculty of Medicine, University of Tsukuba, 1-1-1 Tennoudai, Tsukuba 305-8575, Japan; maruo@md.tsukuba.ac.jp
* Correspondence: hoshisujin@md.tsukuba.ac.jp; Tel.: +81-298-533-148

Abstract: Recently, a minimally invasive treatment for lacrimal passage diseases was developed using dacryoendoscopy. Good visibility of the lacrimal passage is important for examination and treatment. This study aimed to investigate whether image processing can improve the dacryoendoscopic visibility using comb-removal and image-sharpening algorithms. We processed 20 dacryoendoscopic images (original images) using comb-removal and image-sharpening algorithms. Overall, 40 images (20 original and 20 post-processing) were randomly presented to the evaluators, who scored each image on a 10-point scale. The scores of the original and post-processing images were compared statistically. Additionally, in vitro experiments were performed using a test chart to examine whether image processing could improve the dacryoendoscopic visibility in a turbid fluid. The visual score (estimate ± standard error) of the images significantly improved from 3.52 ± 0.26 (original images) to 5.77 ± 0.28 (post-processing images; $p < 0.001$, linear mixed-effects model). The in vitro experiments revealed that the contrast and resolution of images in the turbid fluid improved after image processing. Image processing with our comb-removal and image-sharpening algorithms improved dacryoendoscopic visibility. The techniques used in this study are applicable for real-time processing and can be easily introduced in clinical practice.

Keywords: dacryoendoscopy; lacrimal passage diseases; lacrimal sac; image enhancement; algorithms; image processing; lacrimal passage; dacryocystitis

Citation: Hoshi, S.; Tasaki, K.; Maruo, K.; Ueno, Y.; Mori, H.; Morikawa, S.; Moriya, Y.; Takahashi, S.; Hiraoka, T.; Oshika, T. Improvement in Dacryoendoscopic Visibility after Image Processing Using Comb-Removal and Image-Sharpening Algorithms. *J. Clin. Med.* **2022**, *11*, 2073. https://doi.org/10.3390/jcm11082073

Academic Editors: Vito Romano, Yalin Zheng and Mariantonia Ferrara

Received: 2 February 2022
Accepted: 5 April 2022
Published: 7 April 2022

Publisher's Note: MDPI stays neutral with regard to jurisdictional claims in published maps and institutional affiliations.

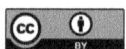

Copyright: © 2022 by the authors. Licensee MDPI, Basel, Switzerland. This article is an open access article distributed under the terms and conditions of the Creative Commons Attribution (CC BY) license (https://creativecommons.org/licenses/by/4.0/).

1. Introduction

Lacrimal passage obstruction may be congenital or acquired [1,2]. Its occurrence is concerning, because it can lead to lacrimal duct infections (such as dacryocystitis [3,4] and chronic conjunctivitis [5]) and significantly reduce the patient's quality of life. Even in the absence of an obvious infection, epiphora due to lacrimal passage obstruction can reduce the vision quality and vision-related quality of life [6,7]. Surgical treatments include dacryocystorhinostomy [8] and the insertion of a silicone tube [9–11] or the Jones tube [12,13]; however, the exact location of the obstruction must be identified for appropriate treatment selection [14–17].

In addition to classical diagnostic methods (such as lacrimal irrigation, blind probing, and dacryocystography), dacryoendoscopy has been recognized as an effective diagnostic tool [18,19]. In dacryoendoscopy, the lacrimal passage is directly visualized using a dacryoendoscope, which is inserted into the lacrimal passage through the lacrimal punctum. This is useful for the diagnosis and treatment of various lacrimal passage diseases, such as congenital [1,20], acquired [10,21], and secondary [22,23] lacrimal duct obstruction; canaliculitis [24]; tissue granulation [25]; and tumors [26]. Fiberscope-type dacryoendoscopes were introduced in the 1990s and had a pixel count of 1800–3000 [27–29]. Subsequently, 6000-pixel dacryoendoscopes were introduced in 2002 [30], while 10,000-pixel and 15,000-pixel dacryoendoscopes were introduced in 2009 [16].

Better visualization of the lacrimal canal with a dacryoendoscope improves the analysis of the lacrimal passage conditions and allows the precise identification of the obstructing lesions, both of which are key to a successful surgery [16,17]. The increase in the number of pixels has led to an improvement in the diagnostic performance of dacryoendoscopes; however, the image quality still requires improvement for an enhanced therapeutic performance [18].

Two main factors limit the quality of fiberscope-type dacryoendoscopic images. One is the limited number of individual fiberlets, which define the number of pixels. The other is the small amount of perfusion fluid that is needed to sufficiently flush away the blood and pus clouding the lacrimal duct. The number of fiberlets and amount of perfusion fluid are determined by the diameter of the dacryoendoscope probe. Increasing the probe diameter can improve the image quality by placing more fiberlets and providing a larger perfusion channel. However, the probe diameters of the current mainstream dacryoendoscopes range from 0.7 mm to 1.1 mm; it is difficult to increase the diameter further due to the small size of the punctum.

We proposed that the imaging quality of fiberscope-type dacryoendoscopes can be improved by image processing. Images obtained from fiberscope-type endoscopes contain black fine mesh noise (a comb artifact), which is caused by the opaque cladding between the fiberlets; this artifact adversely affects the visibility [31,32]. This problem is especially critical in case of dacryoendoscopes, which have a limited number of pixels as compared to the endoscopes used for other organs.

This study aimed to remove the aforementioned comb artifact from dacryoendoscopic images and reduce visibility loss due to blood- or pus-associated opacity in the lacrimal duct by using an algorithm capable of real-time image processing. Thus, we visually evaluated and compared the dacryoendoscopic visibility before and after image processing to assess the usefulness of this algorithm.

2. Materials and Methods

This single-center, observational study was approved by the Ethics Committee of the Faculty of Medicine, University of Tsukuba (R03-101). It adheres to the tenets of the Declaration of Helsinki.

We used images that had already been acquired previously and did not contain any personal information; therefore, patient consent was obtained in an opt-out format.

2.1. Image Samples

The images were arbitrarily extracted from the dacryoendoscopic images acquired and recorded within the scope of standard medical care at the University of Tsukuba Hospital between April 2019 and March 2021.

The dacryoendoscopic images were acquired by five surgeons (T.H., S.H., K.T., H.M. and S.T.). A close-up dacryoendoscope with a focal length of 1.5 mm (LAC-06NZ-HS; MACHIDA Endoscope Co., Ltd., Chiba, Japan) and a high-definition camera (MVH-2010A; MACHIDA Endoscope Co., Ltd., Chiba, Japan) were used for the imaging; this setting produced 16,000-pixel images.

Twenty original images were prepared by arbitrarily extracting five sample images of the canaliculus, lacrimal sac, nasolacrimal duct, and intra-canal materials; the exposure time for each was 10–20 s. In case of the canaliculus, lacrimal sac, and nasolacrimal ducts, images were selected after confirming that the luminal structure was visible and that there was very little or no bleeding- or pus-associated opacity. Images of the intra-canal materials included images of a foreign body straying into the lacrimal canal, those of a silicone tube implanted in the lacrimal canal, and those taken during sheath-guided endoscopic probing [33]. A total of 40 images were subjected to visual evaluation; these comprised the 20 original images and their post-processing versions ($n = 20$).

2.2. Image Processing

The dacryoendoscopic images were processed using comb-removal (WipeFiber®; Logic & Design Inc., Tokyo, Japan, and MACHIDA Endoscope Co., Ltd., Chiba, Japan) and image-sharpening (Medical Image Enhancer: MIEr®; Logic & Design Inc., Tokyo, Japan) algorithms. The image captured by a fiberscope is a collection of small circular images that are captured in turn by the fiberlets, and the fiberlets' boundaries are visible as a comb-structured artifact. This comb-structured artifact is considered the main cause of a reduced visibility during dacryoendoscopy. Comb removal was originally developed as a technique for improving the imaging quality of endoscopes for other organs, such as gastrointestinal endoscopes; however, similar techniques can be applied to dacryoendoscopes. The noise caused by the comb structure appears as a high-frequency component in the spatial frequency domain and can be removed by a low-pass filter. In this study, we used a Gaussian filter, which is a high-performance and an easy-to-implement low-pass filter. Subsequently, the image was sharpened by applying contour enhancement only in the specific frequency region according to the fiberlet diameter, while simultaneously suppressing the restoration of the removed comb structure. The image sharpening process was also used to improve the visibility in low-contrast areas.

The algorithm used in this study could perform real-time image processing; however, real-time processing was not implemented in this study.

2.3. Image Visibility Evaluation

Visual evaluation was performed for all images, and the visibility was scored on a 10-point scale by the evaluator. Three evaluators were presented with the 20 original and the 20 processed images in a random order, one at a time. The images were presented on a 13.3-inch monitor (2560 × 1600-pixel resolution), and the images (>15 cm in diameter) were sequentially displayed on a black background.

The results were analyzed statistically, and comparisons were performed between the images before and after image processing. These comparisons were made separately for all images, including those of the canaliculus, lacrimal sacs, nasolacrimal ducts, and intra-canal materials. A linear mixed-effects model was applied, which included the visibility score as the outcome variable; the processing, image type, and their interaction as the fixed effects; and the image ID and evaluator as the random effects. Subsequently, inferences on the least square mean differences between before and after processing were drawn for all data and each image type. The statistical significance was set at $p < 0.05$. All statistical analyses were performed using the SAS software (version 9.4; SAS Institute, Cary, NC, USA) and SPSS (version 23.0; IBM, Armonk, New York, NY, USA).

2.4. In Vitro Experiments

Image processing comprised comb removal and image sharpening. In vitro experiments were performed to assess the effects of image processing on the deterioration of dacryoendoscopic image quality due to opacity caused by the presence of blood and pus in the lacrimal duct lumen.

We prepared diluted milk saline (DMS), at concentrations of 1%, 2%, and 3%, to simulate turbidity in the lacrimal pathway. We then prepared 50% diluted blood (defibrinated sheep blood, AS ONE Corporation, Osaka, Japan) to simulate hemorrhage in the lacrimal pathway. Saline was used as a control for the test solution. We evaluated the image resolution (line pairs/mm) by imaging a test chart (3M550, Pearl Optical Industry, Tokyo, Japan), as described previously [17].

The test solution was placed on the test chart under a cover glass, and the dacryoendoscope was fixed such that the tip of its probe was positioned 1.5 mm above the test chart.

The images were acquired after confirming that the probe's tip was in contact with the test solution. The power of resolution in each condition from the test chart images were evaluated by two examiners (S.H. and K.T.).

3. Results

Figure 1 shows the original and post-processing images from a representative case; further details are available in Video S1.

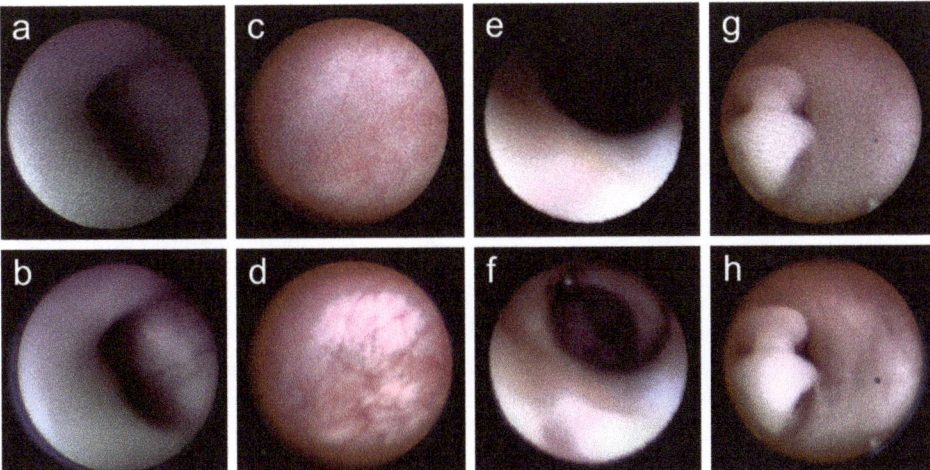

Figure 1. Original and post-processing representative images of the canaliculus (**a,b**), lacrimal sacs (**c,d**), nasolacrimal ducts (**e,f**), and intra-canal materials (**g,h**). The comb-structured artifact was observed in the original images, which were uneven and difficult to observe (**a,c,e,g**). However, in the post-processing images, this artifact was removed by image processing, and the visibility was improved (**b,d,f,h**). The blood vessels in the lacrimal sac mucosa were more highlighted in the processed image than in the original image (**c,d**). On comparing the nasolacrimal duct images, the luminal structures that were obscured in the original image (**e**) were visible in the processed image (**f**).

The comb-structured artifact was observed in the original images, which were uneven and difficult to observe (Figure 1a,c,e,g; Video S1a,c,e,g). However, this artifact was removed by image processing, and the visibility was improved in the post-processing images (Figure 1b,d,f,h; Video S1b,d,f,h).

For example, Figure 1c shows the original image of the lacrimal sac (Figure 1c; Video S1c); the blood vessels in the lacrimal sac mucosa are more highlighted in the corresponding processed image (Figure 1d; Video S1d).

A comparison of the nasolacrimal duct images revealed that the luminal structures that were obscured in the original image (Figure 1e; Video S1e) were visible in the processed image (Figure 1f; Video S1f).

Figure 2 shows a graph comparing the visual scores of all images. The visual score (estimate ± standard error) significantly improved from 3.52 ± 0.26 (original images) to 5.77 ± 0.28 (post-processing images; $p < 0.001$, linear mixed-effects model). Similarly, the visual scores of the original and post-processing images were 2.73 ± 0.45 and 5.07 ± 0.60 for the canaliculus, 4.07 ± 0.47 and 6.33 ± 0.48 for the lacrimal sac, 4.33 ± 0.51 and 6.47 ± 0.47 for the nasolacrimal duct, and 2.93 ± 0.46 and 5.20 ± 0.53 for the intra-canal materials, respectively. After image processing, all scores improved significantly ($p < 0.001$, linear mixed-effects model).

The apparent visibility-improvement effect of image processing was confirmed in the in vitro experiment (Figure 3).

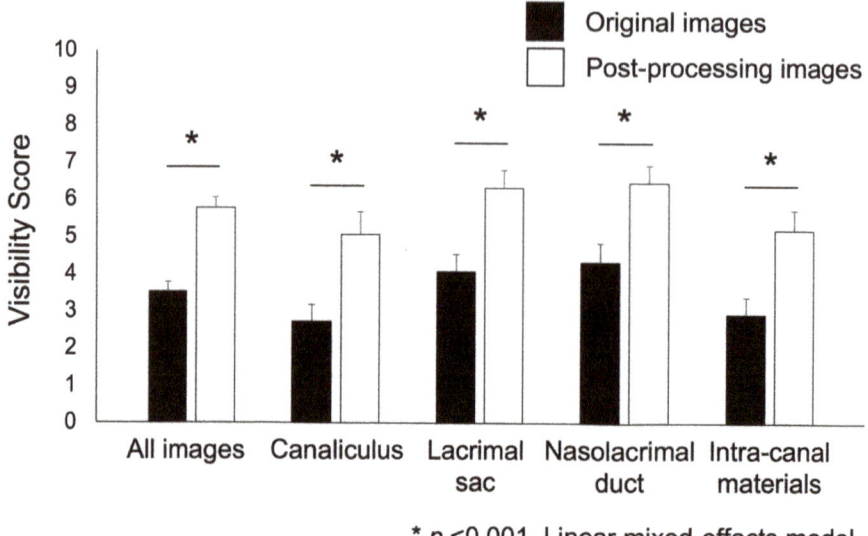

Figure 2. A graph comparing the visual scores of all images before and after image processing, including those of the canaliculus, lacrimal sacs, nasolacrimal ducts, and intra-canal materials.

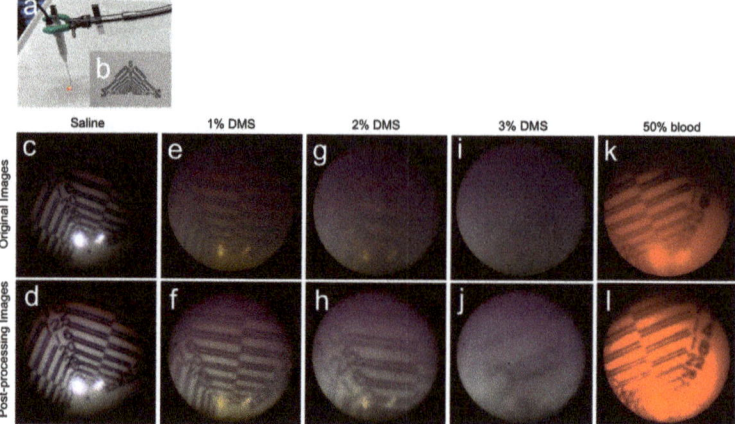

Figure 3. Settings and images of the in vitro experiment conducted to assess the effects of image processing on dacryoendoscopic images, whose quality deteriorated due to opacity caused by blood and pus in the lacrimal duct lumen. The test solution was placed on the test chart with a cover glass, and the endoscope was positioned such that the tip of its probe rested 1.5 mm above the test chart (**a**,**b**). Under saline, the original images (**c**) showed prominent comb artifacts. However, in the processed images (**d**), these comb artifacts were eliminated, and the visibility was improved. The image resolution of the original image was 25 line pairs/mm (**c**), whereas that of the processed image was 28 line pairs/mm (**d**). Images observed with 1%, 2%, and 3% diluted milk saline (DMS) showed an improved contrast and resolution after image processing. The resolutions of the original and post-processing images were as follows: (1) 1% DMS, 10 line pairs/mm (**e**) vs. 22 line pairs/mm (**f**); (2) 2% DMS: 10 line pairs/mm (**g**) vs. 16 line pairs/mm (**h**); and (3) 3% DMS: not evaluable (**i**) vs. 3 line pairs/mm (**j**). The resolution of the original and processed images in 50% blood was 18 line pairs/mm (**k**,**l**).

Under saline, the original image (Figure 3c) showed prominent comb artifacts; however, in the processed image (Figure 3d), the comb artifacts were eliminated, and the visibility was improved. The image resolution of the original image was 25 line pairs/mm (Figure 3c), whereas that of the processed image was 28 line pairs/mm (Figure 3d).

The images observed with 1%, 2%, and 3% DMS showed an improved contrast and resolution after image processing. The resolutions of the original and processed images were as follows: 1% DMS, 10 line pairs/mm (Figure 3e) vs. 22 line pairs/mm (Figure 3f); 2% DMS, 10 line pairs/mm (Figure 3g) vs. 16 line pairs/mm (Figure 3h); and 3% DMS, not evaluable (Figure 3i) vs. 3 line pairs/mm (Figure 3j).

The image observed with 50% blood showed an improved visibility after image processing. However, the resolution barely differed between the original and processed images (18 line pairs/mm (Figure 3k) vs. 18 line pairs/mm (Figure 3l)).

4. Discussion

The image-processing algorithm used in this study improved the dacryoendoscopic visibility for every region of the lacrimal duct lumen. The dacryoendoscope has a small diameter and can deliver a limited amount of light; thus, light cannot reach regions as deep as the nasolacrimal duct. It is often difficult to observe the details in a deep duct (Figure 1e). However, the contrast between components can be improved by image processing. As shown in Figure 1f (post-processing image), it was possible to visualize the details in the luminal structure that were not visible in Figure 1e (original image). Accurate identification of the site of lacrimal passage obstruction is important for its successful treatment with lacrimal endoscopy [16]. Image processing allows a clear visualization of the dimple sign, which indicates an obstruction of the lacrimal duct; this in turn is expected to prevent the creation of false passages and enable an accurate recanalization of the lacrimal duct.

Recently, various microendoscopic transcanalicular therapies have been developed for the management of lacrimal passage obstruction; these include transcanalicular endoscopic dacryoplasty, dacryoendoscopic-assisted nasolacrimal duct intubation [9–11], electrocautery-based techniques [34], and laser or microdrill dacryoplasty [35]. To perform these techniques adequately, it is important to improve the visibility of the dacryoendoscope. Enhancement of the luminal structure images by image processing is expected to improve dacryoendoscopic treatment outcomes for lacrimal passage diseases.

Dacryoendoscopy is attracting increasing attention for performing detailed observations of the lacrimal duct lumen mucosa. Mimura et al., demonstrated that staining of the lacrimal canal mucosa with indigo carmine during dacryoendoscopic examination enabled the assessment of fibrosis and inflammation [36]. In the present study, the blood vessels in the lacrimal sac images were more clearly visible after image processing (Figure 1c,d). Thus, this technique would allow a deeper understanding of lacrimal duct pathologies by enabling a more detailed observation of the lacrimal duct mucosa.

The reduced visibility due to blood- or pus-associated clouding during dacryoendoscopic observation was reportedly improved by using the dacryoendoscope under air perfusion [37]. However, performing lacrimal endoscopy under air perfusion requires a special setting, which is not available commercially and is difficult to establish in general practice. Conversely, the algorithms used in this study can be easily introduced into clinical practice. They can be integrated into an existing video system to perform real-time image processing. In addition, the in vitro experiments performed in our study demonstrated a high image-sharpening effect of these algorithms on the blood- and saline-associated opacity; this is expected to be useful in actual clinical practice.

This study had some limitations. First, the study design did not facilitate the direct evaluation of the improvements in the diagnostic accuracy and treatment outcomes following image processing. Further studies will be needed to clarify whether the proposed algorithms contribute to improved clinical outcomes. Second, other expected benefits, such as a shortened treatment time and reduced surgeon stress, could not be determined due to the study's retrospective nature. Therefore, prospective studies on patients are desirable in order to investigate this. Furthermore, to ensure that this modality benefits the patients, it is important that the image processing device becomes widely available at low additional costs.

5. Conclusions

In conclusion, this study demonstrated that image-processing and image-sharpening algorithms for comb artifact removal could improve the dacryoendoscopic visibility and thus potentially improve the diagnostic accuracy and treatment outcomes in patients with lacrimal passage obstruction.

Supplementary Materials: The following supporting information can be downloaded at: https://www.mdpi.com/article/10.3390/jcm11082073/s1, Video S1: Original and post-processing representative images of the canaliculus (a,b), Video S2: Original and post-processing representative images of the lacrimal sacs (c,d), Video S3: Original and post-processing representative images of the nasolacrimal ducts (e,f), Video S4: Original and post-processing representative images of the intra-canal materials (g,h).

Author Contributions: Conceptualization, S.H. and Y.U.; methodology, S.H. and K.T.; validation, K.M., Y.U. and T.H.; formal analysis, S.H., K.T. and K.M.; investigation, S.H., K.T., H.M., S.M., Y.M. and S.T.; resources, T.O.; data curation, S.H., K.T., K.M., H.M., S.M., Y.M. and S.T.; writing—original draft preparation, S.H.; writing—review and editing, T.O.; supervision, Y.U., T.H. and T.O.; project administration, S.H. All authors have read and agreed to the published version of the manuscript.

Funding: This research received no external funding.

Institutional Review Board Statement: The study was conducted in accordance with the Declaration of Helsinki and approved by the Ethics Committee of the Faculty of Medicine, University of Tsukuba (R03-101; 10 August 2021).

Informed Consent Statement: The study used image samples that had already been acquired and did not contain any personal information; therefore, patient consent was obtained in an opt-out format.

Data Availability Statement: The data presented in this study are available on request from the corresponding author.

Acknowledgments: The authors acknowledge Kimiaki Sato and Masahiro Kobayashi (Logic & Design Inc., Tokyo, Japan) for their technical support during image processing.

Conflicts of Interest: The authors declare no conflict of interest.

References

1. Matsumura, N.; Suzuki, T.; Goto, S.; Fujita, T.; Yamane, S.; Maruyama-Inoue, M.; Kadonosono, K. Transcanalicular Endoscopic Primary Dacryoplasty for Congenital Nasolacrimal Duct Obstruction. *Eye* **2019**, *33*, 1008–1013. [CrossRef] [PubMed]
2. Nakayama, T.; Watanabe, A.; Rajak, S.; Yamanaka, Y.; Sotozono, C. Congenital Nasolacrimal Duct Obstruction Continues Trend for Spontaneous Resolution Beyond First Year of Life. *Br. J. Ophthalmol.* **2020**, *104*, 1161–1163. [CrossRef] [PubMed]
3. Ali, M.J. Metagenomics of the Lacrimal Sac in Primary Acquired Nasolacrimal Duct Obstruction: The Lacriome paper. *Br. J. Ophthalmol.* **2021**, ahead of print. [CrossRef] [PubMed]
4. Khorrami Kashi, A.; Keilani, C.; Nguyen, T.H.; Keller, P.; Elahi, S.; Piaton, J.M. Dacryolithiasis Diagnosis and Treatment: A 25-Year Experience Using Nasal Endoscopy. *Br. J. Ophthalmol.* **2021**, ahead of print. [CrossRef]
5. Hiraoka, T.; Hoshi, S.; Tasaki, K.; Oshika, T. Assessment of Conjunctival Flora in Eyes with Lacrimal Passage Obstruction Before and After Successful Dacryoendoscopic Recanalisation. *Br. J. Ophthalmol.* **2021**, *105*, 909–913. [CrossRef]
6. Tasaki, K.; Hoshi, S.; Hiraoka, T.; Oshika, T. Deterioration of Contrast Sensitivity in Eyes with Epiphora due to Lacrimal Passage Obstruction. *PLoS ONE* **2020**, *15*, e0233295. [CrossRef]
7. Hoshi, S.; Tasaki, K.; Hiraoka, T.; Oshika, T. Improvement in Contrast Sensitivity Function after Lacrimal Passage Intubation in Eyes with Epiphora. *J. Clin. Med.* **2020**, *9*, 2761. [CrossRef]
8. Pakdel, F.; Soleimani, M.; Kasaei, A.; Ameli, K.; Pirmarzdashti, N.; Tari, A.S.; Ghasempour, M.; Banafsheafshan, A. Shifting to Very Early Endoscopic DCR in Acute Suppurative Dacryocystitis. *Eye* **2020**, *34*, 1648–1653. [CrossRef]
9. Curragh, D.S.; Rajak, S.N.; Selva, D. Dacryoendoscopic-Assisted Nasolacrimal Intubation in an Australian Population. *Clin. Exp. Ophthalmol.* **2019**, *47*, 1209–1211. [CrossRef]
10. Lee, S.M.; Lew, H. Transcanalicular endoscopic dacryoplasty in patients with primary acquired nasolacrimal duct obstruction. *Graefes Arch. Clin. Exp. Ophthalmol.* **2021**, *259*, 173–180. [CrossRef]

11. Koh, S.; Ochi, S.; Inoue, Y. Lacrimal Drainage Function after Cheese Wiring of Lacrimal Passage Intubation. *Graefes Arch. Clin. Exp. Ophthalmol.* **2020**, *258*, 1087–1093. [CrossRef] [PubMed]
12. Nowak, R.; Rekas, M.; Ali, M.J. Long-Term Outcomes of StopLoss™ Jones Tube (SLJT) and Minimally Invasive Conjunctivodacryocystorhinostomy. *Graefes Arch. Clin. Exp. Ophthalmol.* **2022**, *260*, 327–333. [CrossRef] [PubMed]
13. Guo, Y.; Rokohl, A.C.; Kroth, K.; Li, S.; Lin, M.; Jia, R.; Heindl, L.M. Endoscopy-Guided Diode Laser-Assisted Transcaruncular StopLoss Jones Tube Implantation for Canalicular Obstructions in Primary Surgery. *Graefes Arch. Clin. Exp. Ophthalmol.* **2020**, *258*, 2809–2817. [CrossRef] [PubMed]
14. Fiorino, M.G.; Quaranta-Leoni, C.; Quaranta-Leoni, F.M. Proximal Lacrimal Obstructions: A Review. *Acta Ophthalmol.* **2021**, *99*, 701–711. [CrossRef]
15. Quaranta-Leoni, F.M.; Fiorino, M.G.; Serricchio, F.; Quaranta-Leoni, F. Management of Proximal Lacrimal Obstructions: A Rationale. *Acta Ophthalmol.* **2021**, *99*, e569–e575. [CrossRef]
16. Sasaki, T.; Sounou, T.; Sugiyama, K. Dacryoendoscopic Surgery and Tube Insertion in Patients with Common Canalicular Obstruction and Ductal Stenosis as a Frequent Complication. *Jpn. J. Ophthalmol.* **2009**, *53*, 145–150. [CrossRef]
17. Sasaki, T.; Sounou, T.; Tsuji, H.; Sugiyama, K. Air-Insufflated High-Definition Dacryoendoscopy Yields Significantly Better Image Quality than Conventional Dacryoendoscopy. *Clin. Ophthalmol.* **2017**, *11*, 1385–1391. [CrossRef]
18. Singh, S.; Ali, M.J. A Review of Diagnostic and Therapeutic Dacryoendoscopy. *Ophthalmic Plast. Reconstr. Surg.* **2019**, *35*, 519–524. [CrossRef]
19. Bae, S.H.; Park, J.; Lee, J.K. Comparison of Digital Subtraction Dacryocystography and Dacryoendoscopy in Patients with Epiphora. *Eye* **2021**, *35*, 877–882. [CrossRef]
20. Fujimoto, M.; Ogino, K.; Matsuyama, H.; Miyazaki, C. Success Rates of Dacryoendoscopy-Guided Probing for Recalcitrant Congenital Nasolacrimal Duct Obstruction. *Jpn. J. Ophthalmol.* **2016**, *60*, 274–279. [CrossRef]
21. Sasaki, T.; Nagata, Y.; Sugiyama, K. Nasolacrimal Duct Obstruction Classified by Dacryoendoscopy and Treated with Inferior Meatal Dacryorhinotomy. Part I: Positional Diagnosis of Primary Nasolacrimal Duct Obstruction with Dacryoendoscope. *Am. J. Ophthalmol.* **2005**, *140*, 1065–1069. [CrossRef] [PubMed]
22. Sasaki, T.; Miyashita, H.; Miyanaga, T.; Yamamoto, K.; Sugiyama, K. Dacryoendoscopic Observation and Incidence of Canalicular Obstruction/Stenosis Associated with S-1, an Oral Anticancer Drug. *Jpn. J. Ophthalmol.* **2012**, *56*, 214–218. [CrossRef] [PubMed]
23. Inomata, D.; Hoshi, S.; Alcântara, C.P.B.C.; Hiraoka, T.; Tasaki, K.; Oshika, T.; Matayoshi, S. Dacryoendoscopic Recanalization of Lacrimal Passage Obstruction/Stenosis After Radioiodine Therapy for Differentiated Thyroid Carcinoma. *Am. J. Ophthalmol. Case Rep.* **2022**, *25*, 101344. [CrossRef] [PubMed]
24. Su, Y.; Zhang, L.; Li, L.; Fan, X.; Xiao, C. Surgical Procedure of Caniculoplasty in the Treatment of Primary Canaliculitis Associated with Canalicular Dilatation. *BMC Ophthalmol.* **2020**, *20*, 245. [CrossRef]
25. Mimura, M.; Ueki, M.; Oku, H.; Sato, B.; Ikeda, T. Evaluation of Granulation Tissue Formation in Lacrimal Duct Post Silicone Intubation and its Successful Management by Injection of Prednisolone Acetate Ointment into the Lacrimal Duct. *Jpn. J. Ophthalmol.* **2016**, *60*, 280–285. [CrossRef]
26. Ali, M.J.; Singh, S.; Ganguly, A.; Naik, M.N. Dacryoendoscopy-Guided Transcanalicular Intralesional Interferon Alpha 2b for Canalicular Squamous Papillomas. *Int. Ophthalmol.* **2018**, *38*, 1343–1346. [CrossRef]
27. Emmerich, K.H.; Meyer-Rüsenberg, H.W.; Simko, P. Endoscopy of the Lacrimal Ducts. *Ophthalmologe* **1997**, *94*, 732–735. [CrossRef]
28. Singh, A.D.; Singh, A.; Whitmore, I.; Taylor, E. Endoscopic Visualisation of the Human Nasolacrimal System: An Experimental Study. *Br. J. Ophthalmol.* **1992**, *76*, 663–667. [CrossRef]
29. Fein, W.; Daykhovsky, L.; Papaioannou, T.; Beeder, C.; Grundfest, W.S. Endoscopy of the Lacrimal Outflow System. *Arch. Ophthalmol.* **1992**, *110*, 1748–1750. [CrossRef]
30. Suzuki, T. Dacryofiberscopy. *Jpn. J. Ophthal. Surg.* **2003**, *16*, 485–491. (In Japanese)
31. Shinde, A.; Matham, M.V. Pixelate removal in an image fiber probe endoscope incorporating comb structure removal methods. *J. Med. Imaging Health Inform.* **2014**, *4*, 203–211. [CrossRef]
32. Waterhouse, D.J.; Luthman, A.S.; Yoon, J.; Gordon, G.S.D.; Bohndiek, S.E. Quantitative Evaluation of Comb-Structure Correction Methods for Multispectral Fibrescopic Imaging. *Sci. Rep.* **2018**, *8*, 17801. [CrossRef] [PubMed]
33. Sugimoto, M. New Sheath-Assisted Dacryoendoscopic Surgery. *J. Eye* **2007**, *24*, 1219–1222.
34. Chen, D.; Ge, J.; Wang, L.; Gao, Q.; Ma, P.; Li, N.; Li, D.Q.; Wang, Z. A Simple and Evolutional Approach Proven to Recanalise the Nasolacrimal Duct Obstruction. *Br. J. Ophthalmol.* **2009**, *93*, 1438–1443. [CrossRef] [PubMed]
35. Mihailovic, N.; Blumberg, A.F.; Rosenberger, F.; Brücher, V.C.; Lahme, L.; Eter, N.; Merté, R.L.; Alnawaiseh, M. Long-Term Outcome of Transcanalicular Microdrill Dacryoplasty: A Minimally Invasive Alternative for Dacryocystorhinostomy. *Br. J. Ophthalmol.* **2021**, *105*, 1480–1484. [CrossRef]
36. Mimura, M.; Alameddine, R.M.; Korn, B.S.; Kikkawa, D.O.; Oku, H.; Sato, B.; Ikeda, T. Endoscopic Evaluation of Lacrimal Mucosa with Indigo Carmine Stain. *Ophthalmic Plast. Reconstr. Surg.* **2020**, *36*, 49–54. [CrossRef] [PubMed]
37. Fujimoto, M.; Uji, A.; Ogino, K.; Akagi, T.; Yoshimura, N. Lacrimal Canaliculus Imaging Using Optical Coherence Tomography Dacryography. *Sci. Rep.* **2018**, *8*, 9808. [CrossRef]

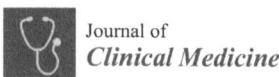

Article

Meibomian Gland Density: An Effective Evaluation Index of Meibomian Gland Dysfunction Based on Deep Learning and Transfer Learning

Zuhui Zhang [1], Xiaolei Lin [2], Xinxin Yu [1], Yana Fu [1], Xiaoyu Chen [1], Weihua Yang [3,*] and Qi Dai [1,4,*]

[1] School of Ophthalmology and Optometry, The Eye Hospital of Wenzhou Medical University, 270 Xueyuanxi Road, Wenzhou 325027, China; zhzhang@eye.ac.cn (Z.Z.); xinxinyu@eye.ac.cn (X.Y.); fuyana@eye.ac.cn (Y.F.); xiaoyuchenny@163.com (X.C.)
[2] Department of Ophthalmology and Visual Science, Eye, Ear, Nose, and Throat Hospital, Shanghai Medical College, Fudan University, Shanghai 200126, China; 19111260013@fudan.edu.cn
[3] Affiliated Eye Hospital, Nanjing Medical University, No.138 Hanzhong Road, Nanjing 210029, China
[4] College of Mathematical Medicine, Zhejiang Normal University, Jinhua 321004, China
* Correspondence: benben0606@139.com (W.Y.); dq@mail.eye.ac.cn (Q.D.); Tel.: +86-13867252557 (W.Y.); +86-18667127070 (Q.D.); Fax: +86-025-8667-7779 (W.Y.); +86-0571-8819-3999 (Q.D.)

Abstract: We aimed to establish an artificial intelligence (AI) system based on deep learning and transfer learning for meibomian gland (MG) segmentation and evaluate the efficacy of MG density in the diagnosis of MG dysfunction (MGD). First, 85 eyes of 85 subjects were enrolled for AI system-based evaluation effectiveness testing. Then, from 2420 randomly selected subjects, 4006 meibography images (1620 upper eyelids and 2386 lower eyelids) graded by three experts according to the meiboscore were analyzed for MG density using the AI system. The updated AI system achieved 92% accuracy (intersection over union, IoU) and 100% repeatability in MG segmentation after 4 h of training. The processing time for each meibography was 100 ms. We discovered a significant and linear correlation between MG density and ocular surface disease index questionnaire (OSDI), tear break-up time (TBUT), lid margin score, meiboscore, and meibum expressibility score (all $p < 0.05$). The area under the curve (AUC) was 0.900 for MG density in the total eyelids. The sensitivity and specificity were 88% and 81%, respectively, at a cutoff value of 0.275. MG density is an effective index for MGD, particularly supported by the AI system, which could replace the meiboscore, significantly improve the accuracy of meibography analysis, reduce the analysis time and doctors' workload, and improve the diagnostic efficiency.

Keywords: meibomian gland dysfunction; meibomian gland density; deep learning; transfer learning; artificial intelligence

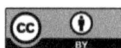

1. Introduction

Meibomian gland dysfunction (MGD) is a chronic, diffuse abnormality of the meibomian glands (MGs), commonly characterized by terminal duct obstruction and/or qualitative/quantitative changes in glandular secretion and also a major cause of dry eye [1,2]. It can cause tear film instability and ocular surface inflammation, resulting in ocular irritation symptoms, and may even damage the cornea and affect visual function in severe cases. In the absence of a gold-standard diagnostic test, finding effective diagnostic parameters for MGD is imperative. Currently, an intuitive index for assessing MGD is the degree of MG atrophy, which is both common and subjective. In addition, morphological changes in the MGs can also predict the severity of MGD [3,4]. Studies have also confirmed that morphological indices of the MGs, such as their length, width, and tortuosity, are related to their function [5,6]. Ban et al. found that MG morphology in the upper eyelid was significantly correlated with the condition of the tear film or ocular surface epithelium [4].

MG atrophy grading has been proven to be an effective diagnostic index for MGD [7–10]. Based on the findings of these studies, further studies used ImageJ and other software to manually label the MG for a quantitative analysis. However, manual labeling of MGs is subject to insurmountable subjective errors and is time-consuming, resulting in low efficiency.

In subsequent studies, image-processing algorithms have become popular research tools for MG image analysis. Some analytical methods showed superiority in MG morphological analysis. Arita et al. reported an image processing system that could analyze the MG morphology and obtain relatively accurate results [11,12]. Llorens-Quintana et al. reported a new methodology for analyzing, in an automated and objective fashion, infrared images of the MG [13]. Ciężar et al. reported that global 2D Fourier transform analysis of infra-red MG images provides values of two new parameters: mean gland frequency and anisotropy in gland periodicity. Their values correlate with MGD [14]. Yeh et al. reported a nonparametric instance discrimination approach that automatically analyses MG atrophy severity from meibography without prior image annotations and categorizes the MG characteristics through hierarchical clustering [15]. However, traditional image algorithms still have some limitations, such as unstable region detection and weak characterization of the extracted features. In addition, the overall evaluation index is based on the dropout grade classification of MGs, and it is impossible to extract and analyze each gland separately [16].

Previous studies on artificial intelligence (AI), such as convolutional neural networks, have proven effective in the automatic evaluation of meiboscore [17–19]. However, these studies focused on MG dropout grade classification and did not segment each MG. Consequently, they could not be further analyzed.

The purpose of this study was to develop an AI-based evaluation system for MG morphology based on deep learning and transfer learning for segmenting each MG and evaluating MG morphological indices accurately. Furthermore, the study also aimed to make it possible to diagnose MGD using MG density, an index that requires many annotations and calculations.

2. Materials and Methods
2.1. Patients and Materials

The subjects used in the AI model training were the same as those in our previous report [20], and a total of 60 randomly selected subjects were recruited. Sixty original annotated meibography images of the upper eyelids were used in this study. Of these, 40 were used as the original training images. A total of 245,760 images were generated from these 40 images as a training set using image enhancement software. Another 20 annotated meibography images were used as validation sets. Subsequently, we adjusted the parameters and trained the AI to apply it to the lower eyelid. Sixty original annotated meibography images of the lower eyelids were used for the validation.

First, 85 eyes from 85 subjects (age, 8–83 years) were enrolled for the AI system analysis and evaluation of the efficacy of MG density for MGD diagnosis. Only one eye of each subject was randomly selected and included for the comprehensive dry eye and MG examination. The exclusion criteria were as follows: (1) history of ocular trauma or surgery; (2) systemic drugs or eye drops affecting MG function or tear film used in the last 2 weeks; (3) contact lenses worn in the last 2 weeks; and (4) ocular or systemic diseases known to affect tear film or MG function. A total of 53 subjects with obstructive MGD (20 males and 33 females; median age, 35.00 (30.00–50.00) years) were included in the MGD group, and 32 healthy subjects (13 males and 19 females; median age, 25.00 (16.25–32.75) years) in the control group.

All 53 subjects with obstructive MGD were diagnosed by two experienced ophthalmologists when any two of the three scores were abnormal: (I) ocular symptom score ≥ 3; (II) lid margin abnormality score ≥ 2; and/or (III) meiboscore ≥ 3 [21]. Subjects diagnosed with obstructive MGD by both ophthalmologists were included in this study. If the ophthalmologists provided different diagnoses, the subjects were excluded from the study.

A total of 4006 meibography images (including 1620 upper eyelids and 2386 lower eyelids) from 2420 randomly selected subjects (age ≥18 years) were used for MG density analysis using the AI system. All 4006 meibography images were graded according to the meiboscore (range, 0–3) by three experienced ophthalmologists, and their majority opinion was obtained. A qualified meibography image needed to meet two requirements: (1) the tarsal plates must be entirely exposed, and (2) the meibography image must be focused correctly and clearly. Unqualified meibography images would interfere with the meiboscore and MG density results. The correlation between MG density obtained by the AI system and meiboscore from ophthalmologists was analyzed.

All subjects were from the Eye Hospital, Wenzhou Medical University. The study was conducted in accordance with the Declaration of Helsinki and was approved by the Research Ethics Committee of the Eye Hospital, Wenzhou Medical University (approval number: 2020-209-K-191). This study is registered on http://www.chictr.org.cn (ChiCTR2100052575, 31 October 2021). Informed consent to publish was obtained from all participants before their inclusion in the study.

2.2. Methods

2.2.1. Data Collection and Processing of Samples

Samples were collected, optimized, and processed using the previously reported method [20]. First, images of both the upper and lower MGs were captured using the Oculus Keratograph 5M (K5M; Oculus, Wetzlar, Germany). Second, these images were optimized, converted to grayscale, and then standardized and normalized.

2.2.2. Network Structure and AI Training

The tarsus segmentation model was based on Mask R-CNN [22]. Based on the pre-trained Mask R-CNN model (https://github.com/matterport/Mask_RCNN, 20 March 2018), we used 100 annotated images of upper and lower tarsus for fine-tuning and obtained fine-tuned model parameters after iterating 200 epochs. Another 20 sample images were used to test the fine-tuned model. Finally, we used the fine-tuned Mask R-CNN model to segment the tarsus.

Transfer learning was used to apply the pretrained model and parameters on ImageNet [23] to our previously reported deep learning model (Figure 1A). The residual neural network (ResNet) exhibits excellent performance in image classification and target detection [24]. The 50-layer ResNet (ResNet50) was replaced with the max-pooling layers of the previous U-net model; however, the upsampling layer remained the same (Figure 1B). We call this the ResNet50_U-net.

Forty annotated meibography images of the upper eyelids were included as the basis for the training set. In each iteration of training, four images of these 40 original meibography images were randomly selected. The data enhancement model (https://github.com/aleju/imgaug#citation, 6 February 2020, Figure 2) was used to enhance the input of four images with random use of algorithms and parameters, with four new images generated. The final version of the model was iterated a total of 61,440 times in all training and generated 245,760 new images as the training set. The amount of data can preliminarily meet the needs of training a deep convolutional neural network.

The original meibography (Figure 3A) was preprocessed to show the glands more clearly (Figure 3B). Compared to the manually annotated result (Figure 3C), the AI system exhibited superior recognition ability (Figure 3D). Figure 4 shows a sample of the original meibography, manual annotation, and AI segmentation of the MGs.

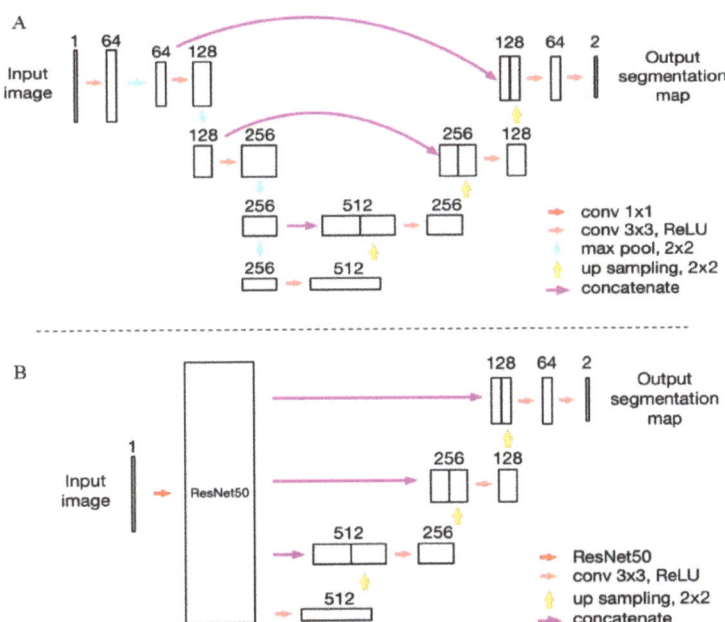

Figure 1. Network Structure. (**A**) The network structure of the modified U-net model as we reported previously; (**B**) the network structure of the ResNet50_U-net model in this study.

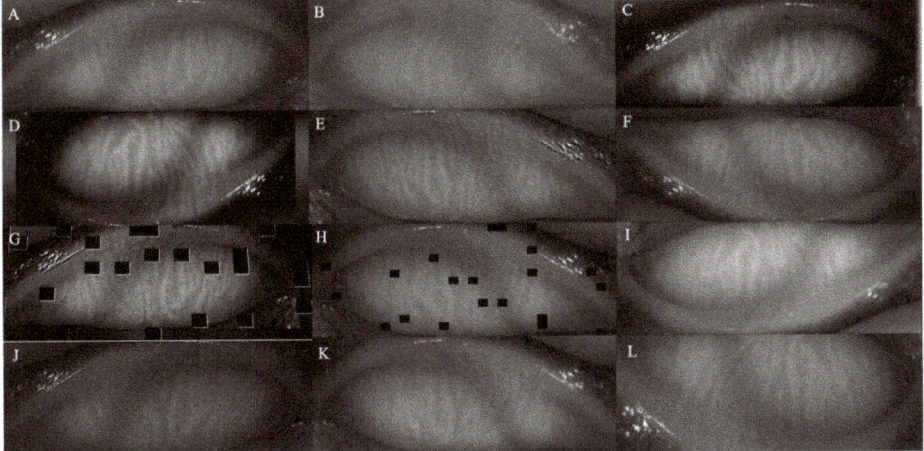

Figure 2. The image enhancement model example. (**A**) Original training image. (**B–L**) Output images with 11 enhancement methods.

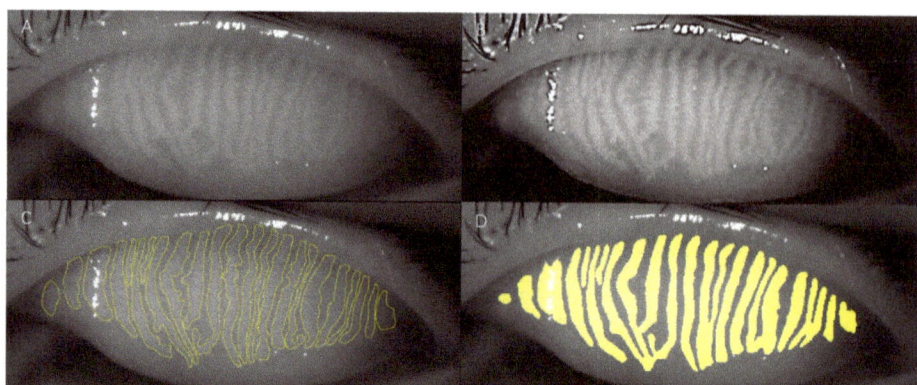

Figure 3. The samples of image processing, annotation and segmentation. (**A**) The original meibography. (**B**) The preprocessed image. (**C**) The manually annotated MGs in yellow outline. (**D**) The segmented MGs by AI system are shown in yellow.

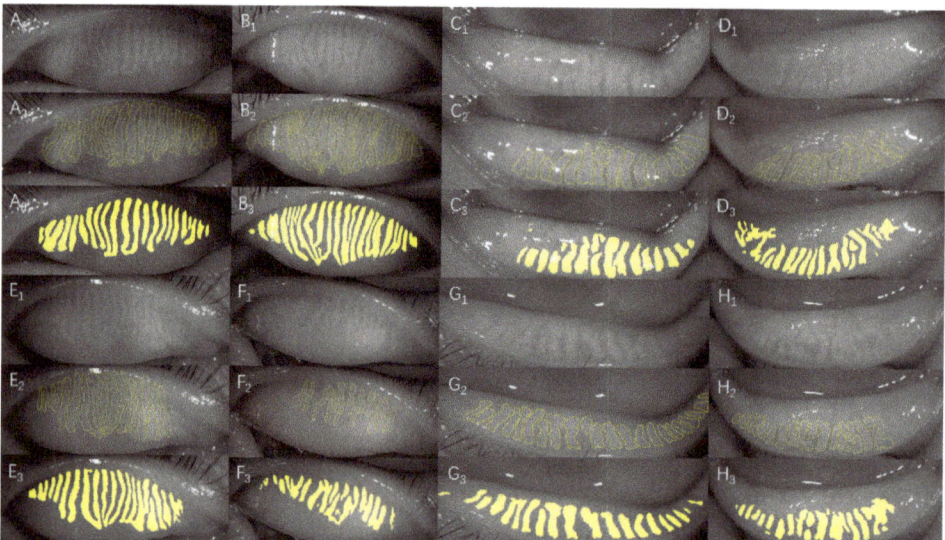

Figure 4. The comparisons of manual annotation and AI automatic segmentation. (A_1, B_1, E_1, F_1) The original meibography of the upper eyelid. (A_2, B_2, E_2, F_2) The manual annotation of the upper eyelid (yellow outline). (A_3, B_3, E_3, F_3) The AI segmentation MGs of the upper eyelid (yellow part). (C_1, D_1, G_1, H_1) the Original meibography of the lower eyelid. (C_2, D_2, G_2, H_2) The manual annotation of the lower eyelid (yellow outline). (C_3, D_3, G_3, H_3) The AI segmentation MGs of the lower eyelid (yellow part).

We used another 20 annotated original upper eyelid meibography images apart from the training set as the validation set. We used the intersection of unions (IoU) to evaluate the accuracy of the MG recognition model (Figure 5). It can be simply understood as the ratio of the intersection of the ground truth (manual annotation) and AI result (AI segmentation) to their union.

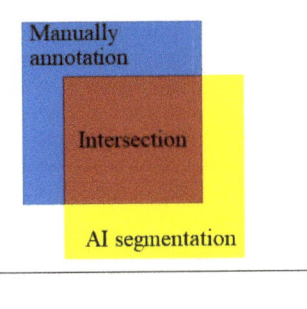

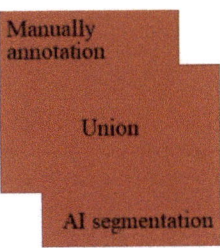

Figure 5. The intersection (green part) of the ground truth (manual annotation, blue part) and the AI result (AI segmentation, yellow part) divided by their union (red part) is IoU.

2.2.3. Clinical Parameters

The clinical assessments were performed sequentially as follows [20]. All subjects completed the Ocular Surface Disease Index (OSDI) questionnaire and were asked whether they had any of the 14 MGD-related ocular symptoms (symptom score) [25]. Images of both the upper and lower MGs were captured using the Keratograph 5M. The central tear meniscus height (TMH) of the lower eyelid was measured 5 s after blinking using the Keratograph 5M. Tear break-up time (TBUT) was measured and corneal fluorescein staining (CFS) was performed after the instillation of fluorescein. TBUT was measured three times, and the mean value was recorded. CFS was graded according to the Baylor grading scheme from 0 to 4 [26]. Four lid margin abnormalities (irregular lid margin, vascular engorgement, plugged meibomian gland orifices, and anterior or posterior replacement of the mucocutaneous junction) were scored from 0 to 4, according to the number of these abnormalities present in each eye [21]. The MG expressibility scores ranged from 0 to 45 by assessing the meibum quality and quantity of the 15 glands on each lower eyelid [27].

2.2.4. MG Indices

To assess the degree of MG dropout, we used the method described by Arita et al. to calculate the meiboscore: 0, no loss of MGs; 1, the lost area was less than one-third of the total area of the MGs; 2, the lost area was between one-third and two-thirds of the total area of the MGs; and 3, the lost area was over two-thirds of the total area of the MGs [9]. The total meiboscore of the upper and lower eyelids ranged from 0 to 6.

MG density was automatically calculated by the AI system using the following formula [28]: the sum of the area of MGs divided by the total area of the tarsus in pixels. $\sum_{i=1}^{n} S_{MG_i}$ = the sum of pixels of all MGs, St = the total pixels of the tarsus.

$$MG\ density = \frac{\sum_{i=1}^{n} S_{MG_i}}{St}$$

2.2.5. Statistical Analysis

The normality of data distributions was analyzed using the Kolmogorov–Smirnov test, and the abnormal data distributions were analyzed using the non-parametric statistical analyses. Values are expressed as the mean ± standard deviation (SD) or (range) or median (interquartile range [IQR]). Either the independent samples t-test or the Mann–Whitney U-test was used to compare differences between MGD subjects and normal control subjects. The generalized estimating equation was used to adjust the age difference. Kruskal–Wallis H-test was used to compare the MG density and the severity score of the meiboscore scale. The correlations between various MG morphological parameters and MG function parameters (i.e., OSDI, TBUT, CFS, lid margin score, meiboscore, and meibum expressibility score) were determined using Pearson's or Spearman's correlation analysis. The χ^2 test was used to compare the sex ratios between the two groups. Receiver operating characteristic (ROC) curve analysis was used to determine the predictive value of MG density for the diagnosis of MGD. A two-sided $p < 0.05$ was considered statistically significant. All statistical analyses were performed using SPSS Statistics 23.0 (IBM, Armonk, NY, USA).

3. Results

3.1. AI Training and Testing

The AI system of Mask R-CNN achieved 93% accuracy (IoU) and 100% repeatability for tarsus segmentation. The AI system of ResNet50_U-net training lasted for 4 h, a significant reduction from the duration of our previous U-Net model training (15 h). Additionally, the ResNet50_U-net model achieved 92% accuracy (IoU) and 100% repeatability for MG segmentation. Subsequently, we adjusted the parameters and trained the AI to automatically segment the lower MGs and achieved the same level of IoU. The processing time of each meibography was 100 ms with a GTX 1070 8G GPU.

3.2. Characteristics

A total of 85 eyes from 85 randomly selected subjects were enrolled for AI system effectiveness testing. These included 53 subjects with obstructive MGD (20 males and 33 females, median age, 35.00 (30.00–50.00) years) and 32 normal volunteers (13 males and 19 females, median age, 25.00 (16.25–32.75) years). Because the age difference between patients with MGD and the normal control group was significant, the generalized estimating equation was used to adjust for age. No significant difference in sex was observed between patients with MGD and normal controls. The baseline characteristics of the 85 subjects are summarized in Table 1.

Table 1. Clinical parameters of the 85 subjects.

Parameter	Normal (n = 32)	MGD (n = 53)	p	p *
Age (years), Median (IQR)	25.00 (16.25–32.75)	35.00 (30.00–50.00)	<0.001	-
Sex (n, male/female)	13/19	20/33	0.794	-
OSDI (0–100), Median (IQR)	4.47 (0.30–12.35)	25.00 (13.24–37.80)	<0.001	<0.001
Symptom score (0–14), Median (IQR)	2.00 (0–4.00)	7.00 (5.00–8.00)	<0.001	<0.001
TBUT (s), Median (IQR)	5.00 (5.00–7.75)	2.50 (1.33–3.67)	<0.001	<0.001
CFS (0–20), Median (IQR)	0 (0–0)	0 (0–0)	0.058	0.021
TMH (mm), Median (IQR)	0.19 (0.16–0.23)	0.20 (0.17–0.24)	0.461	0.871
Lid margin score (0–4), Median (IQR)	0 (0–1.00)	2.00 (1.00–2.00)	<0.001	<0.001
Meiboscore (0–6), Median (IQR)	2.00 (1.00–2.00)	3.00 (2.00–4.50)	<0.001	<0.001
Meibum expressibility score (0–45), Median (IQR)	38.50 (30.00–45.00)	18.00 (5.50–34.50)	<0.001	<0.001

MGD = meibomian gland dysfunction; IQR = interquartile range; OSDI = Ocular Surface Disease Index; TBUT = tear break-up time; CFS = corneal fluorescein staining; TMH = tear meniscus height; Values are expressed as the median (IQR). Mann–Whitney U-test was used to compare differences between MGD subjects and normal control subjects. * p values adjusted for age by generalized estimating equation.

3.3. MG Density and Functions

The MG density in the upper eyelid was significantly correlated with OSDI (r = −0.320, $p = 0.003$), TBUT (r = 0.484, $p < 0.001$), lid margin score (r = −0.350, $p = 0.001$), meiboscore (r = −0.749, $p < 0.001$), and meibum expressibility score (r = 0.425, $p < 0.001$). The MG density in the lower eyelid was significantly correlated with OSDI (r = −0.420, $p < 0.001$), TBUT (r = 0.598, $p < 0.001$), lid margin score (r = −0.396, $p < 0.001$), meiboscore (r = −0.720, $p < 0.001$), and meibum expressibility score (r = 0.438, $p < 0.001$). The MG density in the total eyelid was significantly correlated with OSDI (r = −0.404, $p < 0.001$), TBUT (r = 0.601, $p < 0.001$), lid margin score (r = −0.416, $p < 0.001$), meiboscore (r = −0.805, $p < 0.001$), and meibum expressibility score (r = 0.480, $p < 0.001$). However, there were no significant correlations between MG density and CFS or TMH in upper eyelid, lower eyelid and total eyelid (all $p > 0.05$). These results are shown in Table 2.

Table 2. Correlations of MG density with tear film functions and MG status in 85 subjects.

		OSDI	TBUT	CFS	TMH	Lid Margin Score	Meiboscore	Meibum Expressibility Score
MG density	Upper eyelid	−0.320 †	0.484 ‡	−0.162	−0.059	−0.350 †	−0.749 ‡	0.425 ‡
	Lower eyelid	−0.420 ‡	0.598 ‡	−0.177	−0.058	−0.396 ‡	−0.720 ‡	0.438 ‡
	Total eyelid	−0.404 ‡	0.601 ‡	−0.166	−0.070	−0.416 ‡	−0.805 ‡	0.480 ‡

MG = meibomian gland; OSDI = Ocular Surface Disease Index; TBUT = tear break-up time; CFS = corneal fluorescein staining; TMH = tear meniscus height; Spearman's rank correlation coefficient test. † $p < 0.005$. ‡ $p < 0.001$.

3.4. MG Density with Meiboscore

After analyzing 4006 random meibography images using the AI system, it was observed that the MG density in the upper eyelid was significantly negatively correlated with the meiboscore (r = −0.707, $p < 0.001$), as was that in the lower eyelid (r = −0.472, $p < 0.001$). The corresponding relationship between the MG density and meiboscore is shown in Figure 6.

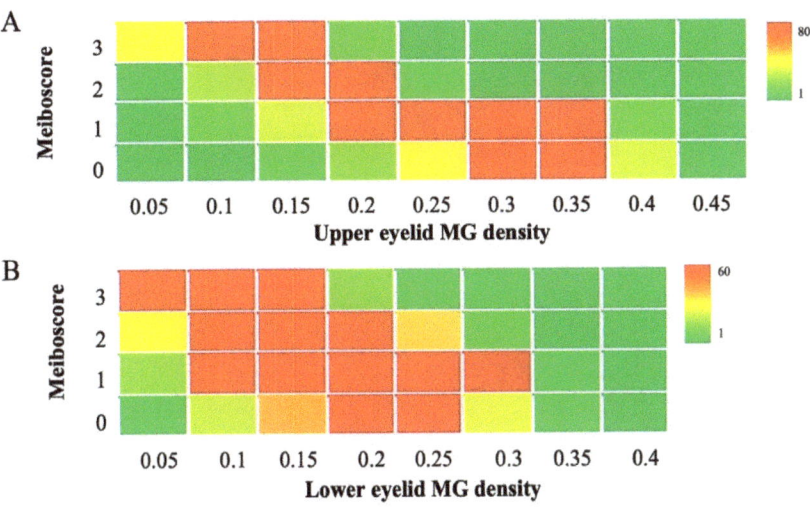

Figure 6. Corresponding relationship between MG density and meiboscore. (**A**) The corresponding relationship between the upper eyelid MG density and meiboscore. (**B**) The corresponding relationship between lower eyelid MG density and meiboscore. The "hot" red areas represent data-intensive areas. The maximum number was 80 and 60 meibography images on the upper eyelid and lower eyelid, respectively. The "cold" green areas are the opposite. The minimum value is 1 meibography image.

3.5. MG Density to Meiboscore

We compared the correspondence between the MG density and meiboscore, as shown in Table 3. The MG density distribution in the upper eyelid on each meiboscore scale was not the same, and the difference was significant (H = 882.932, $p < 0.001$). The MG density distribution in the lower eyelid on each meiboscore scale was not the same, and the difference was significant (H = 596.815, $p < 0.001$). Figure 7 depicts meibography images with varying MG densities and corresponding meiboscores to help readers gain insight into the relationship between MG density and meiboscore.

Table 3. Comparison table of MG density and meiboscore.

	MG Density					
	Upper Eyelid (1620)			Lower Eyelid (2386)		
	Median (IQR)	H-Value	p	Median (IQR)	H-Value	p
Meiboscore 0	0.30 (0.25–0.33)			0.19 (0.14–0.23)		
Meiboscore 1	0.25 (0.21–0.29)	882.932	<0.001	0.17 (0.13–0.21)	596.815	<0.001
Meiboscore 2	0.15 (0.12–0.18)			0.13 (0.10–0.17)		
Meiboscore 3	0.10 (0.06–0.12)			0.07 (0.04–0.11)		

MG = meibomian gland; IQR = interquartile range; p: compare distributions across groups; H-value: test statistic.

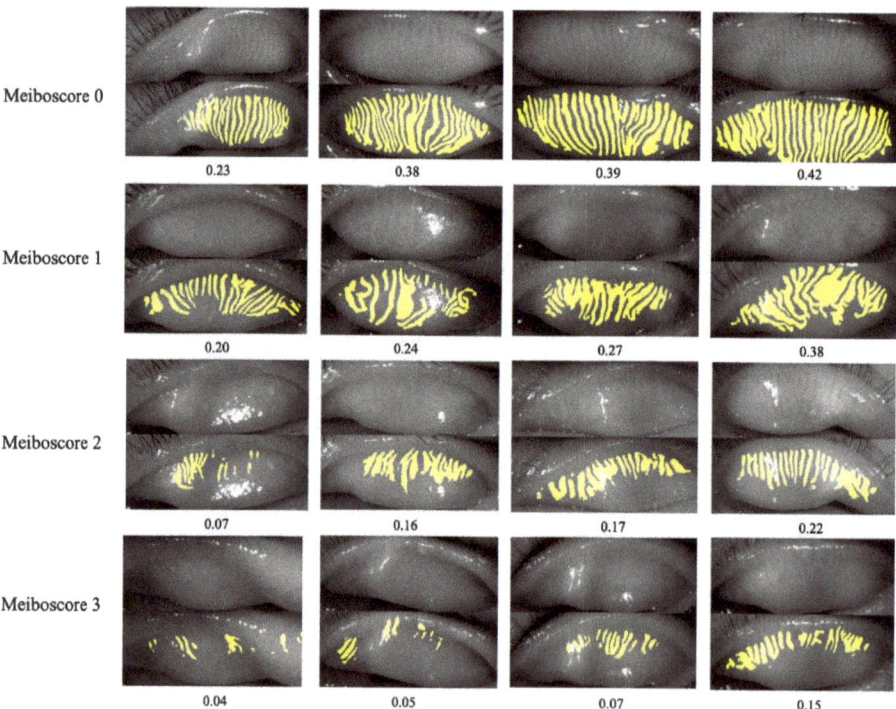

Figure 7. Meibography images with MG densities and meiboscores. Rows 1 to 4 refer to meibography images with meiboscore 0 to 3, respectively. MG density was calculated from the meibography images by our AI system.

3.6. Sensitivity and Specificity of MG Density

Figure 8 shows the results of the ROC curve analyses, which indicated the sensitivity and specificity of MG density for the diagnosis of MGD. The area under the curve (AUC) was 0.836 for MG density in the upper eyelid. The sensitivity and specificity were 73% and 81%, respectively, at a cut-off value of 0.265. The AUC was 0.888 for MG density in the lower eyelid. The sensitivity and specificity were 82% and 88%, respectively, at a cut-off value of 0.255. The AUC was 0.900 for MG density in the total eyelids. The sensitivity and specificity were 88% and 81%, respectively, at a cut-off value of 0.275.

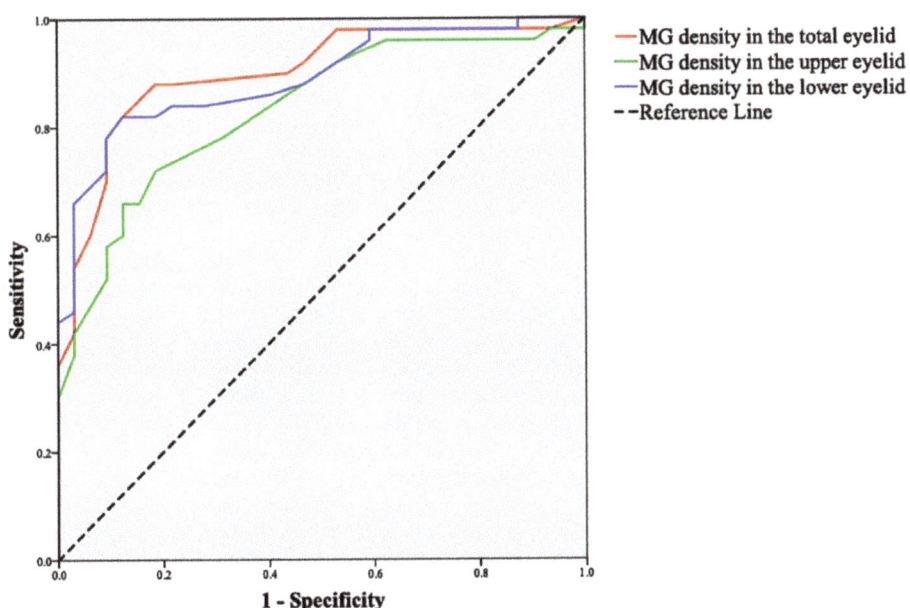

Figure 8. ROC curve analysis of MG density for the diagnosis of MGD.

4. Discussion

Diagnosis of MGD is difficult because most of the diagnostic criteria are subjective and are usually based on a combination of a high meiboscore, dry eye symptoms, and lid margin abnormalities [29]. A comprehensive analysis of MG morphology is the key for determining the severity of MGD. Currently, the most widely used MG morphology criterion is a qualitative MG dropout grading index similar to the meiboscore, and its effectiveness has been proven by a large number of studies. However, the meiboscore and other qualitative grading indices also have the limitations of strong subjectivity and poor repeatability, especially regarding the results adjacent to the grading transition zone. For example, when the MG dropout ratio is 1/3 or 2/3, the meiboscore becomes unstable. This study proposes a novel MG dropout index, the MG density. It is a linear quantitative index that extracts the image of each MG gland and calculates the ratio of the precise gland area relative to the tarsus area. This novel index greatly improves the accuracy compared with the traditional MG atrophy grade method, but it also shows instability and inaccuracy owing to anthropogenic annotation errors, limiting its effectiveness when using manual calculations. This MG density index requires many calculations, which limits its clinical application. AI has a quick mathematical calculation ability and high reliability, which is suitable for calculating MG density. There was no need to control between-group variance and repeatability, such as within-subject SD (SW), within-subject coefficient of variation

(CVw), and intraclass correlation coefficient (ICC), as in our previous study [20,28]. In this study, the AI system achieved a 92% IoU and 100% repeatability.

The AI model used in this study is the latest iteration of the CNN model used in our previous study [20]. To further improve the recognition accuracy of AI systems, a large training dataset is required. To overcome the dilemma of fewer MG images, we selected a data enhancement model to manipulate MG images and a combination of deep and transfer learning for AI model building. Transfer learning techniques attempt to transfer knowledge from previous tasks to a target task when the latter has less high-quality training data. This can be accomplished using a network that has already been pretrained on millions of general-purpose images (ImageNet [30]) without any additional retraining needed for the deep convolutional neural networks on our specific dataset. Using transfer learning, we were able to use a pretrained neural network in our image recognition network, which greatly reduced the dependence on training data and improved the training speed (from 15 h for the U-Net model to 4 h for the ResNet50_U-net model) and accuracy. Transfer learning has been used to study ophthalmic diseases, such as age-related macular degeneration [31] and glaucoma [32]. Although a small number of subjects were used to train AI in this study, the detection accuracy was very high owing to the combination of deep learning and transfer learning.

After comparing the relationship between the MG morphological indices extracted by the AI system and clinical parameters, as previously reported [3,33,34], the AI system in this study revealed that MG dropout was significantly correlated with MGD symptoms, tear film stability, lid margin abnormality, and meibum expressibility. One step further than previous research [7,9,18,19,35,36], our study used MG density instead of meiboscore to evaluate the degree of MG dropout successfully. ROC curve analysis revealed that MG density showed high diagnostic efficiency for MGD. MG density in the total eyelids showed good efficiency, sensitivity, and specificity for the diagnosis of MGD, with a sensitivity and specificity of 88% and 81%, respectively, at a cut-off value of 0.275.

Furthermore, regarding MG atrophy evaluation, a quantitative index based on the continuous numerical result of MG density is a better criterion than a qualitative index based on the MG dropout grade of the meiboscore. It is difficult to provide precise meiboscores when MG atrophy is near the grading transition limits (0%, 33%, and 66%), whereas MG density can be used in such situations. MG density can be used to effectively assess the atrophy condition of the MG in each grading transition area. Simultaneously, we also proposed the corresponding and conversion relation between the MG density and meiboscore by analyzing 4006 meibography images. There was a significant linear correlation between the MG density and meiboscore, especially in the upper eyelid. The MG density of the lower eyelid was slightly less correlated with the meiboscore, which may be related to the fact that the lower palpebral conjunctiva was mistakenly identified as the tarsus by the AI system because of the excessive turnover of the lower eyelid. In the future, based on AI assistance, the quantitative index of MG density can be used to replace the qualitative index of MG dropout, such as the meiboscore.

This study has some limitations. The sample size for AI training was small. Even though we used imgaug, a data enhancement library, which could partially obtain a large amount of information from the original meibography used for AI training and greatly reduce the workload of annotation, it still could not change some basic information of the meibography, such as the number of glands. Therefore, it could not completely replace the newly annotated images. In addition, the sample size for evaluating the diagnostic efficacy of MG density was small. In future studies, the author's team will recruit more subjects for AI system training and testing.

5. Conclusions

MG density is an accurate and effective evaluation index that can completely replace the meiboscore for the quantitative diagnosis of MG dropout. We propose MG density as a novel quantitative index for AI-based diagnosis of MGD. Simultaneously, the AI system can reduce the subjective bias of the observer and doctors' workload, improve efficiency, and assist nonprofessional doctors with MGD diagnosis.

Author Contributions: Conceptualization and writing original draft, Z.Z.; formal analysis, X.L.; investigation, X.Y.; writing—review and editing, Y.F.; data curation, X.C.; supervision, W.Y.; project administration, Q.D. All authors have read and agreed to the published version of the manuscript.

Funding: This research was funded by the Zhejiang Provincial Medical and Health Science Technology Program of Health and Family Planning Commission (grant number: 2022PY074; grant number: 2022KY217), a Project Supported by Scientific Research Fund of Zhejiang Provincial Education Department (Y202147994) and the Nanjing Enterprise Expert Team Project.

Institutional Review Board Statement: The study was approved by the review board of the Eye Hospital of Wenzhou Medical University (approval number: 2020-209-K-191) and adhered to the tenets of the Declaration of Helsinki. This study is registered on http://www.chictr.org.cn (ChiCTR2100052575, 31 October 2021). Informed consent to participate in the study was obtained from a parent or guardian for participants under 18 years old.

Informed Consent Statement: Informed consent to participate in the study was obtained from a parent or guardian for participants under 18 years old.

Data Availability Statement: The datasets generated during and/or analyzed during the current study are available from the corresponding author on reasonable request.

Acknowledgments: The authors are grateful to Jing Ye for technological guidance. They are grateful to Xuewen Chen, Lu Li, Chaoqun Zhang, and Yingyu Mao, who works in the department of dry eye, for their help in collecting data.

Conflicts of Interest: The authors declare no conflict of interest.

References

1. Nichols, K.K.; Foulks, G.N.; Bron, A.J.; Glasgow, B.J.; Dogru, M.; Tsubota, K.; Lemp, M.A.; Sullivan, D.A. The international workshop on meibomian gland dysfunction: Executive summary. *Investig. Ophthalmol. Vis. Sci.* **2011**, *52*, 1922–1929. [CrossRef]
2. Craig, J.P.; Nichols, K.K.; Akpek, E.K.; Caffery, B.; Dua, H.S.; Joo, C.K.; Liu, Z.; Nelson, J.D.; Nichols, J.J.; Tsubota, K.; et al. TFOS DEWS II Definition and Classification Report. *Ocul. Surf.* **2017**, *15*, 276–283. [CrossRef]
3. Giannaccare, G.; Vigo, L.; Pellegrini, M.; Sebastiani, S.; Carones, F. Ocular Surface Workup With Automated Noninvasive Measurements for the Diagnosis of Meibomian Gland Dysfunction. *Cornea* **2018**, *37*, 740–745. [CrossRef]
4. Ban, Y.; Shimazaki-Den, S.; Tsubota, K.; Shimazaki, J. Morphological evaluation of meibomian glands using noncontact infrared meibography. *Ocul. Surf.* **2013**, *11*, 47–53. [CrossRef]
5. Pult, H.; Riede-Pult, B.H.; Nichols, J.J. Relation between upper and lower lids' meibomian gland morphology, tear film, and dry eye. *Optom. Vis. Sci.* **2012**, *89*, E310–E315. [CrossRef]
6. Yin, Y.; Gong, L. Uneven Meibomian Gland Dropout Over the Tarsal Plate and its Correlation With Meibomian Gland Dysfunction. *Cornea* **2015**, *34*, 1200–1205. [CrossRef]
7. Pult, H.; Nichols, J.J. A review of meibography. *Optom. Vis. Sci.* **2012**, *89*, E760–E769. [CrossRef]
8. Srinivasan, S.; Menzies, K.; Sorbara, L.; Jones, L. Infrared imaging of meibomian gland structure using a novel keratograph. *Optom. Vis. Sci.* **2012**, *89*, E788–E794. [CrossRef]
9. Arita, R.; Itoh, K.; Inoue, K.; Amano, S. Noncontact infrared meibography to document age-related changes of the meibomian glands in a normal population. *Ophthalmology* **2008**, *115*, 911–915. [CrossRef]
10. Engel, L.A.; Wittig, S.; Bock, F.; Sauerbier, L.; Scheid, C.; Holtick, U.; Chemnitz, J.M.; Hallek, M.; Cursiefen, C.; Steven, P. Meibography and meibomian gland measurements in ocular graft-versus-host disease. *Bone Marrow Transplant.* **2015**, *50*, 961–967. [CrossRef]
11. Arita, R.; Suehiro, J.; Haraguchi, T.; Shirakawa, R.; Tokoro, H.; Amano, S. Objective image analysis of the meibomian gland area. *Br. J. Ophthalmol.* **2014**, *98*, 746–755. [CrossRef]
12. Xiao, P.; Luo, Z.; Deng, Y.; Wang, G.; Yuan, J. An automated and multiparametric algorithm for objective analysis of meibography images. *Quant. Imaging Med. Surg.* **2021**, *11*, 1586–1599. [CrossRef]
13. Llorens-Quintana, C.; Rico-Del-Viejo, L.; Syga, P.; Madrid-Costa, D.; Iskander, D.R. A Novel Automated Approach for Infrared-Based Assessment of Meibomian Gland Morphology. *Transl. Vis. Sci. Technol.* **2019**, *8*, 17. [CrossRef]
14. Ciężar, K.; Pochylski, M. 2D fourier transform for global analysis and classification of meibomian gland images. *Ocul. Surf.* **2020**, *18*, 865–870. [CrossRef]
15. Yeh, C.H.; Yu, S.X.; Lin, M.C. Meibography Phenotyping and Classification From Unsupervised Discriminative Feature Learning. *Transl. Vis. Sci. Technol.* **2021**, *10*, 4. [CrossRef]

16. Koh, Y.W.; Celik, T.; Lee, H.K.; Petznick, A.; Tong, L. Detection of meibomian glands and classification of meibography images. *J. Biomed. Opt.* **2012**, *17*, 086008. [CrossRef]
17. Wang, J.; Yeh, T.N.; Chakraborty, R.; Yu, S.X.; Lin, M.C. A Deep Learning Approach for Meibomian Gland Atrophy Evaluation in Meibography Images. *Transl. Vis. Sci. Technol.* **2019**, *8*, 37. [CrossRef]
18. Zhou, Y.W.; Yu, Y.; Zhou, Y.B.; Tan, Y.J.; Wu, L.L.; Xing, Y.Q.; Yang, Y.N. An advanced imaging method for measuring and assessing meibomian glands based on deep learning. *Zhonghua Yan Ke Za Zhi* **2020**, *56*, 774–779.
19. Maruoka, S.; Tabuchi, H.; Nagasato, D.; Masumoto, H.; Chikama, T.; Kawai, A.; Oishi, N.; Maruyama, T.; Kato, Y.; Hayashi, T.; et al. Deep Neural Network-Based Method for Detecting Obstructive Meibomian Gland Dysfunction with In Vivo Laser Confocal Microscopy. *Cornea* **2020**, *39*, 720–725. [CrossRef]
20. Dai, Q.; Liu, X.; Lin, X.; Fu, Y.; Chen, C.; Yu, X.; Zhang, Z.; Li, T.; Liu, M.; Yang, W.; et al. A Novel Meibomian Gland Morphology Analytic System Based on a Convolutional Neural Network. *IEEE Access* **2021**, *9*, 23083–23094. [CrossRef]
21. Arita, R.; Itoh, K.; Maeda, S.; Maeda, K.; Furuta, A.; Fukuoka, S.; Tomidokoro, A.; Amano, S. Proposed diagnostic criteria for obstructive meibomian gland dysfunction. *Ophthalmology* **2009**, *116*, 2058–2063.e1. [CrossRef]
22. He, K.; Gkioxari, G.; Dollar, P.; Girshick, R. Mask R-CNN. *IEEE Trans. Pattern. Anal. Mach. Intell.* **2020**, *42*, 386–397. [CrossRef]
23. Deng, J.; Dong, W.; Socher, R.; Li, L.; Kai, L.; Li, F. Imagenet: A large-scale hierarchical image database. In Proceedings of the 2009 IEEE Conference on Computer Vision and Pattern Recognition, Miami, FL, USA, 20–25 June 2009; pp. 248–255.
24. He, K.; Zhang, X.; Ren, S.; Sun, J. Deep Residual Learning for Image Recognition. In Proceedings of the IEEE Conference on Computer Vision and Pattern Recognition, Las Vegas, NV, USA, 27–30 June 2016; pp. 770–778.
25. Markoulli, M.; Duong, T.B.; Lin, M.; Papas, E. Imaging the Tear Film: A Comparison Between the Subjective Keeler Tearscope-Plus™ and the Objective Oculus® Keratograph 5M and LipiView® Interferometer. *Curr. Eye Res.* **2018**, *43*, 155–162. [CrossRef]
26. De Paiva, C.S.; Pflugfelder, S.C. Corneal epitheliopathy of dry eye induces hyperesthesia to mechanical air jet stimulation. *Am. J. Ophthalmol.* **2004**, *137*, 109–115. [CrossRef]
27. Cochener, B.; Cassan, A.; Omiel, L. Prevalence of meibomian gland dysfunction at the time of cataract surgery. *J. Cataract. Refract. Surg.* **2018**, *44*, 144–148. [CrossRef]
28. Lin, X.; Fu, Y.; Li, L.; Chen, C.; Chen, X.; Mao, Y.; Lian, H.; Yang, W.; Dai, Q. A Novel Quantitative Index of Meibomian Gland Dysfunction, the Meibomian Gland Tortuosity. *Transl. Vis. Sci. Technol.* **2020**, *9*, 34. [CrossRef]
29. García-Marqués, J.V.; García-Lázaro, S.; Talens-Estarelles, C.; Martínez-Albert, N.; Cerviño, A. Diagnostic Capability of a New Objective Method to Assess Meibomian Gland Visibility. *Optom. Vis. Sci.* **2021**, *98*, 1045–1055. [CrossRef]
30. Russakovsky, O.; Deng, J.; Su, H.; Krause, J.; Satheesh, S.; Ma, S.; Huang, Z.; Karpathy, A.; Khosla, A.; Bernstein, M.; et al. Imagenet large scale visual recognition challenge. *Int. J. Comput. Vis.* **2015**, *115*, 211–252. [CrossRef]
31. Burlina, P.; Pacheco, K.D.; Joshi, N.; Freund, D.E.; Bressler, N.M. Comparing humans and deep learning performance for grading AMD: A study in using universal deep features and transfer learning for automated AMD analysis. *Comput. Biol. Med.* **2017**, *82*, 80–86. [CrossRef]
32. Asaoka, R.; Murata, H.; Hirasawa, K.; Fujino, Y.; Matsuura, M.; Miki, A.; Kanamoto, T.; Ikeda, Y.; Mori, K.; Iwase, A.; et al. Using Deep Learning and Transfer Learning to Accurately Diagnose Early-Onset Glaucoma From Macular Optical Coherence Tomography Images. *Am. J. Ophthalmol.* **2019**, *198*, 136–145. [CrossRef]
33. Green-Church, K.B.; Butovich, I.; Willcox, M.; Borchman, D.; Paulsen, F.; Barabino, S.; Glasgow, B.J. The international workshop on meibomian gland dysfunction: Report of the subcommittee on tear film lipids and lipid-protein interactions in health and disease. *Investig. Ophthalmol. Vis. Sci.* **2011**, *52*, 1979–1993. [CrossRef]
34. Nelson, J.D.; Shimazaki, J.; Benitez-del-Castillo, J.M.; Craig, J.P.; McCulley, J.P.; Den, S.; Foulks, G.N. The international workshop on meibomian gland dysfunction: Report of the definition and classification subcommittee. *Investig. Ophthalmol. Vis. Sci.* **2011**, *52*, 1930–1937. [CrossRef]
35. Pflugfelder, S.C.; Tseng, S.C.; Sanabria, O.; Kell, H.; Garcia, C.G.; Felix, C.; Feuer, W.; Reis, B.L. Evaluation of subjective assessments and objective diagnostic tests for diagnosing tear-film disorders known to cause ocular irritation. *Cornea* **1998**, *17*, 38–56. [CrossRef]
36. Nichols, J.J.; Berntsen, D.A.; Mitchell, G.L.; Nichols, K.K. An assessment of grading scales for meibography images. *Cornea* **2005**, *24*, 382–388. [CrossRef]

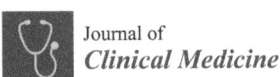

Article

Corneal Findings Associated to Belantamab-Mafodotin (Belamaf) Use in a Series of Patients Examined Longitudinally by Means of Advanced Corneal Imaging

Rita Mencucci [1,†], Michela Cennamo [1], Ludovica Alonzo [1], Carlotta Senni [2], Aldo Vagge [3,4], Lorenzo Ferro Desideri [3,4], Vincenzo Scorcia [5] and Giuseppe Giannaccare [5,*,†]

1. Department of Neurosciences, Psychology, Pharmacology and Child Health, Eye Clinic, University of Florence, 50134 Florence, Italy; rita.mencucci@unifi.it (R.M.); michelacennamo@libero.it (M.C.); ludovica.alonzo@gmail.com (L.A.)
2. Department of Ophthalmology, University Vita-Salute, IRCCS Ospedale San Raffaele, 20132 Milan, Italy; senni.carlotta@hsr.it
3. IRCCS Ospedale Policlinico San Martino, University Eye Clinic of Genoa, 16132 Genova, Italy; aldo.vagge@gmail.com (A.V.); lorenzoferrodes@gmail.com (L.F.D.)
4. Department of Neurosciences, Rehabilitation, Ophthalmology, Genetics, Maternal and Child Health (DiNOGMI), Università di Genova, 16126 Genova, Italy
5. Department of Ophthalmology, University Magna Græcia of Catanzaro, 88100 Catanzaro, Italy; vscorcia@unicz.it

* Correspondence: giuseppe.giannaccare@unicz.it; Tel.: +39-09613647041
† These authors contributed equally to this work.

Abstract: Belantamab mafodotin (belamaf) is a novel antibody–drug conjugate developed for the treatment of patients with relapsed or refractory multiple myeloma (RRMM). Although the drug has demonstrated a good efficacy, corneal adverse events have been reported. In this prospective study, consecutive patients with RRMM who received belamaf infusions were included. The standard ophthalmological visit was implemented with anterior segment (AS)-optical coherence tomography (OCT) and in vivo confocal microscopy (IVCM). Five patients (three males, two females; mean age 66 ± 6.0 years) with MMRR and unremarkable ocular findings at baseline who received belamaf infusion were included. After a median time of 28 days from the first infusion, four of them developed corneal alterations with transient vision reduction to a variable extent. In particular, corneal deposits of microcyst-like epithelial changes (MECs) were detected centrally in one patient and peripherally in three patients. AS-OCT scans showed a bilateral heterogeneous increase in signal intensity, together with hyper-reflective lesions confined within the epithelium in all cases, except for one case in which they also involved the stroma. Corneal maps showed a transient increase in epithelial thickness in the first phase that was followed by a diffuse decrease in the subsequent phase. IVCM scans showed MECs as hyper-reflective opacities located at the level of corneal epithelium, largely intracellular. Multimodal corneal imaging may implement the current clinical scale, helping us to detect corneal abnormalities in patients under belamaf therapy. This workup provides useful data for monitoring over time corneal findings and for optimizing systemic therapy.

Keywords: belantamab mafoditin; belamaf; multiple myeloma; cornea; side effects; vision

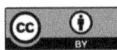

1. Introduction

Ocular surface diseases are common among hematological patients, either due to the underlying diseases or the therapies employed for their treatment [1–3]. Multiple myeloma (MM) is a hematologic cancer characterized by uncontrolled proliferation and subsequent accumulation of malignant plasma cells in bone marrow. Despite the continuous attempt at improving management by investigating new classes of therapeutic agents, unfortunately, MM is still characterized by a poor prognosis. Indeed, a significant number of patients develop relapsed or refractory MM (RRMM) that is resistant to current standard-of-care options, pointing out the widespread problem of an unmet medical need [4].

Belantamab mafodotin (balamaf) is a first-in-class antibody–drug conjugate developed for the treatment of patients with RRMM. It consists of an anti-BMCA mAb conjugated to the microtubule inhibitor monomethyl auristatin F. Belamaf eliminates MM cells by multiple mechanisms of action, including apoptosis, antibody-dependent cell-mediated anti-myeloma responses, accompanied by the release of markers characteristic of immunogenic cell death [5]. Although the drug has demonstrated a deep and durable response in this type of patients, various corneal alterations have been reported so far, making the multidisciplinary management even more challenging.

Herein, we present a series of patients who developed corneal adverse events associated with belamaf use and describe features, clinical outcomes, and potential importance to oncologists as a harbinger of serious ocular sequelae. Furthermore, a multimodal imaging-based diagnostic workup used in this series to detect and monitor over time corneal alterations is presented.

2. Materials and Methods

This is a prospective observational study conducted at the Careggi University Hospital (Florence, Italy) that included consecutive patients who received belamaf infusions at the recommended dose (2.5 mg/kg) every 3 weeks for the treatment of RRMM between January 2021 and March 2021. All patients underwent an ophthalmological visit before starting treatment, including best corrected visual acuity (BCVA) testing, slit lamp evaluation of the cornea with photograph, intraocular pressure measurement and fundoscopy. The standard visit was implemented with a diagnostic workup focused on cornea that included anterior segment (AS)-optical coherence tomography (OCT) for the studying of corneal maps and in vivo confocal microscopy (IVCM). In particular, corneal epithelial thickness was measured in 5 sectors: one central 3 mm diameter and four inner sectors (inferior, superior, nasal, and temporal) within a ring (3–6 mm in diameter). Patients were followed-up for at least 12 months and underwent serial ophthalmological visits before each drug infusion.

3. Results

Overall, five patients (three males, two females; mean age 66 ± 6.0 years) with MMRR were screened for belamaf infusion during the study period. At baseline, all of them presented full vision (mean pre-belamaf BCVA of 20/20) and did not present any remarkable corneal findings; thus, they were treated with belamaf according to drug protocol. Following a mean time of 28 days from the first belamaf infusion, four patients developed corneal alterations with a variable degree of vision reduction (mean post-belamaf BCVA of 20/32). On slit lamp examination, corneal deposits with microcyst-like epithelial changes (MECs) were detected bilaterally in the center of the cornea in one patient and in the peripheral cornea in three patients (Figure 1). Of note, the patient with central MECs complained of blurred vision, while two of the remaining patients with peripheral MECs reported only dry-eye-like symptoms. Two patients switched to a modified therapy regimen, delaying by a week the treatment due to corneal adverse events. In two cases, the epithelial lesions, which were initially small and located in corneal periphery and mid-periphery, migrated towards central cornea, becoming progressively more numerous; afterwards, they slowly decreased in number, as demonstrated both clinically and instrumentally.

AS-OCT scans showed a bilateral heterogeneous increase in signal intensity, together with hyper-reflective lesions corresponding to visible corneal alterations at slit lamp. These lesions were confined within the epithelium, but in one case, they migrated deeper, involving the stroma (Figure 2).

Corneal epithelial maps showed a transient CET increase soon after the first infusion, followed by a progressive decrease during the following infusions ("plateau phase") (Figures 3 and 4).

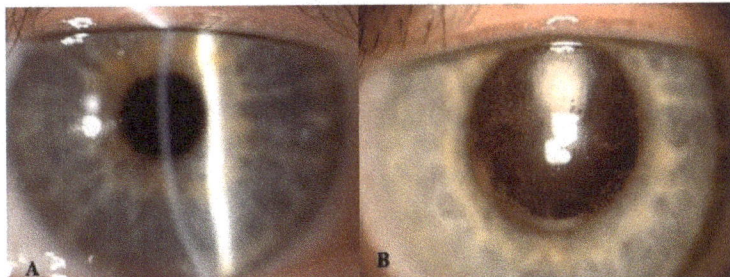

Figure 1. Slit-lamp photograph of the cornea in a patient with belamaf keratopathy. (**A**): Diffuse microcystic-like epithelial changes (MECs) in the central cornea. (**B**): Better visualization of MECs aided by retroillumination and pupil dilation.

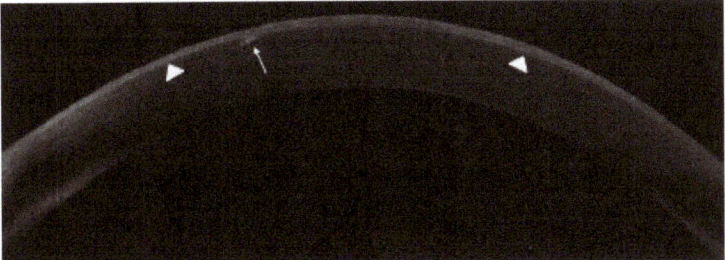

Figure 2. Anterior segment optical coherence tomography (AS-OCT) in a patient with belamaf keratopathy showing heterogeneous, diffuse corneal epithelium hyper-reflectivity corresponding to MECs (arrowheads), with a small hyper-reflective area extending to the anterior stroma associated with a focal interruption of the Bowman layer (arrow).

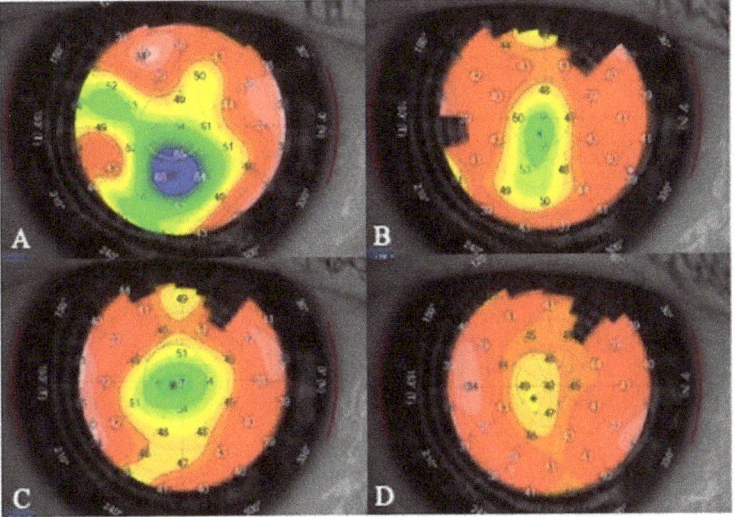

Figure 3. Corneal epithelial thickness (CET) mapping during monthly infusions of belamaf in a patient with belamaf keratopathy. (**A**): Before the second infusion showing a localized transitory CET increase; (**B**–**D**): Progressive reduction in CET over time, respectively, before the third, fourth and fifth infusion ("plateau phase").

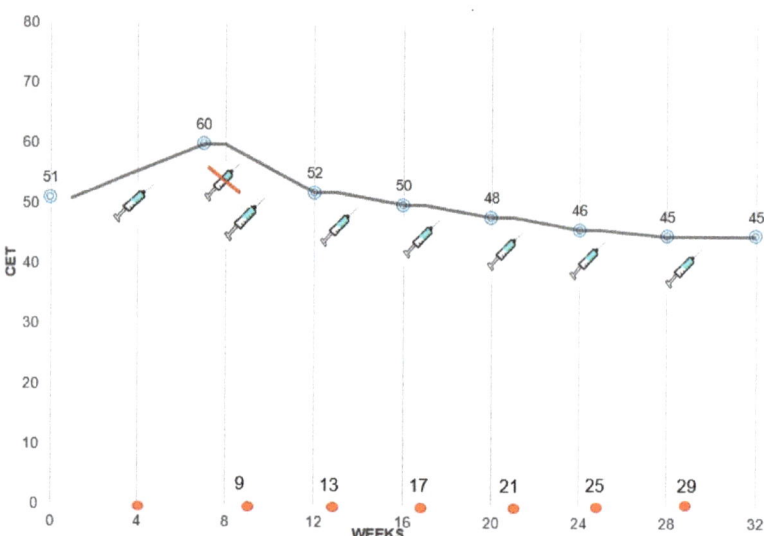

Figure 4. Graph showing the changes of average values of corneal epithelial thickness (CET) measured in 5 sectors according to the infusion of belamaf in a representative patient. After the first dose, an increase in CET with the appearance of central MECs and vision reduction were found. The second dose was therefore delayed by one week. After the third and the fourth dose, a diffuse decrease in CET was assessed, followed by a "plateau phase" after the fifth dose. CET values are expressed in micron.

Using IVCM, MECs appeared as hyper-reflective opacities, sometimes arranged in clusters, resembling a "pseudo-rosette" pattern, located at the level of corneal epithelium, largely intracellular. In particular, in one patient, multiple hyper-reflective deposits were detected inside corneal epithelium at the level of alar and basal corneal cells rather than superficial cells; in another patient, completely asymptomatic, isolated peripheral sub-epithelial opacities were detected that subsequently were also found at the level of anterior stroma by means of IVCM (Figure 5).

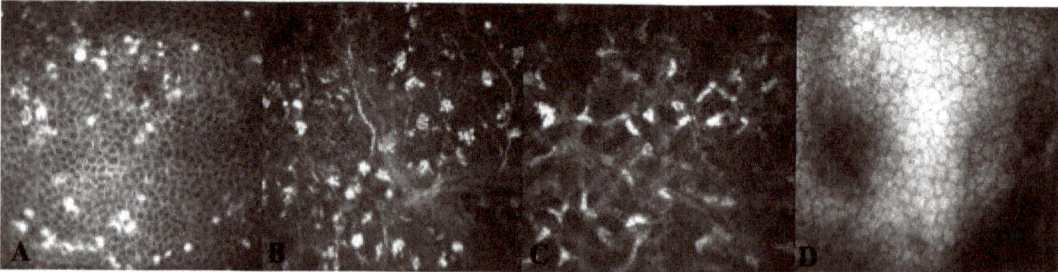

Figure 5. In vivo confocal microscopy (IVCM) of the cornea in a patient with belamaf keratopathy. (**A**): MECs appeared as hyper-reflective (at least predominantly) intracellular opacities present at the level of basal epithelium. (**B**): Hyperreflective lesions arranged in clusters, resembling "pseudo-rosette" pattern at the level of sub-basal nerve plexus. (**C**): Activated keratocyte network detected in the anterior stroma. (**D**): Normal endothelial cells morphology.

4. Discussion

Since the introduction of belamaf therapy for RRMM, a number of corneal side effects have been attributed to its use. These mostly include superficial punctate keratopathy and/or MECs detectable at slit lamp examination. Of note, ocular adverse events such as blurred vision, dry-eye-like symptoms and keratopathy have been reported in 69% to 74% of patients in the DREAMM-1 and DREAMM-2 trials, requiring dose reduction or even interruption in 27% to 46% of cases [6,7]. Remarkably, other off-label drugs previously adopted for the treatment of MM were shown to induce corneal epithelial alterations, probably resulting from drug accumulation in the epithelium and subsequent cellular apoptosis. Among these, depatuximab mafoditin, which acts as an epidermal growth factor receptor inhibitor, caused a reversible corneal epitheliopathy in treated patients, characterized by multiple and diffuse hyper-reflective spots, progressive sub-basal nerve plexus fragmentation and by the appearance of cystic structures at the level of corneal epithelium [8–10].

Belamaf-related corneal alterations usually originate in the peripheral region of the cornea and then gradually migrate towards the center ("centripetal pattern") [4]. The localization of corneal opacities in the central cornea along with the related irregular astigmatism determine changes in vision, including subjective blurred vision. However, a linear relationship between the severity of keratopathy and the reduction in vision has not been observed. More recently, corneal staining patterns suggestive of limbal stem cell deficiency have been described in a cohort of patients receiving prolonged therapy [11].

Corneal toxicity is more likely to occur when the drug is used at higher doses, and the proposed mechanism is thought to derive from the off-target effect of its cytotoxic component (i.e., the microtubule-disrupting monomethyl auristatin-F [MMAF]) [6].

Efforts are being made to understand the etiology behind this clinical entity in order to identify potential mitigation strategies. For this task, multimodal imaging is of crucial importance, as it helps to better characterize the nature of such findings. Of note, the involved areas of corneal epithelium were found to contain hyper-reflective material, rather than microcysts on IVCM. The solid nature of these epithelial lesions is also corroborated by AS-OCT, where they appear once again hyper-reflective. Therefore, this material could potentially represent the accumulation of apoptotic end products in the intercellular spaces of corneal epithelium. Similarly, hyper-reflective lesions on AS-OCT may be the consequence of the accumulation of either pre-apoptotic or degenerated cells caused by the internalization of belantamab [11]. Specifically, it has been hypothesized that belamaf could reach the cornea through limbal vessels or tears and could then undergo cellular uptake into the corneal basal epithelial layer. Once internalized into epithelial cells, it may induce their apoptosis via microtubulin inhibition during their travel from the basal layer towards the surface and the center of cornea [12]. Nevertheless, belamaf deposits were identified also in the sub-Bowman layer, suggesting that other mechanisms of toxicity might also be involved [13].

In order to provide a common standardized and repeatable tool for clinical evaluation, an expert board has recently proposed a keratopathy and visual acuity scale (KVA scale) based on the worst finding of either keratopathy subjectively graded on slit lamp examination (the deeper is the corneal involvement the worst is the grade of the keratopathy) or visual acuity testing. Recommendations for the management of corneal events have been formulated according to the KVA scale as follows: continue treatment at the current dose for grade 1/mild events; delay treatment for grade 2/moderate events until the event improves to a grade 1/mild event or resolves, or for grade 3/4 (severe) events, until these improve to a grade 1/mild event [6].

Our report aimed at describing corneal findings of patients receiving belamaf infusions for RRMM, especially focusing on clinical course monitored by different corneal imaging techniques. Thanks to advances in multimodal corneal imaging including IVCM and AS-OCT, ophthalmologists may benefit from these techniques by easily detecting corneal abnormalities, even at a subclinical stage, and subsequently defining and monitoring over time the entity of corneal involvement [11–14].

Using IVCM, MECs appear as hyper-reflective opacities, sometimes arranged in a "pseudo-rosette" pattern, located within the basal epithelium and the sub-basal nerve plexus; the stroma shows only non-specific signs of inflammation with sporadic activated keratocytes, while the endothelium is typically unaffected; specific lesions at the sub-basal nerve plexus layer were also recently detected and characterized [13]. However, although IVCM is very sensitive to identify potential preclinical findings, it does not provide quantitative measurements of biomarkers useful for monitoring over time corneal changes, especially when few modifications must be detected. Using AS-OCT, corneal alterations can be detected as hyper-reflective lesions, usually located within the corneal epithelium. In one case of our series, it allowed for the identification of lesions located deeper in the stroma (Figure 2). To the best of our knowledge, this AS-OCT finding is reported here for the first time. Furthermore, corneal maps allowed us to measure the thickness of the corneal epithelium that was found to be increased in the initial phase of the keratopathy and then tended to decrease to baseline values (Figure 3) [11].

However, it should be pointed out that, since half of the patients may present objective signs of keratopathy without reporting any symptoms, ophthalmic examination should be performed at baseline and before each dose of the drug in order to detect early corneal changes.

The management of belamaf-induced toxicity requires a multidisciplinary approach involving a hematologist and an ophthalmologist, and the clinical decision should be reached together taking into account the individual benefit/risk ratio according to both ocular and systemic conditions. Overall, single-agent belamaf (2.5 mg/kg) has shown a manageable safety profile. Ocular alterations usually recover spontaneously once treatment is discontinued or may be successfully reversed with dose tapering or by delaying the time interval of suspension between two cycles. This evidence is based on the experience of a DREAMM-2 study that reported the need for drug discontinuation due to keratopathy in only 1 out 95 patients who received the 2.5 mg/kg dose, indicating that patients were able to remain on treatment while these events were monitored [5]. In this regard, the recent flow chart of multidisciplinary approach created by an expert board for managing corneal events with belamaf will assist physician to better cope with this condition [6]. The implementation of the KVA scale with a multimodal corneal imaging may further help to detect corneal abnormalities, even at a subclinical stage, providing useful data for monitoring over time corneal findings and for optimizing belamaf therapy. Although both AS-OCT and IVCM represent two valuable tools for this task, the former examination and, in particular, corneal topography with specific focus on the epithelial map could be incorporated in the current clinical scale (KVA) in order to quantify corneal involvement and provide a reliable biomarker. Furthermore, unlike IVCM, this technique is completely noninvasive and is available in almost the totality of ophthalmic departments.

Future prospective trials are needed to provide more comprehensive information about belamaf-associated keratopathy as well as for identifying the most appropriate diagnostic workup able to optimize therapy in RRMM patients.

Author Contributions: Conceptualization, M.C.; Data curation, L.A., L.F.D. and G.G.; Formal analysis, R.M. and L.A.; Investigation, M.C. and G.G.; Methodology, M.C., C.S., A.V., L.F.D. and G.G.; Project administration, L.F.D.; Resources, C.S.; Supervision, V.S.; Validation, A.V.; Visualization, V.S.; Writing—review & editing, A.V., L.F.D. and V.S. All authors have read and agreed to the published version of the manuscript.

Funding: This research received no external funding.

Institutional Review Board Statement: All subjects gave their informed consent for inclusion before they participated in the study. The study was conducted in accordance with the Declaration of Helsinki. It represents an observational case series deemed not to constitute research, therefore a specific ethics committee/IRB approval was not required.

Informed Consent Statement: Informed consent was obtained from all subjects involved in the study.

Data Availability Statement: The data presented in this study are available on request from the corresponding author. The data are not publicly available due to privacy issues.

Conflicts of Interest: The authors declare no conflict of interes.

References

1. Klintworth, G.K.; Bredehoeft, S.J.; Reed, J.W. Analysis of corneal crystalline deposits in multiple myeloma. *Am. J. Ophthalmol.* **1978**, *86*, 303–313. [CrossRef]
2. Giannaccare, G.; Pellegrini, M.; Bernabei, F.; Scorcia, V.; Campos, E. Ocular surface system alterations in ocular graft-versus-host disease: All the pieces of the complex puzzle. *Graefes Arch. Clin. Exp. Ophthalmol.* **2019**, *257*, 1341–1351. [CrossRef] [PubMed]
3. Chiang, J.C.B.; Zahari, I.; Markoulli, M.; Krishnan, A.V.; Park, S.B.; Semmler, A.; Goldstein, D.; Edwards, K. The impact of anticancer drugs on the ocular surface. *Ocul. Surf.* **2020**, *18*, 403–417. [CrossRef] [PubMed]
4. Farooq, A.V.; Degli Esposti, S.; Popat, R.; Thulasi, P.; Lonial, S.; Nooka, A.K.; Jakubowiak, A.; Sborov, D.; Zaugg, B.E.; Badros, A.Z.; et al. Corneal Epithelial Findings in Patients with Multiple Myeloma Treated with Antibody-Drug Conjugate Belantamab Mafodotin in the Pivotal, Randomized, DREAMM-2 Study. *Ophthalmol. Ther.* **2020**, *9*, 889–911. [CrossRef] [PubMed]
5. Lonial, S.; Nooka, A.K.; Thulasi, P.; Badros, A.Z.; Jeng, B.H.; Callander, N.S.; Potter, H.A.; Sborov, D.; Zaugg, B.E.; Popat, R.; et al. Management of belantamab mafodotin-associated corneal events in patients with relapsed or refractory multiple myeloma (RRMM). *Blood Cancer J.* **2021**, *11*, 103. [CrossRef] [PubMed]
6. Lonial, S.; Lee, H.C.; Badros, A.; Trudel, S.; Nooka, A.K.; Chari, A.; Abdallah, A.-O.; Callander, N.; Lendvai, N.; Sborov, D.; et al. Belantamab mafodotin for relapsed or refractory multiple myeloma (DREAMM-2): A two-arm, randomised, open-label, phase 2 study. *Lancet Oncol.* **2020**, *21*, 207–221. [CrossRef]
7. Trudel, S.; Lendvai, N.; Popat, R.; Voorhees, P.M.; Reeves, B.; Libby, E.N.; Richardson, P.G.; Hoos, A.; Gupta, I.; Bragulat, V.; et al. Antibody–Drug Conjugate, GSK2857916, in Relapsed/Refractory Multiple Myeloma: An Update on Safety and Efficacy from Dose Expansion Phase I Study. *Blood Cancer J.* **2019**, *9*, 37. [CrossRef] [PubMed]
8. Rocha-de-Lossada, C.; Alba Linero, C.; Santos Ortega, A.; Rodríguez Calvo-de-Mora, M.; Rachwani, R.; Borroni, D.; Alba, E.; Benavides Orgaz, M.; Romano, V. Ocular surface toxicity of depatuxizumab mafoditin (ABT-414): Case reports. *Arq. Bras. Oftalmol.* **2021**. [CrossRef]
9. Lee, B.A.; Lee, M.S.; Maltry, A.C.; Hou, J.H. Clinical and Histological Characterization of Toxic Keratopathy from Depatuxizumab Mafodotin (ABT-414), an Antibody-Drug Conjugate. *Cornea* **2021**, *40*, 1197–1200. [CrossRef] [PubMed]
10. Parrozzani, R.; Lombardi, G.; Midena, E.; Londei, D.; Padovan, M.; Marchione, G.; Caccese, M.; Midena, G.; Zagonel, V.; Frizziero, L. Ocular Side Effects of EGFR-Inhibitor ABT-414 in Recurrent Glioblastoma: A Long-Term Safety Study. *Front. Oncol.* **2020**, *10*, 593461. [CrossRef] [PubMed]
11. Bausell, R.B.; Soleimani, A.; Vinnett, A.; Baroni, M.D.; Staub, S.A.; Binion, K.; Jeng, B.H.; Badros, A.Z.; Munir, W.M. Corneal changes after Belantamab mafodotin in multiple myeloma patients. *Eye Contact Lens.* **2021**, *47*, 362–365. [CrossRef] [PubMed]
12. Wahab, A.; Rafae, A.; Mushtaq, K.; Masood, A.; Ehsan, H.; Khakwani, M.; Khan, A. Ocular Toxicity of Belantamab Mafodotin, an Oncological Perspective of Management in Relapsed and Refractory Multiple Myeloma. *Front. Oncol.* **2021**, *11*, 678634. [CrossRef] [PubMed]
13. Marquant, K.; Quinquenel, A.; Arndt, C.; Denoyer, A. Corneal in vivo confocal microscopy to detect belantamab mafodotin-induced ocular toxicity early and adjust the dose accordingly: A case report. *J. Hematol. Oncol.* **2021**, *14*, 159. [CrossRef] [PubMed]
14. Matsumiya, W.; Karaca, I.; Ghoraba, H.; Akhavanrezayat, A.; Mobasserian, A.; Hassan, M.; Regenold, J.; Yasar, C.; Liedtke, M.; Kitazawa, K.; et al. Structural changes of corneal epithelium in belantamab-associated superficial keratopathy using anterior segment optical coherence tomography. *Am. J. Ophthalmol. Case Rep.* **2021**, *23*, 101133. [CrossRef] [PubMed]

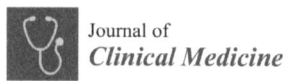

Article

Specular Microscopy of Human Corneas Stored in an Active Storage Machine

Thibaud Garcin [1,2,*], Emmanuel Crouzet [2], Chantal Perrache [2], Thierry Lepine [2,3], Philippe Gain [1,2] and Gilles Thuret [1,2,4]

[1] Ophthalmology Department, University Hospital, 42000 Saint-Etienne, France; philippe.gain@univ-st-etienne.fr (P.G.); gilles.thuret@univ-st-etienne.fr (G.T.)
[2] Corneal Graft Biology, Engineering and Imaging Laboratory, BiiGC, EA2521, Federative Institute of Research in Sciences and Health Engineering, Faculty of Medicine, Jean Monnet University, Rue de la Marandière, 42000 Saint-Etienne, France; e.crouzet@univ-st-etienne.fr (E.C.); chantal.perrache@univ-st-etienne.fr (C.P.); thierry.lepine@institutoptique.fr (T.L.)
[3] Laboratory Hubert Curien, Optics Institute Graduate School, 42000 Saint-Etienne, France
[4] Institut Universitaire de France, Boulevard Saint-Michel, 75005 Paris, France
* Correspondence: t.garcin@univ-st-etienne.fr; Tel.: +33-(0)4-77-12-77-93; Fax: +33-(0)4-77-12-09-95

Abstract: Purpose: Unlike corneas stored in cold storage (CS) which remain transparent and thin, corneas stored in organoculture (OC) cannot be assessed by specular microscopy (SM), because edema and posterior folds occur during storage and prevent from specular reflection. We previously developed an active storage machine (ASM) which restores the intraocular pressure while renewing the storage medium, thus preventing major stromal edema. Its transparent windows allow multimodal corneal imaging in a closed system. Aim: to present SM of corneas stored in this ASM. Methods: Ancillary study of two preclinical studies on corneas stored for one and three months in the ASM. A prototype non-contact SM was developed (CMOS camera, ×10 objective, collimated LED source, micrometric stage). Five non-overlapping fields (935 × 748 µm) were acquired in exactly the same areas at regular intervals. Image quality was graded according to defined categories (American Cornea Donor Study). The endothelial cell density (ECD) was measured with a center method. Finally, $_{SM}$ECD was also compared to Hoechst-stained cell nuclei count ($_{Hoechst}$ECD). Results: The 62 corneas remained thin during storage, allowing SM at all time points without corneal deconditioning. Image quality varied depending on donors and days of control but, overall, in the 1100 images, we observed 55% of excellent and 30% of good quality images. $_{SM}$ECD did not differ from $_{Hoechst}$ECD ($p = 0.084$). Conclusions: The ASM combines the advantages of CS (closed system) and OC (long-term storage). Specular microscopy is possible at any time in the ASM with a large field of view, making endothelial controls easy and safe.

Keywords: active storage machine; cornea; endothelium; endothelial cell density; eye bank; long-term storage; specular microscopy; viable endothelial cell density; image analysis

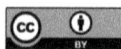

1. Introduction

Short-term cold storage (CS) at 4 °C and long-term organ culture (OC) at 31–37 °C, the two storage methods in use worldwide, have a mandatory step of endothelial assessment. Endothelial cell density (ECD) remains the main quality criterion of a stored cornea because endothelial cells (EC), which ensure the stability of corneal transparency, do not renew in humans and because donor EC die faster during storage [1–5] and in recipients than do native, healthy EC [6].

To acquire images of the EC in these two storage systems, different methods exist. During CS, specular microscopy (SM) can provide non-invasive images of the EC through the wall of the corneal storage-viewing chamber or the vials, because the hyperosmolar medium keeps the cornea thin, and thus, its endothelial surface remains folded very little.

Specular reflection is therefore possible on this nearly smooth surface. During OC, SM is impossible because the cornea quickly becomes edematous (its thickness can double), which induces numerous and deep posterior folds. To see the EC, it is therefore essential to use a transmitted light microscopy method (bright-field or phase-contrast) and to make the EC visible by temporarily dilating the intercellular spaces through a brief exposure to 0.9% sodium chloride, 1.8% sucrose, or hypotonic sodium-balanced salt. This endothelial control is therefore more restrictive and invasive. The two methods are therefore neither interchangeable nor equivalent.

To reproduce a more physiological corneal environment and break the vicious circle of hypotonia—corneal edema—deep posterior folds—endothelial lesion [2,3], we developed an active storage machine (ASM), also called a bioreactor, that reproduces a transcorneal pressure gradient equivalent to the intraocular pressure (IOP) and produces a renewal of the nutrient medium [7]. In two successive ex vivo experiments on pairs of fresh human corneas, we compared the ASM and OC using the same commercial storage medium for 1 month [8] and 3 months [9]. We demonstrated that, contrary to OC, the ASM prevented the corneas from majorly swelling, allowing them to be permanently ready for transplantation with significantly more viable EC than in OC. Furthermore, the better control of corneal thickness in the ASM allowed endothelial controls to be performed by SM.

In our ancillary study of two preclinical studies on corneas stored in the ASM for one and three months, we analyzed the quality of endothelial images obtained by SM.

2. Materials and Methods

2.1. Study Design: Ancillary Study of 1-Month and 3-Month Storage Experiments in the ASM

We analyzed all the SM images obtained on corneas stored in the ASM during the 2 validation studies of this new device [8,9]. All procedures conformed to the tenets of the Declaration of Helsinki for biomedical research involving human subjects. The French Agence de la Biomédecine specifically authorized the retrieval of corneas for these preclinical studies (PFS15-008 and PFS16-010). For the fifty corneas stored in the ASM for one month, EC counts were performed on day (D) 2, 26, and 28. For the twelve corneas stored in the ASM for three months, EC counts were performed on D2, 23, 44, 65, 86, and 88. The complete system of the ASM, control panels excepted, was placed in a 31 °C dry 5% CO_2 incubator. The medium used was CorneaMax, a CE marked OC Dulbecco's Modified Eagle Medium–based medium containing 2% FCS, penicillin, and streptomycin (Eurobio, les Ulis, France). The medium flow rate was set at 2.6 µL/min (normal aqueous humor flow rate) and the transcorneal pressure gradient at 21.5 mmHg (upper limit of normal IOP in humans) with atmospheric pressure as a reference.

In these two studies, we performed a measurement of viable ECD (vECD) by a destructive technique known as triple Hoechst-Ethidium-Calcein-AM staining, which we had previously described, at the end of storage [10,11] (*detailed in part 2.5*). We therefore used the images of the Hoechst staining of all nuclei to obtain a very accurate $_{Hoechst}ECD$ measurement of very large areas. We then compared the SM endothelial counts ($_{SM}ECD$) with the $_{Hoechst}ECD$, which was considered our gold standard.

2.2. Building of a Customized Specular Microscope

A custom SM was built because the 3 commercial eye bank SMs (ebSM) available in our laboratory were not adapted for the ASM. The standard equipment of the HAI EB-2000xyz (HAI, Lexington, KY, USA) and of the EB-10 and Cell-ChekD(+) (KONAN, Nishinomiya, Japan) could not accept the ASM cassette on their stage and/or the working distance of their objective was too short.

Our non-contact SM comprised (Figure 1): an optical bench (Thorlabs, Newton, MA, USA), a CMOS camera (DCC3240M, Thorlabs) equipped with a long working distance (10×/0.25, N Plan,∞/−/B) objective (Leica, Wetzlar, Germany) and driven by Scientific Imaging Thorcam v2.6.7064 software, an LED driver on constant current mode (LEDD1B, Thorlabs), an external LED source (MCWHL5-C2, Thorlabs) mounted and collimated with a diaphragm (SM1D12, Thorlabs) and a plano-convex lens (f30mm LA1805-A, Thorlabs), and a certified micrometric translation XYZ stage (M-UMR5.16A; sensitivity 0.1 μm for the Z axis (SM-13); 1 μm for the XY axis (BM11.10), Newport, Irvine, CA, USA) activated manually and connected to a 3D-printed support intended to receive the ASM. Accuracy in XYZ was verified using calibrated ceramic gage blocks (Mitotoyo, Roissy, France). The resulting field of view of our SM was 935 × 748 μm, with 1280 × 1024 pixels TIFF images' acquisition (2.6Mo). Image calibration was verified using a 10 mm scale with 50 μm divisions (R1L3S1P, Thorlabs).

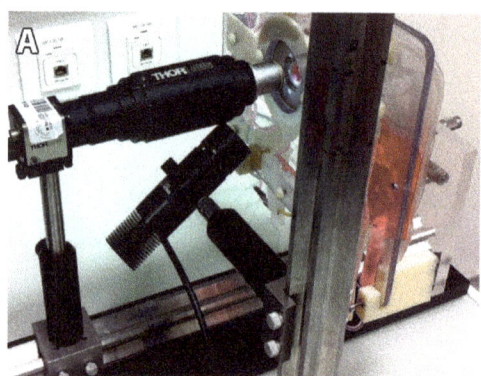
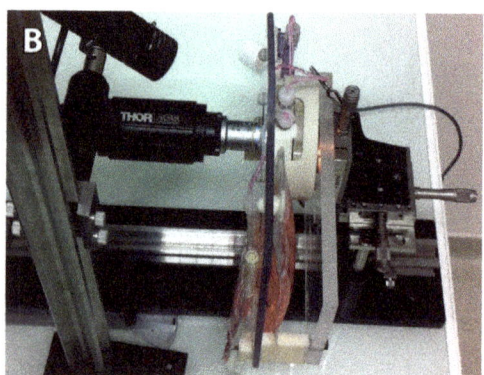
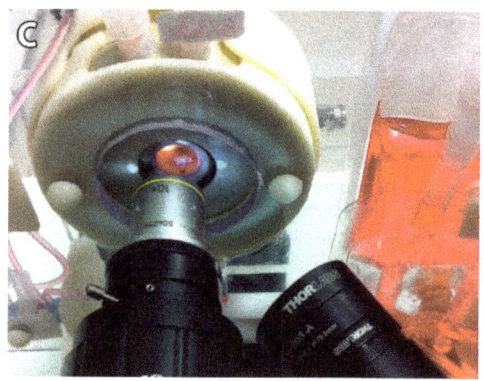
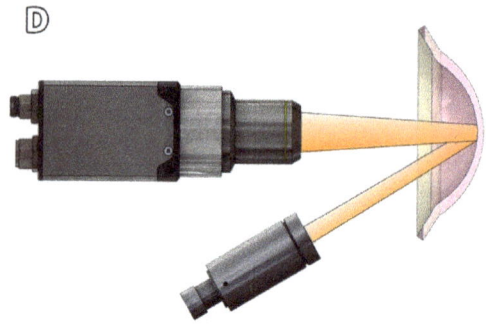

Figure 1. Custom-made specular microscope prototype adapted for our active storage machine (ASM). (**A**) General view of the optical bench, the camera and its objective, the led source, and the 3D-printed support intended to receive the ASM. Note the working distance, the collimated source, and the diaphragm produce a light beam focused on endothelial side of the cornea. (**B**) The ASM could be moved precisely thanks to the micrometric translation XYZ stage. (**C**) Close-up view, with one quadrant. (**D**) Schematic view of specular reflection from endothelial side of the cornea. The collimated source illuminated a corneal area, and the camera recorded the specular reflection.

Although no direct comparison was possible between the 3 commercial microscopes and our prototype, we used an additional cornea stored at 4 °C in Optisol-GS (Bausch & Lomb, Laval, QC, Canada) in a corneal storage viewing chamber (Krolman, Boston, MA, USA) to indirectly compare the surface of the observation fields (Figure 2).

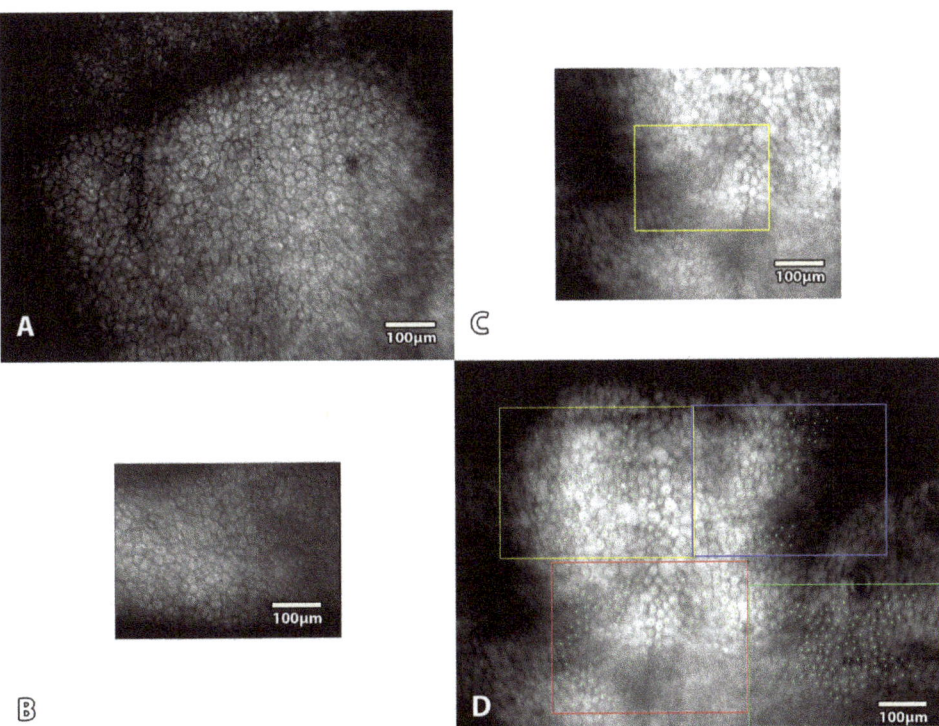

Figure 2. Comparison between our prototype and 3 eye banks' specular microscopes (SM). (**A**) The custom-made prototype SM with 935 × 748 μm and 1280 × 1024 pixels TIFF image. The entire surface could be analyzed. (**B**) The HAI EB-2000xyz had a 368 × 490 μm field of view (480 × 640 pixels BMP image) and analysis (3.9 times smaller). (**C**) The KONAN EB-10 had a 480 × 600 μm field of view (595 × 794 pixels BMP image) and a 280 × 200 μm field of analysis (respectively 2.4 and 12.5 times smaller). (**D**) The KONAN Cell-ChekD(+) had a 1000 × 750 μm field of view (1296 × 972 pixels BMP image) and up to 4 areas of 400 × 300 μm field of analysis (respectively 1.1 times larger but 1.5 times smaller).

2.3. Image Acquisition

Endothelial images were acquired through the endothelial glass window (flat sapphire glass, diameter 23.7 mm, thickness 0.9 mm, France Fourniture Horlogerie, Vence, France) of the ASM without deconditioning the corneas. Both ends of the endothelial chamber tubes were temporarily clamped to maintain pressure inside the endothelial chamber and allow the ASM's removal from the CO_2 incubator (in this experimental version of the ASM, tubes were permeable to gas, and the OC medium used a bicarbonate buffer, making it mandatory to use a 5% CO_2 atmosphere to maintain a physiologic pH).

We standardized the image acquisition: To retrieve specular reflection, the LED source was placed on the endothelial side of the cornea at 31 ± 4° from the camera optical axis. To modulate the contrasts and observe either the EC or the epithelium, the LED source was also specifically inclined on the Y axis (15 ± 4°). The camera software settings were presettled to optimize image quality: pixel clock (20 MHz), fixed frame rate (4.20FPS), fixed exposure time (16.70 ms), pixel data format 8-bit monochrome, gamma software (1.00), automatic image gain, and black level offset auto-adaptation according to each LED source position. Five non-overlapping fields of EC—one in the center and one per quadrant—were acquired inside the 8 central mm (the area usually grafted) (Figure 3). For each cornea, exactly the same area of each field was manually acquired, thanks to our calibrated device, by certified micrometers in this prototype version (position recorded for each cornea), at different periods for the 1-month [8] and 3-month [9] storage periods. Image acquisition took fewer than 10 min.

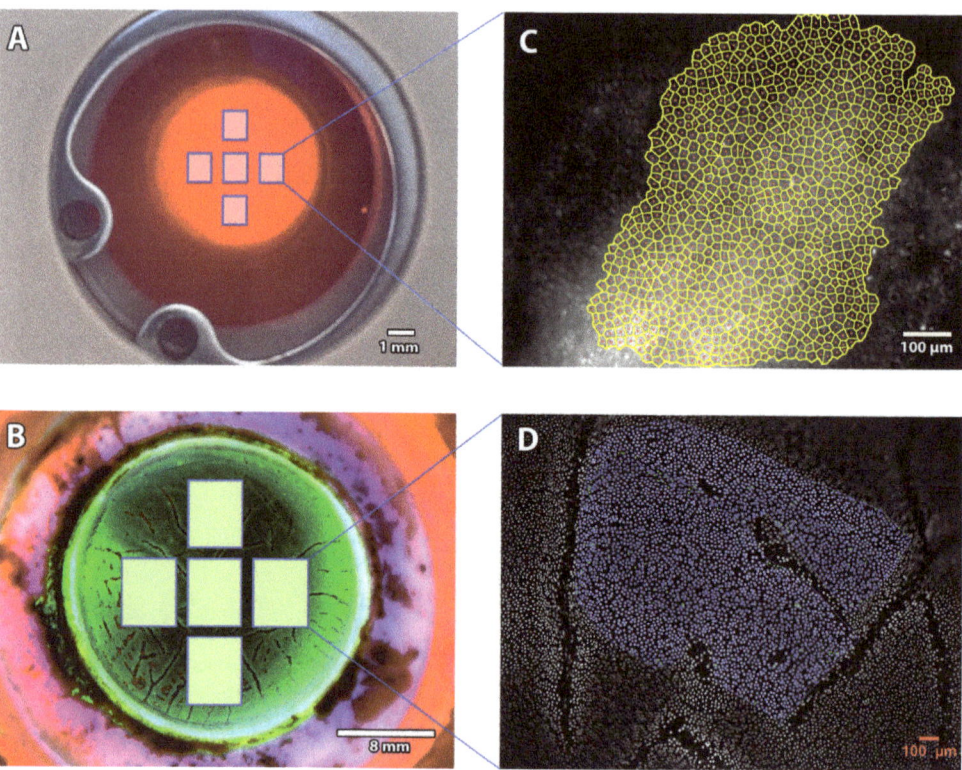

Figure 3. Image acquisition methods. (**A**) Five non-overlapping fields were captured with our non-contact specular microscope. (**B**) Pancorneal triple Hoechst-Etidium-Calcein staining. Five non-overlapping fields were analyzed. In the present study, we used the Hoechst staining image (100% visible nuclei) as a gold standard to analyze the accuracy of specular count. (**C**) Each field was analyzed with validated variable-frame center method [12,13]. (**D**) A close-up view of one of the fields, nuclei of the endothelial cells were counted thanks to the CorneaJ plugin [10,11].

2.4. Image Quality Classification

Endothelial SM images were classified in reference to the Specular Microscopy Ancillary Study (SMAS) of the American Cornea Donor Study [14,15]. We categorized images as either analyzable (subclassified as excellent, good, and fair) or unanalyzable. Briefly, excellent images had at least 50 and as many as 150 cells contiguous to each other that could be counted, with all distinct cell borders, boundaries, and centers across a single image. Good images had at least 50 and as many as 150 cells from variable frames encompassing a minimum of 15 cells contiguous to each other for each variable frame, with sufficient distinct cell borders, boundaries, and centers across a single image. Fair images had at least 50 cells from variable frames encompassing a minimum of 15 cells contiguous to each other for each variable frame, with up to 25% indistinct borders, boundaries, and centers of cells across a single image. Unanalyzable images had an uncountable ECD: fewer than 50 cells with distinct borders, boundaries, and centers from a single image of the endothelium could be counted from variable frames encompassing a minimum of 15 cells contiguous to each other for each variable frame.

2.5. Endothelial Cell Count Methods

To determine the ECD, cells were counted on each field, and the mean of the five was calculated. We used the ImageJ freeware (https://fiji.sc (accessed on 1 November 2016)) with a customized plugin ECD3D [16]. The observer chose areas where EC were most clearly visible and avoided folds when present. The reconstructed full-field image ECD was determined using a validated variable-frame center method [12,13]. Briefly, the center of all EC constituting a continuous group was pointed manually, and the group's boundaries were drawn manually. Cell borders were then automatically reconstructed using Vonoroi segmentation and carefully verified by one skilled observer (TG), who made all necessary corrections. The process was similar to that used in numerous eye banks except for the number of EC manually pointed, which in this study was dramatically elevated (at least 200 EC per field captured—4 times more than in SMAS—and as many as possible in the greatest cell area) to increase cell count reliability [14,15]. The mean ± standard deviation (SD) of the ECD determined in the five fields was calculated for each cornea in the ASM at different time points.

In addition, a final measurement was performed at the end of storage (D28 or D88) in order to determine the vECD by using a triple HEC staining with the CorneaJ plugin for image analysis, as previously reported [10,11]. Pancorneal viability was measured thanks to the mean of five non-overlapping fields of EC acquired inside the 8 central mm (the area usually grafted) by one skilled observer (TG). To assess the accuracy of ECD counted by SM ($_{SM}$ECD), we compared it with ECD measured by counting Hoechst-stained cell nuclei in large variable frames ($_{Hoechst}$ECD) (hereafter referred to as the "histology count") (Figure 3). All specular and Hoechst counts were blinded. They were compared later.

2.6. Statistics

The normality of continuous data distribution was analyzed with the Shapiro-Wilk test, with a non-normality threshold set at 5%. Normally distributed data were described by their mean ± SD. Continuous abnormally distributed variables were summarized as median (10–90 percentiles). The non-parametric Wilcoxon signed-rank test was used when the variable followed an abnormal distribution, and a t-test was used when the variable followed a normal distribution. All tests were two-tailed and paired. Rejection of the null hypothesis was defined as $\alpha < 0.05$. The Holm–Sidak method was used when multiple comparisons occurred (ANOVA). Statistical analyses were performed using SPSS 25.0 (IBM Corp, Armonk, NY, USA).

3. Results

3.1. Baseline Donor Characteristics

Overall, 62 corneas were analyzed: 50 and 12 from one- and three-months' storage, respectively. Donors were 29 females and 35 males, with a mean age of 79 ± 12 years (range 49–97). Mean time from death to procurement was 16 ± 5 h (range 4.30–24). Of the total, 32 eyes (26%) had undergone cataract surgery (same proportion in both groups, ASM and OC).

3.2. Image Quality Classification

Of the 1110 images, 1060 (95%) were analyzable—615 (55%) were excellent, 335 (30%) good, 110 (10%) fair—and 50 (5%) unanalyzable (Figure 4). Seven hundred and fifty images were analyzed for the 1-month study and 360 for the 3-month study. The percentages of the different image quality groups (excellent, good, fair, and unanalyzable) did not differ significantly between the two studies ($p = 0.240$): 59%, 28%, 9%, 4% for the 1-month study; and 47%, 36%, 11%, 6% for the 3-month study. Table 1 shows the details of image quality classification for both studies.

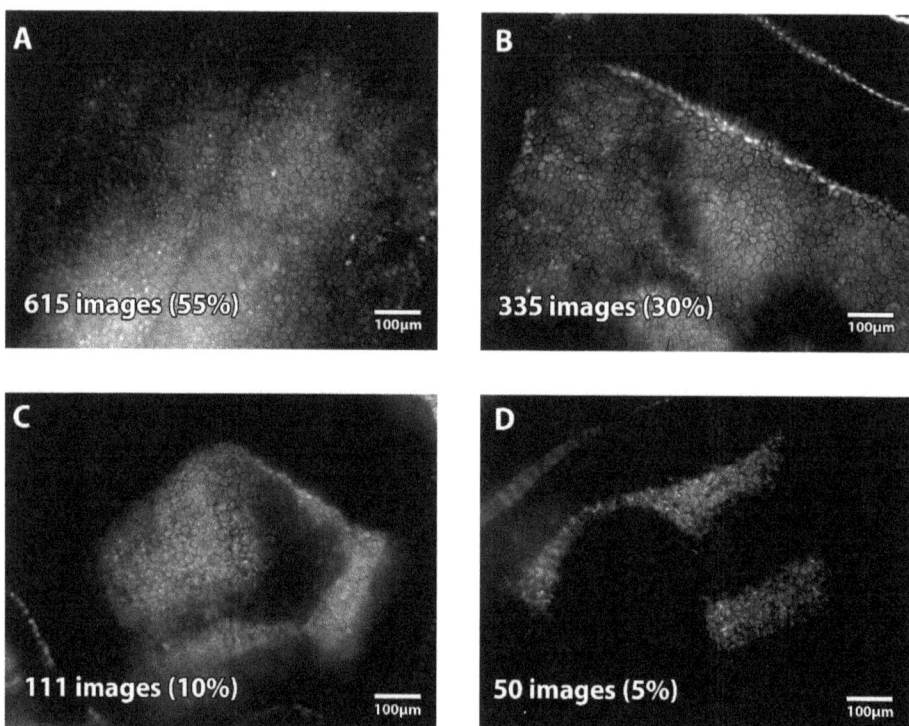

Figure 4. Representative image quality obtained with the prototype specular microscope on corneas stored in the active storage machine. Grading was done using criteria of the Specular Microscopy Ancillary Study [14,15]. (**A**) Excellent-quality image with an ECD of 3022 cell/mm^2. (**B**) Good-quality image with an ECD of 2637 cell/mm^2. (**C**) Fair-quality image with an ECD of 2689 cell/mm^2. (**D**) Unanalyzable image.

Table 1. Image quality classification obtained with specular microscopy of corneas stored in the active storage machine.

	1-Month Study [8]			3-Month Study [9]					1 Month n (%)	3 Months n (%)	Total n (%)
	D2	D26	D28	D2	D23	D44	D65	D86	D88			
n Excellent	146	150	149	26	33	32	30	25	24	445 (59)	170 (47)	615 (55)
n Good	65	70	70	19	20	21	24	23	23	205 (28)	130 (36)	335 (30)
n Fair	27	22	21	10	5	4	4	8	9	70 (9)	40 (11)	110 (10)
n Unanalyzable	12	8	10	5	2	3	2	4	4	30 (4)	20 (6)	50 (5)
TOTAL	250	250	250	60	60	60	60	60	60	750	360	1110

n = number of images analyzed per category; D = day.

3.3. Number of Cells Counted per Image

The mean number of EC counted per image was 1360 ± 433 (range 224–3022), depending on the ECD. In both the 1- and the 3-month studies, the number of counted cells per field/image increased over time (ANOVA, $p < 0.001$). Figure 5 shows an example of the follow-up of the same area at different times during one month. Details for each study are provided in the Supplemental Data (Table S1, Figure S1, Video S1).

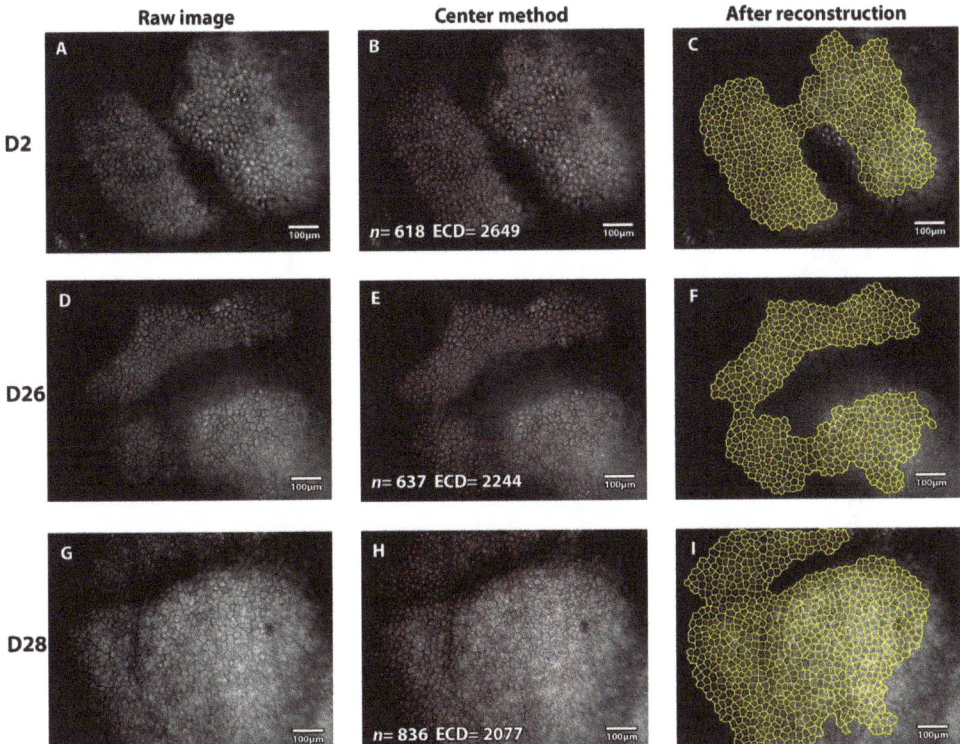

Figure 5. Example of specular microscopy images of the same area of the same cornea stored in the active storage machine for one month. An accurate monitoring of endothelial cell density was possible at day (D) 2, 26, and 28. n = number of cells counted; ECD endothelial cell density in cells/mm^2. At D2, (**A**) raw image with endothelial cells, (**B**) each center was pointed according to the center method, (**C**) cells borders and each center were marked thanks to ImageJ plugin ECD3D [16]. At D26, (**D**) comparative raw image showed larger cells, (**E**) ECD count was determined with the same method, (**F**) reconstruction allowed global view of the studied sample. At D28, (**G**) progressive redistribution of cells occurred, (**H**) more cells were counted on a larger area inside the same field of view (less endothelial folds), (**I**) reconstruction highlighted polymegethism and pleiomorphism.

3.4. Comparison of the SM Counts with the Histology Count

Overall, at the end of storage, $_{SM}$ECD did not significantly differ from $_{Hoechst}$ECD, with 2209 ± 363 versus (vs.) 2251 ± 414 cells/mm^2, respectively (p = 0.084). For the 1-month storage study, ECD were 2299 ± 332 ($_{SM}$ECD) vs. 2344 ± 392 cells/mm^2 ($_{Hoechst}$ECD) (p = 0.138). For the 3-month storage study, ECD were 1831 ± 213 ($_{SM}$ECD) vs. 1863 ± 248 cells/mm^2 ($_{Hoechst}$ECD) (p = 0.081).

3.5. Others Options of the Prototype Specular Microscope

The prototype non-contact SM allowed movie recording in the same area by modulating depth on the Z axis to explore the greatest area of endothelium and to choose the most representative area for each field (Video S2). In addition, epithelial cells could also be observed with the same field of view as the endothelial imaging (Figure 6).

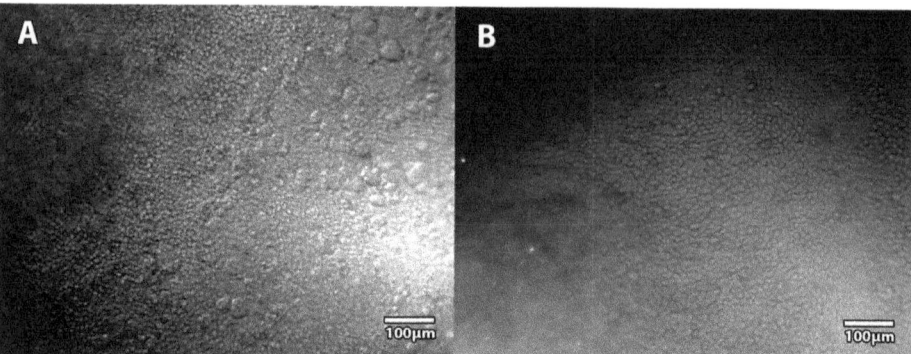

Figure 6. Specular microscopy images of the epithelium of corneas stored in the active storage machine. Thanks to the precision of the Z axis of the microscope stage and the variation of angulation of the LED source, we were able to record epithelium images at different depths: superficial layers (**A**) and more basal layers (**B**).

4. Discussion

The ASM is the first device for corneal graft storage that restores transcorneal pressure gradient equivalent to the IOP while renewing the storage medium. We reported better endothelial survival in the ASM versus the OC and demonstrated its superiority over OC in terms of the preservation of endothelial survival [8,9]. These two initial studies allowed us to transfer the intellectual property to a company that aims to industrialize the ASM so that all the eye banks that wish to use it can do so in the near future. Since the ASM was designed as a totally closed system, it would be inappropriate to have to extract the cornea from the ASM to perform the endothelial controls. Because IOP is involved in the control of corneal hydration ex vivo, the ASM limits the development of stromal edema during long-term storage in a conventional OC medium. In this study carried out before the transfer of the ASM to an industrial company and fully independently of the industrial company, we showed that the endothelium and the epithelium of long-term-stored corneas in the ASM can be observed by SM. To evaluate the quality of the SM images, we used all 1100 images—almost two times as many images as in SMAS [14]—from the two ASM validation studies (1 and 3 months), acquired and analyzed with a standardized method. We decreased sampling fluctuations with at least 200 EC counted per image, meaning 1000 EC counted per cornea at different time points. Our SM counts were reliable: the $_{SM}ECD$ of the last count performed at the end of storage was comparable to the histological count.

The association of the ASM and our prototype SM that we developed has several advantages over existing systems, particularly: (1) The field of view is wider, and the image can be analyzed on its entire surface; (2) The sealed cornea in the ASM and the micrometric stage allow it to have exactly the same position as the ASM along the storage. If the observer wishes, it is thus possible to acquire and analyze, for each cornea, exactly the same endothelial area at different times and to calculate a cell loss rate precisely; (3) With the ASM, it is not necessary to warm up the cornea to see the EC. We showed that SM was possible at any time. When stored at 4 °C, it is essential to warm up the cornea for several hours to acquire satisfactory SM images [17]. It is likely that, at 4 °C, the EC themselves exhibit edema that prevents imaging of cell borders, while the EC are in a more physiological status in the ASM.

During the endothelial controls of corneas in OC, many European eye banks use trypan blue staining to highlight dead EC. However, this counting is not standardized: the staining of the nuclei is often very low, and the count methods do not allow the counting of all the stained cells on a representative surface. The percentage of dead EC is therefore very imprecise. In practice, trypan blue is mainly used to identify large areas of dead cells that may indicate trauma or herpetic infection. Vital staining is impossible in a closed system; thus, it is advisable to repeat EC controls by SM just before corneal graft delivery. Endothelial necrosis at 31–34 °C destroys the endothelium within a few days by cytopathic effect and progression by contiguity, and it will be detected by SM where no EC is visible.

We used the image-quality classification system defined in the SMAS of the CDS, which was referenced in terms of SM image analysis [14]. Interestingly, this prospective study analyzed 688 endothelial images of corneas stored in Optisol-GS, in corneal storage-viewing chambers, submitted by 23 eye banks, acquired with 5 different SM (BioOptics Inc. (Portland, OR, USA); CooperVision (no longer manufactured); HAI Laboratories, Inc. (Lexington, MA, USA); Konan Inc. (Phoenix, AZ, USA); or Tomey (Phoenix, AZ, USA)), and analyzed by a central reading center. They obtained 663 (96%) analyzable images (versus 95% in the present study). However, their image quality seemed inferior, with 6% excellent, 44% good, and 47% fair (versus 55%, 30%, and 10% respectively in our study).

There are limitations to our study. Our experimental prototype SM is not CE-marked or FDA-approved and does not include dedicated cell count software. Conversely, the commercial ebSM are not compatible with the ASM without modifications. It should be possible to adapt the ebSM, requiring FDA or CE approbation: the stages must be modified to receive the ASM cassette, which is much bigger than a conventional corneal storage-viewing chamber; in some cases, the objective must be to adapt its working distance and likely the lighting mode, taking into account the distances between the ASM window and the corneal endothelium. Finally, despite our standardized image acquisition, the settings required rigorous experience to acquire and count images. An all-in-one, more automated commercial version should be developed for routine use in eye banks.

5. Conclusions

Thanks to the control of corneal hydration and the reduction of endothelial folding, corneal grafts stored long-term in our ASM can benefit from endothelial controls with SM at any time, with an image quality comparable to or better than short-term cold-stored corneas.

Supplementary Materials: The following supporting information can be downloaded at: https://www.mdpi.com/article/10.3390/jcm11113000/s1, Table S1: Number of cells counted per image in the 1- and 3-month studies; Figure S1: Time lapse of the same endothelial area during three months in the active storage machine. The same area for each field was precisely acquired repeatedly from Day 2 to Day 86, thanks to the micrometric stage of our specular microscope. Green arrow indicates the redistribution of endothelial cells at the same point of the field. Endothelial cell density decreased over time with larger cells and a progressive slight increase in polymegethism and pleiomorphism; Video S1: Time lapse showing EC redistribution over three months; Video S2: Movie recording example on a defined area.

Author Contributions: Conceptualization, T.G., G.T. and P.G.; data curation, T.G., E.C., C.P. and G.T.; formal analysis, T.G., E.C., C.P., T.L. and G.T.; funding acquisition, G.T. and P.G.; investigation, T.G.; methodology, T.G., G.T. and P.G.; project administration, T.G., G.T. and P.G.; supervision, T.G., G.T. and P.G.; validation, T.G., T.L., G.T. and P.G.; visualization, T.G., T.L., G.T. and P.G.; writing—original draft, T.G. and G.T.; writing—review and editing, T.G., E.C., C.P., T.L., G.T. and P.G. All authors have read and agreed to the published version of the manuscript.

Funding: This research was funded by Agence Nationale de la Sécurité du Médicament (ANSM): research grant 2012 BANCO; EFS 2012 research grant; research grant from Jean Monnet University 2014; Fondation de France Bourse Berthe Fouassier 2016; Fondation Université Jean Monnet 2017; Agence de la Biomédecine research grant 2017; Fondation de l'avenir 2019 project BANCO.

Institutional Review Board Statement: This study was conducted according to the guidelines of the Declaration of Helsinki and approved by the Agence de la Biomédecine (PFS15-008 and PFS16-010).

Informed Consent Statement: Corneas were procured from eligible donors who presented contraindications for clinical use, after obtaining written consent (standard protocol to check no refusal during lifetime (opt-out system)).

Data Availability Statement: The datasets used and/or analyzed during the current study are available from T.G. or G.T. on reasonable request.

Acknowledgments: We are grateful to those who donated their corneas to science and to their families. We thank the hospital coordination team for organ and tissue procurement (JL. Pugniet, T. Peyragrosse, M Barallon, and F. Rogues) for their invaluable expertise during family interviews. We also thank the Agence de la Biomédecine for its institutional support and authorization.

Conflicts of Interest: The authors of this manuscript have conflicts of interest to disclose as described by the Journal of Clinical Medicine. P.G. and G.T. are inventors on "FR1250832/FR2986133B1" and "PCT/US10,18,188,097 B2 29" submitted by University Jean Monnet that covers "Medical device intended for long-term storage of a cornea, or for ex vivo experimentation on a human or animal cornea." P.G. and G.T. are consultants for Laboratoires Théa, Quantel Medical, Sincler, Keranova, and Acusurgical (none related to this study). The other authors have no conflict of interest to disclose.

References

1. Komuro, A.; Hodge, D.O.; Gores, G.J.; Bourne, W.M. Cell death during corneal storage at 4 degrees C. *Investig. Ophthalmol. Vis. Sci.* **1999**, *40*, 2827–2832.
2. Albon, J.; Tullo, A.B.; Aktar, S.; E Boulton, M. Apoptosis in the endothelium of human corneas for transplantation. *Investig. Ophthalmol. Vis. Sci.* **2000**, *41*, 2887–2893.
3. Gain, P.; Thuret, G.; Chiquet, C.; Dumollard, J.M.; Mosnier, J.F.; Burillon, C.; Delbosc, B.; Hervé, P.; Campos, L. Value of two mortality assessment techniques for organ cultured corneal endothelium: Trypan blue versus TUNEL technique. *Br. J. Ophthalmol.* **2002**, *86*, 306–310. [CrossRef] [PubMed]
4. Thuret, G.; Chiquet, C.; Bernal, F.; Acquart, S.; Romanet, J.P.; Mouillon, M.; Hegelhoffer, H.; Burillon, C.; Damour, O.; Maugery, J.; et al. Prospective, randomized clinical and endothelial evaluation of 2 storage times for cornea donor tissue in organ culture at 31 degrees C. *Arch. Ophthalmol.* **2003**, *121*, 442–450. [CrossRef] [PubMed]
5. Kitazawa, K.; Inatomi, T.; Tanioka, H.; Kawasaki, S.; Nakagawa, H.; Hieda, O.; Fukuoka, H.; Okumura, N.; Koizumi, N.; Iliakis, B.; et al. The existence of dead cells in donor corneal endothelium preserved with storage media. *Br. J. Ophthalmol.* **2017**, *101*, 1725–1730. [CrossRef] [PubMed]
6. Armitage, W.J.; Dick, A.D.; Bourne, W.M. Predicting endothelial cell loss and long-term corneal graft survival. *Investig. Ophthalmol. Vis. Sci.* **2003**, *44*, 3326–3331. [CrossRef] [PubMed]
7. Guindolet, D.; Crouzet, E.; He, Z.; Herbepin, P.; Jumelle, C.; Perrache, C.; Dumollard, J.M.; Forest, F.; Peoc'H, M.; Gain, P.; et al. Storage of Porcine Cornea in an Innovative Bioreactor. *Investig. Ophthalmol. Vis. Sci.* **2017**, *58*, 5907–5917. [CrossRef] [PubMed]
8. Garcin, T.; Gauthier, A.; Crouzet, E.; He, Z.; Herbepin, P.; Perrache, C.; Acquart, S.; Cognasse, F.; Forest, F.; Thuret, G.; et al. Innovative corneal active storage machine for long-term eye banking. *Am. J. Transplant.* **2019**, *19*, 1641–1651. [CrossRef] [PubMed]
9. Garcin, T.; Gauthier, A.-S.; Crouzet, E.; He, Z.; Herbepin, P.; Perrache, C.; Acquart, S.; Cognasse, F.; Forest, F.; Gain, P.; et al. Three-month Storage of Human Corneas in an Active Storage Machine. *Transplantation* **2020**, *104*, 1159–1165. [CrossRef] [PubMed]
10. Pipparelli, A.; Thuret, G.; Toubeau, D.; He, Z.; Piselli, S.; Lefèvre, S.; Gain, P.; Muraine, M. Pan-corneal endothelial viability assessment: Application to endothelial grafts predissected by eye banks. *Investig. Ophthalmol. Vis. Sci.* **2011**, *52*, 6018–6025. [CrossRef] [PubMed]
11. Bernard, A.; Campolmi, N.; He, Z.; Thi, B.M.H.; Piselli, S.; Forest, F.; Dumollard, J.M.; Peoc'h, M.; Acquart, S.; Gain, P.; et al. CorneaJ: An imageJ Plugin for semi-automated measurement of corneal endothelial cell viability. *Cornea* **2014**, *33*, 604–609. [CrossRef] [PubMed]
12. Takahashi, E.A. Method for Computing Morphology of Cornea Endothelium Cells. U.S. Patent US5523213A, 4 June 1996.
13. Deb-Joardar, N.; Thuret, G.; Gavet, Y.; Acquart, S.; Garraud, O.; Egelhoffer, H.; Gain, P. Reproducibility of endothelial assessment during corneal organ culture: Comparison of a computer-assisted analyzer with manual methods. *Investig. Ophthalmol. Vis. Sci.* **2007**, *48*, 2062–2067. [CrossRef] [PubMed]
14. Lass, J.H.; Gal, R.L.; Ruedy, K.J.; Benetz, B.A.; Beck, R.W.; Baratz, K.H.; Holland, E.J.; Kalajian, A.; Kollman, C.; Manning, F.J.; et al. An evaluation of image quality and accuracy of eye bank measurement of donor cornea endothelial cell density in the Specular Microscopy Ancillary Study. *Ophthalmology* **2005**, *112*, 431–440. [PubMed]
15. Benetz, B.A.; Gal, R.L.; Ruedy, K.J.; Rice, C.; Beck, R.W.; Kalajian, A.D.; Lass, J.H. Specular microscopy ancillary study methods for donor endothelial cell density determination of Cornea Donor Study images. *Curr. Eye Res.* **2006**, *31*, 319–327. [CrossRef] [PubMed]
16. Jumelle, C.; Garcin, T.; Gauthier, A.S.; Glasson, Y.; Bernard, A.; Gavet, Y.; Klossa, J.; He, Z.; Acquart, S.; Gain, P.; et al. Considering 3D topography of endothelial folds to improve cell count of organ cultured corneas. *Cell Tissue Bank.* **2017**, *18*, 185–191. [CrossRef] [PubMed]
17. Tran, K.D.; Clover, J.; Ansin, A.; Stoeger, C.G.; Terry, M.A. Rapid Warming of Donor Corneas Is Safe and Improves Specular Image Quality. *Cornea* **2017**, *36*, 581–587. [CrossRef] [PubMed]

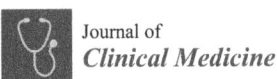

Article

Exploring Retinal Blood Vessel Diameters as Biomarkers in Multiple Sclerosis

Dragana Drobnjak Nes [1], Pål Berg-Hansen [2], Sigrid A. de Rodez Benavent [1], Einar A. Høgestøl [2,3], Mona K. Beyer [4,5], Daniel A. Rinker [2,4], Nina Veiby [1], Mia Karabeg [1,4], Beáta Éva Petrovski [4], Elisabeth G. Celius [2,4], Hanne F. Harbo [2,4] and Goran Petrovski [1,4,*]

[1] Center of Eye Research, Department of Ophthalmology, Oslo University Hospital, 0450 Oslo, Norway; gagid100@hotmail.com (D.D.N.); aune_sigrid@hotmail.com (S.A.d.R.B.); nina.veiby@gmail.com (N.V.); uxgrmi@ous-hf.no (M.K.)
[2] Department of Neurology, Oslo University Hospital, 0372 Oslo, Norway; uxplha@ous-hf.no (P.B.-H.); einar.august@gmail.com (E.A.H.); d.a.rinker@ous-research.no (D.A.R.); uxelgu@ous-hf.no (E.G.C.); h.c.f.harbo@medisin.uio.no (H.F.H.)
[3] Department of Psychology, University of Oslo, 0373 Oslo, Norway
[4] Institute of Clinical Medicine, Faculty of Medicine, University of Oslo, 0372 Oslo, Norway; mona.beyer@lyse.net (M.K.B.); b.e.petrovski@medisin.uio.no (B.É.P.)
[5] Department of Radiology and Nuclear Medicine, Oslo University Hospital, 0379 Oslo, Norway
* Correspondence: goran.petrovski@medisin.uio.no

Abstract: We aimed to determine whether retinal vessel diameters and retinal oxygen saturation in newly diagnosed patients with multiple sclerosis (pwMS) are different from those of a healthy population. Retinal blood vessel diameters were measured using imaging with a spectrophotometric non-invasive retinal oximeter. Twenty-three newly diagnosed untreated relapsing-remitting MS (RRMS) patients (mean age: 32.2 ± 7.5 years, age range = 18–50 years, 56.5% female) were measured and compared to 23 age- and sex-matched healthy controls (HCs) (mean age: 34.8 ± 8.1 years). Patients with Optic Neuritis were excluded. Retinal venular diameter (143.8 µm versus 157.8 µm: mean; $p = 0.0013$) and retinal arteriolar diameter (112.6 µm versus 120.6 µm: mean; $p = 0.0089$) were smaller in pwMS when compared with HCs, respectively. There was no significant difference in the oxygen saturation in retinal venules and arterioles in pwMS (mean: 60.0% and 93.7%; $p = 0.5980$) compared to HCs (mean: 59.3% and 91.5%; $p = 0.8934$), respectively. There was a significant difference in the median low contrast visual acuity (2.5% contrast) between the pwMS and the HC groups ($p = 0.0143$) Retinal arteriolar and venular diameter may have potential as objective biomarkers for MS.

Keywords: retinal vessel diameter; retinal oximetry; multiple sclerosis; fundus imaging

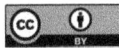

1. Introduction

Multiple sclerosis (MS) is the most common cause of neurological disability in young adults, affecting approximately 2.8 million people worldwide, with variable progression and prognosis [1]. MS is a chronic, immune-mediated disease of the CNS that often results in visual morbidity [2–4]. Early features of MS may include eye motility difficulties and optic neuritis (ON) as presenting ocular sign in 20% of patients, and, as the disease progresses, inter-nuclear ophthalmoplegia [5]. Other ocular conditions, including retinal vasculitis and uveitis, have been associated with MS [6,7].

The retinal ganglion cells (RCGs) and the optic nerve are commonly affected in MS in the form of optic neuritis ON; chronic MS can cause RGC atrophy, which can occur independently from ON [4,8–11].

Retinal involvements in MS have included qualitative changes in the retinal blood vessels, such as histopathological changes remarkable of vascular inflammation in 20% of the patients with MS (pwMS) in post mortem specimens [12], as well as clinical changes remarkable of retinal phlebitis in 16% of pwMS [13].

Quantitative retinal blood vessel metrics are potential markers of MS due to a known clinical relationship between MS and retinal vessel inflammation [13–15], and between MS and RGC loss, which potentially decreases the metabolic demand [16,17]. Structural and physiological abnormalities have been reported in the retina in pwMS [18]. Although retinal vasculitis is common in MS, it is not known if MS is associated with quantitative retinal blood vessel abnormalities.

In MS, low-contrast letter acuity (LCLA) of 2.5% contrast level has proven to be a valuable marker of residual deficits after ON, and serving as a marker of disease progression and an outcome measure in clinical MS research [19]. As visual dysfunction is one of the most common manifestations of MS, and sensitive visual outcome measures are important in examining the effect of treatment.

Spectrophotometric non-invasive retinal oximeter imaging is a technique that generates high-resolution images of the retinal blood vessels; it can measure the oxygen saturation inside the retinal vessels, as well as the vessel diameters. Only a single pilot study exists about the relationship between MS and retinal vessel diameters, which was based on pwMS with history of ON [20].

We hypothesized that the oxygen saturation and retinal vessel diameter in newly diagnosed pwMS would be significantly different from those of HCs.

This study is an important initial step in evaluating measurements of retinal vessel structure as a possible measurable in vivo biomarker of MS, and represents a novel method for assessment of retinal blood vessel metrics in this patient population.

2. Materials and Methods

This is a cross sectional study on pwMS diagnosed and followed at Oslo University Hospital (OUH), Oslo, Norway. In a collaboration between the Departments of Ophthalmology and Neurology at OUH, patients enrolled in Oslo in the MultipleMS study (Horizon 2020 programme, grant agreement 733161) were also referred to an eye examination (in the period 2018–2021). The MS study was approved by the regional committee for research ethics (Ref. 2011/1846-41). Written consent was obtained from the subjects.

The patients were approached to join the study by their treating neurologist, and referred to the ophthalmology department if they consented within two weeks of diagnosis and before starting any disease-modifying therapies. Inclusion criteria were a confirmed diagnosis of MS according to the revised diagnostic McDonald criteria [21,22], as well as age 18–50 years and fluency in Norwegian. Exclusion criteria were no prior ophthalmological, neurological, or psychiatric disease, no head injury, and no substance abuse. Eyes with ON were also excluded from eye examinations. Twenty-three newly diagnosed pwMS were included and compared to twenty-three healthy individuals that were age- and sex-matched. We excluded some of the eyes (1 control, 1 eye from each of 2 different patients) due to missing data or ON.

At the time of diagnosis, all pwMS underwent an MRI of the brain and spine, a lumbar puncture, and detailed neurological examinations, including the Expanded Disability Status Score (EDSS) [23]. EDSS ranges from 0 to 10 in 0.5 unit increments that represent higher levels of disability. EDSS steps 1.0 to 4.5 refer to people with MS who are able to walk without any aid.

Full ophthalmic examination was performed by an experienced ophthalmologist, including indirect ophthalmoscopy. In addition, digital fundus imaging was performed with the fundus camera of the oximeter (Oxymap T1, Oxymapehf., 102 Reykjavik, Iceland), andretinal vessel diameter measurements and oximetry of the retinal blood vessels were performed with using the Oxymap analyses software, as explained later.

Both Corrected Distance Visual Acuity (CDVA) and low contrast letter acuity (LCLA) of 2.5% were measured by an optometrist with an Early Treatment Diabetic Study (ETDRS) visual acuity chart in both eyes and presented as logarithm of the minimum angle of resolution (logMAR) [24]. The recommended test distance of 4 m was respected. The same examination room was used for all study participants and light was lit with approximately 100 lux.

2.1. Oximetry Imaging and Measurements

The retinal oximetry procedure has been described previously [25,26]. The patient was positioned in front of the fundus camera of the oximeter (Oxymap T1, Oxymapehf., Reykjavik, Iceland), and images were taken from both eyes. Two or more fundus photographs centered on the optic disc were taken, and the image with the best quality was used for the analyses. Image quality higher than 6 on the scale from 0 to 10 was considered acceptable. Retinal blood vessel diametersand oxygen saturations were measured by an experienced ophthalmologist (DDN) using the Oxymap analyses software (Oxymap T1, software 2.2.1., version 5436, Reykjavik, Iceland) according to a standardized protocol (Version 21, November 2013; Oxymap Inc., Reykjavik, Iceland) [26,27].

The algorithm for vessel detection and diameter measurements utilizes a supervised classifier that classifies each pixel as belonging to a vessel or background. The algorithm recognizes the pixels in the center of each vessel, evaluates a vessel vector perpendicular to vessel direction, and calculates vessel diameter from the center to the last pixel belonging to the vessel in each direction [28]. Each pixel is approximately 9.3 μm.

Arterioles and venules wider than 8 pixels (74 μm) and longer than 50 pixels (480 μm) were measured in a peripapillary annulus within a standard grid of 1.5 to 3.0 disc diameters from the optic disc center. The right eye from each patient was measured; however, if the image quality was poor or the vessels were ungradable, the left eye was measured instead. The oxygen saturation results are influenced by the vessel diameter, but that is automatically corrected by the analysis software [27].

2.2. Statistics

Data analysis was performed using descriptive statistical analysis; percentage distribution, and mean and standard deviation (SD). In case of non-normality of continuous variables, median and interquartile ranges (IQR, measure of variability) were calculated. Normality of continuous variables was tested on a Q-Q-plot and by the Shapiro–Wilk and Kolmogorov–Smirnov test. When the normality assumption was satisfied, the student t-test was used to compare means of continuous and numerical variables; otherwise, the Mann–Whitney test was used. Homogeneity of variance was analyzed with Levene's test; if the Levene's test was not satisfied, the Welch test was used instead. Chi-square (χ^2) test was used to test the differences of the distribution of categorical variables. Level of significance was set to $p < 0.05$.

Statistical Package for STATA (Stata version 14.0; College Station, TX, USA) was used for the statistical analysis.

3. Results

Some of the eyes (one control, one eye from each of two different patients) were excluded due to missing data or ON. (Table 1).

The retinal venular diameter (mean: 143.8 μm versus 157.8 μm; $p = 0.0013$) and retinal arteriolar diameter (mean: 112.6 μm versus 120.6 μm; $p = 0.0089$) were smaller in pwMS when compared with HCs, respectively (Table 2).

There was no significant difference in the oxygen saturation in retinal venules and arterioles in pwMS (mean: 60.0% and 93.7%, respectively) compared to HCs (mean: 59.3% and 91.5%, respectively) (Table 2).

There was, however, a significant difference in the median low contrast visual acuity (2.5% contrast) between the pwMS and the HC groups ($p = 0.0143$) (Table 2).

Table 1. Subject demographics and study group characteristics.

	Healthy Controls	People with MS
Eyes, n (Patients, n)	45 (23)	44 (23)
Mean Age, years (SD)	34.8 (8.1)	32.2 (7.5)
Female sex, n (%)	13 (56.5)	13 (56.5)
Time since diagnosis, weeks (SD)	-	2 (SD)
Optic Neuritis, n (Patients, n)	0 (0)	2 (2)
EDSS, n (Patients, n): 0; 1.0; 1.5; 2,0; 2.5; 3.0	-	3; 6; 6; 3, 4, 1

EDSS: Expanded Disability Status Scale.

Table 2. Vessel diameters, oxygen saturation, and 2.5% contrast visual acuity in the healthy controls and people with MS.

Variable	Healthy Controls (n = 23)	People with MS (n = 23)	p-Value
Retinal arteriolar diameter (μm) Mean (±SD) 95% CI	120.6 (11.5) 115.4–126–0	112.6 (10.7) 108.1–11.0	0.0013
Retinal venular diameter (μm) Median, Range (IQR)	157.8 (148.0–171.5)	143.8 (123.3–186.8)	0.0089
A-V difference in % Mean (SD) 95% CI	38.3 (14.8) 31.5–45.0	31.8 (12.0) 27.0–37.0	0.0527
Arteriolar O$_2$ saturation (%) Mean (±SD) 95% CI	91.5 (7.3) 88.2–95.0	93.7 (4.2) 92.0–95.5	0.8934
Venular O$_2$ saturation in% Mean (±SD) 95% CI	59.3 (9.5) 55.0–64.0	60.0 (4.6) 92.0–95.5	0.5980
2.5% contrast visual acuity, number of letters Left eye Median, Range (IQR)	31 (27.0–34.0)	23 (18.5–30.0)	0.0143
High contrast visual acuity Right eye /Left eye Mean (±SD) 95% CI	0.43 (0.09) 0.38–0.47/ 0.44 (0.12) 0.38–0.50	0.35 (0.23) 0.25–0.45/ 0.43 (0.24) 0.33–0.53	0.0722 0.04022

Retinal venular diameter was wider in healthy controls (HC) compared with patients with MS groups (Figure 1).

Box chart of 2.5% contrast visual acuity (letters) in the left eye between the healthy controls (HC) and MS patients' groups is presented in Figure 2.

A higher proportion of participants in the study were males. Time since MS diagnosis was 2 weeks. We excluded some of the eyes (one control, one eye from each of two different patients) due to missing data or ON.

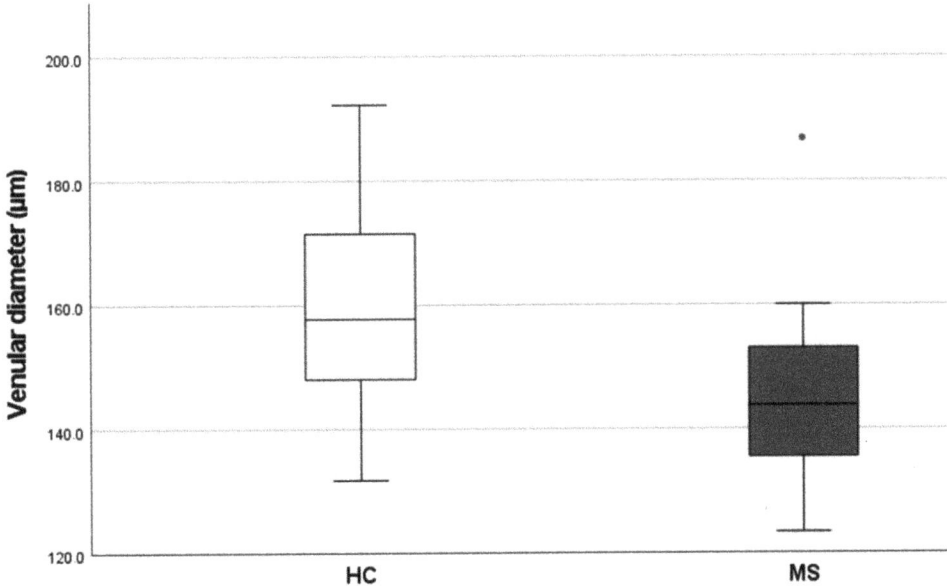

Figure 1. Distribution of retinal venular diameter between the healthy controls (HC) and patients with MS groups. Data presented are in the form of median (IQR: Interquartile range). HC: Healthy Controls; MS: Multiple sclerosis, $p < 0.05$.

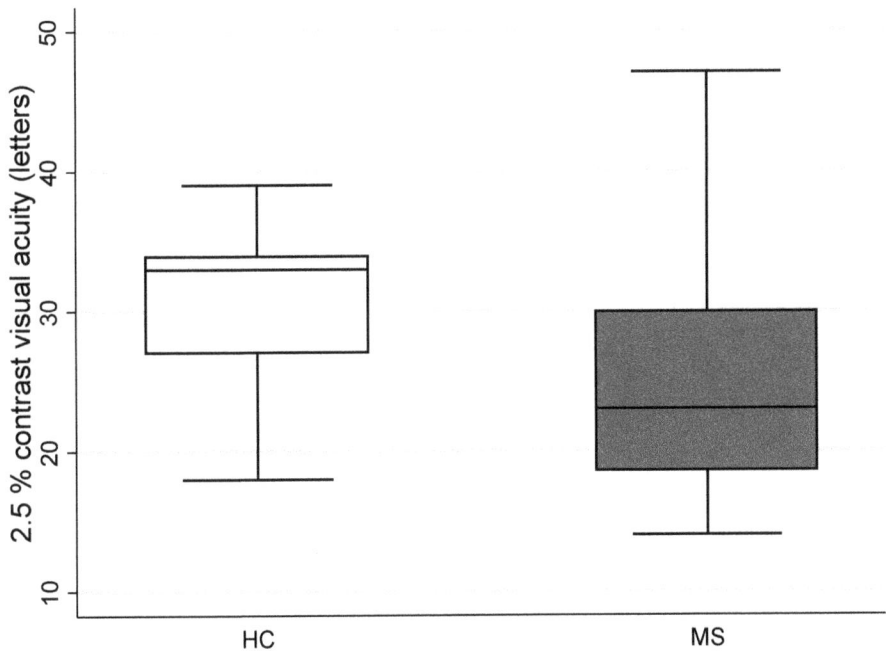

Figure 2. Box chart of 2.5% contrast visual acuity (letters) in the left eye between the healthy controls (HC) and MS patients' groups. Data presented are in the form of median (IQR, Interquartile range). HC: Healthy Controls; MS: Multiple sclerosis, $p < 0.05$.

4. Discussion

This study indicates the existence of narrower retinal vessel diameters in newly diagnosed pwMS compared with HCs. The measurement of the vessel diameter and retinal oximetry has been previously shown to be reliable and repeatable [29], with older age possibly affecting retinal oximetry parameters, which seems irrelevant to the younger population studied here.

A potential explanation for the smaller diameter of retinal vessels in MS subjects may be the presence of RGC loss, leading to lower metabolic demands on the retinal circulation. Wang et al. showed lower ON head blood flow in pwMS with history of ON, compared with both pwMS without a history of ON, and HCs, which stands in support of such a mechanism [29]. Bhaduri et al. used optical coherence tomography (OCT) to show that MS eyes had a lower total blood vessel diameter (BVD) and blood vessel number (BVN) than control eyes [18].

The relationship between the disturbances in cerebral venous outflow and neurological disorders remains an open issue that requires further studies. The high degree of comorbidity between vascular diseases and MS suggest that vascular pathology may be an important factor causing neuronal dysfunction or degeneration in MS [30,31]. There is also evidence suggesting that pwMS are more susceptible to cardiovascular risk factors than HCs, some having demonstrated regional cerebral perfusion abnormalities in these patients [20,30,31].

The decrease in blood vessel diameter has been related to qualitative changes resembling inflammatory pathology in the retinal vessels in MS. Furthermore, retinal phlebitis has been reported to correlate with MS activity, which is similar in pattern to the associations we found for retinal blood vessel diameter [18]. It could be possible that peripapillary changes represent adaptive mechanisms related to present or past phlebitis in the peripheral retina. This evidence is indirect, since the location of the qualitative pathology (in the retinal periphery) is distant from the location of our blood vessel measurements (found around the ON). However, the connected nature of the retinal blood vessels means changes in the proximal vessels are possibly associated with distal pathology. Future studies are needed to compare the clinical and imaging findings in pwMS in order to determine if retinal blood vessel diameter is associated with current or past retinal phlebitis.

There was a significant average difference in low-contrast visual acuity between the HCs and pwMS groups, while no significant difference was found between the oxygen saturation in retinal arterioles and retinal venules in the two groups. There is insufficient knowledge about newly diagnosed MS and its relation to oxygen and vascular supply parameters in the eye. One cohort study on eight pwMS with history of ON found the mean retinal venular oxygen saturation to be higher in pwMS than in HCs [20].

Overall, changes in the retinal vessel diameter, in particular smaller arterioles, have been related to cardiovascular mortality (from coronary heart disease and stroke) [32,33]. In addition, such changes have been found to contribute to the development of diabetic retinopathy, in particular, early stages, and considered to be prognostic markers of the disease [34]. Similarly, we have found that retinal venular oxygen saturation is associated with early stage non-proliferative diabetic retinopathy in type 1 diabetes patients [26].

To our knowledge, our study represents the first application of objective, in vivo ascertainment of retinal oxygenation and vessel diameter in newly diagnosed MS patients, and it confirmed differentiation of parameters measured in controls. A study on newly diagnosed MS patients and retinal oxidative/vascular risk factors has not been performed previously in a Norwegian population, and no large international studies exist either.

Our study has several limitations. It was a pilot study with low number of participants. Blood pressure (BP) was not measured at the same. Retinal venular diameter was not statistically normally distributed, probably due to the low number of participants.

Further studies are needed to confirm our findings, and to explore the implications and biological basis of the decreased blood vessel diameter and vessel density in MS.

5. Conclusions

In conclusion, we found smaller retinal venular and arteriolar diameters in pwMS. If confirmed by longitudinal follow-up, this may be a useful and objective biomarker for neurodegeneration in MS.

Author Contributions: Conceptualization, D.D.N., P.B.-H., E.G.C., H.F.H. and G.P.; methodology, D.D.N., P.B.-H., S.A.d.R.B., E.A.H., M.K.B., D.A.R., N.V., M.K., B.É.P., E.G.C., H.F.H. and G.P.; validation, D.D.N., P.B.-H., E.A.H., M.K.B., N.V., M.K., B.É.P., E.G.C., H.F.H. and G.P.; formal analysis, D.D.N., P.B.-H., E.A.H., M.K.B., N.V., M.K. and B.É.P.; investigation, D.D.N., P.B.-H., S.A.d.R.B., E.A.H., M.K.B., D.A.R., N.V., M.K., E.G.C., H.F.H. and G.P.; resources, D.D.N., P.B.-H., E.G.C., H.F.H. and G.P.; data curation, D.D.N., P.B.-H., E.A.H., M.K.B., M.K., B.É.P., E.G.C., H.F.H. and G.P.; writing—original draft preparation, D.D.N., P.B.-H., S.A.d.R.B., E.A.H., M.K.B., N.V., M.K., B.É.P., E.G.C., H.F.H. and G.P.; writing—review and editing, D.D.N., P.B.-H., S.A.d.R.B., E.A.H., M.K.B., N.V., M.K., B.É.P., E.G.C., H.F.H. and G.P.; visualization, D.D.N. and B.É.P.; supervision, P.B.-H., E.G.C., H.F.H. and G.P.; project administration, P.B.-H., E.G.C., H.F.H. and G.P.; funding acquisition, D.D.N., P.B.-H., E.G.C., H.F.H. and G.P. All authors have read and agreed to the published version of the manuscript.

Funding: This study has been partially funded by the Norwegian Association of the Blind and Partially Sighted.

Institutional Review Board Statement: The MS study was approved by the regional committee for research ethics (Ref. 2011/1846-41).

Informed Consent Statement: Written informed consent has been obtained from the patients to publish this paper.

Data Availability Statement: Data supporting reported results can be provided by the corresponding authors upon request.

Conflicts of Interest: The authors declare no conflict of interest.

References

1. Walton, C.; King, R.; Rechtman, L.; Kaye, W.; Leray, E.; Marrie, R.A.; Robertson, N.; la Rocca, N.; Uitdehaag, B.; van der Mei, I.; et al. Rising prevalence of multiple sclerosis worldwide: Insights from the Atlas of MS, third edition. *Mult. Scler.* **2020**, *26*, 1816–1821. [CrossRef] [PubMed]
2. Costello, F. The afferent visual pathway: Designing a structural-functional paradigm of multiple sclerosis. *ISRN Neurol.* **2013**, *2013*, 134858. [CrossRef] [PubMed]
3. Costello, K. Multiple sclerosis research: Diagnostics, disease-modifying treatments, and emerging therapies. *J. Neurosci. Nurs.* **2013**, *45* (Suppl. S1), S14–S23. [CrossRef] [PubMed]
4. Graham, S.L.; Klistorner, A. Afferent visual pathways in multiple sclerosis: A review. *Clin. Exp. Ophthalmol.* **2017**, *45*, 62–72. [CrossRef]
5. Reulen, J.P.; Sanders, E.A.; Hogenhuis, L.A. Eye movement disorders in multiple sclerosis and optic neuritis. *Brain* **1983**, *106 Pt 1*, 121–140. [CrossRef]
6. Fuest, M.; Rößler, G.; Walter, P.; Plange, N. Retinal vasculitis as manifestation of multiple sclerosis. *Ophthalmologe* **2014**, *111*, 871–875. [CrossRef]
7. Pedraza-Concha, A.; Brandauer, K.; Tello, A.; Rangel, C.M.; Scheib, C. Bilateral Anterior and Intermediate Uveitis with Occlusive Vasculitis as Sole Manifestation of Relapse in Multiple Sclerosis. *Case Rep. Ophthalmol. Med.* **2019**, *2019*, 8239205. [CrossRef]
8. Schmitt, C.; Strazielle, N.; Ghersi-Egea, J.F. Brain leukocyte infiltration initiated by peripheral inflammation or experimental autoimmune encephalomyelitis occurs through pathways connected to the CSF-filled compartments of the forebrain and midbrain. *J. Neuroinflamm.* **2012**, *9*, 1–15. [CrossRef]
9. Petzold, A.; de Boer, J.F.; Schippling, S.; Vermersch, P.; Kardon, R.; Green, A.; Calabresi, P.A.; Polman, C. Optical coherence tomography in multiple sclerosis: A systematic review and meta-analysis. *Lancet Neurol.* **2010**, *9*, 921–932. [CrossRef]
10. Trapp, B.D.; Peterson, J.; Ransohoff, R.M.; Rudick, R.; Mörk, S.; Bö, L. Axonal transection in the lesions of multiple sclerosis. *N. Engl. J. Med.* **1998**, *338*, 278–285. [CrossRef]
11. Balcer, L.J. Clinical trials to clinical use: Using vision as a model for multiple sclerosis and beyond. *J. Neuroophthalmol.* **2014**, *34*, S18–S23. [CrossRef] [PubMed]
12. Kolinko, Y.; Krakorova, K.; Cendelin, J.; Kralickova, Z.T.M. Microcirculation of the brain: Morphological assessment in degenerative diseases and restoration processes. *Rev. Neurosci.* **2015**, *26*, 75–93. [CrossRef] [PubMed]

13. Sepulcre, J.; Murie-Fernandez, M.; Salinas-Alaman, A.; García-Layana, A.; Bejarano, B.; Villoslada, P. Diagnostic accuracy of retinal abnormalities in predicting disease activity in MS. *Neurology* **2007**, *68*, 1488–1494. [CrossRef] [PubMed]
14. Engell, T. Neurological disease activity in multiple sclerosis patients with periphlebitis retinae. *Acta Neurol. Scand.* **1986**, *73*, 168–172. [CrossRef] [PubMed]
15. Kerrison, J.B.; Flynn, T.; Green, W.R. Retinal pathologic changes in multiple sclerosis. *Retina* **1994**, *14*, 445–451. [CrossRef] [PubMed]
16. Harris, A.; Ciulla, T.A.; Chung, H.S.; Martin, B. Regulation of retinal and optic nerve blood flow. *Arch. Ophthalmol.* **1998**, *116*, 1491–1495. [CrossRef] [PubMed]
17. Russo, A.; Costagliola, C.; Rizzoni, D.; Ghilardi, N.; Turano, R.; Semeraro, F. Arteriolar Diameters in Glaucomatous Eyes with Single-Hemifield Damage. *Optom. Vis. Sci.* **2016**, *93*, 504–509. [CrossRef]
18. Bhaduri, B.; Nolan, R.M.; Shelton, R.L.; Pilutti, L.A.; Motl, R.W.; Moss, H.E.; Pula, J.H.; Boppart, S.A. Detection of retinal blood vessel changes in multiple sclerosis with optical coherence tomography. *Biomed. Opt. Express.* **2016**, *7*, 2321–2330. [CrossRef]
19. Balcer, L.J.; Raynowska, J.; Nolan, R.; Galetta, S.L.; Kapoor, R.; Benedict, R.; Phillips, G.; LaRocca, N.; Lynn, H.; Richard, R.; et al. Validity of low-contrast letter acuity as a visual performance outcome measure for multiple sclerosis. *Mult. Scler.* **2017**, *23*, 734–747. [CrossRef]
20. Einarsdottir, A.B.; Olafsdottir, O.B.; Hjaltason, H.; Hardarson, S.H. Retinal oximetry is affected in multiple sclerosis. *Acta. Ophthalmol.* **2018**, *96*, 528–530. [CrossRef]
21. McDonald, W.I.; Compston, A.; Edan, G.; Goodkin, D.; Hartung, H.-P.; Lublin, F.D.; McFarland, H.F.; Paty, D.W.; Polman, C.H.; Reingold, S.C.; et al. Recommended diagnostic criteria for multiple sclerosis: Guidelines from the International Panel on the diagnosis of multiple sclerosis. *Ann. Neurol.* **2001**, *50*, 121–127. [CrossRef] [PubMed]
22. Polman, C.H.; Reingold, S.C.; Banwell, B.; Clanet, M.; Cohen, J.A.; Filippi, M.; Fujihara, K.; Havrdova, E.; Hutchinson, M.; Kappos, L.; et al. Diagnostic criteria for multiple sclerosis: 2010 revisions to the McDonald criteria. *Ann. Neurol.* **2011**, *69*, 292–302. [CrossRef] [PubMed]
23. Kurtzke, J.F. Rating neurologic impairment in multiple sclerosis: An expanded disability status scale (EDSS). *Neurology* **1983**, *33*, 1444–1452. [CrossRef] [PubMed]
24. Stulting, R.D.; Dupps, W.J., Jr.; Kohnen, T.; Mamalis, N.; Rosen, E.S.; Koch, D.D.; Obstbaum, S.A.; Waring, G.O., III; Reinstein, D.Z. Standardized graphs and terms for refractive surgery results. *Cornea* **2011**, *30*, 945–947. [CrossRef]
25. Hardarson, S.H.; Harris, A.; Karlsson, R.A.; Halldorsson, G.H.; Kagemann, L.; Rechtman, E.; Zoega, G.M.; Eysteinsson, T.; Benediktsson, J.A.; Thorsteinsson, A.; et al. Automatic retinal oximetry. *Invest. Ophthalmol. Vis. Sci.* **2006**, *47*, 5011–5016. [CrossRef]
26. Veiby, N.C.B.B.; Simeunovic, A.; Heier, M.; Brunborg, C.; Saddique, N.; Moe, M.C.; Dahl-Jørgensen, K.; Margeirsdottir, H.D.; Petrovski, G. Venular oxygen saturation is increased in young patients with type 1 diabetes and mild nonproliferative diabetic retinopathy. *Acta. Ophthalmol.* **2020**, *98*, 800–807. [CrossRef]
27. Geirsdottir, A.; Palsson, O.; Hardarson, S.H.; Olafsdottir, O.B.; Kristjansdottir, J.V.; Stefánsson, E. Retinal vessel oxygen saturation in healthy individuals. *Invest. Ophthalmol. Vis. Sci.* **2012**, *53*, 5433–5442. [CrossRef]
28. Blondal, R.; Sturludottir, M.K.; Hardarson, S.H.; Halldorsson, G.H.; Stefánsson, E. Reliability of vessel diameter measurements with a retinal oximeter. *Graefes. Arch. Clin. Exp. Ophthalmol.* **2011**, *249*, 1311–1317. [CrossRef]
29. Wang, X.; Jia, Y.; Spain, R.; Potsaid, B.; Liu, J.J.; Baumann, B.; Hornegger, J.; Fujimoto4, J.G.; Wu, Q.; Huang, D. Optical coherence tomography angiography of optic nerve head and parafovea in multiple sclerosis. *Br. J. Ophthalmol.* **2014**, *98*, 1368–1373. [CrossRef]
30. Christiansen, C.F. Risk of vascular disease in patients with multiple sclerosis: A review. *Neurol. Res.* **2012**, *34*, 746–753. [CrossRef]
31. Geraldes, R.; Esiri, M.M.; Perera, R.; Yee, S.A.; Jenkins, D.; Palace, J.; DeLuca, G.C. Vascular disease and multiple sclerosis: A post-mortem study exploring their relationships. *Brain* **2020**, *143*, 2998–3012. [CrossRef] [PubMed]
32. Wang, J.J.; Liew, G.; Klein, R.; Rochtchina, E.; Knudtson, M.D.; Klein, B.E.K.; Wong, T.Y.; Burlutsky, G.; Mitchell, P. Retinal vessel diameter and cardiovascular mortality: Pooled data analysis from two older populations. *Eur. Heart J.* **2007**, *28*, 1984–1992. [CrossRef] [PubMed]
33. Moss, H.E. Retinal vascular changes are a marker for cerebral vascular diseases. *Curr. Neurol. Neurosci. Rep.* **2015**, *15*, 1–9. [CrossRef] [PubMed]
34. Bek, T. Diameter changes of retinal vessels in diabetic retinopathy. *Curr. Diab. Rep.* **2017**, *17*, 1–7. [CrossRef] [PubMed]

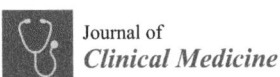

Article

Incidence and Risk Factors for Berger's Space Development after Uneventful Cataract Surgery: Evidence from Swept-Source Optical Coherence Tomography

Zhengwei Zhang [1,2], Jinhan Yao [3], Shuimiao Chang [3], Piotr Kanclerz [4,5], Ramin Khoramnia [6], Minghui Deng [7] and Xiaogang Wang [3,*]

1. Department of Ophthalmology, Wuxi Clinical College, Nantong University, Wuxi 214002, China; weir2008@ntu.edu.cn
2. Department of Ophthalmology, Wuxi No. 2 People's Hospital, Nanjing Medical University, Wuxi 214002, China
3. Department of Cataract, Shanxi Eye Hospital, Shanxi Medical University, Taiyuan 030002, China; yjh961106@163.com (J.Y.); changsm991101@163.com (S.C.)
4. Hygeia Clinic, 80-286 Gdańsk, Poland; p.kanclerz@gumed.edu.pl
5. Helsinki Retina Research Group, University of Helsinki, 00014 Helsinki, Finland
6. The David J. Apple International Laboratory for Ocular Pathology, Department of Ophthalmology, University of Heidelberg, 69120 Heidelberg, Germany; ramin.khoramnia@med.uni-heidelberg.de
7. Department of Cataract, Linfen Yaodu Eye Hospital, Linfen 042000, China; dengminghuimail@163.com
* Correspondence: wangxiaogang@sxmu.edu.cn

Abstract: Background: This study investigates the incidence and risk factors for the development of Berger's space (BS) after uneventful phacoemulsification based on swept-source optical coherence tomography (SS-OCT). Methods: Cataractous eyes captured using qualified SS-OCT images before and after uneventful phacoemulsification cataract surgery were included. Six high-resolution cross-sectional anterior segment SS-OCT images at 30° intervals were used for BS data measurements. BS width was measured at three points on each scanned meridian line: the central point line aligned with the cornea vertex and two point lines at the pupil's margins. Results: A total of 223 eyes that underwent uneventful cataract surgery were evaluated. Preoperatively, only two eyes (2/223, 0.9%) were observed to have consistent BS in all six scanning directions. BS was observed postoperatively in 44 eyes (44/223, 19.7%). A total of 13 eyes (13/223, 5.8%) with insufficient image quality, pupil dilation, or lack of preoperative image data were excluded from the study. A total of 31 postoperative eyes with BS and 31 matched eyes without BS were included in the final data analysis. The smallest postoperative BS width was in the upper quadrant of the vertical meridian line (90°), with a mean value of 280 μm. The largest BS width was observed in the opposite area of the main clear corneal incision, with a mean value >500 μm. Conclusions: Uneven-width BS is observable after uneventful phacoemulsification. Locations with a much wider BS (indirect manifestation of Wieger zonular detachment) are predominantly located in the opposite direction to the main corneal incisions.

Keywords: anterior hyaloid detachment; Berger's space; phacoemulsification; swept-source optical coherence tomography

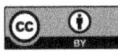

1. Introduction

Berger's space (BS), also termed the vitreolenticular interface, hyaloid–capsular interspace, or patellar fossa, is a space located between the posterior lens capsule and anterior hyaloid of the vitreous. These structures attach in a circular manner via thickened hyalocapsular zonules of the Wieger ligament, the outer limit of which is defined by Egger's line. Growing evidence suggests that BS is a real and clinically significant space in pathological conditions that can be detected using slit-lamp biomicroscopy [1,2]. Further, Weidle [3] identified the presence of BS in infants by filling the space with an ophthalmic viscosurgical device (OVD) after a small posterior capsulotomy during congenital cataract surgery.

In terms of clinical application, to sever attachments and create a wide interspace, Menapace [4] attempted transzonular capsulo-hyaloidal hydroseparation by rinsing the zonular fibers with fluid or additional triamcinolone acetonide (TA) to initiate or complete anterior hyaloid detachment (AHD). This procedure may improve the patency and visibility of BS to augment the control and feasibility of primary posterior laser capsulotomy (PPLC) in femtosecond laser-assisted cataract surgery (FLACS) with an intact anterior hyaloid membrane that acts as a major barrier between the anterior and posterior segments of the eye. In this regard, adequate imaging of the posterior lens capsule and anterior hyaloid membrane is a prerequisite for safe and effective PPLC. Similarly, viscodissection of BS is also greatly important for manual primary posterior capsulorhexis during the surgery of pediatric cataracts, to avoid vitreous prolapse and destabilization of the intraocular lens [5].

Recently, the importance of BS as an anatomical structure for microsurgery has increased. Partial AHD and BS opening are sometimes intentionally induced using hydrostatic pressure to safely and completely remove anterior vitreous hemorrhage [6]. BS can be used as a surgical plane for viscodelamination of the interface between the posterior lens capsule and anterior hyaloid membrane. Lyu et al. [7] reported that retrolental plaques in eyes with pediatric tractional vitreoretinopathy were successfully separated from the posterior lens capsule by blunt tension of cohesive viscoelastic injection into BS with an intact posterior capsule during lens-sparing vitrectomy, because these plaques attach to the anterior hyaloid membrane before invading the BS and posterior lens capsule. Moreover, Kam et al. [8] reported a canal of Petit pneumodissection technique via endoscopy-guided dissection of anatomical planes using filtered air to enable safe and complete separation of the anterior hyaloid of the vitreous from the posterior lens capsule in phakic or pseudophakic eyes. Therefore, both the cataract and vitreoretinal specialist should pay attention to and use this interesting finding to assist or notice the importance of BS or AHD in clinic.

Phacoemulsification is a widely used and safe procedure for the treatment of cataracts. However, rare accidents, such as acute aqueous misdirection syndrome and Descemet membrane detachment, may occur during surgery. In a previous published case of traumatic cataract surgery involving a 41-year-old man with moderate myopia and angle recession in his left eye [9], a large air bubble running into Berger's space (BS) was noticed during the cortex removal procedure. It is, therefore, of importance to cataract surgeons that BS is a noteworthy anatomical structure and has a possible influence on phacoemulsification.

More recently, BS has been visualized intraoperatively during cataract surgery via real-time intraoperative optical coherence tomography (iOCT) attached to femtosecond laser cataract systems [10,11], or with an operating microscope [12]. Detecting BS before and after cataract surgery using advanced noninvasive optical technology is crucial, as these eyes could be at risk of aqueous misdirection [13]. Studies using spectral-domain optical coherence tomography (SD-OCT) with an anterior segment module have identified BS in pseudophakic patients due to the thinner interface of the intraocular lens compared to that of the natural lens [1]. However, it is insufficient to capture images of BS with SD-OCT in most patients with their natural lenses because SD-OCT imaging fails to reach the depth necessary to visualize the interface between the posterior lens capsule and anterior hyaloid.

Compared to SD-OCT, swept-source optical coherence tomography (SS-OCT) employs a longer wavelength and has a greater scanning depth. Accordingly, it is a more appropriate method to evaluate the anterior hyaloid interface [14–17]. Currently, the number of SS-OCT devices commercially available in clinical settings is increasing, which may improve our understanding of the physiology and pathology of BS.

The growing number of published articles has signified increasing interest in this anatomical space in recent years. The main objective of this study was to evaluate the influence of phacoemulsification surgery on the change in the postoperative structure of the hyaloid–capsular interspace using a commercially available SS-OCT device with anterior imaging in a relatively large sample, to further clarify the incidence of pre- and post-BS and potential risk factors for the change in postoperative BS.

2. Materials and Methods

This retrospective observational study included patients who were willing to undergo cataract surgery at Shanxi Eye Hospital between November 2020 and December 2021. The study was registered online on the International Standard Randomized Controlled Trials website (http://www.controlled-trials.com; accessed on 8 November 2021) with the registration number ISRCTN13860301. All participants provided written informed consent for participation in the clinical examination program and to undergo cataract surgery. This study was conducted in accordance with the tenets of the Declaration of Helsinki. The Institutional Review Board of Shanxi Eye Hospital affiliated with Shanxi Medical University approved the protocol (No. 2019LL130).

The medical records of patients with cataracts who consented to surgery were reviewed. Patients undergoing phacoemulsification cataract surgery were enrolled. Inclusion criteria were as follows: diagnosis of cataracts prepared for surgery, dilated pupil size of 7 mm or larger, no pathological alteration in the anterior segment (such as keratoconus, pseudoexfoliation syndrome, or corneal opacity), no retinal diseases impairing visual function, no previous anterior or posterior segment surgery, and no intraoperative or postoperative complications. Multiple parameters were extracted to determine BS and analyze the related factors. All included patients underwent conventional phacoemulsification. Before and after cataract surgery, each patient underwent complete ocular examination, including best-corrected visual acuity (BCVA), non-contact tonometry, slit-lamp examination, and indirect ophthalmoscopy. Axial length was measured using IOLMaster 700 (Carl Zeiss Meditec, Dublin, CA, USA). All included patients underwent anterior segment SS-OCT using the ANTERION device (software version 1.3.4.0; Heidelberg Engineering, Heidelberg, Germany) with a 1300 nm light source [18,19].

SS-OCT anterior segment imaging pre- and post-surgery was performed by the same technician in a semi-dark room without pupillary dilation, with the patient in the seated position, as reported in a previous study [18]. The ANTERION Metrics App in conjunction with a high-resolution SS-OCT imaging device provides 6 high-resolution (axial resolution < 10 μm and lateral resolution < 30 μm) cross-sectional anterior segment images at 30° intervals (0–180°, 30–210°, 60–240°, 90–270°, 120–300°, and 150–330°) centered on the corneal vertex (Figure 1). The quality of each measurement was examined by an expert, and images that revealed BS were used for further analysis. BS width was manually measured at three points on each scanned meridian line: the central point and two point lines aligned with the corneal vertex and pupil margins, respectively (Figure 2). To identify risk factors for the development of BS after surgery, the 31 matched eyes without postoperative BS were selected for comparison analysis.

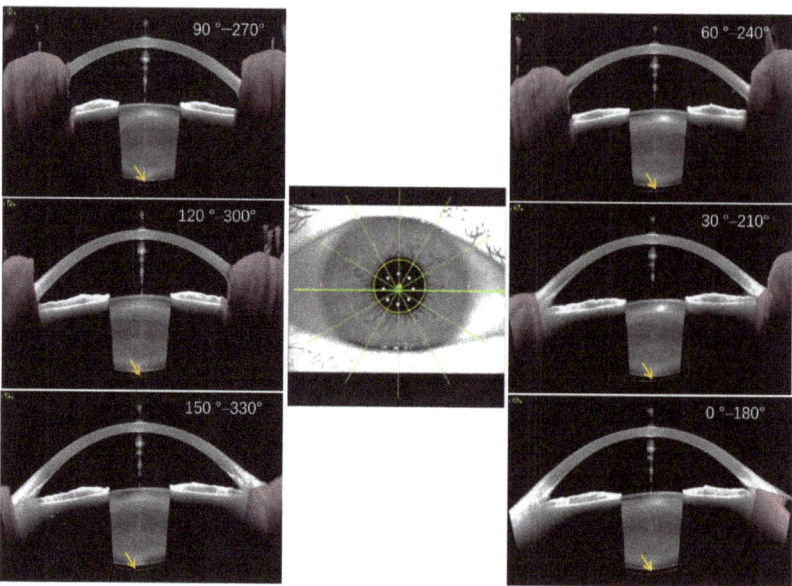

Figure 1. Six high-resolution, cross-sectional anterior segment images with 30° intervals centered on the corneal vertex in a 48-year-old myopic cataract patient with an axial length of 28.70 mm. Yellow arrows indicate Berger's space with a natural lens. Of note, the size of Berger's space in all directions is relatively symmetrical and uniform (around 254 μm).

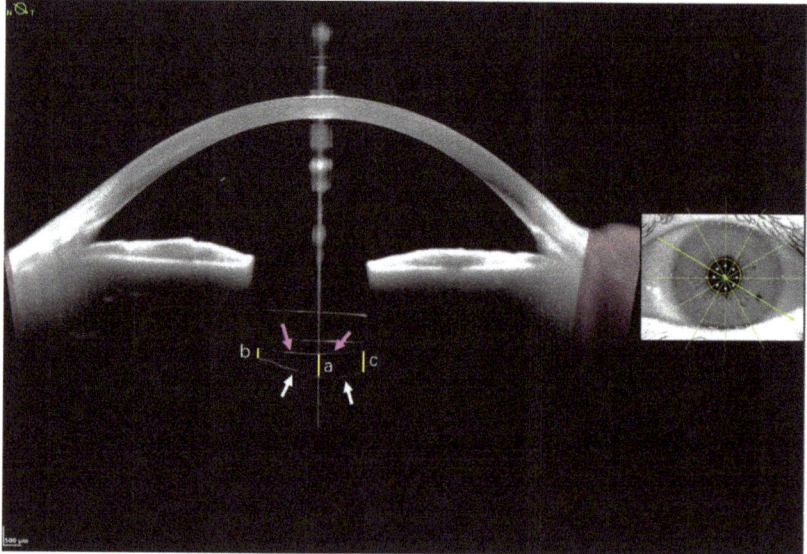

Figure 2. The measurement locations used to determine the width of Berger's space. The width of Berger's space, defined as the vertical distance between posterior lens capsule (pink arrows) and anterior vitreous hyaloid (white arrows), was manually measured at three points of each scanned meridian line: the central point line (**a**) and the two point lines (**b**,**c**) at the margins of the pupil (yellow solid lines).

3. Surgical Procedure

All phacoemulsification surgeries were performed under local anesthesia by a single surgeon (X.G.W.). Phacoemulsification parameters were set as follows: continuous linear mode was used with ultrasound (US) power up to 40%, vacuum was linear to 500 mmHg, and bottle height (recorded as irrigation pressure), to provide passive infusion, was set at 95–110 cm above eye level. A 2.2 mm clear corneal incision was made superior-temporally in the right eye or superior-nasally in the left eye (120°). After the creation of a continuous curvilinear capsulorhexis, phacoemulsification (horizontal phaco-chop technique; angle 30° phaco tip No. DP8730 with outer diameter of 0.9 mm and inner diameter of 0.70–0.5 mm) was followed by aspiration of the cortical remnants using the Stellaris® MICS™ system (Bausch + Lomb, Rochester, NY, USA). A foldable monofocal hydrophobic acrylic intraocular lens (IOL HOYA PY60AD) was implanted into the capsular bag. In all patients, no sutures were used to close the incisions.

4. Statistical Analyses

Statistical analyses were performed using SPSS software (version 21.0, SPSS, Chicago, IL, USA). The normality of the distribution of continuous variables was assessed using a one-sample Kolmogorov–Smirnov test prior to significance testing. Normally distributed data were analyzed with an independent Student's t-test. Non-normally distributed data were analyzed using the Mann–Whitney U-test. Correlations were assessed using Pearson's correlation analysis. All normally distributed values of continuous variables are expressed as the mean ± standard deviation (SD), and non-normally distributed values are expressed as median and interquartile ranges (IQR). All tests were two-tailed with a significance level of 5%.

5. Results

All 223 eyes that underwent uneventful cataract surgery have undergone a preliminary analysis. In 44 eyes (19.7%), BS could be visualized using an SS-OCT device postoperatively; however, 13 eyes were excluded from the study, as the OCT images demonstrated low quality (4 eyes), had pupil dilation (5 eyes), or had no preoperative data (4 eyes). Ultimately, 31 eyes of 30 patients (21 eyes of 20 patients with age-related cataracts, 3 eyes of 3 patients with metabolic cataracts, 3 eyes of 3 patients with complicated cataracts, 2 eyes of 2 patients with glucocorticoid-induced cataracts, 1 eye of 1 case with high myopia, and 1 eye of 1 case with congenital cataracts) with clearly defined BS after uneventful phacoemulsification were included in the study. These results were matched with 31 eyes from 25 patients (16 eyes of 12 patients with age-related cataracts, 9 eyes of 8 patients with metabolic cataracts, 4 eyes of 3 patients with glucocorticoid-induced cataracts, and 2 eyes of 2 patients with high myopia) without preoperative BS to analyze the risk factors for the development of BS. The clinical characteristics of 30 patients with and 25 patients without postoperative BS are presented in Table 1. Preoperative BS was observed in only two eyes (0.9%). No significant differences were observed in age, axial length, lens thickness, and intraocular pressure between eyes with and without BS. BS development was associated with a higher irrigation pressure ($p < 0.001$) and shorter surgery duration ($p = 0.021$).

The mean follow-up time for anterior SS-OCT imaging after cataract surgery was 24.1 days postoperatively. The mean times of OCT imaging for eyes with and without BS were 14.0 days (range, 1–57 days) and 34.2 days (range, 1–395 days) after surgery, respectively. BS persisted for more than 25 days after cataract surgery in 10 of these eyes. The smallest BS width was observed in the upper vertical meridian line (90°), with a mean value of 280 ± 202 µm. The largest BS width was observed in the opposite area of the main clear corneal incision (240°), with a mean value of 557 ± 352 µm (Figures 3 and 4). Hyperreflective postoperative material was noted in BS in six eyes (Figure 5).

Pearson correlation analysis revealed no significant correlation between postoperative BS width at all meridians and ocular parameters (axial length, lens thickness, and intraocular pressure), surgical parameters (surgery time and irrigation pressure), or age (all p values > 0.05).

Table 1. Clinical characteristics of patients with and without postoperative Berger's space (BS).

	With BS	Without BS	p
N	30	25	
Eyes (OD/OS)	31 (18/13)	31 (18/13)	
Age (years)	66.0 ± 14.2	64.1 ± 14.3	0.635 *
Axial length (mm)	23.22 ± 1.14	23.70 ± 1.91	0.239 *
Lens thickness (mm)	4.13 ± 0.50	4.26 ± 0.56	0.443 *
Intraocular pressure (mmHg)			
Before surgery	15.87 ± 2.50	16.81 ± 2.37	0.136 *
After surgery	17.61 ± 1.61	17.03 ± 1.58	0.157 *
Surgical time (min) [†]	12.48 ± 3.95	14.58 ± 2.98	0.021 *
Irrigation pressure (cm H_2O, median (IQR))	110 (110–105)	105 (110–101)	<0.001 [#]

* Independent Student's *t*-test, [#] Mann–Whitney U test. [†] Surgical time was calculated from the beginning of the side incision to the end of the watertight incision closure.

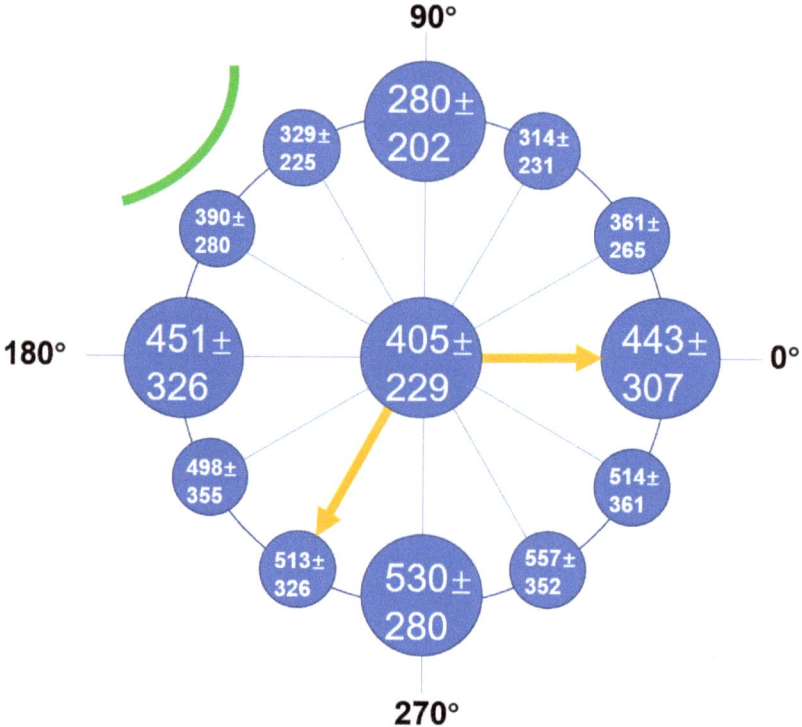

Figure 3. The mean ± standard deviation (SD) width of Berger's space at three points (as illustrated in Figure 2) at each meridian line. The green curved line indicates the main clear corneal incision for the phacoemulsification tip. The region indicated by the two yellow arrows represents the main impact area of irrigation fluid during cataract surgery. The mean width of Berger's space opposite to the main clear corneal incision was the largest, which impacted the influence of irrigation fluid circulations.

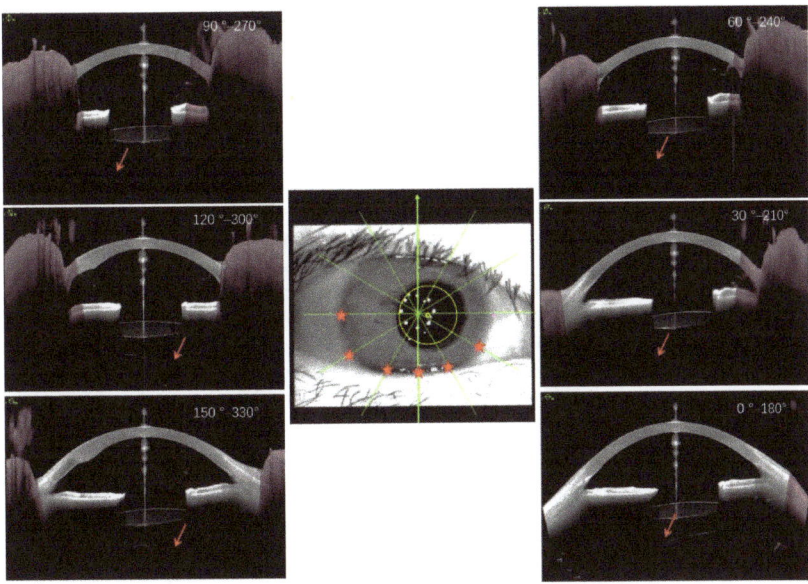

Figure 4. A representative eye postoperatively presented with uneven Berger's space. Berger's space lost its symmetry in all directions and the larger width was predominantly observed in the opposite area of the main clear corneal incision (red arrows in cross-sectional optical coherence tomography (OCT) images and red stars in eye plane image).

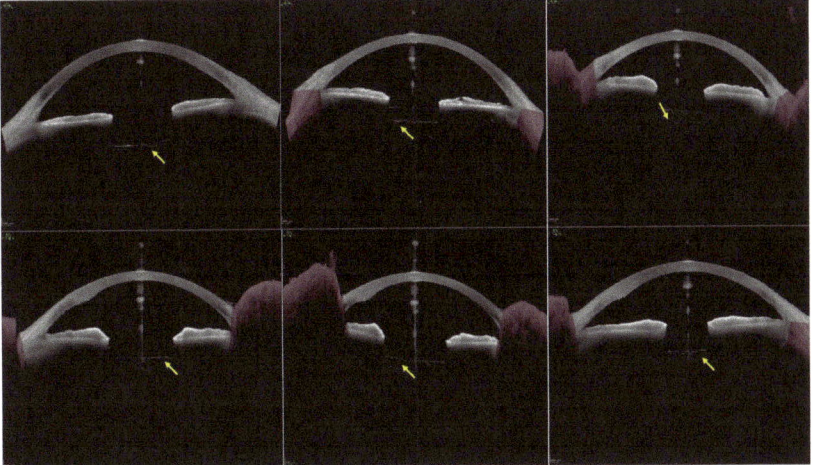

Figure 5. Scattered hyperreflective material (yellow arrows) in Berger's space was observed in six eyes postoperatively in less than 7 days.

6. Discussion

Evidence of direct communication between the anterior chamber and BS during phacoemulsification cataract surgery has been inconclusive. The current findings support the hypothesis that uneventful cataract surgery may induce AHD and provides evidence of the volume characteristics of the created space. We observed that 44 eyes (19.7%) presented with BS after phacoemulsification. A previous study reported that BS can be clearly visualized in 81% of cataract cases immediately after IOL implantation with femtosecond laser-integrated SD-OCT [10]. More recently, Anisimova et al. [20] successfully identified BS in 21 cases (75%) via intraoperative optical coherence tomography (iOCT) during phacoemulsification, and in 23 cases (82%) with SD-OCT postoperatively. This difference may be due to the different characteristics of the included populations, different equipment employed, and different time intervals for scanning. For instance, the study by Anisimova et al. [20] included many patients with pseudoexfoliation syndrome (PEX) whose ciliary zonule was inherently weakened [21]. Of note, BS persisted for more than 25 days (maximum of 57 days) after cataract surgery in 10 eyes in our study, suggesting that AHD cannot recover once it occurs either partially or completely.

In the two eyes with preoperative BS, the size of BS in all directions was relatively symmetrical and uniform (Figure 1). However, BS lost its symmetry in all directions, and the largest width appeared in the area opposite the main corneal incision (Figure 4). This phenomenon could predominantly be due to the impact force of the irrigation fluid flow, which may cause a local crevice of the Wieger ligament in the opposite area through the ciliary zonule, resulting in local AHD (Figure 6). We speculate that BS width is related to the extent of Wieger ligament damage, whereby greater BS width indicates greater extent of Wieger ligament damage.

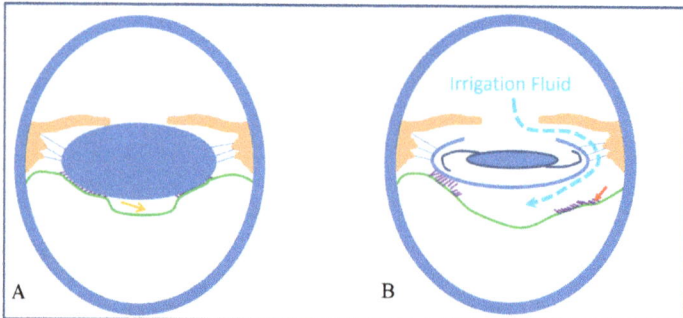

Figure 6. Schematic diagram of Wieger zonular damage and increasing width of Berger's space during phacoemulsification. (**A**) The yellow arrow indicates Berger's space with natural lens before surgery (the green line indicated as the anterior hyaloid of the vitreous; the purple lines indicated the Wieger zonular). (**B**) The curved dash line indicates extensive irrigation fluid through the zonular network, resulting in partial Wieger zonular damage (red arrow).

Phacoemulsification cataract surgery may cause posterior vitreous detachment (PVD) [22,23]. However, there is growing interest in AHD after uneventful cataract surgery [20]. Based on visualization using TA, BS has been recognized as a sac-like structure with a septum located behind the lens that divides BS into a two-thirds temporal and one-third nasal formation [24]. The advent of advanced imaging technology, particularly SS-OCT, has facilitated in vivo visualization of the anatomical structure of the vitreolenticular interface [25].

Despite its rare involvement in ocular pathology, BS can be visualized in certain pathological conditions, such as ocular trauma [26,27], spontaneous vitreous hemorrhage [1], ocular surgeries [3,28,29], pigment dispersion syndrome [30], and idiopathic conditions [31]. Accordingly, BS is an actual space that may constitute a key site of pathology. Shah et al. [32] reported a preterm neonate with type 1 retinopathy of prematurity who presented with hemorrhage in BS immediately after intravitreal bevacizumab injection. The hemorrhage resolved completely at 18 weeks postoperatively, and the crystalline lens remained clear. Therefore, specific attention should be paid to disease or surgical manipulations potentially related to BS.

BS is too narrow to be identified in the presence of a natural crystalline lens, even with modern diagnostic tools. As such, this space is unobservable in most cataract patients preoperatively because the posterior capsule of the lens adheres throughout its extension to the anterior vitreous. As reported in a previous study using SD-OCT with the anterior pole module (Cirrus Lumera 700 Carl Zeiss Meditec), only 3 out of 90 patients presented with BS [25]. Similarly, we only identified 2 eyes with preoperative BS out of 223 eyes using SS-OCT. However, potential BS may develop into an obvious space with varying widths immediately after lens extraction from the capsular bag, accompanied by forward movement of the posterior lens capsule. This would increase the probability of occurrence of BS during and after cataract surgery.

Crucially, BS may be enlarged by excessive irrigation fluid circulation that moves through weakened zonules and incomplete attachment of the Wieger ligament during phacoemulsification. Vasavada et al. [33] reported that using high fluidic parameters during phacoemulsification caused partial AHD with an intact posterior lens capsule. We observed that eyes with BS had higher irrigation pressures ($p < 0.001$, Table 1). However, higher irrigation per se may cause higher pressure and damage to zonular fibers, which facilitates the entry of irrigation fluid into BS. Therefore, in cataract patients with weakened zonular fibers, such as high myopia and PEX, irrigation pressure should be reduced appropriately to mitigate damage to zonules and decrease AHD incidence. Surgeons should also carefully adjust the ratio between the bottle height and flow rate to achieve a balanced state, which may enhance the stability of fluid circulation and safety during surgery.

The presence or increasing width of BS or AHD may lead to complications during or after cataract surgery. Vasavada et al. [33] reported that the use of high bottle heights and aspiration flow rates may have detrimental consequences on the anterior vitreous face, which are clinically undetectable. This causes decompartmentalization and allows the diffusion of infectious microbes and inflammatory mediators through zonules into BS, consequently increasing the risk of vitritis, macular edema, or even endophthalmitis. However, in this study, no significant correlation was identified between BS width and ocular parameters (axial length, lens thickness, and intraocular pressure), surgical parameters (surgery time and irrigation pressure), or age, although eyes with BS had higher irrigation pressure. This could be due to the small sample size, which may have obscured any statistical correlation. Notably, longer surgical time was observed in the group without postoperative BS. This may be attributed to the recording of surgical time as the whole operation time, rather than just the phaco and irrigation/aspiration time. Ideally, a comprehensive consideration of irrigation pressure and surgical time (phaco and irrigation/aspiration) may better reflect the effects of cataract surgery on the vitreolenticular interface.

AHD is associated with increased instability of the posterior lens capsule (due to loss of Wieger ligament fixation), and is a latent risk factor for posterior capsule rupture during the irrigation/aspiration step of phacoemulsification, thereby increasing the risk of posterior capsule rupture. Partial AHD may also partly contribute to the pathogenesis of acute aqueous misdirection syndrome; however, no cases of BS or AHD after phacoemulsification presenting with acute aqueous misdirection syndrome were noted in our study or previous studies [12,20]. Nevertheless, the complex nature of this syndrome may involve changes in the anatomical structure of the anterior vitreolenticular interface as well as the collection of irrigation fluid or OVD in BS.

Previous studies have reported the presence of material in BS after uneventful cataract surgery [20,34]. Lenticular zonular insufficiency or partial AHD may provide access to BS from the anterior chamber during irrigation and aspiration, resulting in the entry of medication, residual lens material, and blood cells into this space. Using iOCT, Anisimova et al. [20] reported the presence of BS and penetration of lens fragments into the hyaloid–capsular interspace. In 767 consecutive phaco cases, Kam et al. [34] identified material in BS in 386 eyes (50.3% of cases), the majority of which was putative lens material (46.5% of all cases), with two cases confirmed by histological investigation. In contrast, another study reported that no retrocapsular lens fragments could be identified cytopathologically after uneventful phacoemulsification [35]. Although we could not confirm that the material (uniformly hyper-reflective signal in SS-OCT images) was in BS in the six eyes analyzed herein, we speculate that the material may be OVD or small residual lens fragments migrating from the anterior chamber through the zonular network and detached Wieger ligament (Figure 5).

Due to its retrospective nature, this study had several limitations. First, the limited field of view was a study limitation due to the lack of mydriasis for imaging. Nonetheless, the effective scan captured useful information from the zone within the pupil diameter, as the iris prevented deeper light propagation. Second, we did not evaluate the stability of the anterior chamber depth during phacoemulsification, which is a factor affecting zonular fiber function.

7. Conclusions

The Berger's space can be visualized by SS-OCT not only before but one day or more than one month after cataract surgery. The presence of postoperative BS may be due to the partial AHD during cataract surgery, and the largest width appeared in the opposite area to the main corneal incision, unlike the size of it in all directions being relatively symmetrical and uniform preoperatively.

Author Contributions: Conceptualization, Z.Z. and X.W.; methodology, X.W.; software, X.W.; validation, J.Y., S.C., M.D. and X.W.; formal analysis, Z.Z. and X.W.; investigation, J.Y., S.C. and M.D.; resources, X.W.; data curation, X.W.; writing—original draft preparation, Z.Z. and X.W.; writing—review and editing, Z.Z., P.K., R.K. and X.W.; visualization, X.W.; supervision, P.K. and R.K.; project administration, X.W., P.K. and R.K.; funding acquisition, Z.Z. and X.W. All authors have read and agreed to the published version of the manuscript.

Funding: This work was supported by the National Natural Science Foundation of China under Grant No. 81971697, and research funding from Shanxi Eye Hospital No. B201804, the Shanxi Scholarship Council of China Grant No. 2021-174 (XGW), and the fund of Wuxi "Double Hundred" Young and Middle-aged Top Medical and Health Talents under Grant No. HB2020030, Research Project of the Wuxi Commission of Health under Grant No. M202131 (ZWZ). All the above-mentioned funding sources had no role in the design of this study, during its execution, analyses, interpretation of the data, or decision to submit results.

Institutional Review Board Statement: This study was conducted in accordance with the tenets of the Declaration of Helsinki. The Institutional Review Board of Shanxi Eye Hospital affiliated with Shanxi Medical University approved the protocol (No. 2019LL130).

Informed Consent Statement: Informed consent was obtained from all subjects involved in the study.

Data Availability Statement: The datasets used during the current study are available from the corresponding author.

Conflicts of Interest: The authors declare no conflict of interest.

References

1. Mares, V.; Nehemy, M.B.; Salomao, D.R.; Goddard, S.; Tesmer, J.; Pulido, J.S. Multimodal Imaging and Histopathological Evaluation of Berger's Space. *Ocul. Oncol. Pathol.* **2020**, *6*, 3–9. [CrossRef] [PubMed]
2. Tolentino, F.I.; Lee, P.F.; Schepens, C.L. Biomicroscopic study of vitreous cavity in diabetic retinopathy. *Arch. Ophthalmol.* **1966**, *75*, 238–246. [CrossRef] [PubMed]
3. Weidle, E.G. Visualization of Berger's space in the living eye. *Ophthalmic Surg.* **1985**, *16*, 733–734. [CrossRef] [PubMed]
4. Menapace, R. Transzonular capsulo-hyaloidal hydroseparation with optional triamcinolone enhancement: A technique to detect or induce anterior hyaloid membrane detachment for primary posterior laser capsulotomy. *J. Cataract Refract. Surg.* **2019**, *45*, 903–909. [CrossRef]
5. Menapace, R. Posterior capsulorhexis combined with optic buttonholing: An alternative to standard in-the-bag implantation of sharp-edged intraocular lenses? A critical analysis of 1000 consecutive cases. *Graefe Arch. Clin. Exp. Ophthalmol.* **2008**, *246*, 787–801. [CrossRef]
6. Ikeda, T.; Sato, K.; Katano, T.; Hayashi, Y. Surgically induced detachment of the anterior hyaloid membrane from the posterior lens capsule. *Arch. Ophthalmol.* **1999**, *117*, 408–409. [CrossRef]
7. Lyu, J.; Zhang, Q.; Zhao, P. Viscodelamination of Localized Retrolental Plaques During Lens-Sparing Vitrectomy in Eyes with Pediatric Tractional Vitreoretinopathy. *Retina* 2020, online ahead of print. [CrossRef]
8. Kam, Y.W.; Funk, R.O.; Barnard, L.; Ajlan, R.S. New Endoscopic Surgical Approach for Anterior Hyaloid Dissection in Phakic and Pseudophakic Patients. *Retina* **2019**, *39* (Suppl. 1), S129–S132. [CrossRef]

9. Dong, J.; Jiang, L.; Sun, B.; Wang, X. Large air bubble in the Berger space during cataract surgery. *JCRS Online Case Rep.* **2021**, *9*, e00051.
10. Dick, H.B.; Schultz, T. Primary posterior laser-assisted capsulotomy. *J. Refract. Surg.* **2014**, *30*, 128–133. [CrossRef] [PubMed]
11. Haeussler-Sinangin, Y.; Schultz, T.; Holtmann, E.; Dick, H.B. Primary posterior capsulotomy in femtosecond laser-assisted cataract surgery: In vivo spectral-domain optical coherence tomography study. *J. Cataract Refract. Surg.* **2016**, *42*, 1339–1344. [CrossRef] [PubMed]
12. Tassignon, M.J.; Ni Dhubhghaill, S. Real-Time Intraoperative Optical Coherence Tomography Imaging Confirms Older Concepts about the Berger Space. *Ophthalmic Res.* **2016**, *56*, 222–226. [CrossRef]
13. Grzybowski, A.; Kanclerz, P. Acute and chronic fluid misdirection syndrome: Pathophysiology and treatment. *Graefe Arch. Clin. Exp. Ophthalmol.* **2018**, *256*, 135–154. [CrossRef] [PubMed]
14. Lains, I.; Wang, J.C.; Cui, Y.; Katz, R.; Vingopoulos, F.; Staurenghi, G.; Vavvas, D.G.; Miller, J.W.; Miller, J.B. Retinal applications of swept source optical coherence tomography (OCT) and optical coherence tomography angiography (OCTA). *Prog. Retin. Eye Res.* **2021**, *84*, 100951. [CrossRef] [PubMed]
15. Montes-Mico, R.; Pastor-Pascual, F.; Ruiz-Mesa, R.; Tana-Rivero, P. Ocular biometry with swept-source optical coherence tomography. *J. Cataract Refract. Surg.* **2021**, *47*, 802–814. [CrossRef]
16. Pujari, A.; Agarwal, D.; Sharma, N. Clinical role of swept source optical coherence tomography in anterior segment diseases: A review. *Semin. Ophthalmol.* **2021**, *36*, 684–691. [CrossRef]
17. Ruminski, D.; Sebag, J.; Toledo, R.D.; Jimenez-Villar, A.; Nowak, J.K.; Manzanera, S.; Artal, P.; Grulkowski, I. Volumetric Optical Imaging and Quantitative Analysis of Age-Related Changes in Anterior Human Vitreous. *Investig. Ophthalmol. Vis. Sci.* **2021**, *62*, 31. [CrossRef]
18. Dong, J.; Wang, X.L.; Deng, M.; Wang, X.G. Three-Dimensional Reconstruction and Swept-Source Optical Coherence Tomography for Crystalline Lens Tilt and Decentration Relative to the Corneal Vertex. *Transl. Vis. Sci. Technol.* **2021**, *10*, 13. [CrossRef]
19. Tana-Rivero, P.; Aguilar-Corcoles, S.; Tello-Elordi, C.; Pastor-Pascual, F.; Montes-Mico, R. Agreement between 2 swept-source OCT biometers and a Scheimpflug partial coherence interferometer. *J. Cataract Refract. Surg.* **2021**, *47*, 488–495. [CrossRef]
20. Anisimova, N.S.; Arbisser, L.B.; Shilova, N.F.; Melnik, M.A.; Belodedova, A.V.; Knyazer, B.; Malyugin, B.E. Anterior vitreous detachment: Risk factor for intraoperative complications during phacoemulsification. *J. Cataract Refract. Surg.* **2020**, *46*, 55–62.
21. Schlötzer-Schrehardt, U.; Naumann, G.O. A histopathologic study of zonular instability in pseudoexfoliation syndrome. *Am. J. Ophthalmol.* **1994**, *118*, 730–743. [CrossRef]
22. Mirshahi, A.; Hohn, F.; Lorenz, K.; Hattenbach, L.O. Incidence of posterior vitreous detachment after cataract surgery. *J. Cataract Refract. Surg.* **2009**, *35*, 987–991. [CrossRef] [PubMed]
23. Park, J.H.; Yang, H.; Kwon, H.; Jeon, S. Risk Factors for Onset or Progression of Posterior Vitreous Detachment at the Vitreomacular Interface after Cataract Surgery. *Ophthalmol. Retin.* **2021**, *5*, 270–278. [CrossRef]
24. Morishita, S.; Sato, T.; Oosuka, S.; Horie, T.; Kida, T.; Oku, H.; Nakamura, K.; Takai, S.; Jin, D.; Ikeda, T. Expression of Lymphatic Markers in the Berger's Space and Bursa Premacularis. *Int. J. Mol. Sci.* **2021**, *22*, 2086. [CrossRef] [PubMed]
25. Santos-Bueso, E. Berger's space. *Arch. Soc. Esp. Oftalmol. (Engl. Ed.)* **2019**, *94*, 471–477. [CrossRef] [PubMed]
26. Li, S.T.; Yiu, E.P.; Wong, A.H.; Yeung, J.C.; Yu, L.W. Management of traumatic haemorrhage in the Berger's space of a 4-year-old child. *Int. Ophthalmol.* **2017**, *37*, 1053–1055. [CrossRef] [PubMed]
27. Gjerde, H.; MacDonnell, T.; Tan, A. Berger's space hemorrhage missing the visual axis. *Can. J. Ophthalmol.* **2020**, *55*, 343. [CrossRef] [PubMed]
28. Salman, A.; Parmar, P.; Coimbatore, V.G.; Meenakshisunderam, R.; Christdas, N.J. Entrapment of intravitreal triamcinolone behind the crystalline lens. *Indian J. Ophthalmol.* **2009**, *57*, 324–325. [CrossRef]
29. Dubrulle, P.; Fajnkuchen, F.; Qu, L.; Giocanti-Auregan, A. Dexamethasone implant confined in Berger's space. *Springerplus* **2016**, *5*, 1786. [CrossRef]
30. Turgut, B.; Turkcuoglu, P.; Deniz, N.; Catak, O. Annular and central heavy pigment deposition on the posterior lens capsule in the pigment dispersion syndrome: Pigment deposition on the posterior lens capsule in the pigment dispersion syndrome. *Int. Ophthalmol.* **2008**, *28*, 441–445. [CrossRef]
31. Tanaka, H.; Ohara, K.; Shiwa, T.; Minami, M. Idiopathic opacification of Berger's space. *J. Cataract Refract. Surg.* **2004**, *30*, 2232–2234. [CrossRef] [PubMed]
32. Shah, P.R.; Sachan, A.; Chandra, P. Retrolental Hemorrhage in Berger's Space after Intravitreal Bevacizumab Injection for Retinopathy of Prematurity. *J. Pediatr. Ophthalmol. Strabismus* **2020**, *57*, e71–e73. [CrossRef] [PubMed]
33. Vasavada, V.; Srivastava, S.; Vasavada, V.; Vasavada, S.; Vasavada, A.R.; Sudhalkar, A.; Bilgic, A. Impact of fluidic parameters during phacoemulsification on the anterior vitreous face behavior: Experimental study. *Indian J. Ophthalmol.* **2019**, *67*, 1634–1637. [CrossRef] [PubMed]
34. Kam, A.W.; Chen, T.S.; Wang, S.B.; Jain, N.S.; Goh, A.Y.; Douglas, C.P.; McKelvie, P.A.; Agar, A.; Osher, R.H.; Francis, I.C. Materials in the vitreous during cataract surgery: Nature and incidence, with two cases of histological confirmation. *Clin. Exp. Ophthalmol.* **2016**, *44*, 797–802. [CrossRef] [PubMed]
35. Liu, D.T.; Lee, V.Y.; Li, C.L.; Choi, P.C.; Lam, P.T.; Lam, D.S. Retrocapsular lens matter in uneventful phacoemulsification: Does it really exist? *Clin. Exp. Ophthalmol.* **2008**, *36*, 31–35. [CrossRef]

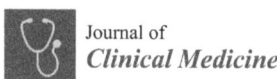

Article

Characteristics of the Ciliary Body in Healthy Chinese Subjects Evaluated by Radial and Transverse Imaging of Ultrasound Biometric Microscopy

Jiawei Ren [1,2,3], Xinbo Gao [1,2,3], Liming Chen [1,2,3], Huishan Lin [1,2,3], Yao Liu [1,2,3], Yuying Zhou [1,2,3], Yunru Liao [1,2,3], Chunzi Xie [1,2,3], Chengguo Zuo [1,2,3,*] and Mingkai Lin [1,2,3,*]

1 State Key Laboratory of Ophthalmology, Guangzhou 510060, China; renjiawei1016@126.com (J.R.); gaoxb@mail.sysu.edu.cn (X.G.); clm222000@163.com (L.C.); linhsh6@mail2.sysu.edu.cn (H.L.); willmakeit@163.com (Y.L.); zhouyuying1220@163.com (Y.Z.); liaoyr5@mail.sysu.edu.cn (Y.L.); 17688806270@163.com (C.X.)
2 Zhongshan Ophthalmic Center, Sun Yat-sen University, Guangzhou 510060, China
3 Guangdong Provincial Key Laboratory of Ophthalmology and Visual Science, Guangzhou 510060, China
* Correspondence: chengguozuo@163.com (C.Z.); linmk@mail.sysu.edu.cn (M.L.)

Citation: Ren, J.; Gao, X.; Chen, L.; Lin, H.; Liu, Y.; Zhou, Y.; Liao, Y.; Xie, C.; Zuo, C.; Lin, M. Characteristics of the Ciliary Body in Healthy Chinese Subjects Evaluated by Radial and Transverse Imaging of Ultrasound Biometric Microscopy. *J. Clin. Med.* 2022, 11, 3696. https://doi.org/10.3390/jcm11133696

Academic Editors: Vito Romano, Yalin Zheng, Mariantonia Ferrara and Tunde Peto

Received: 18 April 2022
Accepted: 21 June 2022
Published: 27 June 2022

Publisher's Note: MDPI stays neutral with regard to jurisdictional claims in published maps and institutional affiliations.

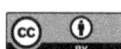

Copyright: © 2022 by the authors. Licensee MDPI, Basel, Switzerland. This article is an open access article distributed under the terms and conditions of the Creative Commons Attribution (CC BY) license (https://creativecommons.org/licenses/by/4.0/).

Abstract: Background: The imaging and analysis of the ciliary body (CB) are valuable in many potential clinical applications. This study aims to demonstrate the anatomy characteristics of CB using radial and transverse imaging of ultrasound biometric microscopy (UBM) in healthy Chinese subjects, and to explore the determining factors. Methods: Fifty-four eyes of 30 healthy Chinese subjects were evaluated. Clinical data, including age, body mass index (BMI), intraocular pressure (IOP), axial length (AL), and lens thickness (LT), were collected. Radial and transverse UBM measurements of the ciliary body were performed. Anterior chamber depth (ACD), ciliary sulcus diameter (CSD), ciliary process length (CPL), ciliary process density (CPD), ciliary process area (CPA), ciliary muscle area (CMA), ciliary body area (CBA), ciliary body thickness (CBT_0, CBT_1, and CBT_{max}), anterior placement of ciliary body (APCB), and trabecular-ciliary angle (TCA) of four (superior, nasal, inferior, and temporal) quadrants were measured. Results: The average CPL was 0.513 ± 0.074 mm, and the average CPA was 0.890 ± 0.141 mm^2. CPL and CPA tended to be longer and larger in the superior quadrant ($p < 0.001$) than in the other three quadrants. Average CPL was significantly correlated with AL (r = 0.535, $p < 0.001$), ACD (r = 0.511, $p < 0.001$), and LT (r = -0.512, $p < 0.001$). Intraclass correlation coefficient (ICC) scores were high for CPL (0.979), CPD (0.992), CPA (0.966), CMA (0.963), and CBA (0.951). Conclusions: In healthy Chinese subjects, CPL was greatest in the superior quadrant, followed by the inferior, temporal, and nasal quadrants, and CPA was largest in the superior quadrant, followed by the tempdoral, inferior, and nasal quadrants. Transverse UBM images can be used to measure the anatomy of the ciliary process with relatively good repeatability and reliability.

Keywords: ciliary body; radial scan; transverse scan; UBM; healthy Chinese subjects

1. Introduction

The ciliary body (CB) is the middle part of the anterior uvea. Anatomically, the CB spans the portion of the eye between the scleral spur and the ora serrata. In the sagittal section, the CB is triangular and divided into two parts: the pars plicata, characterized by a longitudinal radial process called the ciliary process (CP), and the pars plana, which is flat and approximately 4 mm behind the CP [1]. The CB has an important relationship with neighboring structures and has a variety of functions, including aqueous humor production, regulation of aqueous humor output through the uveal sclera pathway, and regulation via the ciliary muscle and suspensory ligament [2]. However, the CB and CP cannot be directly visualized due to the posterior position.

Ultrasound biometric microscopy (UBM) has been widely used to analyze anterior chamber structures, especially the structure behind the iris, such as the CB [3,4]. The UBM imaging and analysis of the CB, based on the radial scan, is valuable in many potential clinical applications, such as analyzing the pathogenesis of different types of angle-closure glaucoma [5–8]; describing the effects of pharmacologic agents on CB [9–11]; revealing the relationship between CBT and refractive error [12]; and assessing the development of uveitis, tumors, and cysts [13–15].

In radial UBM images, only one CB can be seen at one time, and only the pars plana and plicata of the CB can be visualized. In addition, it cannot clearly characterize the morphological features of the CPs due to their irregular arrangement, similar to protuberance. However, a transverse scan of CB is available by UBM. In transverse images, the transducer probe can be aligned with an entire row of CPs to illustrate the complex anatomy of the CB. Such images provide the ability to analyze a group of CPs rather than a single CP as in a radial scan. However, as far as we know, an objective and repeatable protocol of transverse scanning of UBM has never been reported. In this study, we aim to demonstrate the anatomy characteristics of the ciliary body using both radial and transverse scans of UBM in healthy Chinese subjects, and to explore the determining factors for further study of the pathogenesis, prevention, and follow-up of CB-related disease in vivo.

2. Materials and Methods

2.1. Participants

This was a cross-sectional study consisting of healthy Chinese subjects. The research conformed to the Helsinki Declaration's guidelines; was approved by the Ethics Board of the Zhongshan Ophthalmic Center (ZOC), Sun Yat-Sen University; and participants signed informed consents. All subjects underwent detailed ocular examinations, including slit-lamp examination, fundus examination with a 90-diopter lens, and intraocular pressure (IOP) measurement by Goldmann applanation tonometry. Axial length (AL), lens thickness (LT), white-to-white (WTW) corneal diameter, and central corneal thickness (CCT) were measured by the same trained observer (X.G.) via IOL Master 700 (Carl Zeiss Meditec AG, Jena, Germany, version 1.7). High-definition images of the anterior segment and the CB structures were provided by UBM.

The inclusion criteria were: (1) Chinese ethnicity, (2) age $\geq$ 18 years, (3) IOP < 21 mmHg by Goldmann applanation tonometry, and (4) normal optic disc and macular appearance. The exclusion criteria were: (1) any intraocular disease except moderate cataracts, (2) history of ocular trauma, (3) history of eye surgery, (4) ocular surface active inflammation, (5) refractive error exceeding 5.00 diopters of hyperopia/myopia or 2.00 diopters of astigmatism, and (6) systemic disorders that affect visual functions.

2.2. Image Acquisition

UBM imaging was performed using an sw-3200L UBM and 50 MHz linear transducer (Tianjin Suowei Electronic Technology Co., Ltd., Tianjin, China). The highest axial and lateral resolutions of the UBM were no less than 40 μm. All images included in this study were obtained by the same examiner (L.C.). Radial scans were performed in the positions of 9, 12, 3, and 6 o'clock centered over the corneal limbus, and perpendicular sulcus-to-sulcus scans were obtained over the pupil center.

Specifically, transverse scans of UBM images were obtained as follows. The probe was perpendicular to the corneal limbus, and the first and most precise CPs image at the time of disappearance of the ciliary sulcus was obtained from four different quadrants (superior, nasal, inferior, and temporal) of each eye. Measurements of the superior quadrant were performed repeatedly over for 1 h by the same physician while masking the initial results. The images were analyzed by the same observer. Figure 1A–D show the probe directions. Figure 1E shows a transverse (superior) CPs image sample.

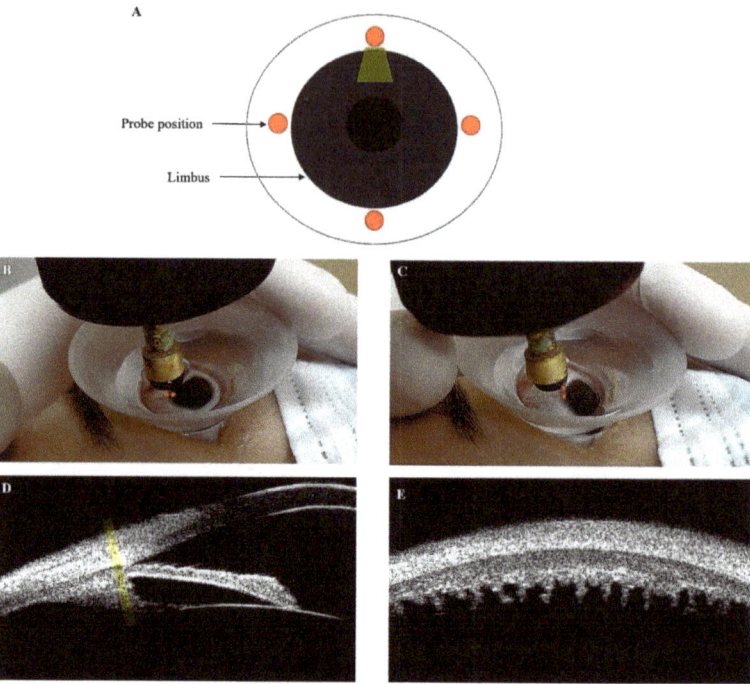

Figure 1. UBM was used to obtain the images of the ciliary body. The ultrasound beam appears in yellow. (**A**) Enface view with the probe position at 9, 12, 3, and 6 o'clock perpendicular to the limbus in red. (**B,C**) These images show the position of probes and eyes when obtaining superior radial and transverse UBM images, respectively. The red arrow shows the direction in which the probe swings during the examination. (**D**) This UBM image shows the relationship of the ultrasound beam to the CB when the transverse scan is performed. (**E**) This image depicts a transverse (superior) UBM image.

2.3. Image Measurement

As Figure 2A shows: (1) the ciliary process length (CPL) was determined by calculating the average length of each individual CP within a 3-mm line in a row; (2) the ciliary process density (CPD) was defined as the overall number of ciliary processes in a 3-mm segment of the transverse CB; (3) the ciliary process area (CPA), ciliary muscle area (CMA), and ciliary body area (CBA) were measured by calculating the area of ciliary processes, ciliary muscle, and CB, respectively, calculating the area within the boundaries of CPs within a 3-mm linear distance using ImageJ software 1.51 (ImageJ Software Inc., Bethesda, MD, USA). The method and the parameters, such as CPL, CPA, CPD, CMA, and CBA of transverse UBM scans, were first defined in this study, so we analyzed the intra-observer reproducibility.

As Figure 2B shows: anterior chamber depth (ACD) was defined as the axial distance between the corneal endothelium and the anterior lens surface. Ciliary sulcus diameter (CSD) was the perpendicular sulcus-to-sulcus distance from 12 to 6 o'clock.

As Figure 2C shows: (1) CBT_0 was the CBT at the point of the scleral spur, and CBT_1 was the CBT at a distance of 1 mm from the scleral spur; (2) maximum CBT (CBT_{max}) was defined as the distance between the innermost point of the CB and the inner surface of the sclera; (3) anterior placement of the ciliary body (APCB) was the distance from the most anterior point of the CB to the vertical line drawn from the inner surface of the scleral spur; (4) the trabecular-ciliary angle (TCA) refers to the angle between the posterior corneal surface and the anterior surface of the CB.

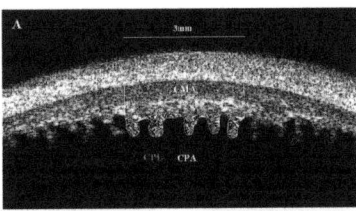
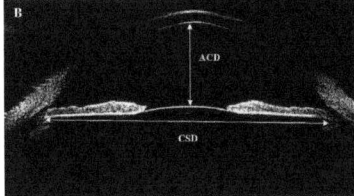
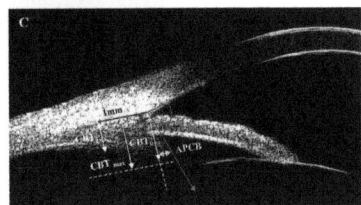

Figure 2. Measurement of ciliary parameters in UBM images. (**A**) Within the boundaries of CPs and a 3-mm linear distance, the ciliary process length (CPL) was measured by calculating the average length of each individual CP. Each individual CPL is shown by the red arrow. The CPD was defined as the number of ciliary processes. The CPA, shown as the shaded area, was measured by calculating the area of ciliary processes. The CMA, the area above the CPA, circled by yellow lines, was measured by calculating the area of the ciliary muscle. The CBA was the sum area of the CPA and the CMA. (**B**) ACD, anterior chamber depth; CSD, ciliary sulcus diameter. (**C**) CBT_0, ciliary body thickness at the point of the scleral spur; CBT_1, ciliary body thickness at a distance of 1 mm from the scleral spur; CBT_{max}, maximum ciliary body thickness; APCB, anterior placement of the ciliary body; TCA, trabecular-ciliary angle.

2.4. Statistical Analysis

All data were imported and sorted by two authors. The statistical analysis and description were performed in SPSS 23 (IBM Corporation, Chicago, IL, USA). One-way analysis of variance (ANOVA) was performed to compare the CPL, CPD, CPA, CMA, CBA, CBT, and APCB in each of the four quadrants. The CPL, CPD, CPA, CMA, CBA, CBT, and APCB values obtained in the four quadrants were averaged, and the Pearson's correlation coefficient test was used to assess the relationships of average CPL, CPD, CPA, CMA, CBA, CBT, and APCB with the following parameters: age, BMI, AL, ACD, LT, and CSD. The intraclass correlation coefficient (ICC) and the Bland–Altman plots were used to analyze the consistency of each parameter for two repeat examinations of the superior CP. $p < 0.05$ was considered to be statistically significant.

3. Results

3.1. Patient Characteristics

Data for this study consisted of 54 eyes of 30 healthy adults. The mean age of the participants was 38.07 ± 12.58 years (range: 18–65 years). Subjects included 14 females and 16 males, with an average BMI of 23.27 ± 3.14 (range: 17.67 to 29.27). Table 1 shows that the mean IOP, CSD, AL, ACD, LT, WTW, and CCT were 14.59 ± 2.13 mmHg, 11.56 ± 0.53 mm, 24.46 ± 1.09 mm, 3.41 ± 0.30 mm, 3.93 ± 0.37 mm, 11.99 ± 0.30 mm, and 528.84 ± 29.81 mm, respectively.

Table 1. Demographic, clinical examination, and ocular biometric parameters of subjects.

Variables	Mean ± SD	Median	Range
Age(years)	38.07 ± 12.58	39	18–65
Female gender%	53.33%	-	-
BMI (kg/m^2)	23.27 ± 3.14	23.27	17.67–29.27

Table 1. Cont.

Variables	Mean ± SD	Median	Range
IOP (mmHg)	14.59 ± 2.13	14.45	10.00–19.70
CSD (mm)	11.56 ± 0.53	11.64	10.07–12.49
AL (mm)	24.46 ± 1.09	24.50	22.45–26.49
ACD (mm)	3.44 ± 0.30	3.40	2.78–4.01
LT (mm)	3.93 ± 0.37	3.96	3.33–4.69
WTW (mm)	11.99 ± 0.30	12.00	11.40–12.70
CCT (μm)	528.84 ± 29.81	527.00	478.00–579.00

SD, standard deviation; BMI, body mass index; IOP, intraocular pressure; CSD, ciliary sulcus diameter; AL axial length; ACD, anterior chamber depth; LT, lens thickness; WTW, white-to-white; CCT, central corneal thickness.

3.2. Intra-Observer Reproducibility of the Parameters in Transverse UBM Scans of CB

Intraclass correlation coefficient (ICC) scores describe the level of absolute agreement between two examinations and provide a measure of reproducibility. In our study, there were 44 images in total. ICC scores were high for CPL (0.979), CPD (0.992), CPA (0.966), CMA (0.963), and CBA (0.951) (Table 2). For all parameters measured, there was good agreement between the two examinations. The mean difference and 95% limits of agreement (LoA) in CPL, CPD, CPA, CMA, and CBA between the first and second examinations were −0.002 (−0.029, 0.024), −0.018 (−0.183, 0.147), 0.001 (−0.064, 0.066), 0.030 (−0.108, 0.169), and 0.031 (−0.140, 0.203), respectively. Differences were plotted against the mean, as shown by the Bland–Altman plots in Figure 3.

Table 2. ICC and 95% LoA results for ciliary body anatomy measured in the superior quadrant from the transverse scan.

Measurement	Mean ± SD		ICC, 95%CI	p	95%LoA	No. of Images
	Examination 1	Examination 2				
CPL (mm)	0.553 ± 0.069	0.555 ± 0.065	0.979(0.962,0.988)	<0.001	−0.029, 0.024	44
CPD (number)	5.641 ± 0.669	5.660 ± 0.645	0.992(0.985,0.995)	<0.001	−0.183, 0.147	44
CPA (mm^2)	0.964 ± 0.127	0.962 ± 0.128	0.966(0.939,0.982)	<0.001	−0.064, 0.066	44
CMA (mm^2)	2.399 ± 0.288	2.368 ± 0.268	0.963(0.923,0.981)	<0.001	−0.108, 0.169	44
CBA (mm^2)	3.362 ± 0.291	3.333 ± 0.297	0.951(0.907,0.974)	<0.001	−0.140, 0.203	44
CBA (mm^2)	3.362 ± 0.291	3.333 ± 0.297	0.951(0.907,0.974)	<0.001	−0.140, 0.203	44

$p < 0.05$, F test of ICC with true value 0; SD, standard deviation; ICC, intraclass correlation coefficient; CI, confidence interval; LoA, limits of agreement; CPL, ciliary process length; CPD, ciliary process density (in 3-mm linear distance); CPA, ciliary process area; CMA, ciliary muscle area; CBA, ciliary body area.

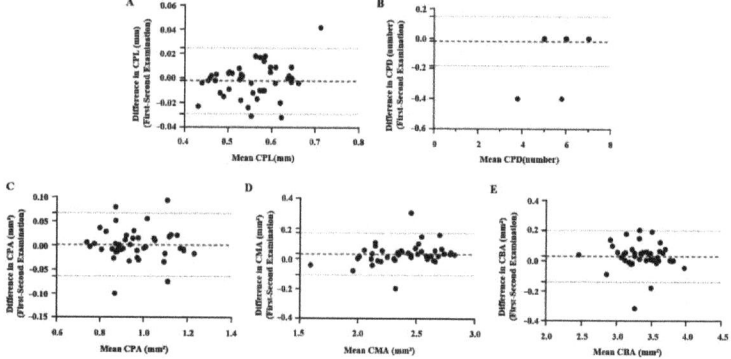

Figure 3. Bland–Altman plots for two repeat examinations of the superior CP. Differences for CPL (A), CPD (B), CPA (C), CMA (D), and CBA (E) generally fell within the repeatability coefficient limit (black dashed line), suggesting that the mean parameter was generally repeatable. The red dashed line shows the mean.

3.3. Anatomy Characteristics of the CB Both from Radial and Transverse Imaging of UBM

Table 3 showed that the average CPL was 0.513 ± 0.074 mm, the average CPA was 0.890 ± 0.141 mm^2, and the average CMA was 2.381 ± 0.280 mm^2 in the four quadrants. The CPL was 0.558 ± 0.070 mm, 0.490 ± 0.062 mm, 0.505 ± 0.075 mm, and 0.498 ± 0.072 mm in the superior, inferior, temporal, and nasal quadrants, respectively. The CPA was 0.964 ± 0.130 mm^2, 0.841 ± 0.112 mm^2, 0.865 ± 0.142 mm^2, and 0.889 ± 0.148 mm^2, whereas the CMA was 2.327 ± 0.312 mm^2, 2.483 ± 0.245 mm^2, 2.355 ± 0.270 mm^2, and 2.361 ± 0.271 mm^2, respectively. There were significant differences in the CPL ($p < 0.001$), CPA ($p < 0.001$), and CMA ($p = 0.019$) among the four different quadrants (Table 3). However, no statistically significant differences in the average CPD, CBA, CBT_0, CBT_1, CBT_{max}, APCB, and TCA ($p > 0.05$) among the four different quadrants were found.

The correlations between average CPL, CPD, CPA, CMA, CBA, CBT_0, CBT_1, CBT_{max}, APCB, TCA, and various other clinical parameters are shown in Table 4. Scatter plots of average CPL and other ocular and systemic parameters are shown in Figure 4. Average CPL was significantly correlated with age ($r = -0.436$, $p = 0.001$), BMI ($r = -0.318$, $p = 0.019$), AL ($r = 0.535$, $p < 0.001$), ACD ($r = 0.512$, $p < 0.001$), LT ($r = -0.512$, $p < 0.001$), and CSD ($r = 0.345$, $p = 0.011$). Average CPD was positively correlated with age ($r = 0.354$, $p = 0.013$) and LT ($r = 0.421$, $p = 0.002$), and negatively correlated with AL ($r = -0.445$, $p = 0.001$), ACD ($r = -0.343$, $p = 0.009$), and CSD ($r = -0.375$, $p = 0.005$). There was no significant correlation between the average CPA and other clinical parameters ($p > 0.05$) or the CBT_{max}. Average CMA showed a significant correlation with age ($r = 0.488$, $p < 0.001$), BMI ($r = 0.349$, $p = 0.010$), AL ($r = -0.279$, $p = 0.041$), and LT ($r = 0.519$, $p < 0.001$), but not with ACD and CSD ($p > 0.05$). Average CBA was not related to AL, ACD, or CSD in all eyes ($p > 0.05$), except for a significant positive correlation with age ($r = 0.439$, $p < 0.001$), BMI ($r = 0.307$, $p = 0.024$), and LT ($r = 0.432$, $p < 0.001$). Average CBT_0 showed a significant correlation with LT ($r = 0.357$, $p = 0.008$), but not with age, BMI, AL, ACD, or CSD ($p > 0.05$). There was only a statistically significant correlation between the average CBT_1 and CSD ($r = 0.287$, $p = 0.035$). Average APCB was significantly correlated with age ($r = 0.483$, $p < 0.001$), AL ($R = -0.513$, $p < 0.001$), ACD ($r = -0.542$, $p < 0.001$), LT ($r = 0.491$, $p < 0.001$), and CSD ($r = -0.566$, $p < 0.001$), but not with BMI ($p > 0.005$). There was a significant correlation between average TCA and age ($r = -0.512$, $p < 0.001$), BMI ($r = -0.352$, $p = 0.009$), AL ($r = 0.464$, $p < 0.001$), ACD ($r = 0.649$, $p < 0.001$), LT ($r = -0.508$, $p < 0.001$), and CSD ($r = 0.569$, $p < 0.001$).

Table 3. Ciliary body and ciliary process parameters measured in the four quadrants.

Quadrant	Average	Superior	Nasal	Inferior	Temporal	p-Value
CPL (mm)	0.513 ± 0.074	0.558 ± 0.070	0.490 ± 0.062	0.505 ± 0.075	0.498 ± 0.072	<0.001
CPD (number)	5.779 ± 0.832	5.596 ± 0.702	5.752 ± 0.790	5.800 ± 0.937	5.969 ± 0.863	0.139
CPA (mm^2)	0.890 ± 0.141	0.964 ± 0.130	0.841 ± 0.112	0.865 ± 0.142	0.889 ± 0.148	<0.001
CMA (mm^2)	2.381 ± 0.280	2.327 ± 0.312	2.483 ± 0.245	2.355 ± 0.270	2.361 ± 0.271	0.019
CBA (mm^2)	3.271 ± 0.292	3.291 ± 0.328	3.323 ± 0.270	3.220 ± 0.282	3.250 ± 0.282	0.272
CBT_0 (mm)	1.053 ± 0.188	1.014 ± 0.175	1.038 ± 0.142	1.054 ± 0.218	1.104 ± 0.203	0.084
CBT_1 (mm)	0.811 ± 0.159	0.849 ± 0.181	0.789 ± 0.124	0.798 ± 0.147	0.811 ± 0.173	0.217
CBT_{max} (mm)	1.248 ± 0.169	1.224 ± 0.153	1.214 ± 0.152	1.261 ± 0.177	1.291 ± 0.183	0.064
APCB (mm)	0.349 ± 0.314	0.322 ± 0.144	0.324 ± 0.138	0.358 ± 0.235	0.392 ± 0.214	0.174
TCA (degree)	79.379 ± 10.020	77.859 ± 8.949	80.635 ± 8.587	80.583 ± 10.684	78.437 ± 11.531	0.343

Values are presented as the mean ± standard deviation; $p < 0.05$, one-way analysis of variance; CPL, ciliary process length; CPD, ciliary process density (in 3-mm linear distance); CPA, ciliary process area; CMA, ciliary muscle area; CBA, ciliary body area; CBT_0, ciliary body thickness at the point of the scleral spur; CBT_1, ciliary body thickness at a distance of 1 mm from the scleral spur; CBT_{max}, maximum ciliary body thickness; APCB, anterior placement of ciliary body; TCA, trabecular-ciliary angle.

Table 4. Correlations between ciliary process, CB parameters, and systemic and ocular parameters.

Variables	Average CPL (mm)		Average CPD (Number)		Average CPA (mm²)		Average CMA (mm²)		Average CBA (mm²)		Average CBT_0 (mm)		Average CBT_1 (mm)		Average CBT_{max} (mm)		Average APCB (mm)		Average TCA (Degree)	
	r	p	r	p	r	p	r	p	r	p	r	p	r	p	r	p	r	p	r	p
Age	−0.436	0.001	0.354	0.013	−0.020	0.884	0.488	<0.001	0.439	<0.001	0.261	0.057	−0.022	0.874	0.154	0.266	0.483	<0.001	−0.512	<0.001
BMI (kg/m²)	−0.318	0.019	0.160	0.246	−0.031	0.823	0.349	0.010	0.307	0.024	0.134	0.335	0.130	0.348	−0.011	0.939	0.229	0.096	−0.352	0.009
AL (mm)	0.535	<0.001	−0.445	0.001	0.202	0.143	−0.279	0.041	−0.170	0.218	−0.074	0.595	0.082	0.554	−0.118	0.396	−0.513	<0.001	0.464	<0.001
ACD (mm)	0.512	<0.001	−0.343	0.011	0.192	0.165	−0.336	0.013	−0.227	0.099	−0.195	0.159	0.126	0.364	−0.076	0.587	−0.542	<0.001	0.649	<0.001
LT (mm)	−0.512	<0.001	0.421	0.002	−0.105	0.450	0.519	<0.001	0.432	<0.001	0.357	0.008	0.081	0.560	0.237	0.085	0.491	<0.001	−0.508	<0.001
CSD (mm)	0.345	0.011	−0.375	0.005	−0.013	0.923	−0.275	0.044	−0.257	0.060	−0.022	0.873	0.287	0.035	0.008	0.954	−0.566	<0.001	0.569	<0.001

$p < 0.05$, Pearson's correlation coefficient. CPL, ciliary process length; CPD, ciliary process density (number in 3-mm linear distance); CPA, ciliary process area; CMA, ciliary muscle area; CBA, ciliary body area; CBT_0, ciliary body thickness at the point of the scleral spur; CBT_1, ciliary body thickness at the distance of 1 mm from scleral spur; CBT_{max}, maximum ciliary body thickness; APCB, anterior placement of ciliary body; TCA, trabecular-ciliary angle; BMI, body mass index; AL, axial length; ACD, anterior chamber depth; LT, lens thickness; CSD, ciliary sulcus diameter.

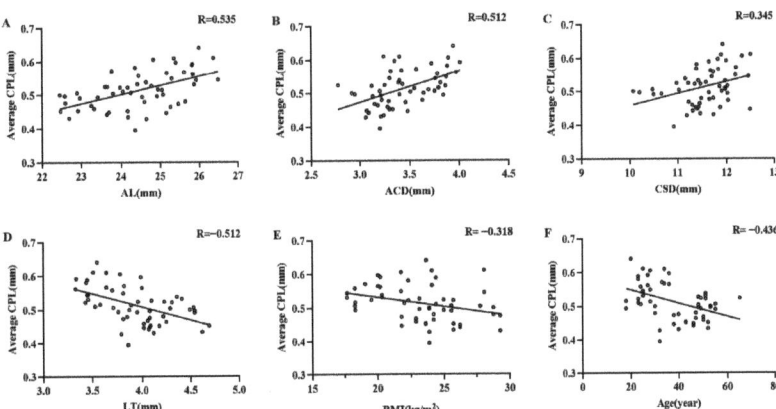

Figure 4. Scatter plots of AL (**A**), ACD (**B**), CSD (**C**), LT (**D**), BMI (**E**), age (**F**), and average CPL in all recruited eyes. The longer the AL, the deeper the ACD, and the larger CSD were, the longer the CPL was. The smaller the BMI and the thinner the LT were, the longer the CPL was. The younger the subject was, the longer the CPL was. The solid line represents the best-fit line.

4. Discussion

The study of CB has gained significant attention because of its involvement in glaucoma and myopia. Several studies have been conducted on humans to provide histological information about the CB, but all have encountered postmortem shrinkage problems [16,17]. UBM can be used to measure any quadrant on living subjects, as it is unaffected by shrinkage. Since its inception, UBM has been used in many clinical and preclinical studies associated with CB-related disease, and it is irreplaceable for the study of the posterior chamber and the innermost structures of the iridociliary region compared to AS-OCT [4,18–20]. To the best of our knowledge, this is the first report that demonstrated the morphology parameters of the CB from both radial and transverse scans in four different quadrants in vivo of Chinese people and the correlations between them with systemic and ocular parameters.

In our study, four quadrantal analyses of the ciliary process revealed that the CPL was longest in the superior quadrant, followed by the inferior, temporal, and nasal quadrants. CPA tended to be larger in the superior quadrant than in the other three quadrants. In contrast to CPL, CMA was largest in the nasal quadrant, followed by the temporal, inferior, and superior quadrants. This may be due to the embryonic development of the eye. Numerous reports about ocular morphology have been published. Retinal nerve fiber layer (RNFL) thickness was found to be thicker in the superior and inferior quadrants, followed by the temporal and nasal quadrants in normal Chinese students aged 6 to 17 years using optical coherence tomography (OCT) [21]. Corneal thickness was lower in the inferotemporal quadrant and higher in the superonasal quadrant using anterior segmental-optical coherence tomography (AS-OCT) [22]. A previous study compared the ciliary body morphology between Caucasians and Chinese individuals aged 40 to 80 years, and found that Chinese individuals had a thinner CBT using UBM [23]. It was reported that CBT_1 was significantly thicker in the superior quadrant than in the nasal, temporal, and inferior quadrants using UBM in Asian subjects aged 11–86 years [24]. However, in our study, no significant difference in CBT_0, CBT_1, and CBT_{max} among the four quadrants was found. The inconsistency may arise from the inclusion of subjects of different races. APCB and TCA were inversely related to anterior rotation of the ciliary body. According to a previous study in Japan, the mean TCA was 79.2 degrees using UBM [3], which is similar to our findings.

Our study provided a new protocol to scan transverse (quadrant) CP images using UBM; in particular, a method to locate the anatomical point to achieve a repeatable fashion. For the first time, we clearly defined CPL as the distance parallel to the long axis of the CP from the farthest end to the midpoint of the line of the bilateral ciliary sulcus according to the morphology. CPD, CPA, CMA, and CBA were all measured within the middle 3-mm linear distance of the transverse CB image. Due to the spherical shape of the eyeball, the surrounding CPs appear deformed in the image at a greater distance. Additionally, if it is at a shorter distance, the number of CPs will be too small, resulting in statistical errors. Therefore, the CPs in the area we chose were the most precise and closest to the actual shape in the scan. To date, there has been no standardized method for reliable measurement of the ciliary process. Only one study published in 2021 obtained CP images of normal human eyes from the temporal pars plicata using UBM, and the ICC values were >0.8 for CP parameters (CPL, CPD, CPA) [25]. However, there was an advantage that all five parameters (CPL, CPD, CPA, CMA, CBA) in our study had ICC values > 0.9, suggesting relatively better repeatability and reliability than the study mentioned above. The reason for this might be that we obtained CP images in our study by focusing the ultrasonic probe perpendicular to the corneal limbus at the time of disappearance of the ciliary sulcus, and this might prove a more reliable method to measure CPs from transverse UBM images.

Additionally, the correlations between parameters of the CP and systemic and ocular parameters in healthy Chinese subjects were revealed, which has not been reported before, as far as we know. In addition, average CPL had a negative correlation with age and BMI, indicating that people who were younger or with lower BMI tended to have a longer CP. In our study, average CPL and average TCA showed a positive correlation with AL and CSD, and showed a negative correlation with LT; average CPD, average CMA, and average APCB showed the opposite correlation. In other words, healthy Chinese subjects, who had smaller eyes with shorter AL, shorter CSD, and thicker lenses, had shorter but denser ciliary processes, thicker ciliary muscle, and more anteriorly located CB, which might provide new inspiration for the occurrence and mechanism of malignant glaucoma in patients with primary angle-closure (PAC) and primary angle-closure glaucoma (PACG). With transverse direction UBM scans, CP can be seen more clearly, which may provide a more accurate way to explore the pathogenesis, and evaluate the surgical prognosis of glaucoma.

In previous studies, CBT_1 was positively correlated with AL in normal subjects [24], and CBT_2 and CBT_3 (2 mm and 3 mm posterior to the scleral spur) were positively correlated with AL in myopic eyes [12]. It was reported that ciliary muscle thickness (CMT_2 and CMT_3, 2 mm and 3 mm posterior to the scleral spur) was increased in myopic eyes compared with nonmyopic eyes, suggesting that a large CB may be associated with a greater contraction of the ciliary muscles to resist equatorial sclera thinning [26,27]. However, a correlation between CBT_0, CBT_1, CBT_{max}, and AL was not found in our study, probably because we used different measured parameters, and the difference was not significant.

As the site of aqueous humor production, the CP is also the site of surgical interventions, such as trans-scleral cyclo-photocoagulation (TSCPC), endoscopic cyclophotocoagulation (ECP), and ultrasound cycloplasty (UCP), which are aimed at destroying the CB to reduce IOP in glaucoma patients [28–30]. Therefore, images of the ciliary process using UBM could provide a more refined observation method to evaluate the morphological changes of the ciliary process in TSCPC-, ECP-, and UCP-treated glaucoma and the relationship between the morphological changes and IOP reduction. The ability to study drug or surgery action on the morphology of the CP itself may offer valuable insights regarding the mechanisms of action.

The main limitation of our study is that the resolution limitations of the UBM technique may have contributed to morphometric errors. The spatial resolution of the UBM is superior in the radial direction compared to the transverse direction. The examination was performed to apply the probe as vertically to the corneal limbus as possible to obtain a precise image. Another significant limitation is the small sample size. Therefore, we need to compensate for the lack of accuracy caused by these limitations by increasing the number of subjects. The third limitation is that we only included Chinese subjects in this study, which limited the generalizability of the results. In order to verify the generalizability of the results, further multiracial studies are warranted to confirm our findings. In addition, even though it does not affect the clinical conclusions, the analysis could be more accurate if the inter-eye correlation was considered.

5. Conclusions

In conclusion, we found a topographical distribution of the ciliary body in healthy Chinese subjects using the application of radial and transverse UBM imaging, and provided more information on the ciliary anatomy. The average CPL and CPA were greatest in the superior quadrant. Given the relatively good repeatability and reliability of ciliary process imaging, further studies should be performed to explore the pathogenesis of CB-related diseases, such as malignant glaucoma, and to evaluate the role of glaucoma interventions aimed at the CB, such as TSCPC, ECP, and UCP.

Author Contributions: Co-first author, J.R. and X.G.; Conceptualization, J.R., X.G. and M.L.; Data curation, X.G.; Funding acquisition, C.Z. and M.L.; Investigation, J.R. and H.L.; Methodology, L.C.; Project administration, M.L.; Supervision, Y.L. (Yao Liu), Y.Z., Y.L. (Yunru Liao) and C.X.; Validation, X.G.; Writing—original draft, J.R.; Writing—review and editing, C.Z. and M.L. All authors have read and agreed to the published version of the manuscript.

Funding: This research was funded by the Natural Science Foundation of Guangdong Province, China (2019A1515011196) and the National Natural Science Foundation of China (81970808).

Institutional Review Board Statement: The study was conducted in accordance with the Declaration of Helsinki, and approved by the Ethics Committee of the Zhongshan Ophthalmic Center (ZOC), Sun Yat-sen University (Ethic ID. 2021KYPJ003).

Informed Consent Statement: Informed consent was obtained from all subjects involved in the study.

Data Availability Statement: The datasets used and/or analyzed during the current study are available from the corresponding author upon reasonable request.

Conflicts of Interest: The authors declare no conflict of interest.

References

1. Kels, B.D.; Grzybowski, A.; Grant-Kels, J.M. Human ocular anatomy. *Clin. Dermatol.* **2015**, *33*, 140–146. [CrossRef] [PubMed]
2. Coca-Prados, M.; Escribano, J. New perspectives in aqueous humor secretion and in glaucoma: The ciliary body as a multifunctional neuroendocrine gland. *Prog. Retin. Eye Res.* **2007**, *26*, 239–262. [CrossRef]
3. Henzan, I.M.; Tomidokoro, A.; Uejo, C.; Sakai, H.; Sawaguchi, S.; Iwase, A.; Araie, M. Ultrasound biomicroscopic configurations of the anterior ocular segment in a population-based study the Kumejima Study. *Ophthalmology* **2010**, *117*, 1720–1728.e1. [CrossRef] [PubMed]
4. Fernández-Vigo, J.I.; Kudsieh, B.; Shi, H.; De-Pablo-Gómez-de-Liaño, L.; Fernández-Vigo, J.; García-Feijóo, J. Diagnostic imaging of the ciliary body: Technologies, outcomes, and future perspectives. *Eur. J. Ophthalmol.* **2022**, *32*, 75–88. [CrossRef] [PubMed]
5. Marchini, G.; Pagliarusco, A.; Toscano, A.; Tosi, R.; Brunelli, C.; Bonomi, L. Ultrasound biomicroscopic and conventional ultrasonographic study of ocular dimensions in primary angle-closure glaucoma. *Ophthalmology* **1998**, *105*, 2091–2098. [CrossRef]
6. Wang, Z.; Chung, C.; Lin, J.; Xu, J.; Huang, J. Quantitative Measurements of the Ciliary Body in Eyes With Acute Primary-Angle Closure. *Investig. Ophthalmol. Vis. Sci.* **2016**, *57*, 3299–3305. [CrossRef] [PubMed]
7. Wang, F.; Wang, D.; Wang, L. Characteristic Manifestations regarding Ultrasound Biomicroscopy Morphological Data in the Diagnosis of Acute Angle Closure Secondary to Lens Subluxation. *BioMed Res. Int.* **2019**, *2019*, 7472195. [CrossRef]
8. Wang, Z.; Huang, J.; Lin, J.; Liang, X.; Cai, X.; Ge, J. Quantitative measurements of the ciliary body in eyes with malignant glaucoma after trabeculectomy using ultrasound biomicroscopy. *Ophthalmology* **2014**, *121*, 862–869. [CrossRef]
9. Alibet, Y.; Levytska, G.; Umanets, N.; Pasyechnikova, N.; Henrich, P.B. Ciliary body thickness changes after preoperative anti-inflammatory treatment in rhegmatogenous retinal detachment complicated by choroidal detachment. *Graefe's Arch. Clin. Exp. Ophthalmol.* **2017**, *255*, 1503–1508. [CrossRef]
10. Mishima, H.K.; Shoge, K.; Takamatsu, M.; Kiuchi, Y.; Tanaka, J. Ultrasound biomicroscopic study of ciliary body thickness after topical application of pharmacologic agents. *Am. J. Ophthalmol.* **1996**, *121*, 319–321. [CrossRef]
11. Arakawa, A.; Tamai, M. Ultrasound biomicroscopic analysis of the human ciliary body after 1 and 2% pilocarpine instillation. *Ophthalmologica* **2000**, *214*, 253–259. [CrossRef]
12. Oliveira, C.; Tello, C.; Liebmann, J.M.; Ritch, R. Ciliary body thickness increases with increasing axial myopia. *Am. J. Ophthalmol.* **2005**, *140*, 324–325. [CrossRef]
13. Gentile, R.C.; Liebmann, J.M.; Tello, C.; Stegman, Z.; Weissman, S.S.; Ritch, R. Ciliary body enlargement and cyst formation in uveitis. *Br. J. Ophthalmol.* **1996**, *80*, 895–899. [CrossRef]

14. Weisbrod, D.J.; Pavlin, C.J.; Emara, K.; Mandell, M.A.; McWhae, J.; Simpson, E.R. Small ciliary body tumors: Ultrasound biomicroscopic assessment and follow-up of 42 patients. *Am. J. Ophthalmol.* **2006**, *141*, 622–628. [CrossRef] [PubMed]
15. Mannino, G.; Malagola, R.; Abdolrahimzadeh, S.; Villani, G.M.; Recupero, S.M. Ultrasound biomicroscopy of the peripheral retina and the ciliary body in degenerative retinoschisis associated with pars plana cysts. *Br. J. Ophthalmol.* **2001**, *85*, 976–982. [CrossRef]
16. Hara, K.; Lütjen-Drecoll, E.; Prestele, H.; Rohen, J.W. Structural differences between regions of the ciliary body in primates. *Investig. Ophthalmol. Vis. Sci.* **1977**, *16*, 912–924.
17. Tamm, E.R.; Lütjen-Drecoll, E. Ciliary body. *Microsc. Res. Tech.* **1996**, *33*, 390–439. [CrossRef]
18. Dada, T.; Gadia, R.; Sharma, A.; Ichhpujani, P.; Bali, S.J.; Bhartiya, S.; Panda, A. Ultrasound biomicroscopy in glaucoma. *Surv. Ophthalmol.* **2011**, *56*, 433–450. [CrossRef] [PubMed]
19. Smith, S.D.; Singh, K.; Lin, S.C.; Chen, P.P.; Chen, T.C.; Francis, B.A.; Jampel, H.D. Evaluation of the anterior chamber angle in glaucoma: A report by the american academy of ophthalmology. *Ophthalmology* **2013**, *120*, 1985–1997. [CrossRef]
20. Janssens, R.; van Rijn, L.J.; Eggink, C.A.; Jansonius, N.M.; Janssen, S.F. Ultrasound biomicroscopy of the anterior segment in patients with primary congenital glaucoma: A review of the literature. *Acta Ophthalmol.* **2021**. Epub ahead of print. [CrossRef]
21. Chen, L.; Huang, J.; Zou, H.; Xue, W.; Ma, Y.; He, X.; Lu, L.; Zhu, J. Retinal nerve fiber layer thickness in normal Chinese students aged 6 to 17 years. *Investig. Ophthalmol. Vis. Sci.* **2013**, *54*, 7990–7997. [CrossRef] [PubMed]
22. Li, Y.; Tan, O.; Brass, R.; Weiss, J.L.; Huang, D. Corneal epithelial thickness mapping by Fourier-domain optical coherence tomography in normal and keratoconic eyes. *Ophthalmology* **2012**, *119*, 2425–2433. [CrossRef]
23. He, N.; Wu, L.; Qi, M.; He, M.; Lin, S.; Wang, X.; Yang, F.; Fan, X. Comparison of Ciliary Body Anatomy between American Caucasians and Ethnic Chinese Using Ultrasound Biomicroscopy. *Curr. Eye Res.* **2016**, *41*, 485–491. [CrossRef] [PubMed]
24. Okamoto, Y.; Okamoto, F.; Nakano, S.; Oshika, T. Morphometric assessment of normal human ciliary body using ultrasound biomicroscopy. *Graefe's Arch. Clin. Exp. Ophthalmol.* **2017**, *255*, 2437–2442. [CrossRef] [PubMed]
25. Li, J.; Drechsler, J.; Lin, A.; Widlus, M.; Qureshi, A.; Stoleru, G.; Saeedi, O.; Levin, M.R.; Kaleem, M.; Jaafar, M.; et al. Repeatability and Reliability of Quantified Ultrasound Biomicroscopy Image Analysis of the Ciliary Body at the Pars Plicata. *Ultrasound Med. Biol.* **2021**, *47*, 1949–1956. [CrossRef]
26. Buckhurst, H.; Gilmartin, B.; Cubbidge, R.P.; Nagra, M.; Logan, N.S. Ocular biometric correlates of ciliary muscle thickness in human myopia. *Ophthalmic Physiol. Opt.* **2013**, *33*, 294–304. [CrossRef]
27. Fernández-Vigo, J.I.; Shi, H.; Kudsieh, B.; Arriola-Villalobos, P.; De-Pablo Gómez-de-Liaño, L.; García-Feijóo, J.; Fernández-Vigo, J. Ciliary muscle dimensions by swept-source optical coherence tomography and correlation study in a large population. *Acta Ophthalmol.* **2020**, *98*, e487–e494. [CrossRef]
28. Khodeiry, M.M.; Sheheitli, H.; Sayed, M.S.; Persad, P.J.; Feuer, W.J.; Lee, R.K. Treatment Outcomes of Slow Coagulation Transscleral Cyclophotocoagulation In Pseudophakic Patients with Medically Uncontrolled Glaucoma. *Am. J. Ophthalmol.* **2021**, *229*, 90–99. [CrossRef] [PubMed]
29. Tóth, M.; Shah, A.; Hu, K.; Bunce, C.; Gazzard, G. Endoscopic cyclophotocoagulation (ECP) for open angle glaucoma and primary angle closure. *Cochrane Database Syst. Rev.* **2019**, *2*, Cd012741. [CrossRef]
30. Giannaccare, G.; Pellegrini, M.; Bernabei, F.; Urbini, L.; Bergamini, F.; Ferro Desideri, L.; Bagnis, A.; Biagini, F.; Cassottana, P.; Del Noce, C.; et al. A 2-year prospective multicenter study of ultrasound cyclo plasty for glaucoma. *Sci. Rep.* **2021**, *11*, 12647. [CrossRef]

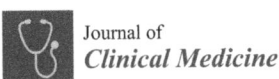

Article

Retromode Imaging Modality of Epiretinal Membranes

Alfonso Savastano [1,2,†], Matteo Ripa [1,2,†], Maria Cristina Savastano [1,2,*], Tomaso Caporossi [1,2], Daniela Bacherini [3], Raphael Kilian [4], Clara Rizzo [5] and Stanislao Rizzo [1,2,6]

1. Ophthalmology Unit, Fondazione Policlinico Universitario Agostino Gemelli IRCCS, 00168 Rome, Italy; asavastano21@gmail.com (A.S.); matteof12@gmail.com (M.R.); tomaso.caporossi@gmail.com (T.C.); stanislao.rizzo@policlinicogemelli.it (S.R.)
2. Ophthalmology Unit, Catholic University "Sacro Cuore", 00168 Rome, Italy
3. Department of Translational Surgery and Medicine, Eye Clinic, University of Florence, Azienda Ospedaliero-Universitaria Careggi, 50134 Florence, Italy; daniela.bacherini@gmail.com
4. Ophthalmology Unit, University of Verona, 37129 Verona, Italy; raphaelkilian8@yahoo.it
5. Ophthalmology Unit, Department of Surgical, Medical, Molecular and Critical Area Pathology, University of Pisa, 56124 Pisa, Italy; clararizzo2@gmail.com
6. Consiglio Nazionale delle Ricerche, Istituto di Neuroscienze, 56127 Pisa, Italy
* Correspondence: mariacristina.savastano@gmail.com
† These authors contributed equally to this work.

Abstract: (1) Purpose: To determine the characteristics of macular epiretinal membranes (ERM) using non-invasive retromode imaging (RMI) and to compare retromode images with those acquired via fundus autofluorescence (FAF) and fundus photography. (2) Methods: Prospective observational case-series study including patients with macular ERM with no other ocular disease affecting their morphology and/or imaging quality. We compared RMI, FAF and fundus photography features by cropping and overlapping images to obtain topographic correspondence. (3) Results: In total, 21 eyes (21 patients) affected by ERM were included in this study. The mean area of retinal folds detected by RMI was significantly higher than that detected by FAF (11.85 ± 3.92 mm^2 and 5.67 ± 2.15 mm^2, respectively, $p < 0.05$) and similar to that revealed by fundus photography (11.85 ± 3.92 mm^2 and 10.58 ± 3.45 mm^2, respectively, $p = 0.277$). (4) Conclusions: RMI appears to be a useful tool in the evaluation of ERMs. It allows for an accurate visualization of the real extension of the retinal folds and provides a precise structural assessment of the macula before surgery. Clinicians should be aware of RMI's advantages and should be able to use them to warrant a wide range of information and, thus, a more personalized therapeutic approach.

Keywords: epiretinal membranes; retromode retinal imaging; confocal scanning laser ophthalmoscope; fundus autofluorescence; personalized medicine

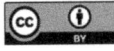

1. Introduction

Epiretinal membranes (ERMs) develop above the internal limiting membrane (ILM) of the retina and represent a relatively common macular finding. Their appearance varies widely from patient to patient, ranging from a translucent wrinkling of the inner retinal surface, all the way to an extensive, thick, epiretinal cellular proliferation [1].

The retinal surgeon benefits greatly from a precise preoperative view of the ERM, which is made possible by continuous advancements in imaging technology.

Thanks to its high-definition cross-sectional scans, optical coherence tomography (OCT) has revolutionized the diagnostic visualization of ERMs [2]. Other common imaging techniques such as fundus autofluorescence (FAF) and enface OCT technology have also been shown to be effective at visualizing ERMs and, in some cases, even at predicting certain post-operative outcomes [3].

The novel retromode imaging (RMI) is a noncontact and a noninvasive imaging method that relies on the newly introduced confocal scanning laser ophthalmoscopic technology. Briefly, there are two kinds of light returning back from the fundus once it is illuminated, a direct reflex and a scattered light. Retromode imaging uses a laterally deviated confocal aperture with a central stop to block the direct light reflex and to collect the backscattered light from one direction [4]. This enables the formation of pseudo-3D images, through the creation of a shadow to one side of the abnormal feature that is being investigated, which eventually enhances the contrast of the lesion. Knowing the ability of infrared lasers to penetrate deeper retinal layers, retromode imaging with infrared laser-technology has been used to evaluate retinal pathological changes in several retinal and choroidal diseases [5].

RMI is performed by a scanning laser ophthalmoscope (SLO) working at an infrared wavelength, which creates a pseudo three-dimensional image with highly contrasting margins of retinal abnormalities (e.g., neurosensory detachments, retinal holes, retinoschisis and intraretinal cystic fluid) [6]. However, to the best of our knowledge, there are no reports describing the retromode imaging of ERMs.

The main outcome of this study was to evaluate morphological features, such as the area of retinal folds and the area of intraretinal cystic spaces, in eyes with ERM. This was achieved by cropping and overlapping images of the ERMs using noninvasive retromode imaging and comparing these to color fundus images. Moreover, we examined the correlation between retromode findings and fundus autofluorescence (FAF).

2. Materials and Methods

The study was performed in accordance with the Declaration of Helsinki and was approved by the Ethics Committee (protocol ID number 3680/20). Written informed consent for participation to the research was obtained from the patients after explanation of the purpose and the process of the study.

We performed a monocentric prospective case-series study enrolling patients with an ERM who attended the ophthalmology unit at the Fondazione Policlinico Universitario A. Gemelli IRCCS, Rome, Italy, from 1 January–1 July 2021.

A comprehensive ocular examination, including measurements of the refractive error (spherical equivalent) and the best correct visual acuity, and a dilated macular examination (through indirect ophthalmoscopy) were performed on the day of enrollment. Patients then received a thorough posterior pole investigation through various imaging techniques (i.e., RMI, FAF, color fundus photography and OCT B-scanning). All scans were performed using the Mirante SLO/OCT (Nidek Co, Gamagori, Japan), providing an image field of 40 degrees, an optical resolution of 16 to 20 μm and an image size of up to 1024×720 pixels. Inclusion criteria were the presence of an epiretinal membrane confirmed via OCT-B scans with no other concomitant intraocular disease. Eyes with a history of ocular trauma, previous intraocular surgery (with the exception of cataract surgery) or any abnormal intraocular findings (i.e., diabetic retinopathy, neovascular age-related macular degeneration, retinal angiomatous proliferation, angioid streaks, pathological myopia, retinal detachment), were excluded from the study. Images with poor quality due to severe cataracts or unstable fixation were also a reason for exclusion.

After the examinations were performed (1–6 months), all included patients underwent surgery for peeling of the ERM. This was performed by two expert vitreo-retinal surgeons, using 23- or 25-gauge pars plana vitrectomy (PPV) (Constellation Vision System, Alcon, Fort Worth, TX, USA) according to the surgeon's choice, as already described by Savastano et al. [7].

2.1. Images Detection

After completing OCT scans of the entire area within the vascular arcades, the fundus was investigated using fundus photography, FAF and retromode imaging. The OCT acquisition protocol consisted of a 6×6 mm (mm) three-dimensional vertical scanning area, centered on the fovea comprising 512×128 scans. Color photos from Nidek Mirante had a 45-degree field of view with a resolution of 1024×720 pixels. Three separate laser wavelengths (red—670 nm, green—532 nm, blue—488 nm) are combined to create color pictures, which are then connected to a specific sensor for each wavelength. A blue-light excitation wavelength of 488 nm (emission > 500 nm) is used to obtain fundus autofluorescence (FAF), whereas the retromode imaging system uses an infrared laser light (790 nm). A right-deviated aperture and a left-deviated aperture were used to obtain two separate retromode pictures per eye. All the tomographic images were acquired, averaging up to 30 frames per image.

2.2. Data Analysis

Image processing was performed using the ImageJ software (National Institutes of Health, MD, USA).

Fundus Autofluorescence, retromode and fundus photography images were cropped and superimposed to have topographic correspondence, and the surface area of each image was measured in square mm^2.

All images were reviewed separately by two authors to identify, record and interpret the various morphologic alterations associated with ERM. In case of disagreement between the two, a third expert would choose which of the measurements was more accurate.

All images were exported as high-quality tiff files and were collected using the REDCap platform (Vanderbilt University), a secure web application for building and managing online surveys and databases [8].

We matched retromode images with color fundus photographs, FAF images and OCT B-scans using various reference points.

The optic nerve's superior and inferior margins and retinal blood vessels on color fundus photography (blue lines and orange lines, respectively) were matched with their counterparts identified on retromode images, as shown in Figure 1. On the other hand, while FAF images were matched to retromode images using the retinal blood vessels alone (orange lines Figure 2), for OCT B-scans we used both the neuroretinal rim (grey lines) and the extension of the ERM itself. Particularly, the ERM margins on OCT images were projected onto the retromode image through *orange lines*, whereas black lines parallel to those originating from the neuroretinal rim were used to project the cystic spaces identified on OCT B-scans to their retromode counterparts (Figure 3).

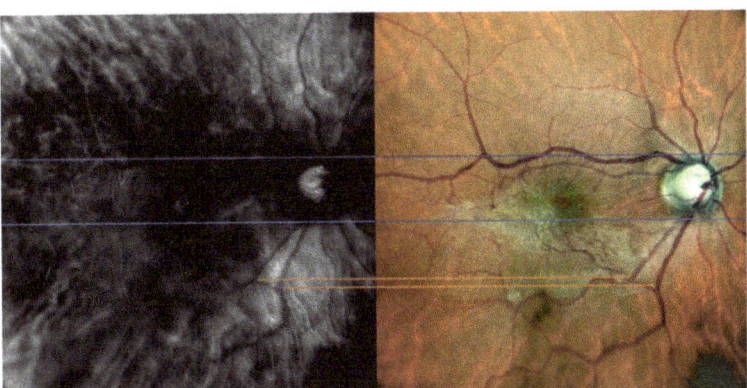

Figure 1. Retromode and fundus photography correspondence: optic nerve vertical outlines' poles (blue lines) and retinal vessels (orange lines) are used as reference points to check for appropriate image matching.

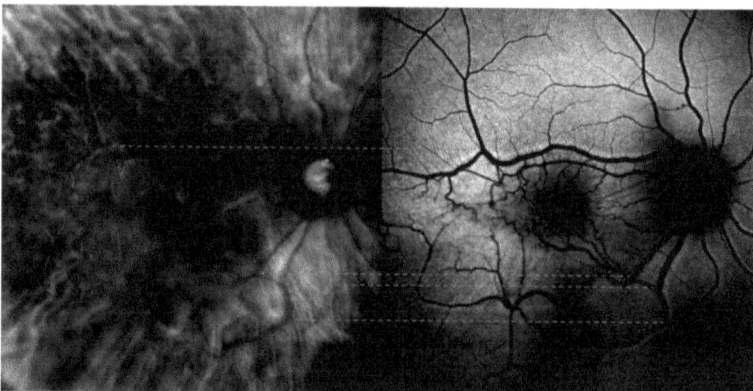

Figure 2. Retromode and fundus autofluorescence (FAF) correspondence: blood vessels on FAF scan (orange lines) are used as reference points to check for appropriate image matching.

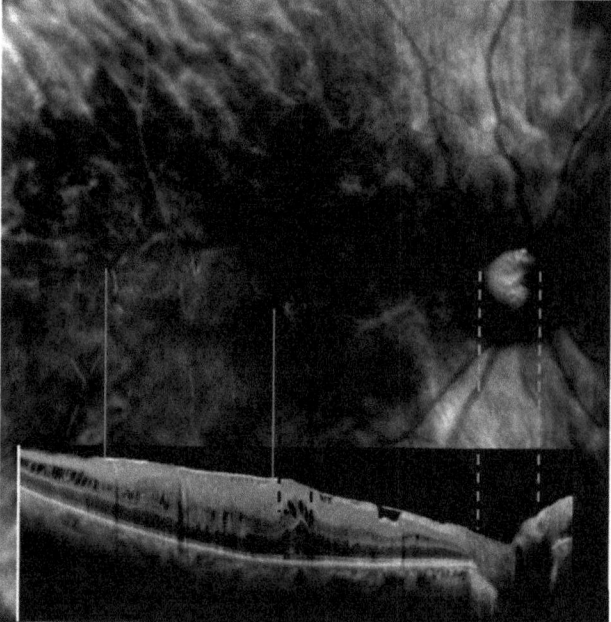

Figure 3. Retromode and SD-OCT correspondence: neuroretinal rim on optical coherence tomography (OCT) scan (grey lines) used as reference points to check for appropriate image matching. Dashed black lines represent the extent of the cystoid spaces.

2.3. Statistical Analysis

All statistical analyses were performed using SPSS version 27 (IBM-SPSS, Chicago, IL, USA). Quantitative variables were expressed as mean and standard deviation (SD), whereas qualitative variables were displayed as percentages. According to the normality test results, the Student's *t*-test was used to compare the independent and paired samples. Pearson's chi-squared test was used to analyze the distribution of the areas of retinal folds among the different multimodal imaging techniques. For each imaging modality, interobserver agreement was calculated using a kappa statistic [9]. The interobserver agreement between the two examiners was not inferior to 0.93 for each comparison. A *p* value of less than 0.5 was considered statistically significant.

3. Results

Twenty-one eyes (21 patients) with an epiretinal membrane were included. Twelve patients (57.1%) were male, nine (42.9%) were female and the mean age was 68.38 ± 7.89 years with a range of 51 to 83 years. Snellen best-corrected visual acuity (BCVA) ranged from 20/320 to 20/25.

The mean area of retinal folds in the FAF images was 5.67 ± 2.15 mm^2 (range 3.12–11.02 mm^2), whereas those in the fundus photographs and RMI were 10.58 ± 3.45 mm^2 (range 5.24–15.62 mm^2) and 11.85 ± 3.91 mm^2 (range 19.98–11.85 mm^2), respectively (Table 1).

Table 1. Demographics and pathological retinal findings of the population of study.

		No. of Patients:	Mean:	SD	Range:
Sex:	Male	12 (57.1%)			
	Female	9 (42.9%)			
Age (years):			68.38	7.89	51–83
FAF folds area (mm^2)			5.67	2.15	3.12–11.02
Fundus photo folds area (mm^2)			10.58	3.45	5.24–15.62
RMI folds area (mm^2)			11.85	3.91	19.98–11.85
B-scan horizontal diameter (μm)			290.52	90.01	100–442
B-scan vertical diameter (μm)			258.57	104.29	100–448
Horizontal B-scan area (μm^2)			0.79	0.44	0.13–1.98

Abbreviations: RMI: retromode imaging; FAF: fundus autofluorescence; μm: micrometer; SD: standard deviation.

Retromode images demonstrated areas of increased reflectance with fingerprint patterns containing radiating retinal striae centered on the fovea (blue arrowheads), along with areas of decreased reflectance with more prominent large choroidal vessels in the pericentral area (dark choroid aspect observed in 5 of 21 eyes) (multiple yellow arrowheads) (Figure 4).

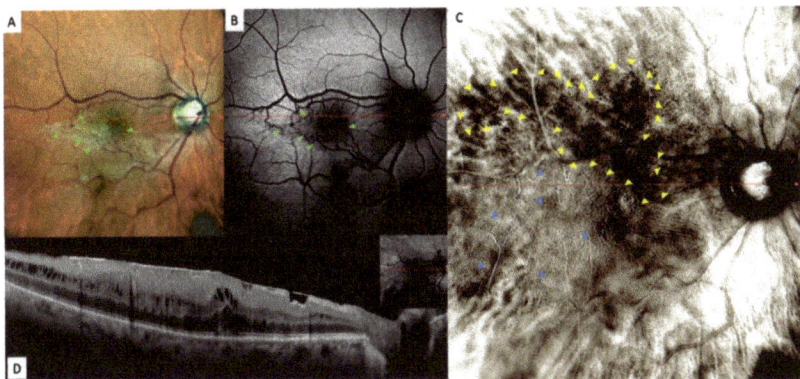

Figure 4. Epiretinal membrane (ERM) in (**A**) confocal scanning laser ophthalmoscopy color fundus photograph (fundus photograph) image, (**B**) fundus autofluorescence (FAF), (**C**) retromode and (**D**) horizontal B-scan. Fundus photography showing the epiretinal proliferation as a whitish light reflex. Retinal folds are well defined in fundus photography and have a fingerprint appearance in retromode imaging analysis. The FAF images showed an irregular-shaped hypoautofluorescence in the macular area.

The areas of increased reflectance, with fingerprint patterns containing radiating retinal striae centered on the fovea in RMI and the retinal folds in the FAF and fundus photography, are displayed in Figure 5.

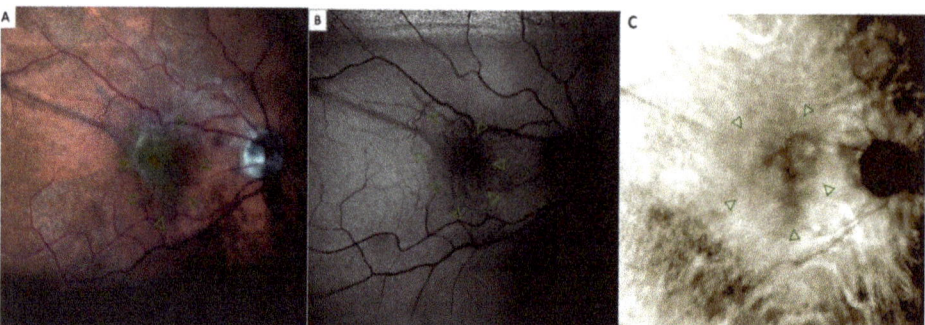

Figure 5. Epiretinal membrane (ERM) in (**A**) confocal scanning laser ophthalmoscopy color fundus photograph, (**B**) fundus autofluorescence (FAF) and (**C**) retromode imaging. The retinal folds are well defined in fundus photography and have a fingerprint appearance in retromode imaging analysis. The FAF image shows an irregular-shaped hypoautofluorescence in the macular area (green arrowheads).

FAF images showed an irregular-shaped area of hypo autofluorescence with distorted retinal vessels (green arrowheads). This area corresponded to the extent of the ERM (Figure 4).

Fundus photography, on the other hand, displayed the epiretinal proliferation as a whitish reflex and evident retinal folds in the macular area that were strictly related to distorted retinal vessels in the FAF images and to fingerprint appearance in the retromode images.

Overall, the lesions in the retromode images seemed more extensive than those in the FAF images. However, retromode imaging showed numerous ovoidal or polygonal cystoid spaces located in only two eyes. Both displayed a large cystoid space beneath the fovea and surrounding small cystic spaces for OCT, and the wider the area of exudation was for RMI, the higher the retinal profile was for optical coherence tomography (OCT).

While examining ERM's pathological findings themselves, in this study we also aimed at investigating the correspondence between retromode images and color fundus photographs. Particularly, we analyzed ERM patterns such as the cystic area (in both retromode and horizontal B-scan images) and the area of retinal folding (on FAF, fundus photograph, retromode, horizontal B-scan). The comparison between the different imaging modalities in the 21 enrolled eyes is shown in Table 2.

There were significant differences between FAF and retro-mode imaging in the detection of retinal folds (i.e., macular traction) ($p < 0.05$).

The mean area of retinal folds detected by RMI was significantly higher than that detected by FAF (11.85 ± 3.92 mm^2 and 5.67 ± 2.15 mm^2, respectively, $p < 0.05$), similar to that detected by fundus photography (11.85 ± 3.92 mm^2 and 10.58 ± 3.45 mm^2, respectively, $p = 0.277$).

Pearson's correlation test revealed a positive correlation between the areas of retinal folds detected by RMI and those detected by fundus photographs, FAF and OCT ($r = -0.90$, $p < 0.001$, $r = -0.63$, $p < 0.001$, $r = -0.35$, $p = 0.003$, respectively).

Table 2. Summary of data detected by multimodal ERM imaging. FAF: fundus autofluorescence; RMI: retromode imaging.

	Cystic Area RMI	Cystic Area Horizontal B-Scan	Folds Area RMI (mm²)	Folds Area FAF (mm2)	Folds Area Fundus Photograph (mm²)
#1	no	no	15.61	10.47	14.52
#2	no	no	9.60	4.02	7.30
#3	no	no	14.52	7.01	13.68
#4	no	no	11.01	3.38	10.18
#5	no	no	8.34	4.90	6.22
#6	no	no	13.24	6.22	12.25
#7	2.2	3.7	15.57	7.19	14.84
#8	2.52	4.9	10.06	5.08	9.46
#9	no	no	18.98	7.10	14.66
#10	no	no	8.09	3.98	7.08
#11	no	no	8.22	4.12	7.21
#12	no	no	11.67	5.22	10.97
#13	no	no	15.99	11.02	15.62
#14	no	no	10.36	5.18	10.01
#15	no	no	19.98	7.28	15.61
#16	no	no	8.47	4.23	7.43
#17	no	no	11.24	5.22	11.17
#18	no	no	13.21	6.73	13.74
#19	no	no	9.67	4.38	8.41
#20	no	no	7.09	3.28	6.58
#21	no	no	6.22	3.12	5.24

Abbreviations: RMI: retromode imaging; FAF: fundus autofluorescence.

4. Discussion

In this study we evaluated the pathological findings related to ERMs using and comparing three imaging techniques: retromode imaging, color fundus photography and fundus autofluorescence.

Thanks to its innovative features, retromode imaging could ease the identification of some ERM features, such as the retinal folds, vessel traction and cystic area, compared to other imaging modalities [4]. The matching between the SD-OCT scans and retromode images of ERMs using pixel-drawing software (ImageJ) has already been described [10]. Indeed, the pseudo-3D effect obtained by filtering the infrared light through a laterally deviated confocal aperture with a central stop creates a directional shadow according to the laterality of the annular aperture and is very effective at detecting retinal folds [4].

Among the classic imaging modalities able to document structural changes caused by ERMs, fundus photography is very useful, as this is a fast, noninvasive and easy test that enables clinicians to gain a direct view of the fundus [11]. Retromode imaging is similar to fundus photography in that it provides a similar field of view and can be performed very quickly in a noninvasive manner. Our comparison between these two techniques indicates a high clinical value of RMI, as it provides a good detection of the involved area. For fundus photography, ERM-related retinal changes are frequently represented by a yellowish/whitish appearance of the membrane associated with vessel tortuosity. retromode imaging can detect the involved macular area in pseudo-3D images with great sensitivity, delivering a more complete view of the anatomical conformation of the retina to the surgeon.

Moreover, monitoring the progression of the hyporeflective areas of the ERM on RMI may be very useful during the follow-up of affected patients, as their enlargement is very easy to detect.

As previously mentioned, retromode images demonstrated areas of increased reflectance with fingerprint patterns, containing radiating retinal striae centered on the fovea. We speculate these may represent areas of splitting of the horizontally oriented internal cone fibers, [12] whereas the areas of decreased reflectance corresponded to the presence of more prominent large choroidal vessels ("dark choroid" aspect). Ahn, S.J. et al. [13] identified a similar finding as well. We observed similar results as in a previous study on myopic patients, but, still, the precise explanation for this remains obscure [12]. One explanation might be that the ERM causes a shadow effect, which obscures the underlying choroid.

RMI enhances the detection quality of ERM's features compared to other common imaging techniques. In our cohort, this technique allowed to better visualize vessel traction and retinal folds compared to the other imaging modalities (FAF and fundus photography, $p < 0.05$). The ERM surface area detected using retromode was significantly larger than that detected by FAF ($p < 0.05$) and quite similar to that detected by fundus photography ($p = 0.277$). These results suggest that retromode imaging may be useful as a supplementary test for ERM detection.

Even though retromode imaging offers several advantages, it also displays some limitations. Above all, in this study, the detection rate of cystoid spaces on RMI was very low (only 2/21 eyes), whereas horizontal B-scanning revealed these lesions to be present in 100% of patients. In fact, the comparison of lesions in retromode imaging is often difficult, as many fundus details were obscured in these images. Moreover, as with most of the newly introduced imaging techniques, another drawback of RMI is its high cost.

Two major limitations of this study are its limited sample size and the fact that all images were manually cropped and superimposed. By comparing the measurements obtained by two retinal experts however, we feel like the risk of measurement errors was limited to the minimum. In the future, automated systems able to precisely compare different imaging modalities would be of help. Moreover, we did not analyze progression of ERMs' associated pathological features and whether RMI features could be able to predict surgical results.

5. Conclusions

In conclusion, this study showed that retromode imaging is a new effective tool that can be used to gain a more accurate visualization of the real extension of an epiretinal membrane. Retromode analysis in cases of ERM allows for a pseudo-3D visualization of epiretinal changes and a 360-degree visualization around the fovea. There is no other imaging modality that can simultaneously provide all this information. Alongside the current imaging modalities, retromode imaging may serve as a useful supplementary test for the preoperative evaluation of ERMs. Clinicians should be aware of RMI's advantages and should be able to use them to warrant a wide range of information and, thus, a more personalized therapeutic approach.

Author Contributions: Conceptualization, A.S., M.C.S., M.R. and S.R.; methodology, M.R.; software, M.R.; validation, M.C.S., S.R. and A.S.; formal analysis, M.R.; investigation, M.R.; resources, A.S., T.C., C.R., D.B., R.K., M.C.S., M.R. and S.R.; data curation, M.R.; writing—original draft preparation, M.R.; writing—review and editing, M.R., A.S. and R.K.; visualization, M.R.; supervision, A.S.; project administration, M.C.S.; funding acquisition, M.C.S. All authors have read and agreed to the published version of the manuscript.

Funding: This research was supported by Ministero della Salute Ricerca Corrente.

Institutional Review Board Statement: The study was conducted in accordance with the Declaration of Helsinki and approved by the Institutional Ethics Committee of Policlinico Agostino Gemelli IRRCS (protocol ID number 3680/20).

Informed Consent Statement: Informed consent was obtained from all subjects involved in the study.

Conflicts of Interest: The authors declare no conflict of interest.

References

1. Inoue, M.; Kadonosono, K. Macular Diseases: Epiretinal Membrane. *Dev. Ophthalmol.* **2014**, *54*, 159–163. [CrossRef] [PubMed]
2. Wilkins, J.R.; Puliafito, C.A.; Hee, M.R.; Duker, J.S.; Reichel, E.; Coker, J.G.; Schuman, J.S.; Swanson, E.A.; Fujimoto, J.G. Characterization of Epiretinal Membranes Using Optical Coherence Tomography. *Ophthalmology* **1996**, *103*, 2142–2151. [CrossRef]

3. Rispoli, M.; Rouic, J.F.L.; Lesnoni, G.; Colecchio, L.; Catalano, S.; Lumbroso, B. Retinal Surface En Face Optical Coherence Tomography: A New Imaging Approach in Epiretinal Membrane Surgery. *Retina* **2012**, *32*, 2070–2076. [CrossRef] [PubMed]
4. Lee, W.J.; Lee, B.R.; Shin, Y.U. Retromode Imaging: Review and Perspectives. *Saudi J. Ophthalmol.* **2014**, *28*, 88–94. [CrossRef] [PubMed]
5. Su, Y.; Zhang, X.; Wu, K.; Ji, Y.; Zuo, C.; Li, M.W.F. The Noninvasive Retro-Mode Imaging of Confocal Scanning Laser Ophthalmoscopy in Myopic Maculopathy: A Prospective Observational Study. *Eye* **2014**, *28*, 998–1003. [CrossRef] [PubMed]
6. Zeng, R.; Zhang, X.; Su, Y.; Li, M.; Wu, K.; Wen, F. The Noninvasive Retro-Mode Imaging Modality of Confocal Scanning Laser Ophthalmoscopy in Polypoidal Choroidal Vasculopathy: A Preliminary Application. *PLoS ONE* **2013**, *8*, e75711. [CrossRef] [PubMed]
7. Savastano, A.; Lenzetti, C.; Finocchio, L.; Bacherini, D.; Giansanti, F.; Tartaro, R.; Piccirillo, V.; Savastano, M.C.; Virgili, S.R. Combining Cataract Surgery with 25-Gauge High-Speed Pars Plana Vitrectomy: Results from a Retrospective Study. *Ophthalmology* **2014**, *121*, 299–304. [CrossRef] [PubMed]
8. Lyon, J.A.; Garcia-Milian, R.; Norton, H.F.; Tennant, M.R. The Use of Research Electronic Data Capture (REDCap) Software to Create a Database of Librarian-Mediated Literature Searches. *Med. Ref. Serv. Q.* **2014**, *33*, 241–252. [CrossRef] [PubMed]
9. Gorelick, M.H.; Yen, K. The Kappa Statistic Was Representative of Empirically Observed Inter-Rater Agreement for Physical Findings. *J. Clin. Epidemiol.* **2006**, *59*, 859–861. [CrossRef] [PubMed]
10. Abràmoff, M.D.; Magalhães, P.J.; Ram, S.J. Image Processing with ImageJ. *Biophotonics Int.* **2004**, *11*, 36–41. [CrossRef]
11. Song, J.H.; Moon, K.Y.; Jang, S.; Moon, Y.R. Comparison of MultiColor Fundus Imaging and Colour Fundus Photography in the Evaluation of Epiretinal Membrane. *Acta Ophthalmol.* **2019**, *97*, e533–e539. [CrossRef] [PubMed]
12. Tanaka, Y.; Shimada, N.; Ohno-Matsui, K.; Hayashi, W.; Hayashi, K.; Moriyama, M.; Yoshida, T.; Tokoro, T.; Mochizuki, M. Retromode Retinal Imaging of Macular Retinoschisis in Highly Myopic Eyes. *Am. J. Ophthalmol.* **2010**, *149*, 635–640.e1. [CrossRef] [PubMed]
13. Ahn, S.J.; Lee, S.U.; Lee, S.H.; Lee, B.R. Evaluation of Retromode Imaging for Use in Hydroxychloroquine Retinopathy. *Am. J. Ophthalmol.* **2018**, *196*, 44–52. [CrossRef] [PubMed]

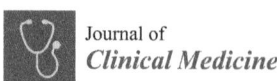

Article

3D Visualization System in Descemet Membrane Endothelial Keratoplasty (DMEK): A Six-Month Comparison with Conventional Microscope

Alberto Morelli [1], Rosangela Ferrandina [2], Eleonora Favuzza [1], Michela Cennamo [1] and Rita Mencucci [1,*]

[1] Eye Clinic, Careggi Hospital, Department of Neurosciences, Psychology, Pharmacology and Child Health (NEUROFARBA), University of Florence, 50134 Florence, Italy; alberto.morelli@unifi.it (A.M.); elefavuzza@gmail.com (E.F.); michelacennamo@libero.it (M.C.)

[2] Department of Biotechnology and Medical-Surgical Sciences, 'Sapienza' University of Rome, 04100 Latina, Italy; rosangela.ferrandina@gmail.com

* Correspondence: rita.mencucci@unifi.it; Tel.: +39-335-627-4390

Abstract: Background: To compare the efficacy and safety of Descemet membrane endothelial keratoplasty (DMEK) surgery using the three-dimensional (3D) display system NGENUITY to DMEK surgery performed with the traditional microscope (TM) in patients affected by Fuchs Endothelial Corneal Disease (FECD). Methods: Retrospective comparative study of 40 pseudophakic eyes of 40 patients affected by FECD who underwent DMEK surgery. Twenty patients (3D group) were operated on using the 3D display system and 20 patients (TM group) were operated on using the traditional microscope. Best spectacle corrected visual acuity (BSCVA), central corneal thickness (CCT), endothelial cell density (ECD) and corneal densitometry (CD) values were documented before and at 1, 3 and 6 months after DMEK. Intra- and postoperative complications were recorded. Results: The baseline assessments did not differ between the two groups ($p > 0.05$). Global surgical time and time to perform descemetorhexis were significantly lower in the TM group ($p = 0.04$ and $p = 0.02$, respectively). BSCVA, CCT, ECD and CD values did not differ significantly in the two groups at all follow-ups ($p > 0.05$). Complication rate was similar between the two groups. Conclusion: Three-dimensional display systems can be securely employed in DMEK surgery considering the satisfactory clinical outcomes, including Scheimpflug CD. Nevertheless, the slightly longer surgical time of the 3D DMEKs may lead to surgeons' hesitancy. The main advantages of the heads-up approach may be the improved ergonomic comfort during surgery and the utility of assistants in surgical training.

Keywords: heads-up surgery; cornea; DMEK; graft surgery; 3D surgery; corneal densitometry

1. Introduction

Endothelial keratoplasty (EK) is the surgical procedure of choice for the treatment of corneal decompensation associated with Fuchs Endothelial Corneal Dystrophy (FECD) [1,2]. Descemet membrane endothelial keratoplasty (DMEK), compared with other EK procedures, shows several advantages, including rapid visual recovery, better anatomical restoration due to the reduced graft thickness (10–15 µm) and minimal light scatter due to minimal interface irregularity [3].

Scheimpflug corneal densitometry (CD) is an objective method for accurately calculating corneal backscatter for defined concentric zones, thus providing an objective measurement for corneal transparency that is widely used after collagen cross-linking and after refractive surgery [4,5]. CD may also provide a feasible and objective method for monitoring corneal transparency after endothelial keratoplasty [6].

DMEK procedures have always been performed using traditional surgical microscopes, but, more recently, 3D visualization systems have also been employed. The term "heads-up" refers to the surgical procedures performed by viewing the 3D microscopic image on a panel display, providing a more natural and ergonomic posture for the surgeon [7]. One of the most used 3D visualization systems in ophthalmology is the NGENUITY 3D visualization system (Alcon, Forth Worth, TX, USA), which was used in our study. It is a modular system that is attached to the traditional microscope, which allows the surgeon to view a 3D stereoscopic image on a panel display using polarized glasses instead of looking at the eyepieces of the microscope.

Such 3D systems were originally employed for vitreoretinal surgery [8–10], but afterwards, their use was extended to anterior segment surgery, especially cataract and corneal graft surgery [11–13]. The use of heads-up procedures in cataract surgery was first described by Weinstock et al., who presented a retrospective analysis comparing surgeries performed using a standard binocular microscope versus a microscope equipped with a 3D visualization system. Excellent results were reported in both groups, with a minimal difference in total surgical time [14]. The use of heads-up in DMEK surgery was described for the first time by Galvis et al., who reported a case of a 68-year-old female with pseudophakic bullous keratopathy [12]. More recently, in 2020, a prospective, single-center, cross-sectional study was conducted at the Rothschild Foundation, Paris, France by Panthier et al. [13]. The study compared DMEK surgeries performed using a standard binocular microscope and the NGENUITY 3D visualization system. Each group included 12 cases: six single DMEK and six combined DMEK and cataract procedures. The authors reported that DMEK using a 3D display system was feasible, but it was more challenging and the total surgical time recorded was longer. However, it was considered certainly useful for instructional courses.

Only a few studies have evaluated the use of 3D systems in endothelial keratoplasty, and, to our knowledge, there are currently no studies in the literature examining corneal densitometry in patients who underwent heads-up DMEK surgery. The purpose of this study was to examine the surgical times, safety and clinical outcomes, including corneal densitometry, of DMEK surgery performed with a 3D system versus a traditional microscope with a six-month follow-up.

2. Materials and Methods

2.1. Design

This single-center, retrospective, controlled study included 40 eyes of 40 patients affected by Fuchs Endothelial Corneal dystrophy (FECD) who underwent DMEK surgery. Procedures were consecutively performed between 1 November 2019 and 28 February 2021 at the Azienda Ospedaliero-Universitaria Careggi, University of Florence, Florence, Italy.

Twenty DMEKs were consecutively performed using the NGENUITY 3D visualization system (3D group) and the other 20 DMEKs were consecutively performed using the traditional surgical microscope, OPMI-Lumera 700 (Carl Zeiss Meditec, Inc., Jena, Germany) (TM group).

This study followed the tenets of the Declaration of Helsinki. Informed consent was obtained from all subjects involved in the study.

Forty patients were included in this study. Inclusion criteria for recipient patients comprised age more than 18 years, uneventful previous cataract surgery at least 3 months before DMEK surgery, endothelial corneal dysfunction from FECD and good candidates for lamellar endothelial transplantation. Only cases with sufficient clinical data at 1, 3 and 6 months were included into the study. Exclusion criteria comprised a history of previous ocular surgery (except for cataract surgery), clinically significant posterior capsular opacity, stromal dystrophies, keratoconus, aphakia, history of ocular trauma, glaucoma, active vascular retinal disease, uveitis, myopia more than 6D, age-related macular degeneration and amblyopia.

2.2. Materials

Alcon NGENUITY is a modular system that consists of a mobile workstation and an Image Capture Module (ICM), a high-definition stereoscopic 3D image capture camera that is mounted on a standard surgical microscope [15]. The ICM collects light from the microscope and generates a stereoscopic image. The stereoscopic images and videos are sent to a 55-inch 3D high-definition (HD) monitor positioned 1.5 m from the surgeon and arranged perpendicular to the direction of his or her gaze. The resolution of the screen is 4K with a 16:9 format. Figure 1 shows the surgeon operating while looking directly at the monitor with the help of special 3D glasses with passive polarization for stereopsis. This allows them to assume the "heads-up" position, in which the head is raised in a neutral position [16].

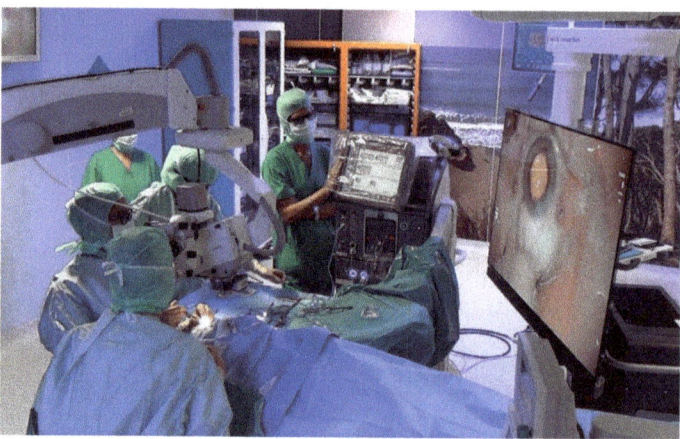

Figure 1. The surgeon operating with a "heads-up" position looking at the 3D monitor with the use of polarized glasses.

The following preoperative donor graft data were collected: donor age (years) and gender, graft endothelial cell density (ECD) (cells/mm^2) measured by Perseus automated endothelial microscopy (CSO Costruzione Strumenti Oftalmici, Florence, Italy), graft thickness (μm) measured by anterior segment OCT Visante (Carl Zeiss Meditech, Dublin, CA, USA) and preservation time until surgery (days).

The following data were collected preoperatively (baseline), and at 1, 3 and 6 months postoperatively: best spectacle-corrected visual acuity (BSCVA), intraocular pressure (IOP) measured by applanation tonometry (Goldmann applanation tonometer, Haag Streit, Bern, Switzerland), central corneal thickness (CCT) obtained by Anterior Segment OCT MS-39 (CSO Costruzione Strumenti Oftalmici, Florence, Italy), endothelial cell density (ECD) measured by Perseus automated endothelial microscopy (CSO Costruzione Strumenti Oftalmici, Florence, Italy), slit lamp biomicroscopy and ocular fundus examination.

Preoperative and postoperative corneal densitometry (CD) values were assessed by a Pentacam device (Oculus GmbH, Wetzlar, Germany). Scheimpflug CD measures the backscattered light in different concentric regions and layers of the cornea. The light scatter is expressed in grayscale units (GSUs) ranging from 0 GSU, which indicates the maximum corneal transparency, to 100 GSUs, which indicates the minimum corneal transparency [17]. CD was performed for total layer (TL, which includes all the corneal layers) at different annular concentric zones: 0–2 mm zone, 2–6 mm zone and 6–10 mm zone. The peripheral 10–12 mm zone was not included in the study because it was, in all cases, beyond the donor grafts' diameter. Moreover, intraoperative and postoperative complications including graft unscrolling failure, primary graft failure, graft rejection, Descemet membrane detachments requiring rebubbling and acute IOP decompensation were recorded.

2.3. Surgery

All DMEK procedures were performed by the same experienced surgeon (R.M.), who received a 2-month training period for 3D-assisted DMEK surgery, performing at least 15 cases before the beginning of this study. In our study, DMEK procedures were performed under locoregional anesthesia with peribulbar block. Pre-cut DMEK grafts were provided by the Eye Bank of Lucca (Italy), after being stripped and placed on their sclerocorneal support. Grafts were immersed in 0.06% trypan blue dye (Vision blue; D.O.R.C, Zuidland, The Netherlands) and trephined by the surgeon to the preferred width by using a Hessburg-Barron donor corneal punch (Barron Precision Instruments, LLC, Grand Blanc, MI, USA).

The recipient's cornea was marked with a trephine to guide the subsequent descemetorhexis and to allow the correct positioning of the graft. A clear corneal incision was made to position an anterior chamber maintainer. Descemetorhexis was performed for the central 8.5 to 9 mm diameter using the inverted Price-Sinskey hook, along the epithelial reference line. The removed flap was positioned on the anterior surface of the recipient's cornea to check its integrity. The pre-cut DMEK graft was carefully detached from the surrounding stroma, immersed in sterile balanced salt solution and aspirated into the glass cartridge of a specific injector (E. Janach S.R.L., Como, Italy). The rolled donor graft was slowly introduced into the recipient's AC through the main incision. The graft was then unfolded and correctly positioned using the Dirisamer technique. Finally, an air bubble was injected in the AC to press the graft against the recipient's stroma.

Patients were discharged the same day of surgery and were instructed to keep a supine position until the air bubble was completely reabsorbed. In the case of ocular hypertension or pupillary block, a small quantity of air was released at the slit lamp. The postoperative management for both groups included topical antibiotics given 4 times a day for the first 2 weeks and dexamethasone eye drops 4 times a day for the first month, which was then incrementally reduced over a 6-month period.

2.4. Statistics

Statistical analysis was performed using SPSS software (V.28.0 for Windows; IBM SPSS, Chicago, IL, USA). Normality of data distribution in both groups was assessed with the Shapiro–Wilk test. Student's t-test was used for the following interval scale parameters: BSCVA, IOP, CCT and CD values. Meanwhile, the Mann–Whitney U test was used for ECD. The χ^2 test was used for categorical variables such as rebubbling rate, intra- and postoperative complication rate. The level of significance was characterized as $p < 0.05$.

3. Results

A total of 40 eyes of 40 patients with a median age of 71.5 years were included in this study.

Patient demographics and corresponding preoperative clinical data are shown in Table 1. No significant differences were found between the two groups ($p > 0.05$).

Table 1. Patient demographics and corresponding preoperative clinical data.

	3D Group		TM Group		
	Mean ± SD (Range)	Absolute Number (%)	Mean ± SD (Range)	Absolute Number (%)	*p* Value
Age (years)	72.6 ± 6.9 (58–87)		68.6 ± 7.4 (54–85)		0.09
Male		7 (35%)		9 (45%)	
Female		13 (65%)		11 (55%)	0.42
Right Eye		9 (45%)		8 (40%)	
Left Eye		11 (55%)		12 (60%)	0.85
BSCVA (logMAR)	0.43 ± 0.21 (0.20–0.90)		0.54 ± 0.42 (0.20–2.00)		0.31
CCT (μm)	641.25 ± 50.2 (585–750)		643.05 ± 46.62 (598–766)		0.90
IOP (mmHg)	14.4 ± 1.4 (12–17)		13.9 ± 1.4 (10–16)		

BSCVA, best spectacle-corrected visual acuity; CCT, central corneal thickness; IOP, intraocular pressure; logMAR, logarithm of the minimum angle of resolution.

Donor graft data as provided by the eye bank are shown in Table 2. They were similar between the two groups ($p > 0.05$).

Table 2. Donor graft data.

	3D Group		TM Group		
	Mean ± SD (Range)	Absolute Number (%)	Mean ± SD (Range)	Absolute Number (%)	p Value
Age (years)	68.7 ± 7.2 (54–76)		64.9 ± 6.8 (45–74)		0.10
Male		7 (35%)		9 (45%)	
Female		13 (65%)		11 (55%)	
ECD (cells/mm^2)	2667.5 ± 192.1 (2300–3000)		2742.8 ± 136.9 (2500–3000)		0.16
Preservation time (days)	27.2 ± 3.3 (22–36)		26.2 ± 2.4 (21–30)		0.30

ECD, endothelial cell density.

Surgical times are shown in Table 3.

Table 3. Surgical times.

	3D Group	TM Group	
	Mean ± SD (Range)	Mean ± SD (Range)	p Value
Total surgical time (min)	24.33 ± 3.56 (17.80–29.60)	22.01 ± 3.58 (15.40–30.40)	0.04
Time to perform descemetorhexis (min)	5.25 ± 2.03 (1.20–8.20)	3.86 ± 1.59 (0.90–7.20)	0.02
Graft unfolding time (min)	4.88 ± 1.38 (2.80–7.20)	4.31 ± 1.31 (2.50–6.90)	0.19

In the 3D group, the total surgical time (24.33 min ± 3.56 min vs. 22.01 min ± 3.58 min, $p = 0.04$) and time to perform descemetorhexis (5.25 min ± 2.03 min vs. 3.86 min ± 1.59 min, $p = 0.02$) were significantly higher than in the TM group, while the graft unfolding time was similar between the two groups (4.88 min ± 1.38 min vs. 4.31 min ± 1.31 min, $p = 0.19$).

All clinical outcome parameters at all follow-ups are shown in Table 4 for each study group.

Table 4. Patient postoperative clinical data.

	Time	3D Group	TM Group	p Value
		Mean ± SD (Range)	Mean ± SD (Range)	
BSCVA (logMAR)	1° month	0.33 ± 0.25 (0.1–1.0)	0.29 ± 0.21 (0.1–1.0)	0.68
	3° month	0.22 ± 0.17 (0–0.6)	0.21 ± 0.19 (0–0.8)	0.86
	6° month	0.20 ± 0.14 (0–0.4)	0.19 ± 0.16 (0–0.6)	0.92
CCT (μm)	1° month	543.1 ± 35.69 (515–657)	542.95 ± 34.99 (520–680)	0.99
	3° month	525.15 ± 20.56 (505–603)	516.95 ± 25.21 (490–600)	0.27
	6° month	516.6 ± 23.66 (495–603)	515.05 ± 32.88 (487–611)	0.87
ECD (cells/mm^2)	1° month	1787.6 ± 300.13 (1250–2302)	1815.9 ± 220.66 (1470–2384)	0.74
	3° month	1711.15 ± 282.87 (1200–2200)	1712.05 ± 197.83 (1300–2200)	0.99
	6° month	1639.4 ± 268.32 (1200–2130)	1654.9 ± 250.76 (1359–2280)	0.85

BSCVA, best spectacle-corrected visual acuity; CCT, central corneal thickness; ECD, endothelial cell density; logMAR, logarithm of the minimum angle of resolution.

Postoperative results for IOP at all follow-ups were similar in both groups ($p > 0.05$). BSCVA in the 3D group was 0.19 ± 0.14 logMAR at 6 months postoperatively, with no significant differences compared with the TM group (0.19 ± 0.15, $p = 0.91$). The mean CCT in the 3D group was 516.60 ± 23.65 μm at 6 months postoperatively, while in the TM group, it was 515.05 ± 32.88 µm, with no significant difference ($p = 0.86$). Endothelial cell density at 6 months postoperatively was 1639.40 ± 268.31 cells/mm2 in the 3D group (ECD loss rate of 38.5%) and 1654.90 ± 250.76 cells/mm^2 in the TM group (ECD loss rate of 39.7%), with no significant difference found ($p = 0.85$).

Table 5 shows the preoperative and postoperative total layer (TL) corneal densitometry (CD) for the different concentric zones. Baseline values in the 3D group were 38.91 ± 9.13 GSU for the 0–2 mm zone, 36.05 ± 77.97 GSU for the 2–6 mm zone and 35.9 ± 5.11 GSU for the 6–10 mm zone, while in the TM group, they were 39.79 ± 10.64 GSU, 37.4 ±6.66 GSU and 36.8 ± 4.27 GSU, respectively, with no statistically significant difference ($p = 0.78$, $p = 0.56$ and $p = 0.55$, respectively). Baseline values showed a significant reduction at 6 months in the 3D group (TL CD values were 20.97 ± 4.39 GSU for the 0–2 mm zone, 21.55 ± 2.58 GSU for the 2–6 mm zone and 23.90 ± 3.52 GSU for the 6–10 mm zone) and in the TM group (TL CD values were 19.92 ± 3.86 GSU for the 0–2 mm zone, 19.85 ± 2.05 GSU for the 2–6 mm zone and 25.30 ± 2.67 GSU for the 6–10 mm zone), showing no statistically significant difference between the two groups ($p = 0.42$, $p = 0.12$ and $p = 0.16$, respectively).

Table 5. Patient preoperative and postoperative corneal densitometry.

		3D Group	TM Group	
	Time	Mean ± SD (Range)	Mean ± SD (Range)	p Value
CD 0–2 mm (GSU)	Baseline	38.91 ± 9.13 (25.7–55.8)	39.79 ± 10.64 (29.0–79.5)	0.78
	1° month	24.53 ± 6.03 (16.0–39.0)	23.03 ± 2.40 (19.0–27.0)	0.40
	3° month	22.78 ± 3.81 (16.0–30.0)	22.38 ± 4.05 (16.0–29.0)	0.75
	6° month	20.98 ± 4.39 (14.0–29.0)	19.93 ± 3.86 (14.0–27.0)	0.43
CD 2–6 mm (GSU)	Baseline	36.05 ± 77.97 (28.0–65.2)	37.4 ±6.66 (30.2–62.3)	0.56
	1° month	23.1 ± 3.7 (19.0–33.0)	21.85 ±2.87 (17.0–19.0)	0.24
	3° month	21.88 ± 2.73 (18.0–28.0)	20.9 ± 2.13 (16.0–25.0)	0.27
	6° month	20.70 ± 2.16 (17.0–25.0)	19.85 ± 2.06 (16.0–24.0)	0.22
CD 6–10 mm (GSU)	Baseline	35.9 ± 5.11 (29.1–45.0)	36.8 ± 4.27 (32.1–44.8)	0.55
	1° month	25.8 ± 4.94 (18.0–37.0)	25.4 ± 2.35 (21.0–29.0)	0.75
	3° month	24.55 ± 3.95 (17.0–33.0)	25.6 ± 2.7 (21.0–31.0)	0.33
	6° month	23.9 ± 3.53 (16.0–30.0)	25.3 ± 2.68 (21.0–30.0)	0.17

CD, corneal densitometry; GSU, grayscale units.

Rebubbling occurred in four cases in both groups (20% rebubbling rate in 3D and TM groups) within the first month, with an uneventful postoperative course. One case of acute IOP decompensation that required air deflation within the first 24 h was recorded in the TM group. No regrafting was needed for both groups.

4. Discussion

DMEK surgery represents one of the most successful treatment options for endothelial disease because of the fast visual recovery combined with the very low incidence of graft failure and graft rejection compared with penetrating keratoplasty [18].

Considering the very low thickness of the graft, it is crucial for the surgeon to have optimal intraoperative visibility and surgical comfort. Consequently, 3D visualization systems may provide an intraoperative detailed view and better surgical ergonomics, thus reducing physical strain, which is known to be widely prevalent among surgeons in ophthalmology [19].

This is, to the best of our knowledge, the first study to investigate the clinical outcomes, including corneal densitometric values, of DMEK surgery in pseudophakic patients with FECD using a 3D system versus a traditional microscope with a 6-month follow-up.

Only a few other studies have investigated the use of 3D visualization systems in corneal transplantation surgery, most of them being case reports [11–13,20]. Mohamed YH et al. reported the first case of corneal surgery using a heads-up system [11]. They performed non-Descemet Stripping Automated Endothelial Keratoplasty (nDSAEK) using 3D technology for a post-traumatic bullous keratopathy and reported a great visual and ergonomic experience. However, the authors stated that frequent focus adjustment was required for a clear stereoscopic view of the flap.

Panthier et al. showed, in a prospective study, the outcomes 3 months after DMEK surgery performed using the NGENUITY 3D visualization system versus a traditional microscope in 24 patients with FECD and pseudophakic bullous keratopathy [13]. The authors found no significant differences in clinical outcomes in the two groups despite the longer surgical times of the 3D group. Nevertheless, they included single DMEK procedures and triple procedures (DMEK combined with phacoemulsification and posterior chamber lens implantation) [13].

The present retrospective study of 40 eyes that underwent DMEK surgery with either a 3D visualization system ($n = 20$) or traditional surgical microscope ($n = 20$) showed a significantly longer global surgical time ($p = 0.04$) and a significantly longer time to perform descemetorhexis ($p = 0.03$) in the 3D group. Nonetheless, the longer surgical time of the 3D group was not crucial as the planned sequence of surgeries of the operating session was not affected in any case.

Conversely, similar outcomes for BSCVA, ECD and CCT values at all follow-ups ($p > 0.05$) could be detected in the 3D group and TM group. We also recorded Scheimpflug CD as an objective parameter for assessing corneal transparency. According to our knowledge, only a few studies analyzing CD after DMEK surgery have been published [5,6,21]. We observed a reduction in CD values in the 6-month follow-up period, with no significant difference in the two groups, implying a similar improvement in corneal clarity after DMEK. Moreover, intraoperative and postoperative complication rates, such as acute IOP decompensation, graft failure and graft rejection rates, were similar between the two groups. Significant graft detachment requiring a rebubbling procedure after DMEK surgery was observed with the same rate of 20% in both groups.

According to our results, 3D-assisted DMEK surgery provided similar outcomes in terms of efficacy and safety compared with DMEK cases performed with a conventional microscope over a 6-month follow-up period.

Furthermore, the surgeon reported better intraoperative ergonomics allowing for a greater degree of freedom during surgery, despite a subtle latency effect (70 ms) due to the processing time of the Image Capture Module, which, nevertheless, did not affect the fluency of the surgeon's maneuvers [22].

The major benefits of a heads-up approach in ophthalmic surgery are described in the literature and they include the more ergonomic position of the operator, the excellent teaching capacity of the 3D image, which is shared in the operating room among all the staff, a wider visual field with a greater image resolution and the possibility to apply digital filters to the 3D image projected on the screen [23–25].

The limitations of our study were the retrospective non-randomized design, the involvement of a relatively small number of patients, as well as the involvement of a single surgeon performing DMEKs. Further multicentric, prospective, randomized studies are warranted to assess the outcomes of heads-up DMEK compared to the surgery performed with the TM.

Moreover, since our study excluded patients with concomitant corneal disorders, complex anterior segment anatomy or a history of previous corneal surgery, we could not investigate the efficacy and safety of 3D-assisted DMEK surgery in complex cases.

In conclusion, we believe that a heads-up approach can be employed to assist DMEK surgery, providing good results in terms of clinical outcomes, despite a slightly longer surgical time. The outstanding teaching capacity as well as the improved comfort provided by the heads-up approach may encourage anterior segment surgeons to implement this new technology for their routine keratoplasty cases, especially in teaching hospitals.

Author Contributions: Conceptualization, R.M., A.M., E.F., M.C. and R.F.; methodology, E.F. and M.C.; data curation, A.M. and R.M.; writing—original draft preparation, R.M., A.M., E.F., M.C. and R.F. All authors have read and agreed to the published version of the manuscript.

Funding: This research received no external funding.

Institutional Review Board Statement: The study was conducted in accordance with the Declaration of Helsinki.

Informed Consent Statement: Informed consent was obtained from all subjects involved in the study.

Data Availability Statement: Data not publicly available.

Conflicts of Interest: The authors declare no conflict of interest.

References

1. Nanavaty, M.A.; Wang, X.; Shortt, A.J. Endothelial keratoplasty versus penetrating keratoplasty for Fuchs endothelial dystrophy. *Cochrane Database Syst. Rev.* **2014**, *2*, CD008420. [CrossRef] [PubMed]
2. Ang, M.; Wilkins, M.R.; Mehta, J.S.; Tan, D. Descemet membrane endothelial keratoplasty. *Br. J. Ophthalmol.* **2016**, *100*, 15–21. [CrossRef] [PubMed]
3. Waldrop, W.H.; Gillings, M.J.; Robertson, D.M.; Petroll, W.M.; Mootha, V.V. Lower Corneal Haze and Aberrations in Descemet Membrane Endothelial Keratoplasty Versus Descemet Stripping Automated Endothelial Keratoplasty in Fellow Eyes for Fuchs Endothelial Corneal Dystrophy. *Cornea* **2020**, *39*, 1227–1234. [CrossRef] [PubMed]
4. Pahuja, N.; Shetty, R.; Subbiah, P.; Nagaraja, H.; Nuijts, R.M.; Jayadev, C. Corneal Densitometry: Repeatability in Eyes with Keratoconus and Postcollagen Cross-Linking. *Cornea* **2016**, *35*, 833–837. [CrossRef] [PubMed]
5. Alnawaiseh, M.; Zumhagen, L.; Wirths, G.; Eveslage, M.; Eter, N.; Rosentreter, A. Corneal Densitometry, Central Corneal Thickness, and Corneal Central-to Peripheral Thickness Ratio in Patients with Fuchs Endothelial Dystrophy. *Cornea* **2016**, *35*, 358–362. [CrossRef] [PubMed]
6. Schaub, F.; Enders, P.; Bluhm, C.; Bachmann, B.O.; Cursiefen, C.; Heindl, L.M. Two-Year Course of Corneal Densitometry after Descemet Membrane Endothelial Keratoplasty. *Am. J. Ophthalmol.* **2017**, *175*, 60–67. [CrossRef] [PubMed]
7. Eckardt, C.; Paulo, E.B. Heads-up surgery for vitreoretinal procedures: An experimental and clinical study. *Retina* **2016**, *36*, 137–147. [CrossRef]
8. Kunikata, H.; Abe, T.; Nakazawa, T. Heads-up macular surgery with a 27-gauge microincision vitrectomy system and minimal illumination. *Case Rep. Ophthalmol.* **2016**, *7*, 265–269. [CrossRef]
9. Skinner, C.C.; Riemann, C.D. 'Heads up' digitally assisted surgical viewing for retinal detachment repair in a patient with severe kyphosis. *Retin. Cases Brief Rep.* **2018**, *12*, 257–259. [CrossRef]
10. Coppola, M.; La Spina, C.; Rabiolo, A.; Querques, G.; Bandello, F. Heads-up 3D vision system for retinal detachment surgery. *Int. J. Retina. Vitr.* **2017**, *3*, 46. [CrossRef]
11. Mohamed, Y.H.; Uematsu, M.; Inoue, D.; Kitaoka, T. First experience of nDASEK with heads-up surgery. *Medicine* **2017**, *96*, e12287. [CrossRef]
12. Galvis, V.; Berrospi, R.D.; Arias, J.D.; Tello, A.; Bernal, J.C. Heads up Descemet membrane endothelial keratoplasty performed using a 3D visualization system. *J. Surg. Case Rep.* **2017**, *2017*, rjx231. [CrossRef]
13. Panthier, C.; Courtin, R.; Moran, S.; Gatinel, D. Heads-up Descemet Membrane Endothelial Keratoplasty Surgery: Feasibility, Surgical Duration, Complication Rates, and Comparison with a Conventional Microscope. *Cornea* **2021**, *40*, 415–419. [CrossRef]
14. Weinstock, R.J.; Diakonis, V.F.; Schwartz, A.J.; Weinstock, A.J. Heads-up cataract surgery: Complication rates, surgical duration, and comparison with traditional microscopes. *J. Refract. Surg.* **2019**, *35*, 318–322. [CrossRef]
15. Moura-Coelho, N.; Henriques, J.; Nascimento, J.; Dutra-Medeiros, M. Three-dimensional Display Systems in Ophthalmic Surgery—A Review. *Eur. Ophthalmic. Rev.* **2019**, *13*, 31. [CrossRef]
16. Berquet, F.; Henry, A.; Barbe, C.; Cheny, T.; Afriat, M.; Benyelles, A.K.; Bartolomeu, D.; Arndt, C. Comparing Heads-Up versus Binocular Microscope Visualization Systems in Anterior and Posterior Segment Surgeries: A Retrospective Study. *Ophthalmologica* **2020**, *243*, 347–354. [CrossRef]
17. Dhubhghaill, S.N.; Rozema, J.J.; Jongenelen, S.; Hidalgo, I.R.; Zakaria, N.; Tassignon, M.J. Normative values for corneal densitometry analysis by Scheimpflug optical assessment. *Investig. Ophthalmol. Vis. Sci.* **2014**, *55*, 162–168. [CrossRef]
18. Ong, H.S.; Ang, M.; Mehta, J. Evolution of therapies for the corneal endothelium: Past, present and future approaches. *Br. J. Ophthalmol.* **2021**, *105*, 454–467. [CrossRef]
19. Weinstock, R.J.; Ainslie-Garcia, M.H.; Ferko, N.C.; Qadeer, R.A.; Morris, L.P.; Cheng, H.; Ehlers, J.P. Comparative Assessment of Ergonomic Experience with Heads-Up Display and Conventional Surgical Microscope in the Operating Room. *Clin. Ophthalmol.* **2021**, *15*, 347–356. [CrossRef]

20. Borroni, D.; Rocha-de-Lossada, C.; Bonci, P.; Rechichi, M.; Rodríguez-Calvo-de-Mora, M.; Rachwani-Anil, R.; Sánchez González, J.M.; Urbinati, F.; Lorente, M.G.; Vigo, L.; et al. Glasses-Assisted 3D Display System-Guided Descemet Membrane Endothelial Keratoplasty Tissue Preparation. *Cornea* **2022**. [CrossRef]
21. Agha, B.; Dawson, D.G.; Kohnen, T.; Schmack, I. Corneal Densitometry after Secondary Descemet Membrane Endothelial Keratoplasty. *Cornea* **2019**, *38*, 1083–1092. [CrossRef]
22. Ta Kim, D.; Chow, D. The effect of latency on surgical performance and usability in a three-dimensional heads-up display visualization system for vitreoretinal surgery. *Graefes. Arch. Clin. Exp. Ophthalmol.* **2022**, *260*, 471–476. [CrossRef]
23. Del Turco, C.; D'Amico Ricci, G.; Dal Vecchio, M.; Bogetto, C.; Panico, E.; Giobbio, D.C.; Romano, M.R.; Panico, C.; La Spina, C. Heads-up 3D eye surgery: Safety outcomes and technological review after 2 years of day-to-day use. *Eur. J. Ophthalmol.* **2022**, *32*, 1129–1135. [CrossRef]
24. Mendez, B.M.; Chiodo, M.V.; Vandevender, D.; Patel, P.A. Heads-up 3D Microscopy: An Ergonomic and Educational Approach to Microsurgery. *Plast. Reconstr. Surg. Glob. Open.* **2016**, *25*, e717. [CrossRef]
25. Bin Helayel, H.; Al-Mazidi, S.; AlAkeely, A. Can the Three-Dimensional Heads-Up Display Improve Ergonomics, Surgical Performance, and Ophthalmology Training Compared to Conventional Microscopy? *Clin. Ophthalmol.* **2021**, *15*, 679–686. [CrossRef]

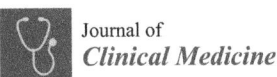

Article

OCT Analysis of Retinal Pigment Epithelium in Myopic Choroidal Neovascularization: Correlation Analysis with Different Treatments

Davide Allegrini [1], Diego Vezzola [1], Alfredo Borgia [1,2], Raffaele Raimondi [1,2,*], Tania Sorrentino [2], Domenico Tripepi [2], Elisa Stradiotto [2], Marco Alì [3], Giovanni Montesano [4] and Mario R. Romano [1,2]

1. Eye Clinic, Humanitas Gavazzeni—Castelli Hospital, Via Giuseppe Mazzini 11, 24128 Bergamo, Italy
2. Department of Biomedical Sciences, Humanitas University, Via Manzoni 113, 20089 Rozzano, Italy
3. Unit of Diagnostic Imaging and Stereotactic Radiosurgery, Centro Diagnostico Italiano, Via Saint Bon 20, 20147 Milan, Italy
4. Optometry and Visual Sciences, University of London, London EC1 0HB, UK
* Correspondence: raffor9@gmail.com

Abstract: *Objective*: The objective of this study was to analyze the status of the retinal pigment epithelium (RPE) by means of the spectral domain optical coherence tomography (SD-OCT) overlying the myopic neovascular lesions in the involutive phase, looking for any correlations between the status of the RPE and the size of the lesions and the type and duration of the treatment. *Methods*: SD-OCT examinations of 83 consecutive patients with myopic choroidal neovascularization (CNV) were reviewed and divided into two groups: group A, patients with CNV characterized by uniformity of the overlying RPE, and group B, patients with CNV characterized by non-uniformity of the overlying RPE. *Results*: The median lesion area, major diameter, and minimum diameter were, respectively, 0.42 mm^2 (0.30–1.01 mm^2), 0.76 mm^2 (0.54–1.28 mm^2), and 0.47 mm^2 (0.63–0.77 mm^2) in group A, and 1.60 mm^2 (0.72–2.67 mm^2), 1.76 mm^2 (1.13–2.23 mm^2), and 0.98 mm^2 (0.65–1.33 mm^2) in group B. These values were lower in group A than in group B ($p < 0.001$). The number of treatments with a period free of disease recurrence for at least 6 months was greater ($p < 0.010$) in group B (6.54 ± 2.82) than in group A (3.67 ± 2.08), and treatments include intravitreal anti-vascular endothelial growth factor injection, photodynamic therapy, or both. *Conclusions*: Our results showed that the size of myopic neovascular lesion influences the development of a uniform RPE above the lesion and therefore the disease prognosis. The presence of uniform RPE was found to be extremely important in the follow-up of patients with myopic CNV, as it influences the duration of the disease and the number of treatments required.

Keywords: medical retina; myopia; CNV; myopic choroidal neovascularization; OCT

1. Introduction

Pathological myopia is one of the leading causes of legal blindness in developed countries, with a prevalence of 2% in the general population; it affects about one-third of all myopes [1]. High myopia is associated with a progressive and excessive elongation of the ocular bulb, which may be accompanied by degenerative changes in the sclera, choroid, Bruch's membrane, retinal pigment epithelium (RPE), neuroretina, and vitreous body [2].

Degenerative processes are localized mainly at the level of myopic staphyloma, and they include geographical atrophy of the RPE and choroid, lacquer cracks in the Bruch's membrane, retinal and subretinal hemorrhages, choroidal neovascularization (CNV), vitreomacular tractions, epiretinal membranes, internal and external foveoschisis, and macular holes.

Among these, the myopic CNVs are associated with the worst visual prognosis with a natural history that reduces visual acuity to less than 1/10 in 90% of the affected eyes at 5 years from the onset of illness [3].

Pathological myopia is the first cause of CNV in subjects less than 50 years old, and a CNV is present in 4–7% of the eyes with myopia above 6 diopters [2,4]. Usually, myopic CNVs develop between the RPE and neuroretina, finding their natural growth space between the rupture of the Bruch's membrane and the atrophy of the overlying RPE that results from it.

The natural history of a CNV, in both human and animal models, is characterized by an initial active phase described by the development of subretinal neovessels that present leakage in fluorescein angiography and that are often associated with retinal and subretinal hemorrhages [5,6]. Subsequently, the CNV shows an evolving scar with the characteristic staining of dye and without signs of leakage. This process is defined as the involution of the CNV [5,7,8], and it is characterized by perilesional atrophy during the last stage of the pathology [3]. Histopathological studies by Miller et al. [9] have demonstrated how the RPE can play a key role in regulating the amount of leakage from neovascular lesions. In particular, it appears that the neovascular lesions in an involutive phase are completely incorporated by the RPE, which proliferates its edges until they are completely covered [9].

The use of spectral-domain optical coherence tomography (SD-OCT) has already been reported in many diseases of the fundus [10–14], including CNV-related diseases [11,15–18]. The SD technology allows a lateral resolution of 5–10 µm. The use of laser scanning ophthalmoscopy technology allows a real-time view of the posterior retinal pole using various wavelengths and simultaneous optical coherence tomography scans of the retino-choroideal complex, allowing the exact localization of tomographic scans on the visible lesions in fundoscopic images.

In this study, we analyzed the status of the RPE by means of the SD-OCT overlying the myopic neovascular lesions in the involutive phase, looking for any correlations between the status of the RPE and the size of the lesions and the type and duration of the treatment.

2. Materials and Methods

2.1. Study Design and Population

All the procedures performed in this study involving human participants were in accordance with the ethical standards of the institutional and/or national research committee and with the 1964 Declaration of Helsinki and its later amendments or comparable ethical standards. The ethical approval was deemed not necessary by the Ethics Committee of Humanitas Gavazzeni, in accordance with Italian law, as our work did not involve particular changes in existing procedures in our clinical practice, and as the drug used is not an experimental product but is widely used and already used at our hospital.

All patients with high myopia with neovascular lesions afferent to the retina were retrospectively analyzed at the clinic of Humanitas Gavazzeni-Castelli.

The inclusion criteria were as follows: (a) patients with a myopic refractive error $\geq$ 6 diopters; (b) evidence of neovascular lesions in fluorescein angiography (FA) and indocyanine green angiography (ICGA); (c) absence of lesion activity for at least 6 months, defined as lack of leakage in FA, unchanged shape and size of the neovascular net in FA and ICGA and absence of new perilesional hemorrhages; (d) treatment-free period for CNV longer than or equal to 6 months; (e) presence of at least 2 linear optical coherence tomography (OCT) scans (horizontal and vertical) overlying the lesion and a standard raster scan involving the CNV; (f) absence of intraretinal edema or subretinal fluid in OCT.

The exclusion criteria were the presence of ongoing inflammatory processes, hereditary diseases, and poor image quality.

After this selection, patients were divided into two groups based on their characteristics. Group A included patients with CNV characterized by uniformity of the overlying RPE (visible as a continuous line with the same reflectivity of the healthy RPE surrounding the lesion and without interruptions either inside or at the junction with the healthy RPE surrounding the lesion). An example is reported in Figure 1A, while group B included patients with CNV characterized by non-uniformity of the overlying RPE (visible as a line with continuity solutions inside it or with lower reflectivity with respect to the RPE around the lesion). An example is shown in Figure 1B.

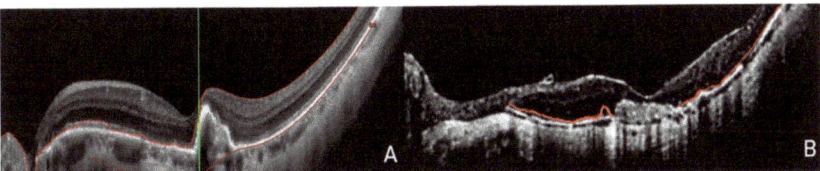

Figure 1. Spectral-domain optical coherence tomography (SD-OCT) images in white mode on a black background to better view the details of the retinal pigment epithelium (RPE). (**A**) The RPE completely covers the myopic choroidal neovascularization (CNV) without interruption of continuity, with the RPE surrounding the lesion clearly visible. (**B**) Neovascular fibrotic injury without evidence of RPE covering it.

Patients' treatments included intravitreal anti-vascular endothelial growth factor injection, photodynamic therapy, or both.

The anti-VEGF that our clinic protocol indicates in the case of myopic CNV is ranibizumab [19].

2.2. Patient's Examination

After detailed ocular anamnesis, each patient underwent baseline examination, which included the best-corrected visual acuity measurement with ETDRS charts before the pupil dilatation.

After dilatation, an indirect ophthalmoscopy with a 90-diopter lens was performed to detect the presence of any perilesional hemorrhages, an infrared (IR) reflectance imaging and fundus autofluorescence (FAF), an FA and ICGA, and an SD-OCT examination with a Spectralis HRA-OCT (Heidelberg Engineering, Heidelberg, Germany). The OCT images were collected with a Spectralis OCT as part of normal clinical practice. The standard protocol at our clinic employs a 30 × 25-degree pattern with horizontal macular B-scans (61 B-scans) (9 averaged scans).

The white-on-black mode of the OCT scans was chosen to best visualize the details of the RPE overlying the neovascular lesion. The presence, location, and type of CNV were evaluated by two masked ophthalmologist graders (DA, AB) on IR, FAF, OCT, FA, and ICGA. All the measurements were made in the same way according to our clinic protocol.

Any disagreement was resolved by open adjudication and, when necessary, consulting a senior retinal specialist (DV or MR). CNV was deemed present if it was detected on at least one imaging modality (namely FA ± ICGA and OCT). The diagnostic agreement between the imaging modalities was then calculated.

Patients were divided into two groups in accordance with the observations of Ding et al. [20]. Group A included patients with choroidal neovascularization (CNV) characterized by uniformity of the overlying retinal pigment epithelium visible as a continuous line with the same reflectivity of the healthy RPE surrounding the lesion and without interruptions either inside or at the junction with the healthy RPE surrounding the lesion. Group B included patients with CNV characterized by non-uniformity of the overlying RPE visible as a line with continuity solutions inside it or with lower reflectivity with respect to the RPE around the lesion.

2.3. Scan Analysis

Spectralis combines the scanning ophthalmoscopy with a high-resolution SD-OCT, and it allows the simultaneous acquisition of OCT scans and images in FA, ICGA, IR, and FAF. The lesion activity was assessed on the basis of the presence of perilesional bleeding, leakage in FA, and intra- or subretinal fluid in OCT and on the basis of the neovascular net extension in FA and ICGA [21].

For each patient, the largest diameter, minor diameter, and lesion area were measured in FA images obtained one minute after intravenous dye injection, using software included in the instrument. In particular, the markings were made manually, pointing precisely at the beginning of the lesion until the first point where restoration of normal anatomical conformation could be detected.

The presence of a hyper-reflecting perilesional ring in IR and autofluorescence in FAF has been evaluated in retinography (Figure 2).

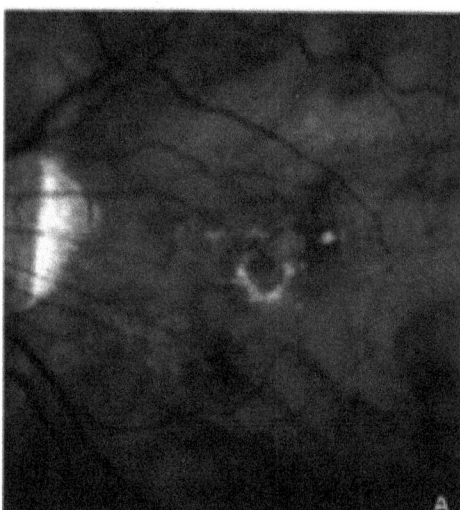 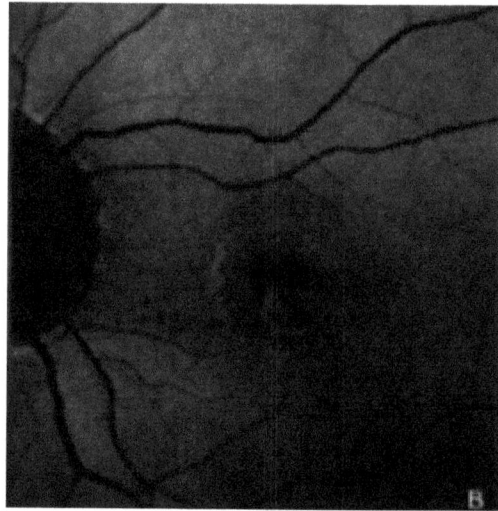

Figure 2. Scanning laser ophthalmoscopy images in infrared (**A**) and autofluorescence (**B**). The perilesional rings are clearly visible.

2.4. Statistical Analysis

Data distribution was evaluated using the Shapiro–Wilk test, and consequently, continuous variables were given as mean and standard deviation (SD) in the case of normal distributation, or median and 25th and 75th percentiles (interquartile range, IQR) in the case of non-normal or non-near-normal distribution.

The intra- and inter-observer correlation coefficients on the evaluation of RPE above the lesion were calculated using the intraclass correlation coefficient (ICC).

The differences between the 2 groups in terms of CNV size, type, and number of treatments and the presence of perilesional ring in IR and FAF were analyzed by ANOVA.

Considering the photodynamic treatment as a possible source of direct damage to the RPE, subgroups were created on the basis of the number of photodynamic therapies (PDTs) performed, and the differences were evaluated using the Fisher test.

A binary logistic regression was then performed for the development of RPE overlying the uniform CNV, considering as independent variables the age of the patients, the presence of perilesional ring in IR and FAF, the dimensions of the CNV, and the treatments performed.

Finally, a subsequent conditional selection of the independent variables was carried out to develop the best regression model.

Statistical analysis was performed using SPSS v.17.0 (IBM SPSS Inc., Chicago, IL, USA), and p-values < 0.05 were considered significant.

3. Results

3.1. Study Population

After the application of the inclusion and exclusion criteria, a total of 83 Caucasian patients with myopic CNV were analyzed. Of this population, 51 patients were included in group A (with uniform RPE) and 32 patients were included in group B (with non-uniform RPE).

Group A consisted of 35 (69%) females and 16 (31%) males with a median age of 66 years (IQR 59–70). Group B consisted of 22 (69%) females and 10 (31%) males, with a median age of 66 years (IQR 57–71). No significant differences in terms of age ($p = 0.949$) and sex ($p = 0.991$) were found. The interval of time between the last treatment and the eye examination was 29 months (13–46 months) in group A and 20 months (10–33 months) in group B, with no significant differences ($p = 0.302$) (Table 1).

Table 1. Comparison between group A and B.

	Group A [#]	Group B [$]	p-Value
N° of patients	51	32	-
Female	35	22	0.991
Age (years)	66 (IQR 59–70)	66 (IQR 57–71)	0.949
N° of eyes (total, L, R)	58 (26 L, 32 R)	32 (14 L, 18 R)	-
Lesion area (mm^2)	0.42 (0.30–1.01)	1.60 (0.72–2.67)	**<0.001**
Major Ø (mm)	0.76 (0.54–1.28)	1.76 (1.13–2.23)	**<0.001**
Minor Ø (mm)	0.47 (0.36–0.77)	0.98 (0.65–1.23)	**<0.001**
N° of treatments	3.67 ± 2.08	6.54 ± 2.82	**<0.010**
Duration of therapy	6.04 ± 8.5	17.2 ± 16.5	**<0.010**
Time from the last treatment (months)	29 (IQR 13–46)	20 (IQR 10–33)	0.302
Ring in infrared	1 (1.72 %)	7 (23.33 %)	**<0.010**
Ring in autofluorescence	6 (10.34 %)	12 (37.5 %)	**<0.010**

[#] Group A included patients with choroidal neovasculariazion (CNV) characterized by uniformity of the overlying retinal pigment epithelium (visible as a continuous line with the same reflectivity of the healthy RPE surrounding the lesion and without interruptions either inside or at the junction with the healthy RPE surrounding the lesion). [$] Group B included patients with CNV characterized by non-uniformity of the overlying RPE (visible as a line with continuity solutions inside it or with lower reflectivity with respect to the RPE around the lesion). Ø, diameter; RPE, retinal pigment epithelium; L, left eye; R, right eye; Max_diam, maximum diameter; Min_diam, minimum diameter. All distributions were reported as mean ± standard deviation, or median and interquartile range (IQR). Significant differences were reported in bold.

3.2. Eye Treatments

Treatments were performed on a total of 90 eyes, of which 58 (26 left, 32 right) belonged to the patients of group A and 32 (14 left, 18 right) belonged to 32 patients of group B.

With regard to the size of the lesion, significantly lower values ($p < 0.001$) of major and minor diameter, and for the lesion area were found than for group B.

Particularly in group A, the median values of major diameter, minor diameter, and lesion area were 0.76 mm (0.54–1.28 mm), 0.47 mm (0.36–0.77 mm), and 0.42 mm (0.30–1.01 mm), respectively; while in group B, the same values were 1.76 mm (1.13–2.23 mm), 0.98 mm (0.65–1.23 mm), and 1.60 mm (0.72–2.67 mm), respectively.

Furthermore, in group B, a significantly greater number of treatments were necessary ($p < 0.010$; number of treatments in Group B 6.54 ± 2.82; Group A 3.67 ± 2.08), such as PDT, intravitreal injections (IVT) of anti-VEGF (vascular endothelial growth factor), or a combination of both treatments, to have a period free of disease recurrence for at least 6 months. Perilesional rings, both in IR ($p < 0.01$) and in FAF ($p < 0.01$), were found to be statistically significant more frequently in group B (N° IR = 7, N° of FAF = 12) compared to group A (N° IR = 1; N° FAF = 6). All the results above are summarized in Table 1.

A subgroup analysis of patients treated with PDT was performed. A total of 37 patients received at least 1 PDT treatment, 15 in group A and 12 in group B. Of these 37 patients, 17 received two or more PDT treatments.

The analysis of subgroups based on the number of PDTs performed showed significant differences only when the number of PDTs was greater than or equal to 2x treatments ($p < 0.05$, Fisher test). No differences were found between the subgroups if only one photodynamic treatment was performed ($p = 0.750$, Fisher test).

Using a general binary logistic regression model, the only significant parameter for the presence of uniform RPE was the lesion size (area and maximum and minimum diameter were associated in consideration of their collinearity).

The conditional selection of the variables showed that the best regression model for the development of uniform RPE is that formed by the size of the neovascular lesion and by the presence of a perilesional ring in IR. These are therefore the only predictors for the presence of uniform RPE overlying the lesion.

The intra- and inter-reader correlation coefficients (ICC) were very good (0.886) and excellent (0.928), respectively.

4. Discussion

Miller's histopathological studies on cynomolgus monkeys observed how RPE tries to cover the laser-generated iatrogenic neovascular lesions [9]. The same study also showed that the activity of these lesions, defined as leakage in late stages of fluorescein angiography, is inversely proportional to the percentage of neovascular tissue covered by RPE, and how the scar lesions, which characterize the involutive process of the CNV, are in fact neovascular membranes completely covered by RPE.

The high definition of the new SD-OCT has allowed the analysis of the details of retinal layers in vivo [22]. Unfortunately, the definition levels are not yet comparable to those of histological preparations, which allow a direct observation of the tissue cells; however, they are sufficient to formulate realistic assumptions.

In the present study, it was observed that the non-uniformity of RPE overlying the lesion was related to a longer history of disease, more treatments, and larger lesion sizes. From these results, we can hypothesize that the RPE is able to cover only part of the large-sized lesions. Therefore, the RPE is not able to block the angiogenic stimulus and then contain the lesions, which allows its growth.

Conditional analysis of the variables confirms that the development of uniform RPE is influenced mostly by the size of the neovascular lesions. The presence of the perilesional ring in IR had a different frequency in the two groups, but with borderline significance in the development of uniform RPE. Those data are in any case of doubtful interpretation given the low prevalence of the IR ring in our sample (Table 1).

There is growing interest in the measurement and study of the morphology of myopic choroidal neovascularization [23].

Results of treatments with PDT are significant [24]. It has already been reported that PDTs can lead to the closure of the vessels of the choriocapillary (easily visible in the ICGA) in the irradiated area and hypo- or hyperfluorescent in FA, depending on the phase of swelling or atrophy of RPE [25]. Histopathological studies of neovascular lesions have confirmed the presence of RPE atrophy three months after photodynamic treatment [26]. Although the current study has considered a small group of patients, results have shown that a single PDT allows the formation of a uniform RPE above the lesion. In addition, the conditional selection of variables has not confirmed that a history of previous PDT can predict the behavior of the RPE. In recent years, PDT has been replaced by intravitreal injections (IVT) of anti-VEGF, which have shown a better visual outcome [27,28].

There are many limitations to our work. First is the narrow sample of patients analyzed and the retrospective nature of the study. Second is the failure to analyze the retinal layers above the RPE (the external retinal layers such as the IS/OS junction and the outer limiting membrane). Third is that the subgroup analysis was carried out on only the PDT group. Furthermore, the location of the lesion (sub-, iuxta-, or extra-foveal), and the visual acuity before and after treatment was not taken into consideration. Finally, the presence of a different therapeutic approach for some patients remains an important bias of our study. It is also interesting to evaluate the changes in the RPE in various phases of the disease in FAF and SD-OCT.

5. Conclusions

The main finding of this study is that the observation of the RPE, through a non-invasive examination such as SD-OCT, can add important prognostic information in order to improve the planning of treatments and follow-up of patients.

With this study, we showed that the size of the myopic neovascular lesion conditions the development of a uniform RPE above the lesion and therefore the disease prognosis.

The presence of uniform RPE was found to be extremely important in the follow-up of patients with myopic CNV, as it influences the duration of the disease and the number of treatments required. A prospective study, with a larger sample and a control group, would be necessary to confirm our results and to establish a standardized treatment protocol for myopic neovascular lesions.

Author Contributions: Conceptualization, D.V. and G.M.; Data curation, D.A.; Formal analysis, R.R.; Investigation, G.M.; Methodology, T.S.; Resources, M.A.; Supervision, E.S. and M.R.R.; Visualization, D.T.; Writing–original draft, R.R.; Writing–review & editing, A.B. All authors have read and agreed to the published version of the manuscript.

Funding: This research received no external funding.

Institutional Review Board Statement: All procedures performed in studies involving human participants were in accordance with the ethical standards of the institutional and/or national research committee and with the 1964 Helsinki declaration and its later amendments or comparable ethical standards.

Informed Consent Statement: Patient consent was waived due to the retrospective nature of this study, and due to the subjects' anonymity and minimal risk to patients.

Data Availability Statement: Database available upon request to corresponding author.

Conflicts of Interest: The authors declare no conflict of interest.

References

1. Wang, N.-K.; Lai, C.-C.; Chou, C.L.; Chen, Y.-P.; Chuang, L.-H.; Chao, A.-N.; Tseng, H.-J.; Chang, C.-J.; Wu, W.-C.; Chen, K.-J.; et al. Choroidal Thickness and Biometric Markers for the Screening of Lacquer Cracks in Patients with High Myopia. *PLoS ONE* **2013**, *8*, e53660.
2. Curtin, B.J.; Karlin, D.B. Axial length measurements and fundus changes of the myopic eye. I. The posterior fundus. *Trans. Am. Ophthalmol. Soc.* **1970**, *68*, 312–334. [PubMed]
3. Yoshida, T.; Ohno-Matsui, K.; Yasuzumi, K.; Kojima, A.; Shimada, N.; Futagami, S.; Tokoro, T.; Mochizuki, M. Myopic choroidal neovascularization: A 10-year follow-up. *Ophthalmology* **2003**, *110*, 1297–1305. [CrossRef]
4. Grossniklaus, H.E.; Green, W.R. Pathologic findings in pathologic myopia. *Retina* **1992**, *12*, 127–133. [CrossRef]
5. Teeters, V.W.; Bird, A.C. A clinical study of the vascularity of senile disciform macular degeneration. *Am. J. Ophthalmol.* **1973**, *75*, 53–65. [CrossRef]
6. Gass, J.D. Biomicroscopic and histopathologic considerations regarding the feasibility of surgical excision of subfoveal neovascular membranes. *Am. J. Ophthalmol.* **1994**, *118*, 285–298. [CrossRef]
7. Gass, J.D. Pathogenesis of disciform detachment of the neuroepithelium. *Am. J. Ophthalmol.* **1967**, *63*, 1–139.
8. Ryan, S.J. Subretinal neovascularization. Natural history of an experimental model. *Arch. Ophthalmol.* **1982**, *100*, 1804–1809. [CrossRef]
9. Miller, H.; Miller, B.; Ryan, S.J. The role of retinal pigment epithelium in the involution of subretinal neovascularization. *Investig. Ophthalmol. Vis. Sci.* **1986**, *27*, 1644–1652.
10. Margolis, R.; Mukkamala, S.K.; Jampol, L.M.; Spaide, R.F.; Ober, M.D.; Sorenson, J.A.; Gentile, R.C.; Miller, J.A.; Sherman, J.; Freund, K.B. The expanded spectrum of focal choroidal excavation. *Arch. Ophthalmol.* **2011**, *129*, 1320–1325. [CrossRef]
11. Haruta, M.; Hangai, M.; Taguchi, C.; Yamakawa, R. Spectral-domain optical coherence tomography of the choroid in choroidal osteoma. *Ophthalmic Surg. Lasers Imaging Retina* **2011**, *42*, e118-21. [CrossRef]
12. Vance, S.K.; Khan, S.; Klancnik, J.M.; Freund, K.B. Characteristic spectral-domain optical coherence tomography findings of multifocal choroiditis. *Retina* **2011**, *31*, 717–723. [CrossRef]
13. Freund, K.B.; Laud, K.; Lima, L.H.; Spaide, R.F.; Zweifel, S.; Yannuzzi, L.A. Acquired Vitelliform Lesions: Correlation of clinical findings and multiple imaging analyses. *Retina* **2011**, *31*, 13–25. [CrossRef]
14. Yehoshua, Z.; Rosenfeld, P.J.; Gregori, G.; Penha, F. Spectral domain optical coherence tomography imaging of dry age-related macular degeneration. *Ophthalmic Surg. Lasers Imaging Retina* **2010**, *41*, S6–S14. [CrossRef]

15. Khan, S.; Engelbert, M.; Imamura, Y.; Freund, K.B. Polypoidal choroidal vasculopathy: Simultaneous indocyanine green angiography and eye-tracked spectral domain optical coherence tomography findings. *Retina* **2012**, *32*, 1057–1068. [CrossRef]
16. Sulzbacher, F.; Kiss, C.; Munk, M.; Deak, G.; Sacu, S.; Schmidt-Erfurth, U. Diagnostic evaluation of type 2 (classic) choroidal neovascularization: Optical coherence tomography, indocyanine green angiography, and fluorescein angiography. *Am. J. Ophthalmol.* **2011**, *152*, 799–806. [CrossRef]
17. Giani, A.; Luiselli, C.; Esmaili, D.D.; Salvetti, P.; Cigada, M.; Miller, J.W.; Staurenghi, G. Spectral-domain optical coherence tomography as an indicator of fluorescein angiography leakage from choroidal neovascularization. *Investig. Ophthalmol. Vis. Sci.* **2011**, *52*, 5579–5586. [CrossRef]
18. Golbaz, I.; Ahlers, C.; Stock, G.; Schütze, C.; Schriefl, S.; Schlanitz, F.; Simader, C.; Prünte, C.; Schmidt-Erfurth, U.M. Quantification of the therapeutic response of intraretinal, subretinal, and subpigment epithelial compartments in exudative AMD during anti-VEGF therapy. *Investig. Ophthalmol. Vis. Sci.* **2011**, *52*, 1599–1605. [CrossRef]
19. Costagliola, C.; Semeraro, F.; dell'Omo, R.; Romano, M.R.; Russo, A.; Aceto, F.; Mastropasqua, R.; Porcellini, A. Effect of intravitreal ranibizumab injections on aqueous humour concentrations of vascular endothelial growth factor and pigment epithelium-derived factor in patients with myopic choroidal neovascularisation. *Br. J. Ophthalmol.* **2015**, *99*, 1004–1008. [CrossRef]
20. Ding, X.; Zhan, Z.; Sun, L.; Yang, Y.; Li, S.; Zhang, A.; Luo, X.; Lu, L. Retinal pigmental epithelium elevation and external limiting membrane interruption in myopic choroidal neovascularization: Correlation with activity. *Graefe's Arch. Clin. Exp. Ophthalmol.* **2018**, *256*, 1831–1837. [CrossRef]
21. Verteporfin in Photodynamic Therapy (VIP) Study Group1234. Photodynamic therapy of subfoveal choroidal neovascularization in pathologic myopia with verteporfin: 1-year results of a randomized clinical trial—VIP report No. 1. *Ophthalmology* **2001**, *108*, 841–852. [CrossRef]
22. Michels, S.; Schmidt-Erfurth, U. Sequence of Early Vascular Events after Photodynamic Therapy. *Investig. Ophthalmol. Vis. Sci.* **2003**, *44*, 2147–2154. [CrossRef] [PubMed]
23. Wang, X.; Yang, J.; Liu, Y.; Yang, L.; Xia, H.; Ren, X.; Hou, Q.; Ge, Y.; Wang, C.; Li, X. Choroidal Morphologic and Vascular Features in Patients with Myopic Choroidal Neovascularization and Different Levels of Myopia Based on Image Binarization of Optical Coherence Tomography. *Front. Med.* **2022**, *8*, 791012. [CrossRef] [PubMed]
24. Rinaldi, M.; Semeraro, F.; Chiosi, F.; Russo, A.; Romano, M.R.; Savastano, M.C.; dell'Omo, R.; Costagliola, C. Reduced-fluence verteporfin photodynamic therapy plus ranibizumab for choroidal neovascularization in pathologic myopia. *Graefe's Arch. Clin. Exp. Ophthalmol.* **2017**, *255*, 529–539. [CrossRef]
25. Parodi, M.B.; Da Pozzo, S.; Ravalico, G. Angiographic features after photodynamic therapy for choroidal neovascularisation in age related macular degeneration and pathological myopia. *Br. J. Ophthalmol.* **2003**, *87*, 177–183. [CrossRef]
26. Schnurrbusch, U.E.; Welt, K.; Horn, L.C.; Wiedemann, P.; Wolf, S. Histological findings of surgically excised choroidal neovascular membranes after photodynamic therapy. *Br. J. Ophthalmol.* **2001**, *85*, 1086–1091. [CrossRef]
27. Yoon, J.U.; Byun, Y.J.; Koh, H.J. Intravitreal anti-VEGF versus photodynamic therapy with verteporfin for treatment of myopic choroidal neovascularization. *Retina* **2010**, *30*, 418–424. [CrossRef]
28. Ikuno, Y.; Nagai, Y.; Matsuda, S.; Arisawa, A.; Sho, K.; Oshita, T.; Takahashi, K.; Uchihori, Y.; Gomi, F. Two-year visual results for older Asian women treated with photodynamic therapy or bevacizumab for myopic choroidal neovascularization. *Am. J. Ophthalmol.* **2010**, *149*, 140–146. [CrossRef]

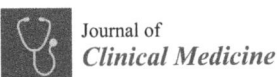

Article

Assessment of Corneal Angiography Filling Patterns in Corneal Neovascularization

Luca Pagano [1,2,*,†], Haider Shah [1,†], Kunal Gadhvi [1], Mohammad Ahmad [1], Nardine Menassa [1,3], Giulia Coco [4], Stephen Kaye [1,3] and Vito Romano [3,5,6]

1. St. Paul's Eye Unit, Royal Liverpool University Hospital, Liverpool L7 8XP, UK
2. Department of Biomedical Sciences, Humanitas University, Pieve Emanuele, 20090 Milan, Italy
3. Department of Eye and Vision Science, Institute of Life Course and Medical Sciences, University of Liverpool, Liverpool L7 8TX, UK
4. Department of Clinical Science and Translational Medicine, University of Rome Tor Vergata, 00133 Rome, Italy
5. Eye Unit, Department of Medical and Surgical Specialties, Radiological Sciences, and Public Health, University of Brescia, Viale Europa 15, 25123 Brescia, Italy
6. Eye Unit, ASST Spedali Civili di Brescia, Piazzale Spedali Civili, 1, 25123 Brescia, Italy
* Correspondence: luca.pagano91@hotmail.it
† These authors contributed equally to this work.

Abstract: The purpose of the paper is to describe vascular filling patterns in corneal neovascularization (CoNV) and evaluate the effect of corneal lesion location, CoNV surface area and multi-quadrant CoNV involvement on the filling pattern. It is a retrospective study of patients who were investigated for CoNV using fluorescein angiography (FA) or indocyanine green angiography (ICGA) between January 2010 and July 2020. Angiography images were graded and analyzed multiple independent corneal specialists. The corneal surface was divided into four quadrants and patient information was obtained through electronic records. A total of 133 eyes were analyzed. Corneal lesions were located on the peripheral (72%) or central (28%) cornea. Central lesions were associated with multi-quadrant CoNV more frequently than peripheral lesions ($p = 0.15$). CoNV located within the same quadrant of the corneal lesion was often first to fill (88.4%). In multi-quadrant CoNV, the physiological inferior–superior–nasal–temporal order of filling was usually respected (61.7%). Central lesions resulted in larger CoNV surface area than peripheral lesions ($p = 0.09$). In multi-quadrant CoNV, the largest area of neovascularization was also the first to fill in (peripheral lesion 74%, central lesion 65%). Fillings patterns in healthy corneas have previously been reported. Despite CoNV development, these patterns are usually respected. Several factors that may influence filling patterns have been identified, including corneal lesion location, CoNV surface area and aetiology of CoNV. Understanding filling patterns of neovascularization allows for the identification of areas at higher risk of developing CoNV, aiding in earlier detection and intervention of CoNV.

Keywords: corneal neovascularization; corneal vessels; CoNV; vessels filling pattern; ISNT rule

1. Introduction

A unique property of the healthy cornea is its angiogenic privilege. This characteristic is sustained by local pro- and anti-angiogenic factors [1]. Insults, such as inflammation, infection or surgery, may disrupt this balance, resulting in corneal neovascularization (CoNV). New vessels typically arise from the marginal corneal vascular arcades (MC); however, they can arise from conjunctival, episcleral and iris vessels [2]. This pathological process leads to a loss of corneal transparency, localised lipid sequestration and chronic inflammation.

CoNV plays a key role in corneal transplantation and the presence of CoNV is a leading cause of corneal graft failure [3]. New vessels and accompanying lymphatics deliver allo-antigens to host lymphoid tissue, resulting in a loss of immune privilege, thus facilitating allograft rejection [4]. Prompt identification and treatment of CoNV is important in reducing the risk of corneal graft rejection and improving outcomes. Current therapies include topical or localized delivery of anti-angiogenic factors and/or mechanical disruption of vessels with modalities such as fine needle diathermy [5,6].

Although CoNV may be appreciated with slit lamp biomicroscopy, accurately defining the anatomical origin and distribution of the new vessels, as well as monitoring progression, is challenging, and not all vessels are clinically detected. Currently, anterior segment angiography is the only dynamic examination that can facilitate the analysis of normal and abnormal corneal vasculature [7,8]. Both fluorescein (FA) and indocyanine green angiography (ICGA) have been utilized—the latter providing excellent angiographic detail, even in the presence of scarring, as it is not subject to leakage [2]. Effective utilization of angiography can allow for early identification and better delineation of neovascularization, thus potentiating accurate risk assessment prior to corneal grafting, as well as aiding in treatments such as fine needle diathermy [9].

Despite being an important component of assessing CoNV, there is limited information on angiographic filling patterns. Zheng et al. described an ordered filling pattern of inferior–superior–nasal–temporal (ISNT pattern) in healthy marginal corneal arcades (MCA) [2]. There is no information, however, on the filling patterns of diseased corneas with CoNV. The purpose of this study, therefore, was to define the angiographic filling patterns of neovascularized corneas. Better understanding of filling patterns may help identify areas of the cornea at higher risk of CoNV and guide treatment.

2. Materials and Methods

2.1. Study Population

The images of patients who presented with corneal lesions with accompanying CoNV who had undergone FA and ICGA at The Royal Liverpool University Hospital between January 2010 and July 2020 were included. Data collection was initially performed from the Heidelberg OCT software and subsequently from electronic patient records. All scans categorized as 'anterior segment angiography" on the Heidelberg OCT software were included. Angiographies demonstrating 1 or more quadrants of CoNV were studied. Anterior segment angiography performed for conjunctival lesions with localized extension onto the cornea, such as ocular surface malignancy and pterygium, were excluded. Low-quality images were excluded as detailed below. Clinical details and patients' demographics were obtained from patients' electronic records. No identifiable information was recorded. Ethical approval was obtained by the Stanmore Ethics Committee (15/LO/2166) and the study was conducted in accordance with the tenets of the Declaration of Helsinki.

2.2. Analysis of Images

Image quality was first assessed by 2 independent ophthalmologists and qualitatively graded from 0 to 4 (0 = no discernible vessels, 1 = poor vessel delineation, 2 = good vessel delineation, 3 = very good vessel delineation, 4 = excellent vessel delineation). Only images graded as 2 and above by both observers were included [7]. Patients were also excluded if discrimination of the order of CoNV filling was not possible due to blinking or loss of focus in the images/videos.

Each cornea was divided into 4 quadrants (superior, inferior, nasal and temporal) by super-imposing a cross image (Figure 1). The location of the corneal lesion was recorded as either central or peripheral if the lesion was close to or adjacent to the limbus. Peripheral lesions were grouped according to which quadrant they were located in. FA and ICGA images and videos were reviewed by 2 independent ophthalmologists (cornea specialists) to assess: (1) the location and order of CoNV filling patterns (Figure 2) and (2) the extent of CoNV. The origin of CoNV was determined by its point of origin from the MCA. All images were assessed in the same environmental condition with dim room light and maximum computer screen lighting.

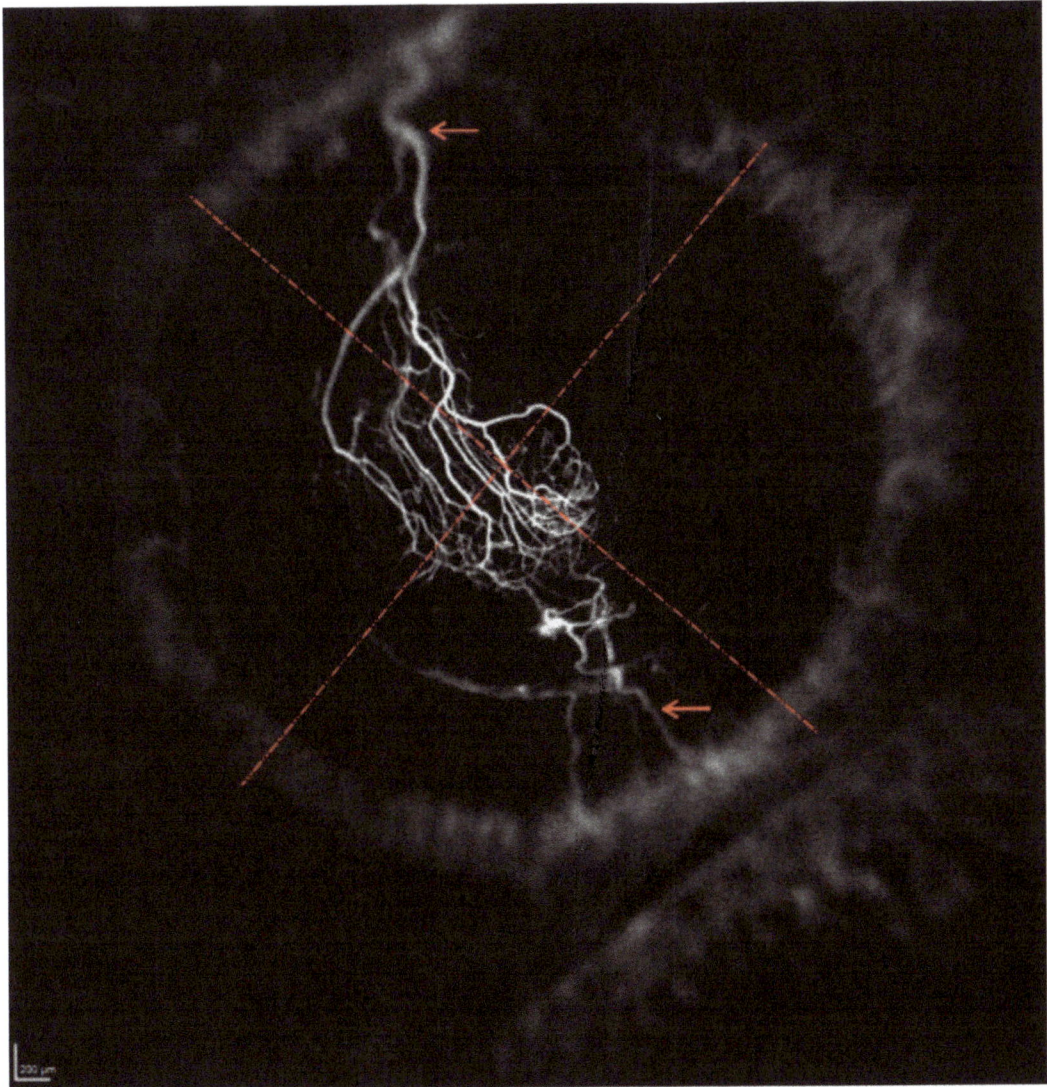

Figure 1. Division of cornea into four quadrants with a super-imposed cross image (dashed). The origin of the ConV is highlighted by arrows.

2.3. Statistical Analysis

Data are presented as the mean ± standard deviation (SD), or as a percentage for categorical variables.

The Chi-squared test was used to determine statistical differences between groups. The statistical analyses were performed using STATA 14.0 (StataCorp, College Station, TX, USA), and a p-value of less than 0.05 was considered statistically significant.

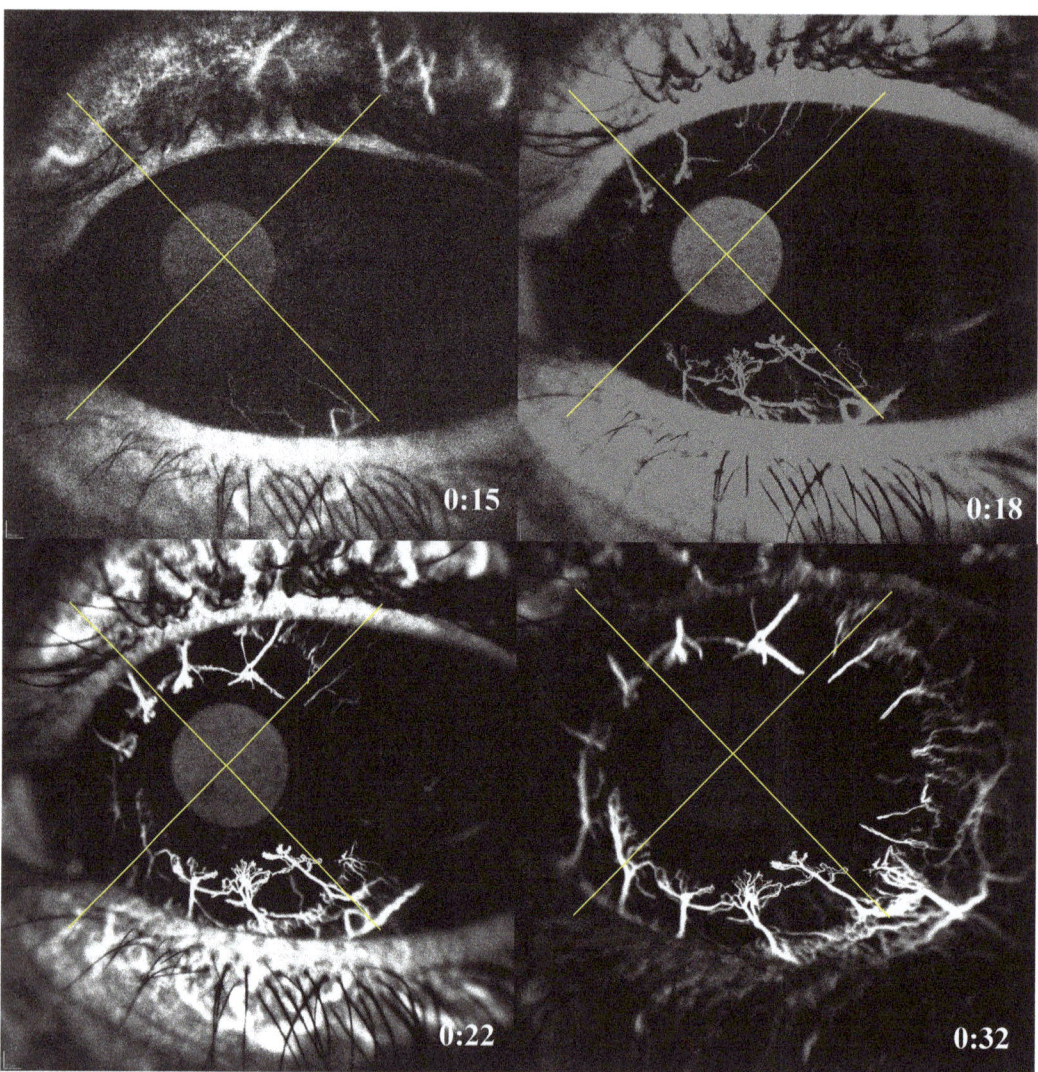

Figure 2. Indocyanine angiography showing a corneal neovascularization following the ISNT rule. The patient had a left eye penetrating keratoplasty that was followed by intensive 360° neovascularization. (**Top left**) shows that the first quadrant to fill is the inferior at 15 s, followed by (**top right**) the superior quadrant at 18 s, then the nasal quadrant at 22 s (**bottom left**) and ultimately the temporal quadrant at 32 s (**bottom right**).

3. Results

In total, 133 eyes of 130 patients were included. There was a 1:1 ratio of males (n = 66) and females (n = 67), with a mean age of 59.8 ± 18.1 years (range: 19–91 years).

3.1. Lesion and CoNV Location

Corneal lesions were peripheral in 95/133 cases (71.4%) and central in 38 cases (28.6%). Causes of CoNV (Table 1) included microbial keratitis in 76/133 cases (57.1%), of which 43/133 (32.3%) were bacterial and 33/133 (24.8%) were herpetic. Ocular surface disorders accounted for 35/133 (26.3%) cases—these included limbal stem cell deficiency (n = 6/133, 4.5%), allergic eye disease (n = 5/133, 3.8%), previous pterygium removal (n = 6/133, 4.5%), chemical injury (n = 2/133, 1.5%), mucous membrane pemphigoid (n = 2, 1.5%), central neurotrophic ulcer (n = 2, 1.5%), exposure keratopathy (n = 1, 0.8%) and ocular surface disorders with no known cause (n = 11, 8.3%). Previous penetrating keratoplasty accounted for 11 cases (8.3%) (Table 1). In 11 cases (8.3%), a cause for CoNV was not specified.

Table 1. Disease and number of quadrants of corneal neovascularization (CoNV).

Cause	CoNV Quadrants Involvement (n)			
	1	2	3	4
Keratitis (n = 76)	47 (62%)	16 (21%)	8 (10%)	5 (7%)
Ocular surface disease (n = 35)	22 (63%)	6 (17%)	2 (6%)	5 (14%)
Previous graft (n = 11)	10 (91%)	-	1 (9%)	-

In 86 eyes (64.7%), the CoNV was confined to one quadrant, 23 eyes (17.3%) had involvement of two quadrants, 12 (9%) had three quadrants and 12 (9%) had all four quadrants involved (Table 2). The number of quadrants involved was not different per different CoNC cause ($p = 0.68$). There was a trend for central lesions to be associated with multi-quadrant CoNV more frequently than peripheral lesions (44.7% vs. 31.6%, $p = 0.15$). For central lesions, the CoNV was fairly evenly distributed amongst four quadrants with the inferior quadrant involved in 20/38 (52.6%) cases, the superior involved in 22/38 (57.9%) cases, the nasal involved in 17/38 (44.7%) cases and temporally involved in 12/38 (31.6%) cases (Figure 2). For peripheral corneal lesions, the CoNV was co-located in the same quadrant as the lesion in most cases but with some extension into adjacent quadrants (Table 2).

Table 2. Number of quadrants with CoNV for peripheral and central lesions.

Location	CoNV Quadrants Involvement (n)			
	1	2	3	4
Central (n = 38)	55% (21)	18% (7)	16% (6)	10% (4)
Peripheral (n = 95)	68% (65)	17% (16)	6% (6)	8% (8)

3.2. Order of Filling of CoNV

The quadrant containing the corresponding corneal lesion was the first to fill in 84/95 (88.4%) cases, second to fill in 9/95 (9.5%) cases and third to fill in 2/95 (2.1%) cases. In cases where the first quadrant to fill did not correspond with the location of the lesion, the inferior quadrant would typically fill first (7/11 cases, 64%). For CoNV located in more than one quadrant (47 cases), a pattern of order of filling occurred: inferior, superior, nasal and then temporal (ISNT) in 61.7% of cases.

Specifically, when two quadrants of CoNV were present, the ISNT filling was respected in 69.5% of cases, 50.0% with three quadrants and 58.3% with CoNV involving four quadrants, irrespective of lesion location (Figure 3). For peripheral lesions, CoNV tended to be confined to the same quadrant; therefore, for the analysis of the filling pattern, this was limited to central lesions. Infections were associated with a more random filling pattern, respecting the ISNT rule only in 51.7% of cases (15/29), compared to the other causes, which respected the ISNT rule in 77.7% of cases (14/18). Limiting the analysis to ocular surface inflammation only, this increased to 81.8% (9/11). The inferior quadrant was significantly more likely to fill first followed by the superior and nasal followed by the temporal (Table 3).

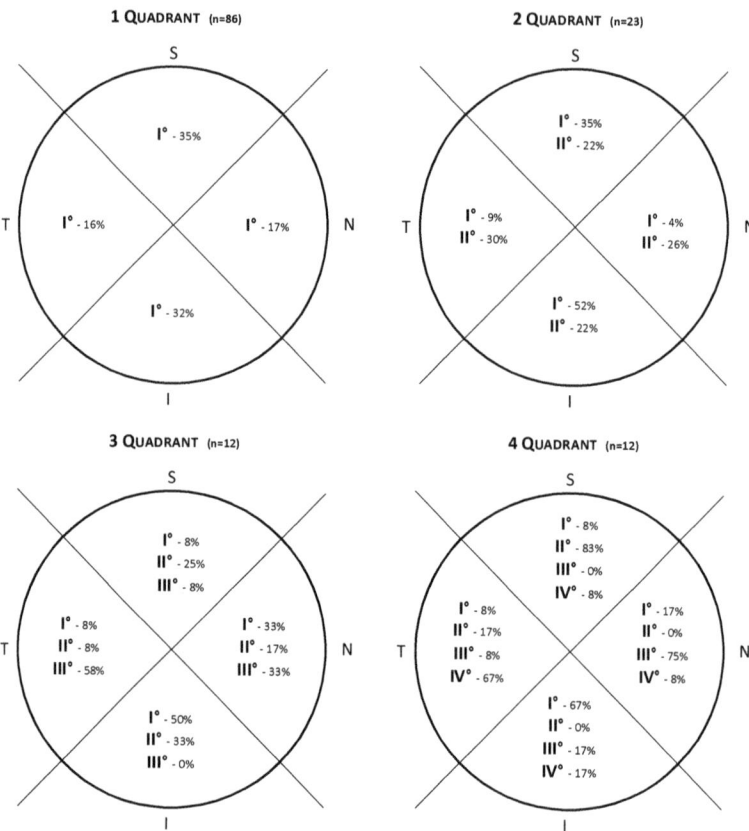

Figure 3. Diagram showing the filling patterns in neovascularization involving one, two, three and all four quadrants. Taking the four quadrants diagram as an example, the inferior quadrant is the first to fill in 67%, the superior quadrant fills second in 83% of cases, the nasal quadrant fills third in 75% of cases and the temporal quadrant is the last to fill in 67% of cases.

Table 3. Agreement of ISNT rule with respect to CoNV filling patterns for central lesions.

		Inferior	Superior	Nasal	Temporal	Total	p-Value
1st quadrant	Yes	15	11	7	5	38	$p = 0.041$
	No	23	27	31	33	114	
2nd quadrant	Yes	3	10	5	2	20	$p = 0.017$
	No	17	10	15	18	60	
3rd quadrant	Yes	1	1	5	2	9	$p = 0.09$ (NS)
	No	8	8	4	7	27	
4th quadrant	Yes	1	0	0	3	4	$p = 0.046$
	No	3	4	4	1	12	

NS = non-statistically significant.

4. Discussion

CoNV is associated with visual loss and is an important consideration in the management of patients, such as in corneal transplantation. Understanding angiographic filling patterns increases our understanding of angiogenesis and may improve approaches to treatment. Angiography has proven superior in detecting early signs of CoNV or in revealing more extensive CoNV than slit lamp examination only [10]. Practically, it facilitates directing treatment at likely feeder vessels such as with fine needle diathermy [6,11–13]. Specifically, in such cases, our protocol includes identifying the afferent vessels with angiography, cutting it with a needle at the slit lamp and cauterizing it with a thermal cautery (electrolysis needle in our practice). Our previously reported results suggest that angiographically guided FND is effective in reducing the area of CoNV [11].

Prior to assessing angiography, it is important to recognize the type of corneal lesion present and specific areas at high risk of CoNV. In peripheral corneal lesions, there is a high likelihood that CoNV is contained within the same quadrant. In contrast, with central corneal lesions, a diffuse pattern of CoNV is often present with multi-quadrant involvement often only evident with corneal angiography. Central lesions tend to be associated with larger surface areas of CoNV as compared to peripheral lesions (2.23 ± 1.5 mm^2 vs. 2.96 ± 2.0 mm^2). The large areas of involvement with central lesions suggest a greater, or at least less localized, angiogenic response compared to a lesion in the peripheral cornea.

Zheng et al. described MCA filling patterns in healthy corneas, in which the inferior quadrant would typically fill first, followed by the superior, nasal and then temporal quadrant (ISNT pattern of filling) [2]. The ISNT pattern, identified previously in healthy corneas, was also noted in this study—wherein approximately 60% of pathological corneas also respected the ISNT filling pattern. The reasons for such a filling pattern are not entirely clear. It is possible that vascular differences may be due to the variation in vascular supply in different quadrants. Alternatively, eyelid blinking may provide a pump-like mechanism, facilitating filling of the inferior and superior arcades to a greater extent than the lateral and medial. Anatomical variations that exist, however, might explain why this is not seen in all cases. The ISNT rule may explain some common findings, e.g., conditions, such as corneal arcus, which tends towards inferior and superior corneal margins first. It is not clear whether following or not the ISNT rule can have different prognostic implications and would require further studies to investigate.

When used in assessment of pathological corneas, this study highlights central lesions as potentially higher risk of ill-defined, larger areas of neovascularization [14]. Angiography will help delineate the location and extent of CoNV in such cases.

Although we have been able to identify key patterns in angiography of corneal pathologies, we note that several limitations arose during the analysis. Corneal angiography is a dynamic study, requiring trained technicians to obtain reproducible high-quality images, and trained clinicians to assess such images. Although observations are subjective, we aimed to minimize this by involving several independent trained observers and keeping the splitting of the quadrants standardized. Furthermore, angiographic techniques may not identify deep capillaries in the presence of masking by superficial leakage and they provide two-dimensional projections from all visualized layers rather than true three-dimensional vessel mapping. OCT-angiography (OCT-A) technologies offer a non-invasive approach that could analyze vessels throughout the entire depth of the cornea and provide simultaneous structural imaging of the cornea itself [15]. However, unlike dye-based angiography, OCT-A cannot differentiate afferent vs. efferent vessels.

We appreciate that anterior segment angiography is not readily available at many facilities; however, it is becoming an increasingly recognized tool for corneal specialists, and this study aims to allow for improved interpretation and accuracy when implementing this investigation. OCT-A technologies have the potential to provide a wider adoption, even though in the current state, those systems are less precise in capturing small vessels in CoNV complexes [16], and validation studies are needed for segmentation software [17].

The focus of this study was primarily analysis of filling patterns in pathological corneas. Anatomical variations may occur between patients; therefore, in patients with unilateral disease, using the healthy other eye as a control may be beneficial. We also note grouping of 'central lesions' encompasses a much wider array of pathologies as compared to the 'peripheral lesions.' No apparent differences were found between different causes of central lesions.

5. Conclusions

We identified several factors that may influence filling patterns for corneal neovascularization, including corneal lesion location, CoNV surface area and etiology of CoNV. Understanding key patterns of neovascularization may help with understanding their angiogenesis and identifying areas at higher risk, aiding in earlier detection and intervention of CoNV.

Author Contributions: Conceptualization, L.P., H.S., K.G., M.A., N.M., S.K. and V.R.; Methodology, S.K.; Formal analysis, L.P., H.S., M.A., G.C. and S.K.; Investigation, M.A.; Data curation, L.P., H.S., K.G. and V.R.; Writing—original draft, L.P. and H.S.; Writing—review & editing, L.P., H.S., K.G., M.A., N.M., G.C., S.K. and V.R.; Supervision, S.K. and V.R.; Project administration, V.R. All authors have read and agreed to the published version of the manuscript.

Funding: This research received no external funding.

Institutional Review Board Statement: The study was conducted in accordance with the Declaration of Helsinki, and approved by the Ethics Committee of Stanmore ethics committee (protocol code 15/LO/2166 and date of approval 5 January 2018).

Informed Consent Statement: Informed consent was obtained from all subjects involved in the study.

Data Availability Statement: The data presented in this study are available on request from the corresponding author.

Conflicts of Interest: The authors declare no conflict of interest.

References

1. Cursiefen, C.; Schlötzer-Schrehardt, U.; Küchle, M.; Sorokin, L.; Breiteneder-Geleff, S.; Alitalo, K.; Jackson, D. Lymphatic vessels in vascularized human corneas: Immunohistochemical investigation using LYVE-1 and podoplanin. *Investig. Opthalmol. Vis. Sci.* **2002**, *43*, 2127–2135.
2. Zheng, Y.; Kaye, A.E.; Boker, A.; Stewart, R.K.; Tey, A.; Ahmad, S.; Willoughby, C.; Bron, A.J.; Kaye, S.B. Marginal Corneal Vascular Arcades. *Investig. Opthalmol. Vis. Sci.* **2013**, *54*, 7470–7477. [CrossRef] [PubMed]
3. Di Zazzo, A.; Kheirkhah, A.; Abud, T.B.; Goyal, S.; Dana, R. Management of high-risk corneal transplantation. *Surv. Ophthalmol.* **2017**, *62*, 816–827. [CrossRef] [PubMed]
4. Chauhan, S.K.; Dohlman, T.H.; Dana, R. Corneal Lymphatics: Role in Ocular Inflammation as Inducer and Responder of Adaptive Immunity. *J. Clin. Cell Immunol.* **2014**, *5*, 1000256. [CrossRef] [PubMed]
5. Palme, C.; Romano, V.; Brunner, M.; Vinciguerra, R.; Kaye, S.B.; Steger, B. Functional Staging of Corneal Neovascularization Using Fluorescein and Indocyanine Green Angiography. *Transl. Vis. Sci. Technol.* **2018**, *7*, 15. [CrossRef] [PubMed]
6. Romano, V.; Steger, B.; Brunner, M.; Ahmad, S.; Willoughby, C.; Kaye, S.B. Method for Angiographically Guided Fine-Needle Diathermy in the Treatment of Corneal Neovascularization. *Cornea* **2016**, *35*, 1029–1032. [CrossRef] [PubMed]
7. Romano, V.; Steger, B.; Ahmad, M.; Coco, G.; Pagano, L.; Ahmad, S.; Zhao, Y.; Zheng, Y.; Kaye, S.B. Imaging of vascular abnormalities in ocular surface disease. *Surv. Ophthalmol.* **2022**, *67*, 31–51. [CrossRef] [PubMed]
8. Anijeet, D.R.; Zheng, Y.; Tey, A.; Hodson, M.; Sueke, H.; Kaye, S.B. Imaging and Evaluation of Corneal Vascularization Using Fluorescein and Indocyanine Green Angiography. *Investig. Opthalmol. Vis. Sci.* **2012**, *53*, 650–658. [CrossRef] [PubMed]
9. Romano, V.; Steger, B.; Kaye, S.B. Fine-Needle Diathermy Guided by Angiography. *Cornea* **2015**, *34*, e29–e30. [CrossRef] [PubMed]
10. Kirwan, R.P.; Zheng, Y.; Tey, A.; Anijeet, D.; Sueke, H.; Kaye, S.B. Quantifying Changes in Corneal Neovascularization Using Fluorescein and Indocyanine Green Angiography. *Am. J. Ophthalmol.* **2012**, *154*, 850–858.e2. [CrossRef] [PubMed]
11. Spiteri, N.; Romano, V.; Zheng, Y.; Yadav, S.; Dwivedi, R.; Chen, J.; Ahmad, S.; Willoughby, C.E.; Kaye, S.B. Corneal Angiography for Guiding and Evaluating Fine-Needle Diathermy Treatment of Corneal Neovascularization. *Ophthalmology* **2015**, *122*, 1079–1084. [CrossRef] [PubMed]
12. Romano, V.; Spiteri, N.; Kaye, S.B. Angiographic-Guided Treatment of Corneal Neovascularization. *JAMA Ophthalmol.* **2015**, *133*, e143544. [CrossRef] [PubMed]
13. Steger, B.; Romano, V.; Kaye, S.B. Corneal Indocyanine Green Angiography to Guide Medical and Surgical Management of Corneal Neovascularization. *Cornea* **2016**, *35*, 41–45. [CrossRef] [PubMed]
14. Liu, S.; Romano, V.; Steger, B.; Kaye, S.B.; Hamill, K.J.; Willoughby, C.E. Gene-based antiangiogenic applications for corneal neovascularization. *Surv. Ophthalmol.* **2018**, *63*, 193–213. [CrossRef] [PubMed]
15. Nicholas, M.P.; Mysore, N. Corneal neovascularization. *Exp. Eye Res.* **2021**, *202*, 108363. [CrossRef] [PubMed]

16. Brunner, M.; Romano, V.; Steger, B.; Vinciguerra, R.; Lawman, S.; Williams, B.; Hicks, N.; Czanner, G.; Zheng, Y.; Willoughby, C.E.; et al. Imaging of Corneal Neovascularization: Optical Coherence Tomography Angiography and Fluorescence Angiography. *Investig. Opthalmol. Vis. Sci.* **2018**, *59*, 1263–1269. [CrossRef] [PubMed]
17. Ong, H.S.; Tey, K.Y.; Ke, M.; Tan, B.; Chua, J.; Schmetterer, L.; Mehta, J.S.; Ang, M. A pilot study investigating anterior segment optical coherence tomography angiography as a non-invasive tool in evaluating corneal vascularisation. *Sci. Rep.* **2021**, *11*, 1212. [CrossRef] [PubMed]

Disclaimer/Publisher's Note: The statements, opinions and data contained in all publications are solely those of the individual author(s) and contributor(s) and not of MDPI and/or the editor(s). MDPI and/or the editor(s) disclaim responsibility for any injury to people or property resulting from any ideas, methods, instructions or products referred to in the content.

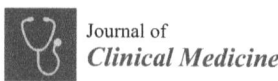

Article

Effect of Low-Temperature Preservation in Optisol-GS on Preloaded, Endothelium-Out DMEK Grafts

Alessandro Ruzza [1], Stefano Ferrari [1,*], Matteo Airaldi [2,*], Vito Romano [2,3] and Diego Ponzin [1]

1. Fondazione Banca degli Occhi del Veneto, 30174 Venice, Italy
2. Department of Medical and Surgical Specialties, Radiological Sciences, and Public Health, Ophthalmology Clinic, University of Brescia, 25121 Brescia, Italy
3. Eye and Vision Science, Institute of Life Course and Medical Sciences, University of Liverpool, Liverpool L3 5TR, UK
* Correspondence: stefano.ferrari@fbov.it (S.F.); matteo.m.airaldi@gmail.com (M.A.)

Abstract: The aim of the study was to assess different temperature ranges for the preservation of pre-loaded Descemet Membrane Endothelial Keratoplasty (DMEK) grafts in the DMEK RAPID Mini device. Methods: Three groups of 15 DMEK grafts (five per group) were pre-loaded in the DMEK RAPID Mini and preserved in Optisol-GS for 72 h at different temperatures: group A at >8 °C, group B between 2–8 °C and group C at <2 °C. After stripping and preservation, the viability of the endothelium, cell loss and morphology were assessed through light microscopy following trypan blue and alizarin red staining. Results: Overall mortality was 4.07%, 3.97% and 7.66%, in groups A, B and C, respectively, with percentages of uncovered areas of 0.31%, 1.36% and 0.20% (all $p > 0.05$). Endothelial cell density variation was 5.51%, 3.06% and 2.82% in groups A, B and C, respectively ($p = 0.19$). Total Endothelial Cell Loss (ECL) was 4.37%, 5.32% and 7.84% in groups A, B and C, respectively ($p = 0.39$). Endothelial cell morphology was comparable in all three groups. Conclusions: In the DMEK RAPID Mini, low temperatures (<2 °C) may affect the quality of pre-loaded grafts, inducing a higher ECL after 72 h of preservation, although no significant differences among groups could be proved. Our data would suggest maintaining grafts loaded in the DMEK RAPID Mini at temperatures between 2–8 °C for appropriate preservation.

Keywords: DMEK; eye bank; preloaded; temperature

1. Introduction

Eye banks are playing a crucial role in the development of more standardized and surgeon-friendly techniques for preparing, loading, transporting and delivering grafts for Descemet Membrane Endothelial Keratoplasty (DMEK) [1–4]. In the early years of the development of this technique, surgeons had to prepare the grafts autonomously just before transplantation, increasing surgical time and exposing themselves to the risk of graft preparation failure. Owing to the experience gained by eye banks in the preparation of grafts for Descemet Stripping Automated Endothelial Keratoplasty, the separation of the Descemet Membrane (DM) from the stroma, the trephination at the desired diameter, and loading of the graft into the injector are better off carried out by technicians routinely involved in such preparations [5–7].

In the eye bank, the DM can be loaded inside the injector either with the corneal endothelium folded outwards (ENDO-OUT configuration) or inwards (ENDO-IN configuration). Once separated completely from the posterior stroma, the DM naturally adopts a scrolled, ENDO-OUT configuration, an effect likely due to the different degrees of elasticity of the anterior and posterior surfaces of the DM [8]. Instead, in the ENDO-IN configuration, the membrane is folded in the opposite way to its natural scrolling tendency. Folding can take several minutes to be carried out, but once inside the patient's eye, it requires minimal time for unfolding, since it is perceived as an unnatural conformation [9]. Despite such

Citation: Ruzza, A.; Ferrari, S.; Airaldi, M.; Romano, V.; Ponzin, D. Effect of Low-Temperature Preservation in Optisol-GS on Preloaded, Endothelium-Out DMEK Grafts. *J. Clin. Med.* **2023**, *12*, 1026. https://doi.org/10.3390/jcm12031026

Academic Editor: Francisco Javier Ascaso

Received: 4 December 2022
Revised: 16 January 2023
Accepted: 24 January 2023
Published: 28 January 2023

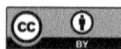

Copyright: © 2023 by the authors. Licensee MDPI, Basel, Switzerland. This article is an open access article distributed under the terms and conditions of the Creative Commons Attribution (CC BY) license (https://creativecommons.org/licenses/by/4.0/).

differences, both techniques have been reported to lead to comparable results in terms of visual outcomes and it is up to the surgeon's expertise and skill to decide which one to use for DMEK [10,11].

Eye banks have been collaborating with surgeons to provide pre-trephined and pre-loaded membranes preserved either with ENDO-IN or ENDO-OUT configurations. To improve such preparations, efforts are being made to minimize Endothelial Cell Loss (ECL) associated with preparation [2,3,12,13], loading [11,14–16], preservation and transportation [1,17–21] and, finally, injection [10,11,14,15,22] of DMEK grafts.

While no dedicated device is so far available for membranes folded inwards, the DMEK RAPID Mini system (Geuder AG, Heidelberg, Germany) has recently received CE marking for the transportation of pre-loaded, ENDO-OUT grafts [17]. This system was initially designed for corneal tissues preserved in organ culture (OC) and stored at intervals ranging from room temperature to 31 °C. However, the majority of eye banks outside Europe use cold storage (CS) as the preferred method for preservation, with corneal tissues placed in single small vials and kept in a refrigerator at 2–8 °C. The DMEK RAPID Mini has been recently adapted for CS. The idea behind the CS of DMEK grafts is that cold temperature reduces cellular demand for metabolic energy [23,24]. However, concerns regarding the shorter conservation time and possibly higher endothelial cell mortality associated with hypothermia exist [24–26], highlighting the need for a deeper understanding of the effects of different low-temperature ranges on endothelial viability in preloaded DMEK grafts.

The aim of this study was, therefore, to evaluate the effects of preservation at different low-temperature ranges on corneal endothelial cells viability, simulating the transport of pre-loaded DMEK grafts in the DMEK RAPID Mini device.

2. Materials and Methods

Donor corneal tissues unsuitable for transplantation due to poor endothelial cell counts, procured by Fondazione Banca degli Occhi del Veneto Onlus (Venice, Italy) were used for the research purposes and the validation studies described in this manuscript, according to the realms of the law 91/99 and after an informed consent form was signed by the donor's next of kin.

2.1. Tissue Preparation

In this study, we used fifteen corneas (n = 15) retrieved from the morgue and preserved in Cold X Medium (homemade medium) at 4 °C for up to 3 days. The membranes were prepared following a standard stripping protocol as previously reported [2], using a 9.5 mm diameter punch (Moria, Antony, France) and leaving a small area of peripheral adhesion between DM and stroma. After the stripping step, all tissues were stained with 0.25% Trypan Blue dye (Gibco, NY, USA) and evaluated by light microscopy (Axiovert, Zeiss, Oberkochen, Germany). If deemed acceptable, the grafts were punched again with an 8.25 mm punch and completely detached from the stroma. The corneal concavity was completely filled with Optisol-GS (Rochester, NY, USA). Having enough space, the membranes roll up on themselves assuming a cylindrical shape and exposing the endothelium outwards. The membranes were then loaded into the DMEK RAPID Mini device as previously described [17]. Briefly, the DMEK RAPID Mini device consists of a front plug connected to the tip of an injector from one side and to a silicone tube on the other. A 5 mL syringe is attached to the silicone tube connector. The whole system must be filled with Optisol-GS, to avoid any air bubble formation. The folded membrane is sucked into the device by means of a syringe vacuum through the posterior part of the injector. The back of the injector is then blocked using the rear plug. In this study, the whole system was fixed in the transportation holder and finally placed in the dedicated vial filled with Optisol-GS.

The tissues were divided into three groups (A, B and C) and stored at different temperatures, as described below:

- Group A: >8 °C storage (n = 5);
- Group B: 2–8 °C storage in a "transport simulation" condition (n = 5);

- Group C: <2 °C storage (*n* = 5).

Transport simulation was performed by leaving the pre-loaded tissues on a laboratory shaker (Duomax 1030, Heidolph, Schwabach, Germany) placed inside a temperature-monitored refrigerator for the entire duration of the experiment. All the membranes were preserved for 72 h.

2.2. Tissue Evaluation and Study Outcomes

The tissues were analyzed after the stripping step (T0). The membranes were stained with trypan blue dye and evaluated by means of light microscopy (Primovert; Zeiss, Jena, Germany) using a hypotonic analysis solution (HAS) to highlight the intercellular borders and to assess Endothelial Cell Density (ECD), cell mortality rate, acellular areas (extensive blue-stained portions on the membrane with no traces of endothelial cells). To be included in this study, tissues had to have an ECD > 1700 cells/mm^2, a mortality rate lower than 2.5% and percentages of uncovered areas lower than 1% at T0.

After 72 h of preservation (T72), the membranes were carefully extracted from the injector, gently placed and unfolded on a glass slide, stained with trypan blue dye and immersed in hypotonic analysis solution to perform the second light microscopy evaluation.

In general, trypan blue positive cells appear within the corneal endothelium as a result of different possible discomfort events or situations, such as poor initial quality of the tissue, long post-mortem time, long storage time, stressful storage conditions, iatrogenic trauma, etc. All these conditions lead to changes in the cell membrane permeability, allowing the dye to stain the cellular nuclei. These cells are considered dead and ready to detach from the Descemet membrane. Uncovered (or acellular) areas are a natural consequence of cellular deaths or are caused by severe mechanical traumas leading to cell detachment (Figure 1).

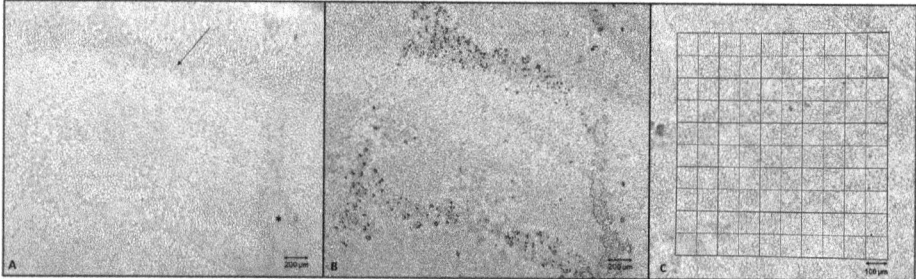

Figure 1. (**A**) Group B, 40× magnification, Trypan Blue and Alizarin Red, after 72 h of preservation. Cornea with trypan blue positive cells (arrow) on folds and de-cellularized areas (asterisk) displayed by dye suffusion onto Descemet's membrane. (**B**) Same tissue but stained by Alizarin red dye which only stains the Descemet's membrane, clearly showing the cell margins and the uncovered areas, confirming what observed with the Trypan Blue staining. (**C**) 100× magnification, Trypan Blue, archive photo. Trypan blue positive cells localized on the Descemet folds. To perform the mortality assessment, the reticle is overlayed to the image and then the number of small squares covering the areas are counted. To get the percentage, this value is referred to the whole surface of the membrane.

To estimate the ECD and the extent of damaged areas, the cells in five 1 mm^2 squares of a 10 × 10 mm reticule inserted in the eyepiece of an inverted microscope were counted manually at 100× magnification. The number of trypan blue positive cells allowed us to determine the percentage of cell death and uncovered areas (Figure 1) in relation to membrane surface diameters of 9.5 mm (70.85 mm^2) and 8.25 mm (53.43 mm^2). For the confirmation of uncovered areas, Alizarin red (5%; ThermoFisher Scientific, Waltham, MA, USA) was topically applied, and the tissues were incubated for 5 min at RT away from bright light. The tissues were then re-evaluated under the light microscope.

The overall mortality was obtained by calculating the difference between the mortality detected at T72 (post-preservation) and the mortality found at T0 (post-stripping). The overall uncovered areas were calculated using the same method. By doing so, the damage that occurred during the stripping phase could be excluded from the final data evaluation, which will be only referred to in the conservation phase. Total ECL was obtained by combining these two values (overall uncovered areas plus overall mortality).

2.3. Statistical Analysis

Descriptive data were summarized using the mean (standard deviation) and percentages where appropriate.

The normal distribution of outcomes was checked by means of Shapiro–Wilk tests and visual inspection of Q-Q plots.

One-way ANOVA was used to compare the effect of the 3 temperature groups on ECD, mortality rate and uncovered areas at T0 and at T72, as well as ECD variation, overall mortality, overall uncovered area and total ECL between T0 and T72. Homogeneity of variance and covariance was confirmed by means of Levene's test and Box's M-test, respectively.

Post hoc pairwise *t*-tests with Bonferroni correction were used for comparisons between groups in case of a significant ANOVA result.

A *p*-value of 0.05 was considered statistically significant. All analyses were conducted using R software version 4.2.2 (R Project for Statistical Computing, Vienna, Austria; R Foundation for Statistical Computing; 2022, https://cran.rproject.org accessed on 3 December 2022).

3. Results

Membranes with similar biological features were used for all the groups (Table 1).

Table 1. Post-stripping and post-preservation endothelial cell density, mortality rate and uncovered areas in Group A (storing for 72 h post-stripping in Optisol-GS at >8 °C), Group B (2–8 °C) and Group C (<2 °C).

N	Preservation	Post Stripping (T0)			Post Preservation (T72)		
		ECD (cells/mm^2)	Mortality (%)	Uncovered Areas (%)	ECD (cells/mm^2)	Mortality (%)	Uncovered Areas (%)
1	>8 °C	2100	0	0	2000	0.37	0
2	>8 °C	2100	0	0	2000	0.60	0
3	>8 °C	2300	0.14	0.64	2100	8.89	0
4	>8 °C	2000	0.47	0	1900	7.48	0.60
5	>8 °C	2300	0.71	0.16	2200	4.31	1.11
6	2–8 °C	1800	1.19	0	1800	7.10	3.74
7	2–8 °C	2300	1.27	0	2300	6.50	0
8	2–8 °C	2000	0.96	0	1900	2.38	0.76
9	2–8 °C	2000	0.78	0	1900	3.09	0.97
10	2–8 °C	2450	0.90	0.35	2320	5.87	1.66
11	<2 °C	2200	0.79	0	2100	10.67	0.50
12	<2 °C	2200	1.23	0	2100	5.37	0.24
13	<2 °C	2000	0.35	0	1900	15.74	0
14	<2 °C	2000	0.21	0.06	2000	4.31	0
15	<2 °C	1900	0.10	0.64	1900	4.87	0.83

ECD, Endothelial Cell Density; N, number.

After stripping (T0), in Group A the mean ± SD ECD was 2160 ± 134 cells/mm^2, the mortality rate was 0.26 ± 0.31% and the percentage of uncovered areas was of 0.16 ± 0.27%. In Group B, the average ECD was 2110 ± 260 cells/mm^2, the mortality rate was 1.02 ± 0.21% and the percentage of uncovered areas was of 0.07 ± 0.16%. In Group C, the average ECD was 2060 ± 134 cells/mm^2, the mortality rate was 0.54 ± 0.47% and the percentage of uncovered areas was of 0.14 ± 0.28% (Table 2).

Table 2. Average values and differences in Endothelial Cell Density, Mortality and Uncovered Areas at T0 and T72.

	Groups			
	A, n = 5 Mean (SD)	B, n = 5 Mean (SD)	C, n = 5 Mean (SD)	p *
Post-stripping (T0)				
ECD (cells/mm^2)	2160 (134)	2110 (261)	2060 (134)	0.7
Mortality (%)	0.26 (0.31)	1.02 (0.21)	0.54 (0.47)	0.01
Pairwise comparison [#]:				
Group A vs. Group B				0.01
Group A vs. Group C				0.23
Group B vs. Group C				0.09
Uncovered areas (%)	0.16 (0.27)	0.07 (0.16)	0.14 (0.28)	0.84
Post-extraction (T72)				
ECD (cells/mm^2)	2040 (114)	2044 (246)	2000 (100)	0.9
Mortality (%)	4.33 (3.88)	4.99 (2.12)	8.19 (4.93)	0.27
Uncovered areas (%)	0.34 (0.50)	1.43 (1.42)	0.32 (0.36)	0.12
T0–T72 difference				
ECD Variation (%)	5.51 (1.79)	3.06 (2.80)	2.82 (2.58)	0.19
Overall Mortality (%)	4.07 (3.76)	3.97 (1.97)	7.66 (4.95)	0.25
Overall Uncovered areas (%)	0.31 (0.44)	1.36 (1.42)	0.20 (0.20)	0.1
Total Endothelial Cell Loss (%)	4.37 (3.86)	5.32 (2.90)	7.84 (4.94)	0.39

ECD, Endothelial Cell Density; n, number; SD, standard deviation. * One-way ANOVA. [#] Post hoc pairwise comparison with t-test using Bonferroni correction.

At T0, only the mortality rate was significantly different among the three groups (ANOVA, $p = 0.01$). The post hoc pairwise comparison showed that the mortality rate was significantly greater in group B compared to group A ($p = 0.01$).

The average storage temperature recorded by the probes in the refrigerator was 9.3 °C in group A, 5.1 °C in group B and 1.3 °C in group C. After preservation (T72), in Group A the mean ± SD ECD we found was 2040 ± 114 cells/mm^2, mortality was 4.33 ± 3.88% and the percentage of uncovered areas was of 0.34 ± 0.50%. In Group B, the ECD was 2044 ± 246 cells/mm^2, mortality was 4.99 ± 2.12% and the percentage of uncovered areas was 1.43 ± 1.42%. In Group C, the ECD was 2000 ± 100 cells/mm^2, mortality was 8.19 ± 4.93% and the percentage of uncovered areas was 0.32 ± 0.36%.

At T72, no significant difference in ECD, mortality rate or uncovered areas could be identified (all $p > 0.05$).

The mean ± SD ECD variation between T0 and T72 was 5.51 ± 1.79%, 3.06 ± 2.80% and 2.82 ± 2.58% in Group A, B and C, respectively ($p = 0.19$). Likewise, no difference was found in Overall Uncovered Areas ($p = 0.1$). In group C, Overall Mortality (7.66 ± 4.95%) and Total ECL (7.84 ± 4.94%) were higher than in group A (4.07 ± 3.76% and 4.37 ± 3.86%) and group B (3.97 ± 1.97% and 5.32 ± 2.90%). However, these differences were not statistically significant ($p = 0.25$ and $p = 0.39$).

Boxplot graphical representations of the distribution of mortality rate, uncovered areas and total ECL at T0 and T72 in the three groups are shown in Figure 2.

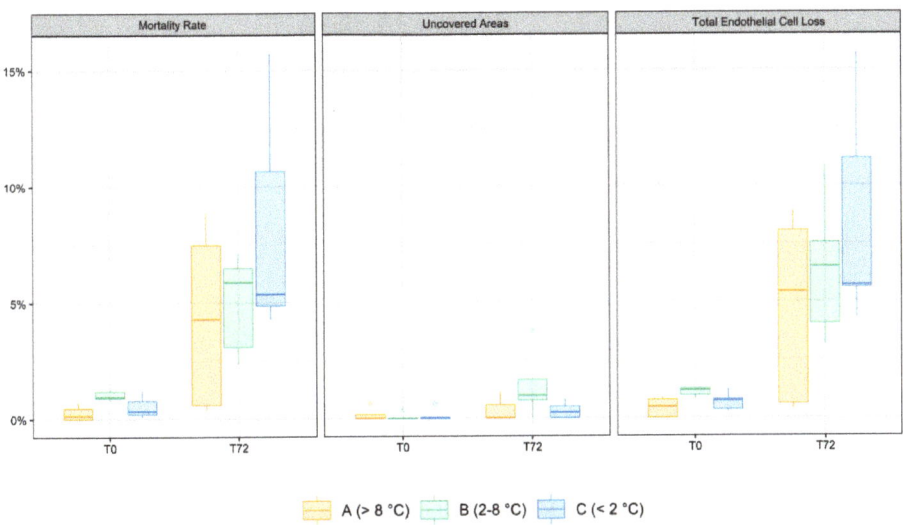

Figure 2. Boxplots displaying the distribution of mortality rate, uncovered areas and total Endothelial Cell Loss (ECL) in the three groups at T0 and T72. The solid lines represent the median, the boxes span the 25th and 75th quantile, the whiskers of the boxes extend to 1.5 times the interquartile range, and solid dots represent outliers. Only mortality rate was significantly different among the three groups at T0, and post hoc pairwise comparison showed that it was significantly greater in group B compared to group A ($p = 0.01$). At T72, mortality rate and total ECL showed a trend for inversely proportional correlation to temperature, although these differences did not reach statistical significance.

Light Microscopy Samples

In all groups, well-defined areas of trypan blue positive cells (Figure 3A) located in different parts of the membrane and especially in the mid-periphery, could be identified. These linear stress marks could be attributable to friction, stripping and/or handling of the grafts. However, three tissues in Group C displayed scattered mortality with the presence of small acellularized areas (Figure 3B,C), likely due to widespread cellular sufferance caused by the low storage temperature conditions (Figure 3D).

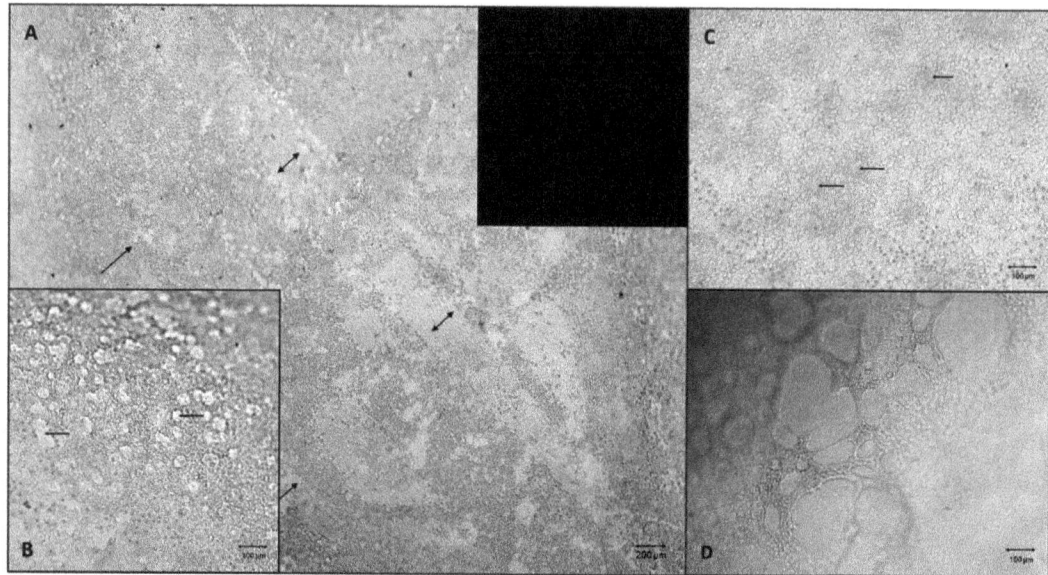

Figure 3. (**A**) Group C, 40× magnification, Trypan Blue/V9, after 72 h of storage, blending of two images. Long area (approximately 5 mm) of localized mortality with well-defined margins (arrows) located in the middle periphery of the membrane. This shape of mortality was also observed on membranes stored in other groups. (**B**,**C**) Group C, 100× magnification, Trypan Blue/V9, after 72 h of storage. Diffuse presence of Trypan Blue positive cells and uncovered areas (arrows) homogeneously distributed throughout the Descemet membrane endothelial surface. (**D**) 100× magnification, Trypan Blue/sucrose, preserved at 4 °C, archive photo (2010). After being retrieved from the morgue, the tissue was preserved in a vial with tissue culture medium and mistakenly put in direct contact with an ice pocket. After 12 h of preservation, the endothelium showed circular areas with absence of cells and a high percentage of scattered mortality throughout the endothelial surface.

4. Discussion

In this study, DMs were exposed to three different temperature ranges to verify the best conditions for cell survival during preservation in Optisol-GS within a DMEK RAPID Mini device in the endothelium folded outwards configuration. At the end of the experiment, a higher mortality and higher total ECL were detected in Group C (preservation at <2 °C) compared to that seen in Group B (2–8 °C) and A (>8 °C), although these differences did not reach statistical significance.

Along with preservation time, the temperature is a crucial parameter for appropriate corneal tissue preservation, especially when the isolated Descemet Membrane, and its endothelium, are preserved [24]. The findings of this study seem to confirm that storage temperature plays an important role in maintaining endothelial cell viability [23]. Low temperatures (<2 °C) can disrupt the cellular junctions leading to plasmatic membrane breakage and, consequently, increase the cell mortality rate [27,28]. Low storage temperatures have also been shown to affect cellular metabolism [25,26], thus reducing the endothelium's ability to reorganize and replenish the exposed areas as a consequence of cellular death. Conversely, a rearrangement of the endothelial mosaic can be observed following a metabolic activation triggered by storage at higher temperatures, as shown in previous studies on epithelial cells [29,30]. This could explain why a progressive ECD variation was found in tissues preserved at different temperatures, such as in Group A compared to Group C, an effect likely due to endothelial repair reactivation caused by increased temperatures [31]. Finally, studies on cultured endothelial cells show that the oxidative stress generated by low storage temperatures might be particularly damaging to the mitochondria-rich endothelial cell [24,32]. Mitochondria are, in fact, abundant in the highly interdigitated apical complexes of endothelial cells, indicative of their crucial role in active fluid transport and cellular adhesion [33]. Cold storage conditions paradoxically enhance the formation of reactive oxygen species, promoting adhesion loss and non-apoptotic cell death of mitochondria-rich endothelial cells [32–34].

To date, two main storage systems of corneal tissue have been developed: cold storage, mainly used in America and Asia, maintains the cornea between 2 °C and 8 °C for a maximum of 14 days, while Organ Culture preservation, which uses room temperature up to 31–37 °C for storage of corneas, can preserve the tissues for up to 28 days [1,18,23]. The advantages of cold storage (no microbiology, no serum, less cost and storing space, ease of transport) must be weighed against those of organ culture, which is more technically difficult and time-consuming but can support cell metabolism under physiologic conditions and maintain cell viability for longer periods of time [20,23,24,30,31].

In this study, the preservation of corneal tissue was performed in Optisol-GS, the most widely employed medium for CS [23]. Other studies have employed organ culture medium for the storage and analysis of preloaded DMEK grafts stored in the DMEK RAPID system, with results comparable to ours. In particular, Wojcik and colleagues found a total ECL of 3.3–11.5% after storage and transport at room temperature in the DMEK RAPID device with tissue culture medium (TCM) supplemented with Dextran, a commonly used deswelling agent [17]. Català and colleagues found a total ECL of 16.7% and uncovered areas of 8% after transportation at an ambient temperature of endothelium-out DMEK grafts in the DMKE RAPID device employing analogous TCM and 6% Dextran [18].

As DMEK continues to evolve, optimization of the preparatory steps leading to surgery will represent more and more a key area for development. The efforts to minimize ECL in the preparation, storing and shipping of preloaded grafts are paramount given its prominent role in early postoperative ECL. In fact, preoperative ECD has been directly correlated with 6-month post-DMEK ECD, which in turn was found to be a key predictor of late endothelial failure. Specifically, a 6-month ECD count of less than ~830 cells/mm^2 has been associated with a significantly lower 5-year graft survival rate in a study by Vasiliauskaitė and colleagues [35]. Given the multifactorial, high variability in tolerance to the cellular stress caused by stripping and preservation [1,3], the authors suggest that identification and exclusion by Eye Banks of "low-performing" grafts may ensure that only grafts with good tolerance to manipulation and, therefore, with higher postoperative, ECD counts get transplanted [35].

Limitations of this study could be attributed to damage to the endothelium not related to hypothermic storage, which could have confounded our results. In the pre-loaded, ENDO-OUT configuration, the membrane is left free to roll up and then vacuumed through a tubing system connected to a syringe and can be accommodated in a larger space as compared to the devices for ENDO-IN membranes. Since the graft spontaneously rolls up with the endothelium folded outwards, corneal endothelial cells may be exposed to a certain degree of friction against the internal walls of the injector, especially during the injection phase when the diameter of the funnel is reduced [1]. Furthermore, some of the variability in the degree of overall mortality could also be influenced by the unpredictable folding of the DMs, spontaneously assuming configurations such as the double scroll shape [36,37], and consequently exposing different regions of the endothelium. However, we observed well-defined areas of trypan blue positive cells, located in different peripheral areas of the membrane, across all three different groups, meaning that the effects of friction, stripping and/or handling of the DMs have most likely equally affected all tissues in our study. Indeed, the degree of ECL is in line with previous studies using the DMEK RAPID system [17,18] or other alternative devices used for transporting preloaded and pre-stripped grafts for DMEK [15,21,38].

Finally, given the small sample size available, we might have been underpowered to detect significant differences among the three groups (Post Hoc Power range = 0.1–0.85).

5. Conclusions

In conclusion, to preserve the quality of isolated DMEK grafts folded in the ENDO-OUT configuration in the DMEK RAPID Mini device in Optisol-GS, it is recommended to keep the grafts at temperatures between 2 to 8 °C. Lower temperatures can alter the morphological characteristics of the endothelium and possibly increase cell mortality. Conversely, no major issue has been observed with higher temperatures as long as these are kept below room temperature to avoid fungal growth [39].

Author Contributions: Conceptualization, A.R. and S.F.; methodology, A.R.; formal analysis, M.A.; investigation, A.R. and S.F.; writing—original draft preparation, A.R. and M.A.; writing—review and editing, S.F., V.R. and D.P.; visualization, A.R. and M.A. All authors have read and agreed to the published version of the manuscript.

Funding: This research received no external funding.

Institutional Review Board Statement: Not applicable.

Informed Consent Statement: Informed consent was signed by the donor's next of kin.

Data Availability Statement: Data is contained within the article.

Conflicts of Interest: The authors declare no conflict of interest.

References

1. Romano, V.; Parekh, M.; Ruzza, A.; Willoughby, C.E.; Ferrari, S.; Ponzin, D.; Kaye, S.B.; Levis, H.J. Comparison of Preservation and Transportation Protocols for Preloaded Descemet Membrane Endothelial Keratoplasty. *Br. J. Ophthalmol.* **2018**, *102*, 549–555. [CrossRef] [PubMed]
2. Parekh, M.; Ruzza, A.; Romano, V.; Favaro, E.; Baruzzo, M.; Salvalaio, G.; Grassetto, A.; Ferrari, S.; Ponzin, D. Descemet Membrane Endothelial Keratoplasty Learning Curve for Graft Preparation in an Eye Bank Using 645 Donor Corneas. *Cornea* **2018**, *37*, 767–771. [CrossRef] [PubMed]
3. Parekh, M.; Borroni, D.; Ruzza, A.; Levis, H.J.; Ferrari, S.; Ponzin, D.; Romano, V. A Comparative Study on Different Descemet Membrane Endothelial Keratoplasty Graft Preparation Techniques. *Acta Ophthalmol.* **2018**, *96*, e718–e726. [CrossRef] [PubMed]
4. Pagano, L.; Gadhvi, K.A.; Parekh, M.; Coco, G.; Levis, H.J.; Ponzin, D.; Ferrari, S.; Virgili, G.; Kaye, S.B.; Edwards, R.T.; et al. Cost Analysis of Eye Bank versus Surgeon Prepared Endothelial Grafts. *BMC Health Serv. Res.* **2021**, *21*, 801. [CrossRef]
5. Busin, M.; Scorcia, V.; Patel, A.K.; Salvalaio, G.; Ponzin, D. Pneumatic Dissection and Storage of Donor Endothelial Tissue for Descemet's Membrane Endothelial Keratoplasty: A Novel Technique. *Ophthalmology* **2010**, *117*, 1517–1520. [CrossRef]
6. Parekh, M.; Ruzza, A.; Salvalaio, G.; Ferrari, S.; Camposampiero, D.; Busin, M.; Ponzin, D. Descemet Membrane Endothelial Keratoplasty Tissue Preparation from Donor Corneas Using a Standardized Submerged Hydro-Separation Method. *Am. J. Ophthalmol.* **2014**, *158*, 277–285.e1. [CrossRef]
7. Muraine, M.; Gueudry, J.; He, Z.; Piselli, S.; Lefevre, S.; Toubeau, D. Novel Technique for the Preparation of Corneal Grafts for Descemet Membrane Endothelial Keratoplasty. *Am. J. Ophthalmol.* **2013**, *156*, 851–859. [CrossRef]
8. Mohammed, I.; Ross, A.R.; Britton, J.O.; Said, D.G.; Dua, H.S. Elastin Content and Distribution in Endothelial Keratoplasty Tissue Determines Direction of Scrolling. *Am. J. Ophthalmol.* **2018**, *194*, 16–25. [CrossRef]
9. Yu, A.C.; Myerscough, J.; Spena, R.; Fusco, F.; Socea, S.; Furiosi, L.; De Rosa, L.; Bovone, C.; Busin, M. Three-Year Outcomes of Tri-Folded Endothelium-In Descemet Membrane Endothelial Keratoplasty With Pull-Through Technique. *Am. J. Ophthalmol.* **2020**, *219*, 121–131. [CrossRef]
10. Price, M.O.; Lisek, M.; Kelley, M.; Feng, M.T.; Price, F.W. Endothelium-in Versus Endothelium-out Insertion With Descemet Membrane Endothelial Keratoplasty. *Cornea* **2018**, *37*, 1098–1101. [CrossRef]
11. Parekh, M.; Ruzza, A.; Ferrari, S.; Ahmad, S.; Kaye, S.; Ponzin, D.; Romano, V. Endothelium-in versus Endothelium-out for Descemet Membrane Endothelial Keratoplasty Graft Preparation and Implantation. *Acta Ophthalmol.* **2017**, *95*, 194–198. [CrossRef]
12. Borroni, D.; Gadhvi, K.; Wojcik, G.; Pennisi, F.; Vallabh, N.A.; Galeone, A.; Ruzza, A.; Arbabi, E.; Menassa, N.; Kaye, S.; et al. The Influence of Speed During Stripping in Descemet Membrane Endothelial Keratoplasty Tissue Preparation. *Cornea* **2020**, *39*, 1086–1090. [CrossRef] [PubMed]
13. Jardine, G.J.; Holiman, J.D.; Stoeger, C.G.; Chamberlain, W.D. Imaging and Quantification of Endothelial Cell Loss in Eye Bank Prepared DMEK Grafts Using Trainable Segmentation Software. *Curr. Eye Res.* **2014**, *39*, 894–901. [CrossRef] [PubMed]
14. Downes, K.; Tran, K.D.; Stoeger, C.G.; Chamberlain, W. Cumulative Endothelial Cell Loss in Descemet Membrane Endothelial Keratoplasty Grafts From Preparation Through Insertion With Glass Injectors. *Cornea* **2018**, *37*, 698–704. [CrossRef]

15. Shen, E.; Fox, A.; Johnson, B.; Farid, M. Comparing the Effect of Three Descemet Membrane Endothelial Keratoplasty Injectors on Endothelial Damage of Grafts. *Indian J. Ophthalmol.* **2020**, *68*, 1040–1043. [CrossRef] [PubMed]
16. Schallhorn, J.M.; Holiman, J.D.; Stoeger, C.G.; Chamberlain, W. Quantification and Patterns of Endothelial Cell Loss Due to Eye Bank Preparation and Injector Method in Descemet Membrane Endothelial Keratoplasty Tissues. *Cornea* **2016**, *35*, 377–382. [CrossRef] [PubMed]
17. Wojcik, G.; Parekh, M.; Romano, V.; Ferrari, S.; Ruzza, A.; Ahmad, S.; Ponzin, D. Preloaded Descemet Membrane Endothelial Keratoplasty Grafts With Endothelium Outward: A Cross-Country Validation Study of the DMEK Rapid Device. *Cornea* **2021**, *40*, 484–490. [CrossRef] [PubMed]
18. Català, P.; Vermeulen, W.; Rademakers, T.; van den Bogaerdt, A.; Kruijt, P.J.; Nuijts, R.M.M.A.; LaPointe, V.L.S.; Dickman, M.M. Transport and Preservation Comparison of Preloaded and Prestripped-Only DMEK Grafts. *Cornea* **2020**, *39*, 1407–1414. [CrossRef] [PubMed]
19. Parekh, M.; Ruzza, A.; Ferrari, S.; Ponzin, D. Preservation of Preloaded DMEK Lenticules in Dextran and Non-Dextran-Based Organ Culture Medium. *J. Ophthalmol.* **2016**, *2016*, 5830835. [CrossRef]
20. Parekh, M.; Ruzza, A.; Gallon, P.; Ponzin, D.; Ahmad, S.; Ferrari, S. Synthetic Media for Preservation of Corneal Tissues Deemed for Endothelial Keratoplasty and Endothelial Cell Culture. *Acta Ophthalmol.* **2021**, *99*, 314–325. [CrossRef]
21. Parekh, M.; Romano, V.; Hassanin, K.; Testa, V.; Wongvisavavit, R.; Ferrari, S.; Willoughby, C.; Ponzin, D.; Jhanji, V.; Sharma, N.; et al. Delivering Endothelial Keratoplasty Grafts: Modern Day Transplant Devices. *Curr. Eye Res.* **2022**, *47*, 493–504. [CrossRef] [PubMed]
22. Romano, V.; Ruzza, A.; Kaye, S.; Parekh, M. Pull-through Technique for Delivery of a Larger Diameter DMEK Graft Using Endothelium-in Method. *Can. J. Ophthalmol. J. Can. Ophthalmol.* **2017**, *52*, e155–e156. [CrossRef] [PubMed]
23. Parekh, M.; Salvalaio, G.; Ferrari, S.; Amoureux, M.-C.; Albrecht, C.; Fortier, D.; Ponzin, D. A Quantitative Method to Evaluate the Donor Corneal Tissue Quality Used in a Comparative Study between Two Hypothermic Preservation Media. *Cell Tissue Bank.* **2014**, *15*, 543–554. [CrossRef]
24. Parekh, M.; Peh, G.; Mehta, J.S.; Ahmad, S.; Ponzin, D.; Ferrari, S. Effects of Corneal Preservation Conditions on Human Corneal Endothelial Cell Culture. *Exp. Eye Res.* **2019**, *179*, 93–101. [CrossRef] [PubMed]
25. Zagórski, Z. Experimental Studies on the Growth of Cultured Epithelium and Endothelium of Rabbit Cornea Exposed to Low Temperature. *Pol. Med. Sci. Hist. Bull.* **1976**, *15*, 253–259.
26. Redbrake, C.; Salla, S.; Frantz, A.; Reim, M. [Energy metabolism of the human cornea in various culture systems]. *Klin. Monatsbl. Augenheilkd.* **1997**, *210*, 213–218. [CrossRef] [PubMed]
27. Doughman, D.J.; Van Horn, D.; Rodman, W.P.; Byrnes, P.; Lindstrom, R.L. Human Corneal Endothelial Layer Repair during Organ Culture. *Arch. Ophthalmol.* **1976**, *94*, 1791–1796. [CrossRef] [PubMed]
28. McCartney, M.D.; Wood, T.O.; McLaughlin, B.J. Freeze-Fracture Label of Functional and Dysfunctional Human Corneal Endothelium. *Curr. Eye Res.* **1987**, *6*, 589–597. [CrossRef] [PubMed]
29. Jackson, C.J.; Pasovic, L.; Raeder, S.; Sehic, A.; Roald, B.; de la Paz, M.F.; Tønseth, K.A.; Utheim, T.P. Optisol-GS Storage of Cultured Human Limbal Epithelial Cells at Ambient Temperature Is Superior to Hypothermic Storage. *Curr. Eye Res.* **2020**, *45*, 1497–1503. [CrossRef] [PubMed]
30. Raeder, S.; Utheim, T.P.; Utheim, O.A.; Nicolaissen, B.; Roald, B.; Cai, Y.; Haug, K.; Kvalheim, A.; Messelt, E.B.; Drolsum, L.; et al. Effects of Organ Culture and Optisol-GS Storage on Structural Integrity, Phenotypes, and Apoptosis in Cultured Corneal Epithelium. *Investig. Ophthalmol. Vis. Sci.* **2007**, *48*, 5484–5493. [CrossRef]
31. Nejepinska, J.; Juklova, K.; Jirsova, K. Organ Culture, but Not Hypothermic Storage, Facilitates the Repair of the Corneal Endothelium Following Mechanical Damage. *Acta Ophthalmol.* **2010**, *88*, 413–419. [CrossRef] [PubMed]
32. Wahlig, S.; Peh, G.S.L.; Adnan, K.; Ang, H.-P.; Lwin, C.N.; Morales-Wong, F.; Ong, H.S.; Lovatt, M.; Mehta, J.S. Optimisation of Storage and Transportation Conditions of Cultured Corneal Endothelial Cells for Cell Replacement Therapy. *Sci. Rep.* **2020**, *10*, 1681. [CrossRef] [PubMed]
33. Vallabh, N.A.; Romano, V.; Willoughby, C.E. Mitochondrial Dysfunction and Oxidative Stress in Corneal Disease. *Mitochondrion* **2017**, *36*, 103–113. [CrossRef] [PubMed]
34. Naguib, Y.W.; Saha, S.; Skeie, J.M.; Acri, T.; Ebeid, K.; Abdel-rahman, S.; Kesh, S.; Schmidt, G.A.; Nishimura, D.Y.; Banas, J.A.; et al. Solubilized Ubiquinol for Preserving Corneal Function. *Biomaterials* **2021**, *275*, 120842. [CrossRef] [PubMed]
35. Vasiliauskaitė, I.; Quilendrino, R.; Baydoun, L.; van Dijk, K.; Melles, G.R.J.; Oellerich, S. Effect of Six-Month Postoperative Endothelial Cell Density on Graft Survival after Descemet Membrane Endothelial Keratoplasty. *Ophthalmology* **2021**, *128*, 1689–1698. [CrossRef]
36. Marty, A.-S.; Burillon, C.; Desanlis, A.; Damour, O.; Kocaba, V.; Auxenfans, C. Validation of an Endothelial Roll Preparation for Descemet Membrane Endothelial Keratoplasty by a Cornea Bank Using "No Touch" Dissection Technique. *Cell Tissue Bank.* **2016**, *17*, 225–232. [CrossRef]
37. Fogla, R.; Thazethaeveetil, I.R. A Novel Technique for Donor Insertion and Unfolding in Descemet Membrane Endothelial Keratoplasty. *Cornea* **2021**, *40*, 1073–1078. [CrossRef]

38. Ho, J.; Jung, H.; Banitt, M. Quantitative and Qualitative Differences in Endothelial Cell Loss Between Endothelium-In Versus Endothelium-Out Loading in Descemet Membrane Endothelial Keratoplasty. *Cornea* **2020**, *39*, 358–361. [CrossRef]
39. Brothers, K.M.; Shanks, R.M.Q.; Hurlbert, S.; Kowalski, R.P.; Tu, E.Y. Association Between Fungal Contamination and Eye Bank-Prepared Endothelial Keratoplasty Tissue: Temperature-Dependent Risk Factors and Antifungal Supplementation of Optisol-Gentamicin and Streptomycin. *JAMA Ophthalmol.* **2017**, *135*, 1184–1190. [CrossRef]

Disclaimer/Publisher's Note: The statements, opinions and data contained in all publications are solely those of the individual author(s) and contributor(s) and not of MDPI and/or the editor(s). MDPI and/or the editor(s) disclaim responsibility for any injury to people or property resulting from any ideas, methods, instructions or products referred to in the content.

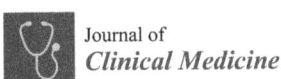

Article

Recovery of Corneal Innervation after Treatment in Dry Eye Disease: A Confocal Microscopy Study

Alberto Barros [1,2], Javier Lozano-Sanroma [1,2], Juan Queiruga-Piñeiro [1,2], Luis Fernández-Vega Cueto [1,2,3,*], Eduardo Anitua [4], Ignacio Alcalde [1,2,*] and Jesús Merayo-Lloves [1,2,3]

1. Instituto Universitario Fernández-Vega, Fundación de Investigación Oftalmológica, Universidad de Oviedo, 33012 Oviedo, Spain
2. Instituto de Investigación Sanitaria del Principado de Asturias (ISPA), 33011 Oviedo, Spain
3. Department of Surgery and Medical-Surgical Specialities, Universidad de Oviedo, 33006 Oviedo, Spain
4. Biotechnology Institute (BTI), 01007 Vitoria, Spain
* Correspondence: lfvc@fernandez-vega.com (L.F.-V.C.); nacho.alcalde@fio.as (I.A.); Tel.: +34-985-240-141 (L.F.-V.C & I.A.)

Abstract: Purpose: To analyze the changes in corneal innervation by means of in vivo corneal confocal microscopy (IVCM) in patients diagnosed with Evaporative (EDE) and Aqueous Deficient Dry Eye (ADDE) and treated with a standard treatment for Dry Eye Disease (DED) in combination with Plasma Rich in Growth Factors (PRGF). Methods: Eighty-three patients diagnosed with DED were enrolled in this study and included in the EDE or ADDE subtype. The primary variables analyzed were the length, density and number of nerve branches, and the secondary variables were those related to the quantity and stability of the tear film and the subjective response of the patients measured with psychometric questionnaires. Results: The combined treatment therapy with PRGF outperforms the standard treatment therapy in terms of subbasal nerve plexus regeneration, significantly increasing length, number of branches and nerve density, as well as significantly improving the stability of the tear film ($p < 0.05$ for all of them), and the most significant changes were located in the ADDE subtype. Conclusions: the corneal reinnervation process responds in a different way depending on the treatment prescribed and the subtype of dry eye disease. In vivo confocal microscopy is presented as a powerful technique in the diagnosis and management of neurosensory abnormalities in DED.

Keywords: corneal nerves; corneal confocal microscopy; dry eye disease

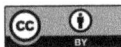

1. Introduction

The cornea is one of the most densely innervated tissues in the human body, mainly by sensory and autonomic nerve fibers. In addition to the importance of its sensory functions, corneal nerves help maintain the functional integrity of the ocular surface by releasing trophic substances that promote epithelial homeostasis and by activating circuits in the brainstem that stimulate tear production and blinking [1]. Damage to these nerve endings, whether mechanical in the case of eye surgery, or caused by ocular and systemic diseases, can lead to long-term damage to the integrity of the ocular surface [1,2].

Dry Eye Disease (DED) is one of the most common diseases in ocular surface consultationss worldwide [3], and it is accompanied by discomfort or pain sensations [4]. The Tear Film and Ocular Surface Society (TFOS) Dry Eye Workshop (DEWS) II [4] defined DED as a multifactorial disease of the ocular surface characterized by a loss of homeostasis of the tear film, and accompanied by ocular symptoms, in which tear film instability and hyperosmolarity, ocular surface inflammation and damage, and neurosensory abnormalities play etiological roles [4]. Two main subtypes of dry eye have been described [5]. In evaporative dry eye (EDE), tear hyperosmolarity is the result of excessive tear film evaporation in the presence of normal tear function, while in aqueous deficient dry eye

(ADDE) hyperosmolarity is due to reduced tear secretion in the presence of a normal evaporation rate [6].

There is a growing interest in the study of neurosensory alterations of corneal innervation related with DED [6]. In vivo corneal confocal microscopy (IVCM) is a safe and noninvasive technique for the study and analysis of corneal innervation. Recently, several studies have used IVCM to analyze changes in the subbasal nerve plexus in DED [7–9], and also to evaluate the differences in this innervation between different types of dry eye [10,11]. This technique has been previously used to analyze corneal innervation in different ocular conditions, such as corneal dystrophies [12], trauma [13], infections [14], or in systemic diseases such as diabetes [15,16]. More recently, IVCM has been used to evaluate changes in the subbasal nerve plexus of patients affected by neurodegenerative diseases, such as Fibromyalgia [17,18], Parkinson's disease [19,20], Multiple sclerosis [21–23] and even to evaluate small fiber neuropathy after viral infection with Sars-CoV-2 [24].

DEWS II established treatment strategies for DED to address tear film insufficiency (artificial tears), alterations of the palpebral margin (lid hygiene), inflammation (corticosteroids [25] immunosuppressants and immunomodulators such as Cyclosporine A, Tacrolimus and Lifitegrast [26]). Surgical approaches and nutritional supplements (diets, vitamin supplements) are also used to treat DED [27].

Artificial tears composed of blood derivatives have been gaining prominence in the treatment of DED, most notably Autologous Serum (AS), which was the first derivative of a patient's own blood to be used for the treatment of DED [28,29]. In recent years, a type of blood-based eye drops has been described, known as PRGF–Endoret® (BTI, Vitoria, Spain), which is a plasma rich in growth factors, including epidermal growth factor (EGF), transforming growth factor–β1(TGF-β1), platelet-derived growth factor (PDGF), insulin-like growth factor I (IGF-I), vascular endothelial growth factor (VEGF), nerve growth factor (NGF), and fibronectin among others. In contrast to AS, PRGF–Endoret® is formulated without inflammatory cells such as leukocytes [30,31]. PRGF treatments have shown regenerative effects on the ocular surface epithelium in neurotrophic keratitis [32], persistent epithelial defects [33], and postoperative processes [34,35]. In addition, the safety and efficacy of PRGF for the treatment of DED have been previously demonstrated [36,37] and a clinical trial using PRGF–Endoret® compared with AS in the treatment of moderate and severe dry eye is currently under way, with results expected in 2023 [38].

However, little is known about the effect of PRGF treatment on the recovery of corneal innervation.

The purpose of this study was to analyze the changes in corneal innervation in patients diagnosed with evaporative and aqueous deficient dry eye and treated with a standard treatment for dry eye disease in combination with plasma rich in growth factors.

2. Methods

This observational retrospective, longitudinal study was conducted in accordance with the Declaration of Helsinki and approved by the Committee on Ethics in Medical Research of the Principality of Asturias with the code number 2022.167 of 11 May 2022. It follows the Strengthening the Reporting of Observational Studies in Epidemiology (STROBE). Prior to data collection, patients were informed about the purpose of the study and the procedures were read and signed by them.

Eighty-three patients with a diagnosis of DED were recruited in this study. Inclusion criteria were Ocular Surface Disease Index (OSDI) score over 13, indicating moderate grade or higher of the disease, and tear break up time less than 10 s.

In addition, subjects who had a Schirmer's test of less than 5.5 mm were included in the subgroup of predominantly aqueous deficient dry eye (ADDE), while those above 5.5 mm were included in the predominantly—evaporative dry eye group (EDE) [6,39].

Other eye diseases that could indirectly affect corneal integrity were exclusion criteria (glaucoma, macular degeneration, previous ocular surgery procedures or corneal infections such as herpes virus, bacterial or fungal keratitis, adenovirus, and Acanthamoeba). Patients presenting systemic diseases that could cause alterations in corneal innervation such as Diabetes, Fibromyalgia, Parkinson, dysautonomia, etc. were also excluded.

2.1. In Vivo Confocal Microscopy (IVCM)

Patients were examined using a Heidelberg® Retina Tomograph III confocal microscope equipped with the Rostock Cornea Module (Heidelberg Engineering, Heidelberg, Germany) with a 670 nm wavelength Helium-Neon diode laser, 63x objective and numeric aperture of 0.9.

Before the beginning of the examination with the IVCM, topical anesthetic (Tetracaine 0.1% + Oxibuprocaíne; Alcon Cusí) was applied to the eye and a sterile cap (TomoCap©, Heidelberg Engineering) was attached to the lens of the microscope and a high viscosity gel (Recugel®, Baush & Lomb®, Vaughan, ON, Canada) was used as a bonding agent between the cap and the lens.

One eye of each patient was randomly selected (randomizer.org, accessed on 6 September 2022) and images of the corneal nerves of the selected eye were taken using the section mode in the central and paracentral cornea.

A total of 15 to 25 images of five non overlapping areas of each eye were selected.

The examination addressed the analysis of the entire corneal thickness from the epithelium to the anterior stroma, in order to make sure that the level of the sub basal nerve plexus was swept. The size of the images obtained was 384×384 pixel, which corresponds to an area of 400×400 μm.

The images were analyzed and quantified automatically with ACCMetrics© software (MA Dabbah, Imaging science and Biomedical engineering, Manchester, UK) [40,41].

This software reported the measurements of the following seven parameters: Corneal Nerve Fiber Density (CNFD), which shows the total number of nerves per mm^2; Corneal Nerve Branch Density (CNBD), the number of first branches originating from primary axons per mm^2; Corneal Nerve Fiber Length (CNFL), which measures the total length of all nerve fibers and branches in mm/mm^2; Corneal Total Branch Density (CTBD), the total number of branches/mm^2; Corneal Nerve Fiber Area (CNFA) in mm^2/mm^2; Corneal Nerve Fiber Width (CNFW), which shows the average nerve fiber width of the sub basal plexus in mm/mm^2, and Corneal Nerve Fractal Dimension (CNFrD), which is an indicator of the structural complexity of the corneal nerve image (Figure 1).

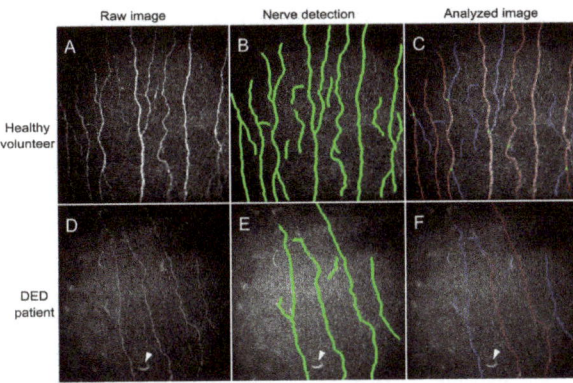

Figure 1. Examples IVCM image analysis using ACCMetrics© software. (**A–C**) show an image from a healthy cornea. (**D–F**) show the analysis process in the cornea of a DED patient. Note the differences in nerve fiber number and thickness between healthy (**A**) and DED (**D**) raw images (as obtained directly from the microscope). ACCMetrics© software detects nerve fibers (traces marked in green in (**B,E**) automatically and segregates traces in primary axons (red), first branches (blue) and the points of branching (green dots) in the analyzed images for quantification((**C,F**). Arrowheads in (**D–F**) show one dendritic cell in DED patient images.

The same images were also analyzed using the cell counter plugin of FIJI© image analysis software (ImageJ 1.53c: NIH, Bethesda, MD, USA) with the objective of quantify the incidence of neuromas (total number of neuromas per frame), beaded axons (count of the number of nerves which presented beaded axons per frame), and number of dendritic cells per frame of the central cornea. This part of the measurements was carried out in a semi-automatic way, in which the operator marked the presence of each of the disturbances in each image, and the Cell Counter plugin automatically calculated the total numbers [42].

The images were analyzed by a single experienced researcher. The final value used for each parameter was the average of the measure of all selected images of each patient.

To avoid any mistake in the classification of selected IVCM morphological alterations, once a pathological sign of the three items mentioned previously was located, the corneal structure was examined in detail with the aim of differentiating them from similar anatomical structures [43,44].

Both types of analysis with ACCMetrics® and ImageJ® software were applied to each of the images from all patients. The average of the values obtained for each parameter were used for statistical analysis.

2.2. Tear Film Break Up Time

To assess tear film stability, a drop of preservative-free 2% sodium fluorescein was instilled into the lower fornix of the patient's eye. The eye was then observed at the slit lamp at low magnification and the patient was urged to blink several times and keep the eyelids open until dark areas were observed within the green staining provided by the fluorescein. The time between the last blink and the appearance of the dark areas was recorded.

2.3. Schirmer Test

To quantify tear production, the Schirmer test (Katena®, Denville, NJ, USA) was performed on all patients by placing the paper strips on the temporal part of the inner edge of the lower eyelid for 5 min after instillation of a drop of topical anesthetic to minimize reflex tearing [45,46]. After 5 min, the millimeters of impregnated strip were measured.

2.4. Diagnostic Questionnaires

The presence of symptoms of ocular surface disease as well as their perceived severity, were assessed with the Ocular Surface Disease Index (OSDI) and the severity and intensity scales of the Symptoms Analysis in Dry Eye (SANDE).

2.5. Treatment

The patients were divided into two groups according to the treatment therapy prescribed by the ocular surface unit of Fernández-Vega Ophthalmological Institute.

Thirty-two patients were treated with a DED treatment therapy consisting of a corticosteroid regimen with Fluorometholone 0.1% (FML®, Allergan©) in a descending pattern of 4 times a day for one week, three times a day for one week, twice a day for one week and once a day for one week, combined with ocular surface hydration with Trehalose 3% and sodium hyaluronate 0.15% (Thealoz Duo®, Thea, Milan, Italy) 4 times a week and eyelid hygiene once a day, both until the follow-up visit. This group was named as the standard treatment group.

Fifty-one patients were treated with the same treatment therapy as the previous group, plus an ocular surface regeneration treatment consisting of Plasma Rich in Growth Factors 4 times a day until 3 months.

According to manufacturer's instructions, blood from this treatment group was collected into 9-mL tubes with 3.8% (wt/v) sodium citrate or in serum collection tubes (Z Serum Clot activator, Vacuette, GmbH, Kremsmünster, Austria). Blood samples were centrifuged at $580\times g$ for 8 min at room temperature in an Endoret System centrifuge (BTI Biotechnology Institute, S.L., Miñano, Alava, Spain); the whole plasma column over the buffy coat was collected using Endoret ophthalmology kit (BTI Biotechnology Institute, S.L.,

Miñano, Alava, Spain) avoiding the layer containing leukocytes. Platelets and leukocytes counts were performed with a hematology analyzer (Micros 60, Horiba ABX, Montpellier, France). Plasma preparations were incubated with Endoret activator (BTI Biotechnology Institute©, S.L., Miñano, Alava, Spain) at 37 °C for 1 h and PRGF supernatants were filtered, aliquoted and stored at 80 °C until use. All procedures were performed under sterile conditions inside a laminar flow hold. The patients were instructed to keep the PRGF eye drops dispensers at −20 °C for a maximum of 3 months [47–49]. This group was named PRGF treatment group.

All patients repeated the same tests at the follow-up visit.

2.6. Statistical Analysis

The SPSS statistical software v. 22 for Windows (SPSS Inc., Chicago, IL, USA) was used for the analysis of the data. Values were expressed as mean ± standard error of the mean (SEM). Normality of the sample was checked with the Kolmogórov–Smirnov and Shapiro Wilk tests according to the sample size. The Student's *t*-test and the Wilcoxon test were used to compare the means of the different study variables of paired samples according to the distribution of the data. In addition, the effect size was calculated with Cohen's *d* for each of the variables in all study groups.

3. Results

This observational, longitudinal, and retrospective study involved 83 patients with diagnosis of Dry Eye Disease who have visited the Fernández-Vega Ophthalmological Institute between January 2020 and April 2022. Table 1 shows the demographic data; no statistically significant differences were found from the inclusion criteria for both groups.

Table 1. Demographics and inclusion criteria.

	Standard Treatment		PRGF Treatment		
	n/Mean	±SEM	n/Mean	±SEM	*p* Value
Number of subjects	32	-	51	-	-
Age	55.13	2.08	56.08	2.29	0.766
Sex distribution (female/male)	23/9	-	39/12	-	0.639
Previous OSDI Score	36.12	3.38	43.17	3.52	0.219
Previous Break Up Time	5.27	0.58	4.93	0.47	0.581
Time of treatment (months)	4.75	0.62	4.80	0.55	0.621

3.1. General Results

3.1.1. Corneal Nerve Quantification

As shown in Table 2, the automatic analysis of corneal nerves using ACCMetrics® software showed that the morphology of the subbasal nerve plexus was not significantly altered in the standard group. The data revealed an increase in nerve branching (CNBD and CTBD) and fractal dimension (CNFrD), which was not significant in any of the parameters. The rest of the values extracted from the automatic analysis such as CNFD, CNFL, CNFW, CNFA saw slightly decreased values at follow-up with respect to the baseline visit, without being statistically significant for any of the morphological parameters.

The PRGF treatment group showed an evident increase in CNFD and CNFL ($p < 0.001$), CNBD, CNFA and Fractal Dimension ($p < 0.005$) and CTBD ($p < 0.05$).

Corneal Nerve Fiber Width did not show any differences.

3.1.2. Morphological Alterations and Cell Infiltration

The semi-automatic analysis of IVCM images using FIJI® software showed a significant reduction in the presence of dendritic cells for the standard treatment group ($p < 0.05$), as well as in the count of Axonal Beads for both groups ($p < 0.005$ for standard treatment group and $p < 0.05$ for PRGF treatment group).

Although the presence of neuromas was low in both groups, the changes observed were not significant after treatment.

Table 2. General results.

	Standard Treatment				PRGF Treatment			
	Baseline	Follow-Up			Baseline	Follow-Up		
	Mean (±SEM)	Mean (±SEM)	p Value	Effect Size	Mean (±SEM)	Mean (±SEM)	p Value	Effect Size
OSDI SCORE	36.119 ± 3.386	25.456 ± 3.680	0.002 *	0.412	43.169 ± 3.520	31.553 ± 2.926	0.005 *	0.366
SCHIRMER (mm)	7.193 ± 1.277	5.875 ± 1.159	0.194	0.136	5.340 ± 0.561	6.125 ± 0.738	0.685	0.121
FBut (sec)	5.269 ± 0.588	4.875 ± 0.595	0.654	0.087	4.935 ± 0.468	6.106 ± 0.463	0.003 *	0.262
SANDE Frequency	65.000 ± 4.512	41.093 ± 4.455	0.000 *	0.666	70.102 ± 4.196	39.591 ± 3.263	0.000 *	0.820
SANDE Severity	56.719 ± 4.113	34.687 ± 4.312	0.000 *	0.654	65.510 ± 3.557	35.102 ± 3.142	0.000 *	0.915
CNFD (n/mm^2)	19.572 ± 1.188	19.340 ± 1.615	0.859	0.020	13.827 ± 1.019	17.556 ± 1.162	0.000 *	0.338
CNBD (n/mm^2)	22.874 ± 2.728	24.672 ± 2.925	0.432	0.079	17.440 ± 2.092	23.796 ± 2.762	0.002 *	0.257
CNFL (mm/mm^2)	13.087 ± 0.590	12.965 ± 0.677	0.832	0.024	10.177 ± 0.537	11.863 ± 0.603	0.000 *	0.293
CTBD (n/mm^2)	38.181 ± 3.751	41.022 ± 4.118	0.466	0.190	32.257 ± 3.158	40.925 ± 4.148	0.012 *	0.233
CNFA (mm^2/mm^2)	0.0059 ± 0.0003	0.0057 ± 0.0003	0.607	0.078	0.0053 ± 0.0003	0.0057 ± 0.0003	0.004 *	0.123
CNFW (mm/mm^2)	0.0213 ± 0.0002	0.0215 ± 0.0002	0.400	0.091	0.0222 ± 0.0003	0.0220 ± 0.0002	0.368	0.060
CNFrD	1.4638 ± 0.009	1.4684 ± 0.006	0.801	0.072	1.4331 ± 0.010	1.4500 ± 0.009	0.004 *	0.229
Dendritic cells (n/frame)	4.9519 ± 1.810	2.3541 ± 1.252	0.039 *	0.209	3.1908 ± 0.549	2.5806 ± 0.545	0.077	0.110
Neuroma (n/frame)	0.1984 ± 0.075	0.0519 ± 0.034	0.064	0.315	0.1465 ± 0.049	0.0692 ± 0.042	0.104	0.167
Axonal Beads (n/frame)	0.6694 ± 0.147	0.1669 ± 0.561	0.002 *	0.564	0.3890 ± 0.078	0.1278 ± 0.052	0.008 *	0.389

OSDI (Ocular Surface Disease Index); FBut (Fluorescein Break Up Time); SANDE (Symptom Assesment in Dry Eye); CNFD (Corneal Nerve Fiber Density); CNBD (Corneal Nerve Branch Density); CNFL (Corneal Nerve Fiber Length); CTBD (Corneal Total Branch Density); CNFA (Corneal Nerve Fiber Area); CNFW (Corneal Nerve Fiber Width); CNFrD (Corneal Nerve Fractal Dimension). Asterisks (*) in the table indicate statistical differences ($p < 0.05$).

3.1.3. Tear Film and Ocular Surface Disease Questionnaires

The assessment of tear quantity with the Schirmer test did not show statistically significant differences in either treatment group at the follow-up visit. Tear stability measured with the Fluorescein Break Up Time was significantly increased in the PRGF treatment group ($p < 0.005$) compared to the standard treatment group ($p = 0.654$).

The OSDI score decreased significantly for both the standard treatment group ($p < 0.005$) and the PRGF combination therapy group ($p = 0.005$). The SANDE frequency and severity questionnaire score were also significantly decreased for both treatment groups ($p < 0.001$).

3.2. Subtypes of Dry Eye Disease

To study the response of corneal innervation according to the type of dry eye, the sample was divided into EDE and ADDE according to the measurement of tear quantity.

3.2.1. Difference between Subtypes of Dry Eye Disease

Baseline data were compared to identify differences between the two subtypes of dry eye disease studied. The CNFD values for the ADDE subtype was 15.007 ± 8.122 fibers per mm, while for the EDE group it was 18.218 ± 5.99 ($p = 0.066$). CNBD was 18.766 ± 16.323 branches per mm in the ADDE and 21.129 + 13.541 ($p = 0.339$) for the evaporative subgroup. For CNFL the values for the ADDE were 10.784 ± 4.228 mm per mm, and 12.185 ± 3.130 ($p = 0.147$) for the EDE. Differences were also not statistically significant for both groups in neuromas ($p = 0.195$), dendritic cells ($p = 0.700$) and axonal beadings ($p = 0.861$). For the ADDE group, the psychometric questionnaires showed an OSDI of 41.337 ± 23.638, SANDE frequency of 65.943 ± 28.673 and SANDE intensity of 60.188 ± 25.850, while for the EDE group the values were OSDI 38.400 ± 20.648 ($p = 0.748$), SANDE frequency 71.142 ± 26.297 ($p = 0.326$) and SANDE intensity of 65.535 ± 21.745 ($p = 0.420$).

3.2.2. Evaporative Dry Eye Subtype

Fifteen patients of this subtype of Dry Eye were treated with PRGF while fourteen patients were treated with the standard treatment group.

Baseline values were compared according to the assigned treatment, finding no significant differences for any of the treatment groups ($p = 0.363$ for CNFD, $p = 0.692$ for CNBD, $p = 0.233$ for CNFL, $p = 0.234$ for Schirmer, $p = 0.870$ for Fbut, $p = 0.847$ for dendritic cell count, $p = 0.477$ for neuromas count, $p = 0.533$ for Beadings count, $p = 0.486$ for OSDI score, $p = 477$ for neuromas count, $p = 0.533$ for Beadings count, and $p = 0.062$ for SANDE intensity questionnaire) apart from the SANDE frequency questionnaire which showed significant differences in baseline values according to treatment groups ($p = 0.027$).

As shown in Figure 2, nerve parameters such as density, length and number of branches increased slightly in the PRGF-treated group at the follow-up visit but were not statistically significant. The same values decreased for the standard treatment group, being significant for CNFD ($p < 0.05$) and for CNFL ($p = 0.01$).

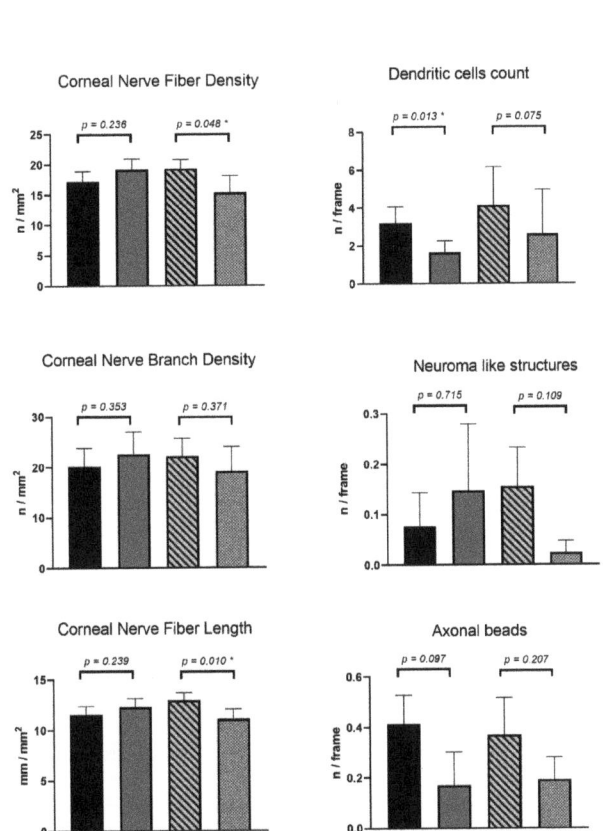

Figure 2. Corneal nerve quantification and morphological alterations Evaporative Dry Eye subtypes according to groups of treatment. Asterisks (*) in the graphs indicate statistical differences between groups ($p < 0.05$).

The morphological alterations of nerves (neuromas and beadings) and cell infiltration (dendritic cells) showed no relevant differences in any of the parameters analyzed, apart from the dendritic cell count in the PRGF treatment group ($p < 0.05$). Although not significant, a certain increase in the presence of neuromas was observed at the follow-up visit for the PRGF treatment group.

Focusing on the tear film and psychometric questionnaires, results in Figure 3 showed that tear film volume was reduced was reduced for both treatment therapies, with the reduction being statistically significant for the standard treatment group ($p = 0.045$).

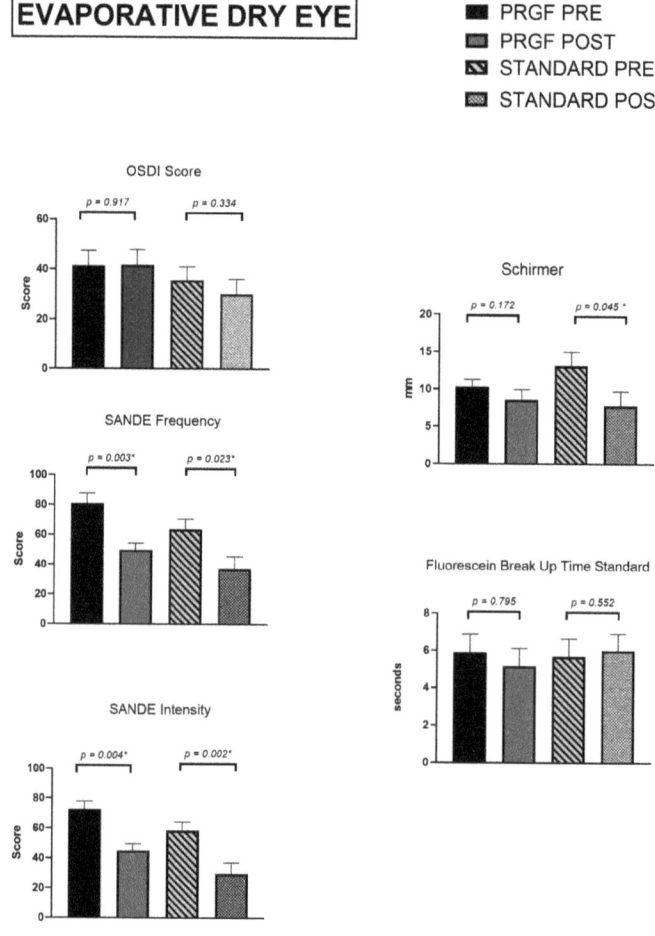

Figure 3. Tear film and psychometric questionnaires for Evaporative Dry Eye Subtype. Asterisks (*) in the graphs indicate statistical differences between groups ($p < 0.05$).

Tear break-up time did not change significantly for either treatment group at the follow-up visit.

The OSDI questionnaire remained significantly unchanged at the follow-up visit in both the standard and combined PRGF treatment groups.

For the SANDE frequency and intensity questionnaires, reductions were significant for both groups of treatment at the follow-up visit ($p < 0.005$).

3.2.3. Aqueous Deficient Dry Eye Subtype

Thirty-three patients of this subtype of Dry Eye were treated with PRGF while eighteen patients were treated with the standard treatment group. Data for one patient in the PRGF treatment group was estimated as a missing value because no post-treatment tear volume value was available.

As in the EDE subtype, baseline values were compared according to treatment type and no significant differences were found for CNBD ($p = 0.148$), FBut ($p = 0.749$), Schirmer ($p = 0.232$), dendritic cell count ($p = 0.916$), neuromas ($p = 0.619$), OSDI score ($p = 0.286$), SANDE frequency ($p = 0.798$) and SANDE intensity ($p = 0.250$). However, significant differences in these values were identified for CNFD ($p = 0.001$), CNFL ($p = 0.003$) and axonal beads count ($p = 0.013$).

In this subtype of DED, Figure 4 shows a statistically significant increase for length, density, and number of nerve branches ($p < 0.05$ for all of them) after combined treatment with PRGF, compared to the standard group, which also showed an increase, without statistical significance.

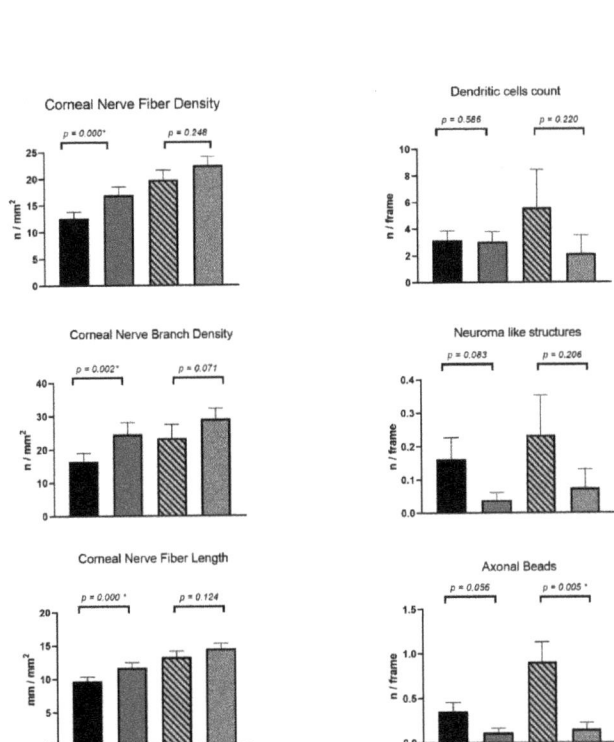

Figure 4. Corneal nerve quantification and morphological alterations ADDE subtype according to groups of treatment. Asterisks (*) in the graphs indicate statistical differences between groups ($p < 0.05$).

In the case of morphological alterations and presence of inflammation, axonal beads significantly decreased in the standard treatment group ($p = 0.05$). No other relevant differences were observed in any of the parameters analyzed, although their values decreased at the follow-up visit in both treatment subgroups.

The tear film study showed (Figure 5) an increase for the combined PRGF treatment subgroup and the standard treatment subgroup, but this was not significant for either of them.

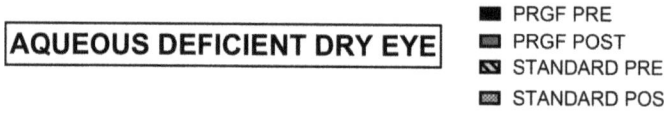

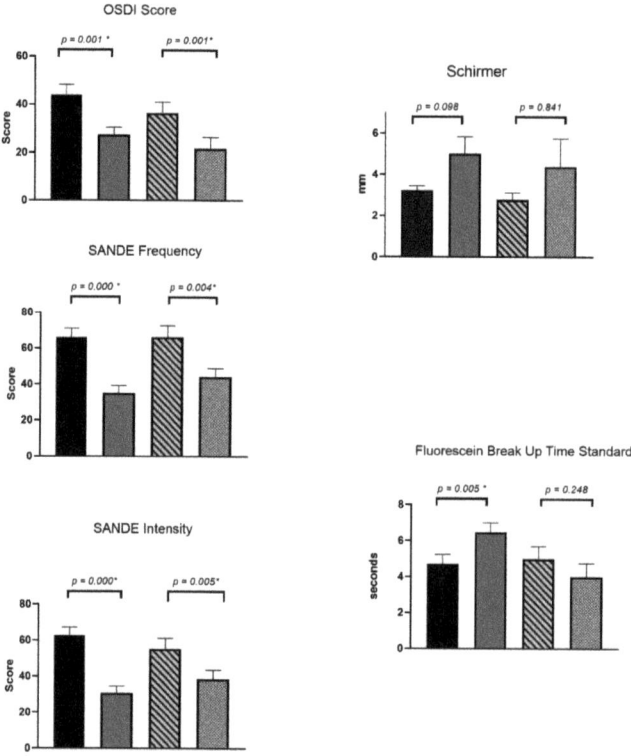

Figure 5. Tear film and psychometric questionnaires for Aqueous Deficient Dry Eye. Asterisks (*) in the graphs indicate statistical differences between groups ($p < 0.05$).

An increase in tear break-up time was found in the PRGF subgroup ($p = 0.005$) while the same value decreased slightly for the standard treatment subgroup ($p = 0.248$).

As for the psychometric questionnaires, both OSDI and SANDE frequency and intensity had significantly reduced values at the follow-up visit, with $p < 0.005$ for each of them in both treatment subgroups.

3.3. Effect Size

To answer the question of how big the change in the analyzed variables after each of the treatments was, the effect size was calculated for each of them according to the subtype of DED, comparing the values obtained at the baseline visit with those at the follow-up visit. (Table 3).

Table 3. Effect size according to the subtype of DED.

	Evaporative Dry Eye		Aqueous Deficient Dry Eye	
	Standard Treatment	PRGF Treatment	Standard Treatment	PRGF Treatment
CNFD	0.366 ↓	0.288 ↑	0.263 ↑	0.413 ↑
CNBD	0.135 ↓	0.111 ↑	0.253 ↑	0.308 ↑
CNFL	0.402 ↓	0.162 ↑	0.243 ↑	0.322 ↑
Dendritic cells	0.130 ↓	0.432 ↓	0.258 ↓	0.054 ↓
Neuromas	0.141 ↓	0.117 ↑	0.282 ↓	0.321 ↓
Beadings	0.277 ↓	0.184 ↓	0.756 ↓	0.379 ↓
Break Up Time	0.096 ↑	0.052 ↓	0.274 ↓	0.464 ↑
Schirmer	0.521 ↓	0.261 ↓	0.272 ↑	0.379 ↑
OSDI Score	0.183 ↓	0.015 ↑	0.539 ↓	0.509 ↓
SANDE Frequency	0.661 ↓	1.398 ↓	0.663 ↓	0.874 ↓
SANDE Intensity	0.822 ↓	1.235 ↓	0.506 ↓	0.948 ↓

Arrows indicate the trend of the effect with respect to baseline values.

For the EDE subtype, the standard treatment had a negative effect for CNFD, CNBD and CNFD, and for nerve length was at the edge of the medium size. With PRGF treatment, the effect size, although low, was positive for the same variables.

As for morphological alterations of the subbasal nerve plexus in this type of DED, the effect size was negative for all of them, apart from neuromas in the PRGF treatment group, although with a low effect. The effect size value was at the limit of the medium consideration for dendritic cells in the PRGF treatment group.

The tear film study did not reveal a significant effect size on tear break-up time. However, a negative effect of medium size on tear quantity—quantified by Schirmer's test—was observed for the standard treatment group.

No significant effect size was observed in both treatment groups for the OSDI score, while for the SANDE questionnaires this value was medium-high for both groups and higher for the PRGF treatment group.

In the aqueous deficient dry eye subtype, the two treatment groups had a positive effect on CNFD, CNBD and CNFL, with Cohen's d being higher for the PRGF treatment group for these three variables. The effect was negative for all of the three subbasal nerve plexus morphological alterations studied, with a value of 0.756—medium-high effect size—for axonal bead count in the standard treatment group.

Tear analysis for this dry eye subtype showed higher Cohen's d values in the PRGF treatment group. Note the negative effect for BUT in the standard treatment group.

The effect size was medium for the OSDI score in both treatment groups and for the SANDE questionnaires in the standard treatment group, while in the PRGF treatment group the effect found was high.

4. Discussion

We conducted a study including 83 eyes of 83 patients diagnosed with DED to compare the changes in corneal innervation when treated with a standard treatment and the same treatment in combination with plasma rich in growth factors.

The results of the study suggested that the combined treatment therapy with PRGF outperforms the standard treatment therapy in terms of subbasal nerve plexus regeneration, significantly increasing length, number of branches and nerve density, as well as significantly improving the stability of the tear film analyzed with fluorescein BUT.

Our findings were consistent with previous studies analyzing the response of corneal innervation to different topical treatments.

The positive effect of hematic derivatives on the ocular surface has been studied repeatedly. Fox et al. [28] described in 1984 an improvement in the symptomatology and objectivity of fifteen patients treated with artificial tears made from the patient's serum, which had not improved with conventional artificial tears. These results were also confirmed by other authors, including a randomized clinical trial [50], which is consistent with our results in a significant decrease in OSDI, improvement in BUT and also found no significant changes in the Schirmer's measurement.

The effect that hematic derivatives induce in corneal innervation has also been the subject of previous studies. In this regard, there has been some discrepancy between publications. Giannaccare et al. [51] found a significant increase in CNFD, CNFL and CNFrD in patients treated with peripheral allogenic blood serum and umbilical cord blood serum in their prospective study, although with a short follow-up period. On the other hand, Mahelkova's prospective work [52] found no differences in subbasal plexus nerve fibers in patients treated with autologous serum tears. These discrepancies may be explained by the difference in measuring devices, the cause of the DED, the sample size or the type of hematic derivative.

PRGF–Endoret® is an autologous platelet plasma rich in growth factors, standardized to reduce the proinflammatory cytokines in its formulation by removing leukocytes and by a heating treatment [53]. This feature would help to treat DED, as it is associated with a chronic inflammatory process [54].

Due to the high concentration in growth factors, PRGF-based eye drops promote a range of biological events, including cell proliferation, migration, and differentiation, while protecting against microbial contamination on the ocular surface [47,55,56]. A higher concentration of most growth factors was found in PRGF formulations than in AS [57]. Among growth factors, NGF has been shown to stimulate corneal epithelium proliferation and promote subbasal nerve plexus regeneration [58].

Our results showed no statistically significant differences in the subbasal nerve plexus between the two DED subtypes analyzed, with smaller values for ADDE. Other studies found significant reductions in corneal nerves in ADDE versus EDE using a semi-automated quantification method that reports higher values for these parameters than we obtained with the technique used in our study [10]. However, when we grouped our sample into the two dry eye subtypes according to the treatment prescribed, we found significant differences in the baseline values of CNFD and CNFL of the ADDE, with lower values in the subgroup of combined treatment with PRGF. This treatment subgroup also had higher OSDI and SANDE values and previous studies found a negative correlation between OSDI and CNFD [59].

This may be explained by the fact that in professional practice within the ocular surface unit, the ophthalmologist could have prescribed combined treatment with plasma rich in growth factors to patients who showed a higher subjective severity as measured by psychometric questionnaires, based on his previous experience and research in this field [32,35,55,60].

On the other hand, we found no significant changes in corneal innervation at the follow-up visit in the standard treatment group, and even a slight decrease in CNFL and CNFD. There are some discrepancies between previous studies regarding how corticosteroid [61,62] and immunomodulation-based treatments [63,64] affect the subbasal nerve plexus in DED. Reduction in subbasal nerves, as seen in cases of DED treated with cyclosporine A [64], may be explained by reduced NGF production and other cytokines, such as IL-1 and TNF-α. Although it is known that these treatments act by intervening in the inflammatory process associated with the disease, their mechanisms of action on corneal innervation remains unclear.

Consistent with a reduction of inflammation, we observed a significant reduction in the dendritic cell count in the standard treatment group. Villani et al. [62] also found no significant changes in the subbasal nerve plexus in their open-label and masked study, using a semi-automated nerve fiber quantification system. This study and that of Li Bei [65] are also consistent with ours in the reduction of dendritic cells after treatment with topical steroids.

The DEWS established at its first meeting in 2007 that hyperosmolarity and tear film instability are the starting point for the development of dry eye disease [66] The main cause of EDE is known to be tear film disruption accompanied by Meibomian gland dysfunction, and reduced tear secretion secondary to age-related degeneration of the lacrimal gland is the main cause of lacrimal secretion deficit dry eye [6]. It is therefore difficult to draw the line between dry eye due to a lack of secretion and evaporative dry eye, so it would be more accurate to talk about which is the predominant category in each case [5].

Our results suggest that the combined treatment with PRGF in DED contributes to the creation of the ocular surface regeneration scenario, in which corneal regeneration is promoted [3,67]. When this regenerative scenario occurs in ADDE, it induces an improvement in the stability and quantity of the tear film, as well as anti-inflammatory agents and growth factors, which create the perfect context for the corneal reinnervation process, and we observed a significant increase in this process compared to the group treated with standard treatment.

However, when the scenario occurs in EDE, the treatment also contributes to the regeneration of the ocular surface, but without solving one of the main problems which is the alteration of the eyelids and dysfunction of the Meibomian glands, which will continue to generate a situation of evaporative excess and instability of the tear film, which are described as one of the main pathogenic factors of the vicious circle in ocular surface disease [67].

As a limitation of the study, in the analyzed sample, all the patients were prescribed for eyelid hygiene protocol, but the condition of the eyelids was not monitored, so it could not be concluded whether the alterations at this level were resolved at the follow-up visit. This may explain why the most significant changes at the level of the sub basal nerve plexus are in the ADDE and raises the need for future studies quantifying the status of the eyelids and the degree of Meibomian gland dysfunction. Moreover, all the patients included in our study had a BUT below 10 s, so all had an evaporative component, and were subsequently grouped according to the reduction in tear secretion, so our study is limited by not having subjects with BUT greater than 10 s accompanied by low Schirmer values. The sample size, although in line with other published studies, can be considered small and unrepresentative and our study is also limited in this aspect, so prospective studies with larger samples are needed.

5. Conclusions

The corneal reinnervation process responds in a different way depending on the treatment prescribed and the subtype of dry eye disease. This process can be monitored and quantified non-invasively and in vivo using confocal microscopy, which is presented as a technique that can be useful in the diagnosis and management of one of the five main pathogenic factors of ocular surface diseases, of which DED is one of the most important; this can contribute to personalized treatment therapies for the disease.

Author Contributions: Conceptualization, J.M.-L. and L.F.-V.C.; methodology, A.B., J.Q.-P. and J.L.-S.; software, A.B; validation, L.F.-V.C., J.M.-L. and I.A.; formal analysis, A.B.; investigation, A.B.; resources, L.F.-V.C.; data curation, A.B., J.Q.-P. and J.L.-S.; writing—original draft preparation, A.B.; writing—review and editing, A.B. and I.A.; visualization, I.A.; supervision, E.A., I.A. and J.M.-L.; project administration, L.F.-V.C.; funding acquisition, L.F.-V.C. and J.M.-L. All authors have read and agreed to the published version of the manuscript.

Funding: This research was funded by a grant RD21/0002/0041 (Instituto de Salud Carlos III).

Institutional Review Board Statement: The study was conducted in accordance with the Declaration of Helsinki and approved by the Committee on Ethics in Medical Research of the Principality of Asturias with the code number 2022.167 of 11 May 2022.

Informed Consent Statement: Informed consent was obtained from all subjects involved in the study.

Data Availability Statement: All the obtained data used to support the findings of this study are available from the corresponding author upon reasonable request.

Acknowledgments: The authors want to especially acknowledge the devoted work of medical and technical staff at the Instituto Oftalmológico Fernández-Vega and for valuable comments and guidance of the research team at the Fundación de Investigación Oftalmológica.

Conflicts of Interest: The authors declare that there is no conflict of interest.

References

1. Marfurt, C.F.; Cox, J.; Deek, S.; Dvorscak, L. Anatomy of the Human Corneal Innervation. *Exp. Eye Res.* **2010**, *90*, 478–492. [CrossRef] [PubMed]
2. Müller, L.J.; Marfurt, C.F.; Kruse, F.; Tervo, T.M. Corneal Nerves: Structure, Contents and Function. *Exp. Eye Res.* **2003**, *76*, 521–542. [CrossRef] [PubMed]
3. Rolando, M.; Merayo-Lloves, J. Management Strategies for Evaporative Dry Eye Disease and Future Perspective. *Curr. Eye Res.* **2022**, *47*, 813–823. [CrossRef] [PubMed]
4. Craig, J.P.; Nichols, K.K.; Akpek, E.K.; Caffery, B.; Dua, H.S.; Joo, C.K.; Liu, Z.; Nelson, J.D.; Nichols, J.J.; Tsubota, K.; et al. TFOS DEWS II Definition and Classification Report. *Ocul. Surf.* **2017**, *15*, 276–283. [CrossRef] [PubMed]
5. Wolffsohn, J.S.; Arita, R.; Chalmers, R.; Djalilian, A.; Dogru, M.; Dumbleton, K.; Gupta, P.K.; Karpecki, P.; Lazreg, S.; Pult, H.; et al. TFOS DEWS II Diagnostic Methodology Report. *Ocul. Surf.* **2017**, *15*, 539–574. [CrossRef]
6. Bron, A.J.; de Paiva, C.S.; Chauhan, S.K.; Bonini, S.; Gabison, E.E.; Jain, S.; Knop, E.; Markoulli, M.; Ogawa, Y.; Perez, V.; et al. TFOS DEWS II Pathophysiology Report. *Ocul. Surf.* **2017**, *15*, 438–510. [CrossRef]
7. Matsumoto, Y.; Ibrahim, O.M.A. Application of in Vivo Confocal Microscopy in Dry Eye Disease. *Invest. Ophthalmol. Vis. Sci.* **2018**, *59*, DES41–DES47. [CrossRef]
8. Said, D.G.; Liu, Y.; Chou, Y.; Dong, X.; Liu, Z.; Jiang, X.; Hao, R.; Li, X. Corneal Subbasal Nerve Analysis Using In Vivo Confocal Microscopy in Patients with Dry Eye: Analysis and Clinical Correlations. *Cornea* **2019**, *38*, 1253–1258. [CrossRef]
9. Ma, B.; Xie, J.; Yang, T.; Su, P.; Liu, R.; Sun, T.; Zhou, Y.; Wang, H.; Feng, X.; Ma, S.; et al. Quantification of Increased Corneal Subbasal Nerve Tortuosity in Dry Eye Disease and Its Correlation with Clinical Parameters. *Transl. Vis. Sci. Technol.* **2021**, *10*, 26. [CrossRef]
10. Cox, S.M.; Kheirkhah, A.; Aggarwal, S.; Abedi, F.; Cavalcanti, B.M.; Cruzat, A.; Hamrah, P. Alterations in Corneal Nerves in Different Subtypes of Dry Eye Disease: An in Vivo Confocal Microscopy Study. *Ocul. Surf.* **2021**, *22*, 135–142. [CrossRef]
11. Matsumoto, Y.; Ibrahim, O.M.A.; Kojima, T.; Dogru, M.; Shimazaki, J.; Tsubota, K. Corneal In Vivo Laser-Scanning Confocal Microscopy Findings in Dry Eye Patients with Sjögren's Syndrome. *Diagnostics* **2020**, *10*, 497. [CrossRef]
12. Ahuja, Y.; Baratz, K.H.; McLaren, J.W.; Bourne, W.M.; Patel, S.V. Decreased Corneal Sensitivity and Abnormal Corneal Nerves in Fuchs Endothelial Dystrophy. *Cornea* **2012**, *31*, 1257–1263. [CrossRef]
13. Pal-Ghosh, S.; Tadvalkar, G.; Stepp, M.A. Alterations in Corneal Sensory Nerves During Homeostasis, Aging, and After Injury in Mice Lacking the Heparan Sulfate Proteoglycan Syndecan-1. *Invest. Ophthalmol. Vis. Sci.* **2017**, *58*, 4959–4975. [CrossRef] [PubMed]
14. Chopra, R.; Mulholland, P.J.; Hau, S.C. In Vivo Confocal Microscopy Morphological Features and Cyst Density in Acanthamoeba Keratitis. *Am. J. Ophthalmol.* **2020**, *217*, 38–48. [CrossRef]
15. Zhao, H.; He, Y.; Ren, Y.R.; Chen, B.H. Corneal Alteration and Pathogenesis in Diabetes Mellitus. *Int. J. Ophthalmol.* **2019**, *12*, 1939–1950. [CrossRef]
16. Tummanapalli, S.S.; Issar, T.; Kwai, N.; Poynten, A.; Krishnan, A.V.; Willcox, M.; Markoulli, M. Association of Corneal Nerve Loss with Markers of Axonal Ion Channel Dysfunction in Type 1 Diabetes. *Clin. Neurophysiol.* **2020**, *131*, 145–154. [CrossRef]
17. Oudejans, L.; He, X.; Niesters, M.; Dahan, A.; Brines, M.; van Velzen, M. Cornea Nerve Fiber Quantification and Construction of Phenotypes in Patients with Fibromyalgia. *Sci. Rep.* **2016**, *6*, 23573. [CrossRef]
18. Klitsch, A.; Evdokimov, D.; Frank, J.; Thomas, D.; Saffer, N.; Meyer Zu Altenschildesche, C.; Sisignano, M.; Kampik, D.; Malik, R.A.; Sommer, C.; et al. Reduced Association between Dendritic Cells and Corneal Sub-Basal Nerve Fibers in Patients with Fibromyalgia Syndrome. *J. Peripher. Nerv. Syst.* **2020**, *25*, 9–18. [CrossRef]
19. Badian, R.A.; Allgeier, S.; Scarpa, F.; Andréasson, M.; Bartschat, A.; Mikut, R.; Colonna, A.; Bellisario, M.; Utheim, T.P.; Köhler, B.; et al. Wide-Field Mosaics of the Corneal Subbasal Nerve Plexus in Parkinson's Disease Using in Vivo Confocal Microscopy. *Sci. Data* **2021**, *8*, 306. [CrossRef]
20. Jeziorska, M.; Atkinson, A.; Kass-Iliyya, L.; Kobylecki, C.; Gosal, D.; Marshall, A.; Malik, R.A.; Silverdale, M. Small Fibre Neuropathy in Parkinson's Disease: Comparison of Skin Biopsies from the More Affected and Less Affected Sides. *J. Parkinsons Dis.* **2019**, *9*, 761–765. [CrossRef]
21. Petropoulos, I.N.; Kamran, S.; Li, Y.; Khan, A.; Ponirakis, G.; Akhtar, N.; Deleu, D.; Shuaib, A.; Malik, R.A. Corneal Confocal Microscopy: An Imaging Endpoint for Axonal Degeneration in Multiple Sclerosis. *Invest Ophthalmol. Vis. Sci.* **2017**, *58*, 3677–3681. [CrossRef] [PubMed]

22. Bitirgen, G.; Akpinar, Z.; Uca, A.U.; Ozkagnici, A.; Petropoulos, I.N.; Malik, R.A. Progressive Loss of Corneal and Retinal Nerve Fibers in Patients with Multiple Sclerosis: A 2-Year Follow-up Study. *Transl. Vis. Sci. Technol.* **2020**, *9*, 37. [CrossRef]
23. Testa, V.; de Santis, N.; Scotto, R.; della Giustina, P.; Ferro Desideri, L.; Cellerino, M.; Cordano, C.; Inglese, M.; Uccelli, A.; Vagge, A.; et al. Corneal Epithelial Dendritic Cells in Patients with Multiple Sclerosis: An in Vivo Confocal Microscopy Study. *J. Clin. Neurosci.* **2020**, *81*, 139–143. [CrossRef] [PubMed]
24. Barros, A.; Queiruga-Piñeiro, J.; Lozano-Sanroma, J.; Alcalde, I.; Gallar, J.; Fernández-Vega Cueto, L.; Alfonso, J.F.; Quirós, L.M.; Merayo-Lloves, J. Small Fiber Neuropathy in the Cornea of Covid-19 Patients Associated with the Generation of Ocular Surface Disease. *Ocul. Surf.* **2022**, *23*, 40–48. [CrossRef] [PubMed]
25. Kallab, M.; Szegedi, S.; Hommer, N.; Stegmann, H.; Kaya, S.; Werkmeister, R.M.; Schmidl, D.; Schmetterer, L.; Garhöfer, G. Topical Low Dose Preservative-Free Hydrocortisone Reduces Signs and Symptoms in Patients with Chronic Dry Eye: A Randomized Clinical Trial. *Adv. Ther.* **2020**, *37*, 329–341. [CrossRef]
26. Leonardi, A.; van Setten, G.; Amrane, M.; Ismail, D.; Garrigue, J.-S.; Figueiredo, F.C.; Baudouin, C. Efficacy and Safety of 0.1% Cyclosporine a Cationic Emulsion in the Treatment of Severe Dry Eye Disease: A Multicenter Randomized Trial. *Eur. J. Ophthalmol.* **2016**, *26*, 287–296. [CrossRef]
27. Giannaccare, G.; Pellegrini, M.; Sebastiani, S.; Bernabei, F.; Roda, M.; Taroni, L.; Versura, P.; Campos, E.C. Efficacy of Omega-3 Fatty Acid Supplementation for Treatment of Dry Eye Disease: A Meta-Analysis of Randomized Clinical Trials. *Cornea* **2019**, *38*, 565–573. [CrossRef]
28. Fox, R.I.; Chan, R.; Michelson, J.B.; Belmont, J.B.; Michelson, P.E. Beneficial Effect of Artificial Tears Made with Autologous Serum in Patients with Keratoconjunctivitis Sicca. *Arthritis Rheum.* **1984**, *27*, 459–461. [CrossRef]
29. Shtein, R.M.; Shen, J.F.; Kuo, A.N.; Hammersmith, K.M.; Li, J.Y.; Weikert, M.P. Autologous Serum-Based Eye Drops for Treatment of Ocular Surface Disease: A Report by the American Academy of Ophthalmology. *Ophthalmology* **2020**, *127*, 128–133. [CrossRef]
30. Anitua, E.; Muruzabal, F.; de la Fuente, M.; Riestra, A.; Merayo-Lloves, J.; Orive, G. PRGF Exerts More Potent Proliferative and Anti-Inflammatory Effects than Autologous Serum on a Cell Culture Inflammatory Model. *Exp. Eye. Res.* **2016**, *151*, 115–121. [CrossRef]
31. Anitua, E.; Muruzabal, F. PRGF in Equine Corneal Cells: A Standardised Protocol Is the Key to Achieve Accurate Results. *Equine Vet. J.* **2018**, *50*, 274–275. [CrossRef]
32. Sanchez-Avila, R.M.; Merayo-Lloves, J.; Riestra, A.C.; Fernandez-Vega Cueto, L.; Anitua, E.; Begoña, L.; Muruzabal, F.; Orive, G. Treatment of Patients with Neurotrophic Keratitis Stages 2 and 3 with Plasma Rich in Growth Factors (PRGF-Endoret) Eye-Drops. *Int. Ophthalmol.* **2018**, *38*, 1193–1204. [CrossRef]
33. Lopez-Plandolit, S.; Morales, M.C.; Freire, V.; Etxebarria, J.; Duran, J.A. Plasma Rich in Growth Factors as a Therapeutic Agent for Persistent Corneal Epithelial Defects. *Cornea* **2010**, *29*, 843–848. [CrossRef]
34. Ibares-Frias, L.; Gallego-Munoz, P.; Orive, G.; Anitua, E.; Cantalapiedra-Rodriguez, R.; Merayo-Lloves, J.; Martinez-Garcia, M.C. Potential Effect of Plasma Rich in Growth Factors-Endoret in Stromal Wound Healing in Additive Surgery. *Ophthalmic. Res.* **2020**, *63*, 203–212. [CrossRef]
35. Sanchez-Avila, R.M.; Merayo-Lloves, J.; Fernandez, M.L.; Rodriguez-Gutierrez, L.A.; Jurado, N.; Muruzabal, F.; Orive, G.; Anitua, E. Plasma Rich in Growth Factors for the Treatment of Dry Eye after LASIK Surgery. *Int. J. Mol. Sci.* **2018**, *60*, 80–86. [CrossRef]
36. Merayo-Lloves, J.; Sanchez-Avila, R.M.; Riestra, A.C.; Anitua, E.; Begoña, L.; Orive, G.; Fernandez-Vega, L. Safety and Efficacy of Autologous Plasma Rich in Growth Factors Eye Drops for the Treatment of Evaporative Dry Eye. *Ophthalmic. Res.* **2016**, *56*, 68–73. [CrossRef]
37. Lopez-Plandolit, S.; Morales, M.C.; Freire, V.; Grau, A.E.; Duran, J.A. Efficacy of Plasma Rich in Growth Factors for the Treatment of Dry Eye. *Cornea* **2011**, *30*, 1312–1317. [CrossRef]
38. Jongkhajornpong, P.; Numthavaj, P.; Anothaisintawee, T.; Lekhanont, K.; Mckay, G.; Attia, J.; Thakkinstian, A. Comparison of Treatment Efficacy between 100% Platelet-Rich Plasma and 100% Serum Eye Drops in Moderate-to-Severe Dry Eye Disease: A Randomised Controlled Trial Protocol. *BMJ Open* **2021**, *11*, 479. [CrossRef]
39. Willcox, M.D.P.; Argueso, P.; Georgiev, G.A.; Holopainen, J.M.; Laurie, G.W.; Millar, T.J.; Papas, E.B.; Rolland, J.P.; Schmidt, T.A.; Stahl, U.; et al. TFOS DEWS II Tear Film Report. *Ocul. Surf.* **2017**, *15*, 366–403. [CrossRef]
40. Dabbah, M.A.; Graham, J.; Petropoulos, I.; Tavakoli, M.; Malik, R.A. Dual-Model Automatic Detection of Nerve-Fibres in Corneal Confocal Microscopy Images. *Med. Image Comput. Comput. Assist. Interv.* **2010**, *13*, 300–307. [CrossRef]
41. Petropoulos, I.N.; Manzoor, T.; Morgan, P.; Fadavi, H.; Asghar, O.; Alam, U.; Ponirakis, G.; Dabbah, M.A.; Chen, X.; Graham, J.; et al. Repeatability of in Vivo Corneal Confocal Microscopy to Quantify Corneal Nerve Morphology. *Cornea* **2013**, *32*, 83–89. [CrossRef] [PubMed]
42. O'brien, J.; Hayder, H.; Peng, C. Automated Quantification and Analysis of Cell Counting Procedures Using ImageJ Plugins. *J. Vis. Exp.* **2016**, *117*, e54719. [CrossRef]
43. Stepp, M.A.; Pal-Ghosh, S.; Downie, L.E.; Zhang, A.C.; Chinnery, H.R.; Machet, J.; di Girolamo, N. Corneal Epithelial "Neuromas": A Case of Mistaken Identity? *Cornea* **2020**, *39*, 930–934. [CrossRef] [PubMed]
44. Moein, H.R.; Akhlaq, A.; Dieckmann, G.; Abbouda, A.; Pondelis, N.; Salem, Z.; Müller, R.T.; Cruzat, A.; Cavalcanti, B.M.; Jamali, A.; et al. Visualization of Microneuromas by Using in Vivo Confocal Microscopy: An Objective Biomarker for the Diagnosis of Neuropathic Corneal Pain? *Ocular. Surf.* **2020**, *18*, 651–656. [CrossRef]

45. Li, N.; Deng, X.-G.; He, M.-F. Comparison of the Schirmer I Test with and without Topical Anesthesia for Diagnosing Dry Eye. *Int. J. Ophthalmol.* **2012**, *5*, 478–481. [CrossRef]
46. Tsubota, K.; Kaido, M.; Yagi, Y.; Fujihara, T.; Shimmura, S. Diseases Associated with Ocular Surface Abnormalities: The Importance of Reflex Tearing. *Br. J. Ophthalmol.* **1999**, *83*, 89–91. [CrossRef]
47. Anitua, E.; Muruzabal, F.; de la Fuente, M.; Merayo, J.; Duran, J.; Orive, G. Plasma Rich in Growth Factors for the Treatment of Ocular Surface Diseases. *Curr. Eye Res.* **2016**, *41*, 875–882. [CrossRef]
48. Anitua, E.; de la Fuente, M.; Riestra, A.; Merayo-Lloves, J.; Muruzábal, F.; Orive, G. Preservation of Biological Activity of Plasma and Platelet-Derived Eye Drops After Their Different Time and Temperature Conditions of Storage. *Cornea* **2015**, *34*, 1144–1148. [CrossRef]
49. Anitua, E.; de la Fuente, M.; Muruzabal, F.; Riestra, A.; Merayo-Lloves, J.; Orive, G. Plasma Rich in Growth Factors (PRGF) Eye Drops Stimulates Scarless Regeneration Compared to Autologous Serum in the Ocular Surface Stromal Fibroblasts. *Exp. Eye Res.* **2015**, *135*, 118–126. [CrossRef]
50. Celebi, A.R.C.; Ulusoy, C.; Mirza, G.E. The Efficacy of Autologous Serum Eye Drops for Severe Dry Eye Syndrome: A Randomized Double-Blind Crossover Study. *Graefes Arch. Clin. Exp. Ophthalmol.* **2014**, *252*, 619–626. [CrossRef]
51. Giannaccare, G.; Pellegrini, M.; Bernabei, F.; Moscardelli, F.; Buzzi, M.; Versura, P.; Campos, E.C. In Vivo Confocal Microscopy Automated Morphometric Analysis of Corneal Subbasal Nerve Plexus in Patients With Dry Eye Treated With Different Sources of Homologous Serum Eye Drops. *Cornea* **2019**, *38*, 1412–1417. [CrossRef]
52. Mahelkova, G.; Jirsova, K.; Seidler Stangova, P.; Palos, M.; Vesela, V.; Fales, I.; Jiraskova, N.; Dotrelova, D. Using Corneal Confocal Microscopy to Track Changes in the Corneal Layers of Dry Eye Patients after Autologous Serum Treatment. *Clin. Exp. Optom.* **2017**, *100*, 243–249. [CrossRef]
53. Anitua, E.; Muruzabal, F.; de la Fuente, M.; Merayo-Lloves, J.; Orive, G. Effects of Heat-Treatment on Plasma Rich in Growth Factors-Derived Autologous Eye Drop. *Exp. Eye Res.* **2014**, *119*, 27–34. [CrossRef]
54. Periman, L.M.; Perez, V.L.; Saban, D.R.; Lin, M.C.; Neri, P. The Immunological Basis of Dry Eye Disease and Current Topical Treatment Options. *J. Ocul. Pharmacol. Ther.* **2020**, *36*, 137–146. [CrossRef]
55. Anitua, E.; Muruzabal, F.; Alcalde, I.; Merayo-Lloves, J.; Orive, G. Plasma Rich in Growth Factors (PRGF-Endoret) Stimulates Corneal Wound Healing and Reduces Haze Formation after PRK Surgery. *Exp. Eye Res.* **2013**, *115*, 153–161. [CrossRef]
56. Anitua, E.; Sanchez, M.; Merayo-Lloves, J.; de la Fuente, M.; Muruzabal, F.; Orive, G. Plasma Rich in Growth Factors (PRGF-Endoret) Stimulates Proliferation and Migration of Primary Keratocytes and Conjunctival Fibroblasts and Inhibits and Reverts TGF-Beta1-Induced Myodifferentiation. *Invest. Ophthalmol. Vis. Sci.* **2011**, *52*, 6066–6073. [CrossRef]
57. Anitua, E.; Muruzabal, F.; Tayebba, A.; Riestra, A.; Perez, V.L.; Merayo-Lloves, J.; Orive, G. Autologous Serum and Plasma Rich in Growth Factors in Ophthalmology: Preclinical and Clinical Studies. *Acta Ophthalmol.* **2015**, *93*, e605–e614. [CrossRef]
58. Lambiase, A.; Manni, L.; Bonini, S.; Rama, P.; Micera, A.; Aloe, L. Nerve Growth Factor Promotes Corneal Healing: Structural, Biochemical, and Molecular Analyses of Rat and Human Corneas. *Invest Ophthalmol. Vis. Sci.* **2000**, *41*, 1063–1069.
59. Tepelus, T.C.; Chiu, G.B.; Huang, J.; Huang, P.; Sadda, S.V.R.; Irvine, J.; Lee, O.L. Correlation between Corneal Innervation and Inflammation Evaluated with Confocal Microscopy and Symptomatology in Patients with Dry Eye Syndromes: A Preliminary Study. *Graefe's Arch. Clin. Exp. Ophthalmol.* **2017**, *255*, 1771–1778. [CrossRef]
60. Merayo-Lloves, J.; Rushton, J.O. Effects of Three Blood Derived Products on Equine Corneal Cells, an in Vitro Study. *Equine Vet. J.* **2018**, *50*, 356–362. [CrossRef]
61. Kheirkhah, A.; Dohlman, T.H.; Amparo, F.; Arnoldner, M.A.; Jamali, A.; Hamrah, P.; Dana, R. Effects of Corneal Nerve Density on the Response to Treatment in Dry Eye Disease. *Ophthalmology* **2015**, *122*, 662–668. [CrossRef] [PubMed]
62. Villani, E.; Garoli, E.; Termine, V.; Pichi, F.; Ratiglia, R.; Nucci, P. Corneal Confocal Microscopy in Dry Eye Treated with Corticosteroids. *Optom. Vis. Sci.* **2015**, *92*, e290–e295. [CrossRef] [PubMed]
63. Levy, O.; Labbé, A.; Borderie, V.; Hamiche, T.; Dupas, B.; Laroche, L.; Baudouin, C.; Bouheraoua, N. Increased Corneal Sub-Basal Nerve Density in Patients with Sjögren Syndrome Treated with Topical Cyclosporine A. *Clin. Exp. Ophthalmol.* **2017**, *45*, 455–463. [CrossRef] [PubMed]
64. Iaccheri, B.; Torroni, G.; Cagini, C.; Fiore, T.; Cerquaglia, A.; Lupidi, M.; Cillino, S.; Dua, H.S. Corneal Confocal Scanning Laser Microscopy in Patients with Dry Eye Disease Treated with Topical Cyclosporine. *Eye* **2017**, *31*, 788–794. [CrossRef]
65. Li, B.; Tian, Y.; Wang, S. The Correlation of Cytokines and Sensory Hypersensitivity in Mild Dry Eye Patients Characterized by Symptoms Outweighing Signs—PubMed. Available online: https://pubmed.ncbi.nlm.nih.gov/32476816/ (accessed on 23 January 2023).
66. Lemp, M.A.; Baudouin, C.; Baum, J.; Dogru, M.; Foulks, G.N.; Kinoshita, S.; Laibson, P.; McCulley, J.; Murube, J.; Pflugfelder, S.C.; et al. The Definition and Classification of Dry Eye Disease: Report of the Definition and Classification Subcommittee of the International Dry Eye WorkShop (2007). *Ocul Surf* **2007**, *5*, 75–92. [CrossRef]
67. Aragona, P.; Giannaccare, G.; Mencucci, R.; Rubino, P.; Cantera, E.; Rolando, M. Modern Approach to the Treatment of Dry Eye, a Complex Multifactorial Disease: A P.I.C.A.S.S.O. Board Review. *Br. J. Ophthalmol.* **2021**, *105*, 446–453. [CrossRef]

Disclaimer/Publisher's Note: The statements, opinions and data contained in all publications are solely those of the individual author(s) and contributor(s) and not of MDPI and/or the editor(s). MDPI and/or the editor(s) disclaim responsibility for any injury to people or property resulting from any ideas, methods, instructions or products referred to in the content.

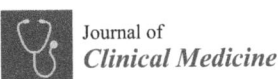

Article

Does PLEX® Elite 9000 OCT Identify and Characterize Most Posterior Pole Lesions in Highly Myopic Patients?

Pablo Arlanzon-Lope *, Miguel Angel. Campos, Ivan Fernandez-Bueno and Rosa M. Coco-Martin

Retina Group, Instituto de Oftalmobiologia Aplicada (IOBA), Universidad de Valladolid, 47011 Valladolid, Spain
* Correspondence: parlanzonl@ioba.med.uva.es; Tel.: +34-983-423559

Abstract: High myopia (HM) is defined as an axial length (AL) ≥ 26 mm that may result in various pathologies that constitute pathologic myopia (PM). The PLEX® Elite 9000 (Carl Zeiss AC, Jena, Germany) is a new swept-source optical coherence tomography (SS-OCT) underdevelopment that allows wider, deeper and more detailed posterior-segment visualization; it can acquire ultra-wide OCT angiography (OCTA) or new ultra-wide high-density scans in one image. We assessed the technology's ability to identify/characterize/quantify staphylomas and posterior pole lesions or image biomarkers in highly myopic Spanish patients and estimate the technology's potential to detect macular pathology. The instrument acquired 6 × 6 OCTA, 12 × 12 or 6 × 6 OCT cubes, and at least two high-definition spotlight single scans. A hundred consecutive patients (179 eyes; age, 51.4 ± 16.8 years; AL, 28.8 ± 2.33 mm) were recruited in one center for this prospective observational study. Six eyes were excluded because images were not acquired. The most common alterations were perforating scleral vessels (88.8%), classifiable staphyloma (68.7%), vascular folds (43%), extrafoveal retinoschisis (24%), dome-shaped macula (15.6%), and more uncommonly, scleral dehiscence (4.46%), intrachoroidal cavitation (3.35%), and macular pit (2.2%). The retinal thickness of these patients decreased, and the foveal avascular zone increased in the superficial plexus compared with normal eyes. SS-OCT is a novel potent tool that can detect most main posterior pole complications in PM and may provide us with a better understanding of the associated pathologies; some pathologies were identifiable only with this new kind of equipment, such as perforating scleral vessels, which seem to be the most common finding and not so frequently related to choroidal neovascularization, as previously reported.

Keywords: pathologic myopia; OCT; Plex Elite 9000

1. Introduction

According to the International Myopia Institute (IMI), any refractive defect whose spherical equivalent is −0.50 diopter (D) or less is considered to be myopia, while high myopia (HM) is defined as a refractive error of −6 D or less or an axial length (AL) exceeding 26 mm [1,2]. However, pathologic myopia (PM) is defined as an axial HM with either staphyloma or myopic maculopathy (MM), the latter of which includes myopic macular degeneration (MMD), tractional maculopathy (TM), or dome-shaped macula (DSM) [3,4].

Staphyloma was defined by Spaide as an outpouching of the ocular globe wall in which the curvature radius is smaller compared to that of the surrounding area [5]. In 1977, Curtin defined 10 types of staphylomas using funduscopy to show the one that affects the posterior pole and the inferior lesion type was the most common [6]. Ohno-Matsui later proposed six types of staphylomas using fundus photographs and three-dimensional magnetic resonance [7]. Eyes with staphyloma have a high risk of having MMD, which would include diffuse or patchy macular atrophy with/without lacquer cracks that can be observed via optical coherence tomography (OCT) imaging as defects in Bruch's membrane and active choroidal neovascularization (CNV) and subsequent Fuch's spots [8].

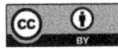

Several authors have proposed classifications of MM. First, Curtin and Karlin proposed a classification including the following categories: chorioretinal atrophy, Fuch's spot, optic nerve damage, lacquer cracks, and posterior staphyloma [9]. Later, Avila et al. [10] proposed a classification using five levels. Ohno-Matsui et al. [11] then proposed the international classification and grading system for MM called META-PM, which has been widely used and is based on retinographies. This classification has the following categories: 0 corresponds to a normal fundus appearance, 1 to tessellated fundus, 2 to diffuse atrophy, 3 to patchy atrophy without foveal involvement, and 4 to macular atrophy. The presence of any of these three plus lesions (lacquer cracks, CNV, and Fuch's spot) also indicates PM [11]. However, this classification does not consider the tractional component of MM, which is an important cause of visual loss in PM [12]; thus, Ruiz-Medrano et al. proposed the ATN classification using both fundus and OCT images where A indicates atrophic, T tractional, and N neovascular classifications. There are different levels for each component and the final classification is the combination of the three [4]. Finally, a DSM or the presence of a ridge-shaped macula (RSM) in cases of inferior staphylomas has also been included in the IMI OCT classification as a feature of MM [3], with RSM defined as macular elevation in only one meridian across the fovea and differing from DSM, which is an area of elevation [13].

Structural OCT is a useful method to study PM features and the best method to identify tractional maculopathy [14]. In addition, one of the most important causes of visual loss in PM is CNV [15,16], and recently, OCT angiography (OCTA) has shown good sensitivity for detecting it [17,18]. Thus, structural OCT and OCTA are important for detecting macular pathologies that are otherwise difficult to identify.

It is difficult to estimate the prevalence of PM/MM and the related lesions because large population studies with large patient samples are needed. A recent review found that studies that use different definitions of MM and different diagnostic techniques are mainly conducted in Asian populations, and the prevalence of HM varied from 1.5% to 8% and the prevalence of MM from 0.2% to 10.7% [19]. However, two population studies in Germany and Russia showed prevalence rates of MM of 0.5% and 1.3%, respectively. The prevalence of HM is high in Spain and one of the highest in Europe, although it is even higher in Asian populations [20]. A study published in 2010 found that MP was the second most common cause of visual impairment in a nursing home [21]. In addition, our previous study showed differences between our population and Asian populations [22].

Concerning studies that use OCT, Ruão et al. found that patchy retinal atrophy is the most frequent finding (79.1%), followed by CNV (69.1%) and TM (53.7%) in a hospital sample of patients with HM from the Iberian Peninsula [23]. However, it is necessary to acknowledge that HM is associated with reduced signal strength spectral-domain OCT and it is more likely to produce unreliable OCT measurements [24].

The purpose of the current study was to assess whether wide-field SS-OCT and OCTA images reinforced by funduscopy/retinography allow the identification and characterization of staphyloma and the most posterior pole lesions or image biomarkers in a series of Spanish patients with HM. We also wanted to estimate the frequency of observations of the previously described pathological features and study the potential high-definition swept-source OCT (SS-OCT), which is still being developed, for detecting macular pathologies.

2. Materials and Methods

This longitudinal observational study of a single-center, prospective cohort followed the tenets of the Helsinki Declaration of 1964 (last amendment, 2013). The Clinical Research Ethics Committee of the Valladolid East Health Area approved the study. All patients understood the specifics of the study and provided informed consent.

A sample of consecutive patients with HM was recruited at the Institute of Applied Ophthalmobiology (IOBA), an eye institute of the University of Valladolid. Patients were included if they were older than 18 years, Caucasian, and had an AL ≥ 26 mm. Patients were excluded if they had any other retinal pathology not attributable to HM, significant media opacities that prevented good-quality images, or those who had undergone surgery during the previous 3 months.

Family and past medical antecedents were gathered, including previous ocular pathologies and surgeries. Visual acuity (VA) was tested using an Early Treatment Diabetic Retinopathy Study panel and recorded as the logarithmic of the minimum angle of resolution (logMAR) scale. A phenylephrine (100 mg/mL) and a tropicamide (10 mg/mL drop) was instilled in each eye. The AL was measured using the IOLMaster 500 (Carl Zeiss AC, Jena, Germany). Keratometry, anterior chamber depth, and white-to-white distance were also recorded as control variables. Central retinography was later performed using either Topcon 3D (Topcon Corporation, Tokyo, Japan) or Topcon Triton DRI (Topcon Corporation). Finally, several protocol scans using the PLEX® Elite 9000 OCT (Carl Zeiss AC) were performed. These included a 6 × 6 OCTA scan centered on the macula and a 12 × 12 HD51 scan centered on the macula; however, if the quality precluded it, a 6 × 6 HD51 scan was performed instead. A total of 120 6 × 6 HD51 scans and 59 12 × 12 scans were taken. Finally, at least 2 single HD spotlight line scans (90 and 180 degrees, 16 mm) were performed. To better characterize the type of staphyloma in some patients, extra scans were taken at 135° in their right eyes and 45° in their left eyes. All tests were performed by two equally trained operators (PAL and MAC).

The presence of staphyloma was assessed using OCT. The staphylomas were classified in a similar manner to the Ohno-Matsui criterion [7]. In addition, the following lesions were identified using OCT: lacquer cracks were defined as linear Bruch defects with OCT and retinography; atrophic maculopathy was defined as extensive Bruch's defect with OCT; if there were CNV or Fuch´s spot they were usually visible with OCTA, where active CNV may associate hemorrhage and/or exudation signs, whereas in its scar phase flow is less likely to be detected and that has the typical blackened appearance of Fuch's spots on retinography [3,4]. Tractional maculopathy is defined by the T dominion of the ATN classification that on OCT images is shown as a split between the inner and outer retina within the staphyloma defined as foveoschisis or extrafoveal retinoschisis, which may be associated with lamellar holes or epiretinal membranes; however, preretinal membranes are often hard to distinguish from inner laminar membrane detachment in high myopia [3,4]. DSM/RSM is recognized as an inward bulge of the macula within the chorioretinal posterior concavity of the eye at the macular location in OCT that is sometimes associated with serous macular detachment [3]. Presence of peripapillary atrophy was subclassified by us as (1) myopic conus, (2) circumpapillary atrophy, (3) circumpapillary atrophy involving the macula, or (4) extensive circumpapillary atrophy involving the fovea. A tilted disk was considered to be present if the optic nerve entered the eye at an oblique angle, usually infero-nasal, while being rotated along its anterior–posterior axis [25]. We also looked for rare findings, such as macular pits defined as a sharp retina, RPE, choroid and scleral outpouching usually located within an area of patchy macular atrophy; choroidal cavitation defined as an absence of the choroidal space that is preferably located adjacent to the optic disc; scleral dehiscence defined as full-thickness scleral defects, together with outward displacement of the retina; vascular folds defined as paravascular inner retinal cleavage due to the traction of the vessels within a staphyloma detected on OCT; and perforating scleral vessels (PSV) defined as hypofluorescent vessel-like areas breaking through the sclera and reaching the choroid, demonstrating the relationship between them and other macular lesions [26–28]. The foveal avascular zone (FAZ) area and its perimeter at the superficial and deep retinal plexus were then manually measured using the caliper tool in the 6 × 6 OCTA macula-centered scans, where the segmentation was automatically performed by the software. The retinal thickness was measured manually from the external limiting membrane to the Bruch–retinal pigmented epithelium (B-RPE) complex. The choroidal thickness was measured from the B-RPE complex to the choroidal–scleral junction. The scleral thickness was measured from the choroidal–scleral junction to the end of the visible sclera. The vertical HD spotlight scan that produced the measurements was performed by one researcher (PAL). The presence of the cilioretinal artery was evaluated using retinography and classified according to the criterion of Meng et al. [29].

The appropriate sample size was calculated for estimating the proportion of staphyloma that was considered as the principal variable. A sample size of 100 eyes was obtained to estimate an expected proportion of 0.5 with an accuracy of 0.1 and a statistical power and significance level of 80% and 0.05, respectively.

Data were collected in an Excel sheet (MS, Redmond, WA, USA) and statistical analysis was performed using the Statistical Package for the Social Sciences version 23 (IBM, Armonk, NY, USA) for Windows. Quantitative variables are expressed as the mean ± standard deviation (SD) and categorical variables as percentages.

3. Results

A total of 179 eyes of 100 patients were studied (68.7% women; age, 50.58 ± 14.98 years; VA, 0.18 ± 0.29 logMAR; AL, 28.83 ± 2.34 mm). A total of 6 of the 21 excluded eyes were rejected due to poor-quality OCT images, and the rest did not fulfil the inclusion criteria (mainly second eyes with AL < 26 mm of anisometropic patients). Of the six eyes excluded for poor images, the reasons for exclusion were poor fixation for very low VA (four eyes), intraocular lens opacification (one eye), and endotropia (one eye).

Staphyloma was detected in the OCT images in 123 (68.7%) eyes, and it was possible to classify all of them. The types of staphylomas detected and classified based on OCT imaging are presented in Figure 1.

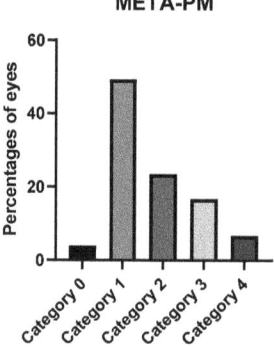

Figure 1. Types of detected staphylomas.

The most common types of staphyloma were the wide and the narrow macular types, followed by the nasal and peripapillary types and the least common were the inferior and other types. The images of each type of staphyloma are presented in Figure 2.

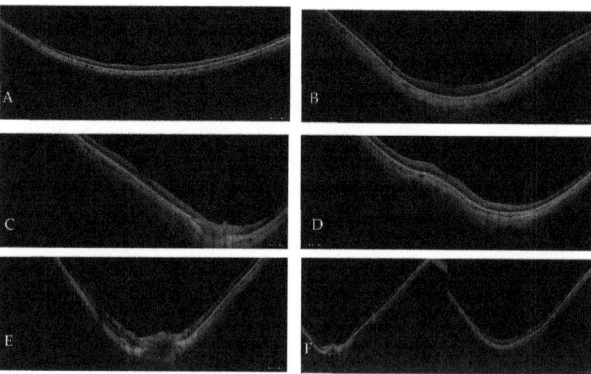

Figure 2. Types of staphylomas: (**A**) wide macular; (**B**) narrow macular; (**C**) nasal; (**D**) inferior; (**E**) peripapillary, and (**F**) other types. All images are horizontal in orientation except D.

Atrophic maculopathy grading according to the META-PM classification is presented in Figure 3.

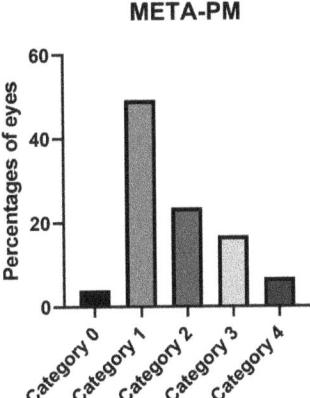

Figure 3. Percentage of eyes in the categories of the META-PM classification.

The number of eyes in each category of the ATN classification is shown in Table 1.

Table 1. Number of Eyes in Each ATN Category.

Atrophic Classification	No. of Eyes	Tractional Classification	No. of Eyes	Neovascular Classification	No. of Eyes
A0	7	T0	160	N0	136
A1	87	T1	6	N1	12
A2	41	T2	9	N2a	7
A3	32	T3	2	N2s	27
A4	12	T4	2		

The number of eyes in each atrophic category is correlated with the META-PM classification because their criteria are identical. We obtained 29 possible combinations, resulting in a mixture of the three categories. The most frequent combinations were as follows: 78 eyes with A1T0N0 (43.57%), 27 eyes with A2T0N0 (15.08%), and 13 eyes with A3T0N2 (7.26%). According to this classification, 125 eyes (69.8%) from our sample had PM.

The results obtained when using the IMI OCT classification are shown in Table 2.

Table 2. Number of Eyes in Each Category of the IMI OCT Classification.

IMI OCT Classification	No. of Eyes
No MM	88
Ia	19
Ib	27
II	12
III	5
IIIa	17
IIIb	11

Lacquer cracks identified as linear Bruch membrane defects (BMD) on structural OCT frames were found in 18 eyes (10.11%) (Figure 4), whereas 7 eyes showed signs of active CNV at the time of the study (Figure 5), and 32 (17.88%) showed identifiable inactive CNV, the so-called Fuch's spot (Figure 6). The mean subfoveal choroidal thickness of the eyes with CNV was 75.66 ± 38.5 µm (range, 27–133 µm). When evaluating the CNV location, 2 (33.33%) eyes were subfoveal and 4 (66.67%) perifoveal, whereas 11 (33.33%)

eyes had a subfoveal Fuch's spot, 21 (63.63%) had a perifoveal spot and 1 eye demonstrated a spot > 3 mm from the fovea.

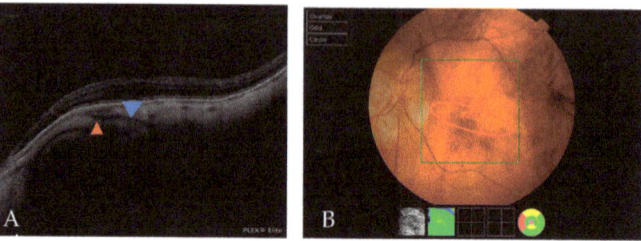

Figure 4. (**A**) An OCT scan that shows a BMD caused by a lacquer crack (blue arrowhead). The red arrowhead indicates a PEV reaching the choroid. (**B**) A fundus image of the same patient, in which the red circle indicates a lacquer crack.

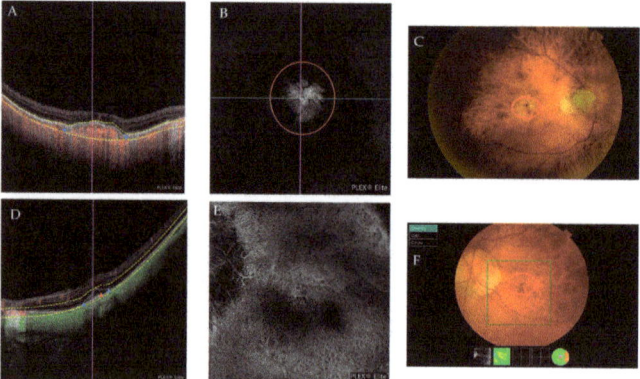

Figure 5. (**A–C**) Multimodal imaging from the same patient with a Fuch's spot. (**A**) The blue arrowheads indicate the limits of the CNV. (**B**) The outer retina to the choriocapillaris (ORCC) on the OCTA images with a tailing artifact removed from the en-face image. The red circle indicates the CNV. (**C**) The red circle indicates the position of the CNV obtained via retinography. (**D,E**) Multimodal imaging from the same patient presenting with active CNV. (**D**) An OCT scan that shows signs of CNV activity with retinal thickening due to subretinal fluid and small intraretinal cysts (red arrowhead). Its limits are indicated by the blue arrowheads. (**E**) En-face ORCC from an OCTA image of the same patient. (**F**) The red circle indicates the presence of the membrane and blood in this patient's retinography.

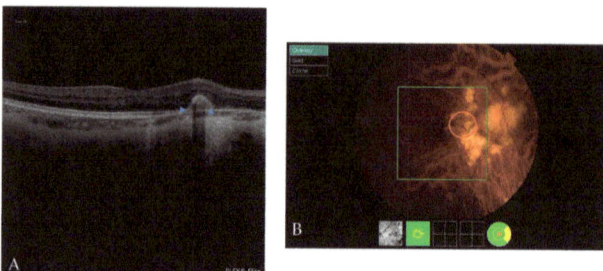

Figure 6. Multimodal image of a Fuch´s spot. (**A**) An OCT scan shows a Fuch´s spot (blue arrowheads). (**B**) The red circle indicates the Fuch´s spot in the retinography.

A BMD associated with patchy or macular atrophy was found in 42 (23.46%) eyes. A BMD associated with peripapillary atrophy was found in 83 (46.37%) eyes (Figure 7).

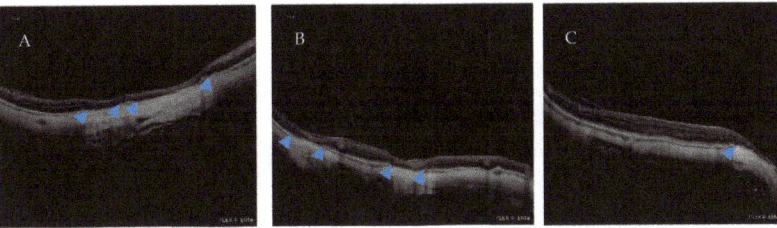

Figure 7. (**A**) An OCT scan of the BMDs associated with patchy atrophy. (**B**) An OCT scan of a BMD involving the fovea. (**C**) An OCT scan of a BMD associated with peripapillary atrophy. Blue arrowheads indicate the presence of BMDs.

A total of 45 eyes (24%) had extrafoveal retinoschisis, of which 20 (46.5%) had inner and outer retinoschisis, 11 (25.64%) had inner retinoschisis only, and 6 had purely outer retinoschisis. Two eyes had either inner or outer retinoschisis and a lamellar hole and two eyes had both inner and outer retinoschisis and a lamellar hole (Figure 8).

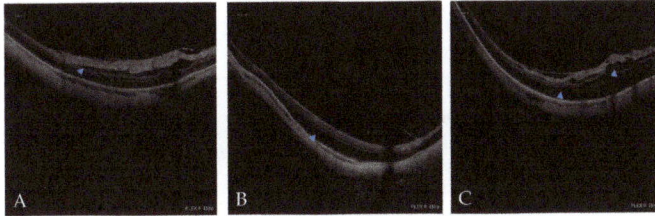

Figure 8. (**A**) An OCT scan of inner retinoschisis. (**B**) An OCT scan of outer retinoschisis. (**C**) An OCT scan of inner and outer retinoschisis. Blue arrowheads indicate the presence of retinoschisis.

We also found that 28 (15.6%) eyes had a DSM. Only one eye had associated subretinal fluid and OCTA excluded the presence of CNV (Figure 9). We also found a RSM in six eyes, as defined by the IMI OCT classification, four of which were found via vertical scans and were associated with inferior staphyloma.

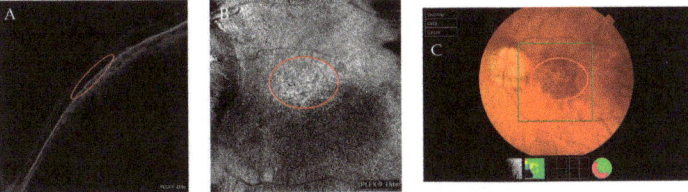

Figure 9. Multimodal images of a DSM. (**A**) In an OCT scan, the red circle indicates the presence of subretinal fluid. (**B**) In an en-face image, the red circle indicates a hyperreflective area correlated with the subretinal fluid. (**C**) In a retinography image, the red circle indicates the area where subretinal fluid is present.

We also evaluated the optic nerve head in the retinography scan and found that 70 (39.1%) eyes had a tilted optic nerve head. Myopic conus was present in 73 (40.72%) eyes; 59 eyes (80.08%) had it temporally, 10 nasally and 3 inferiorly, and 1 had a myopic conus exceeding one quadrant. More extensive peripapillary atrophy was present in 83 eyes (46.37%), and of them, 60 eyes (72.29%) had minor circumpapillary atrophy, 20 eyes (24.1%)

had atrophy extending toward the macular area, and 3 eyes had atrophy extending toward the fovea.

Four eyes had a macular pit, two of which were associated with scleral dehiscence (Figures 10 and 11).

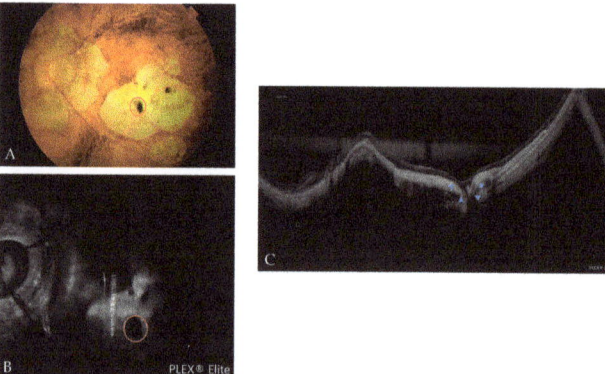

Figure 10. Multimodal images of a macular pit with scleral dehiscence. (**A**) In a fundus photograph, the red circle indicates a grayish and black lesion that is correlated with the pit. (**B**) In an OCT reflectance image, the red circle indicates an area of hyporeflectance correlated with the pit. (**C**) In an OCT scan, the blue arrowheads indicate the pit with scleral dehiscence.

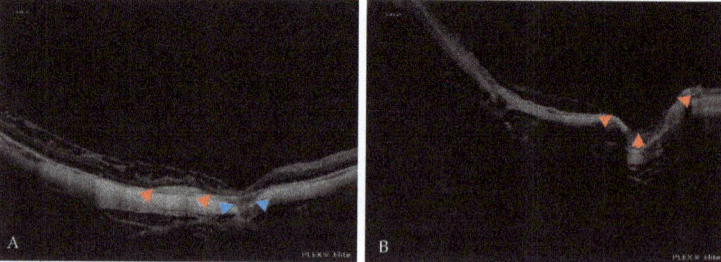

Figure 11. (**A**) In an OCT scan, the blue arrowheads indicate scleral dehiscence. The red arrowheads indicate a Fuch´s spot. (**B**) In an OCT scan, the red arrowheads indicate the macular pit.

Six eyes had scleral dehiscence without a macular pit. Scleral dehiscence and macular pits were both found in areas of chorioretinal atrophy. Choroidal cavitation was detected in six eyes (Figure 12).

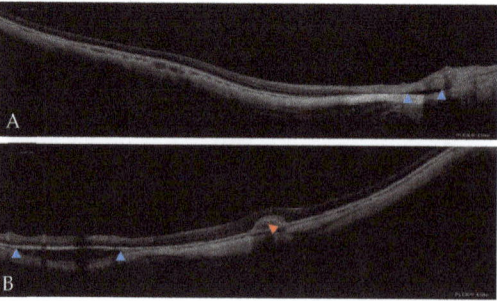

Figure 12. In the OCT scans, the blue arrowheads indicate intrachoroidal cavitation (ICC). (**A**) A small ICC is near the optic nerve head. (**B**) A large ICC is in the vicinity of the CNV (red arrowhead).

Seventy-seven eyes (43%) had vascular folds in the HD51 scan (Figure 13). PSV were detected in 159 eyes (88.8%) and 16 of them were related to a Fuch´s spot and 4 eyes with active CNV. Seven eyes had PSV with lacquer cracks.

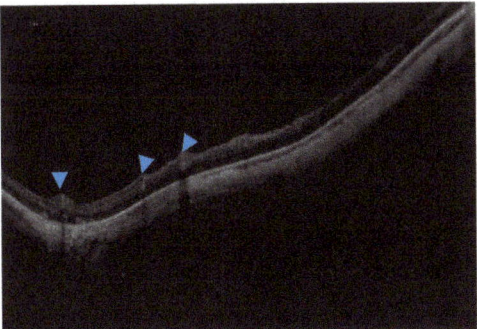

Figure 13. In an OCT scan, the blue arrowheads indicate vascular folds.

Concerning the retinal, choroidal, and scleral foveal thicknesses, six eyes were excluded due to their inability to detect the fovea, mainly because of macular atrophy (Figure 14).

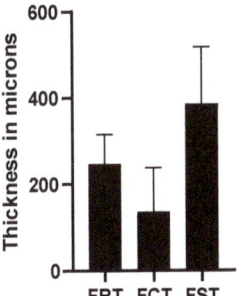

Figure 14. Retina, choroidal, and scleral foveal thicknesses. FRT = foveal retinal thickness; FCT = foveal choroidal thickness; FST = foveal scleral thickness.

Only 132 eyes were evaluated to measure the FAZ and its perimeter due to segmentation errors at the superficial plexus and 127 for the deep plexus. The results from those eyes are shown in Figure 15.

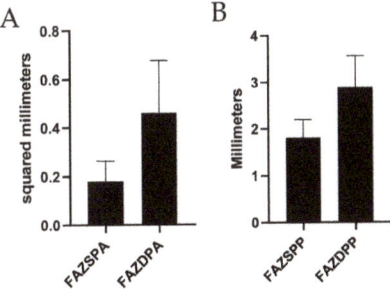

Figure 15. The mean area (**A**) and perimeter (**B**) for superficial and deep plexuses in the FAZ. FAZSPA = foveal avascular zone and superficial plexus area; FAZSPP = foveal avascular zone and superficial plexus perimeter; FAZDPA = foveal avascular zone and deep plexus area; FAZDPP = foveal avascular zone and deep plexus perimeter.

Only 166 fundus retinographies could be analyzed to study the cilioretinal arteries due to problems of focus or loss of transparency that made the task difficult. We found a cilioretinal artery in 20 eyes (12.04%), and the different types of cilioretinal arteries are presented in Figure 16.

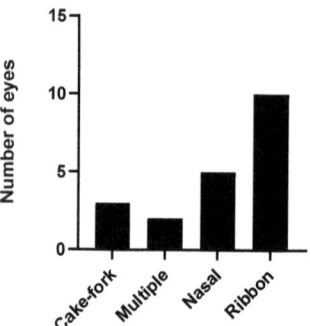

Figure 16. Number of eyes with each type of cilioretinal artery.

Table 3 shows a comparison among other studies of FAZ measurements. Table 4 shows a comparison among different studies of the retinal, choroidal, and scleral foveal thicknesses.

Table 3. Comparison of the FAZ Measurements among Different Studies.

Authors and Countries	Xiuyan et al. [30] China	Lee et al. [31] Republic of Korea	Arlanzón et al. Spain (Present Study)
No. of eyes	154	30	179
Baseline age (years) mean ± SD	21.80 ± 1.32	55.5 ± 13.5	50.58 ± 14.98
Mean spherical equivalent ± SD	−4.06 ± 2.26 D	−9.98 ± 5.03 D	−6.74 ± 6.44D
SPFAZA (mm)	0.1835 ± 0.0477	0.37 ± 0.15	0.18 ± 0.084
DPFAZA (mm)	0.3299 ± 0.0601	0.43 ± 0.16	0.46 ± 0.217

SPFAZA = superficial plexus foveal avascular zone area; DPFAZA = deep plexus foveal avascular zone area.

Table 4. Comparison of Retinal, Choroidal and Scleral Layer Thicknesses among Different Studies.

Authors and Countries	Xiuyan et al. [30] China	Liu et al. [32] China	Park et al. [33] Republic of Korea	Wong et al. [34] Singapore	Maruko et al. [35] Japan	Hayashi et al. [36] Japan	Tan et al. [37] China	Arlanzón et al. Spain (Present Study)
No. of eyes	154	30	237	92	58	75	38	179
Baseline age (years) mean ± SD	21.80 ± 1.32	24.43 ± 3.43	63.0 ± 11.6	60.2 ± 8.4	65.5 ± NA	62.3 ± 11.3	NA	50.58 ± 14.98
Mean spherical equivalent ± SD in diopter	−4.06 ± 2.26	−7.85 ± 1.37	−15.4 ± 5.4	−12.5 ± 5.1	−12.8 ± 3.6	−12.9 ± 4.1	−7.35 ± 1.1	−6.74 ± 6.44
Retinal thickness (μm)	252.14 ± 17.33	240.91 ± 13.36	NA	NA	206 ± 92	NA	NA	247.06 ± 68.87
Choroidal thickness (μm)	232.16 ± 56.65	NA	29.2 ± 21.7 with staphyloma 46.9 ± 39.3 without staphyloma	82.0 ± 57.12 in mild MMD 31.5 ± 0.5 in severe MMD	52 ± 38	NA	253.8 ± 71.0	135.95 ± 102.44
Scleral thickness (μm)	NA	NA	268.7 ± 95.9 with staphyloma 316.2 ± 76.5 without staphyloma	297.0 ± 73.8 in mild MMD 261.6 ± 78.5 in severe MMD	335 ± 130	284.0 ± 70.4	NA	385.40 ± 131.41

MMD = myopic macular degeneration; NA = not applicable; SD = standard deviation.

4. Discussion

In this study, multimodal imaging was used to detect the main complications of the eyes with PM. We used structural SS-OCT and SS-OCTA supported by retinography to detect macular lesions related to PM. To our knowledge, this is the largest study that uses a Caucasian sample and focuses on a high number of lesions, which is important, as Spanish PM cohorts may not behave in the same way as Asian cohorts [22]. Our study highlights the importance and potential of the use of widefield SS-OCT to detect less frequently reported complications in PM, such as macular pits, choroidal cavitations, scleral dehiscence, PSV, or vessel folds.

We evaluated the presence of staphyloma using HD spotlight 16 mm line scans with which we could identify and define the size, location, and limits of staphylomas in many patients, which are difficult to assess with other OCT tools whose scan size may be smaller or produce mirror artifacts that make image interpretation difficult. The percentage of patients with staphyloma is smaller compared to an early study published by our group (92.7%) [22]. This may be explained by the fact that our previous study recruited patients only from the retina unit, which may have introduced bias toward more severe pathology; this study included patients from other specialties, such as refractive surgery, and the findings were not only based on the OCT assessment performed in the present study, which also might have affected the results. In the study of Haarman et al. [38], a prevalence rate of up to 43% of posterior staphyloma was found, which was more common with older age. This number is smaller than ours, but the study of Haarman et al. was based on the general population. Our results are slightly lower than those of Shinohara et al. [39] (75% of eyes in an Asian sample), but the authors also found that the wide macular and narrow macular types were most prevalent, similar to the results of our study and to that of Frisina et al. [40], who also found wide macular and narrow macular types to be the most common types of staphyloma in a Caucasian HM sample.

A multimodal approach to detect lacquer cracks is advised, mainly because lacquer cracks are sometimes small defects that can be missed by OCT [41]; thus, we evaluated the presence of lacquer cracks by combining retinography and OCT that are viewed as linear BMDs. The percentage of lacquer cracks found in the current study is similar to our previous results [22] and slightly lower than that found by Fang et al. (14.7%) [42] in an Asian sample, whereas Park et al. [33] found higher values (24.5%); however, the AL in their sample was longer than ours, which may explain the differences.

We used OCT and OCTA to detect CNV and Fuch's spot. However, it is difficult sometimes to distinguish between the two, since flow can also be detected by OCTA in some Fuch's spots. The neovascular vessels also may be difficult to detect in the en-face image of OCTA due to the extreme retinal thinning in patients with PM, changes in the curvature of the posterior pole, and the presence of segmentation errors. In fact, a differential diagnosis must often be carried out considering the patient's symptomatology. The percentage reported in this study is similar to our previous study [22]. Fang et al. [42] found higher percentages in their PM cohort of 26.9%, but a smaller value in their overall HM and PM cohorts of 17.3%. Our results also are higher than those of Park et al. [33] of 7.6%, although their mean AL was also longer. When comparing the results of atrophic maculopathy to those obtained in the previous study published by our group [22], we also found that category 1 was the most frequently found category. The main difference arises in category 3, as our previous study found a higher percentage for this category, which may be explained again by the differences in the recruitment origin that have been previously mentioned. Our results differed significantly from those of Ruão et al. [23], in that they found a prevalence for patchy atrophy (category 3 in our study) of 79.9% compared to our value of 16.8%. They also found higher values for CNV, which was present in 61.9% of their eyes, since their recruitment was carried out in the macula unit of a large hospital, which also may have introduced bias toward the presence of more severe symptomatic pathology. A comparison of the results obtained in our study with large population studies with different designs may not be valuable [19].

We found that 69.8% of our sample had MM, as defined by the META-PM classification, which differs from that obtained by Haarman et al. [38], who found a prevalence of 25.9% in a Dutch HM sample. The differences may be due to the different ethnicities and the fact that our sample had a longer AL; their recruitment process also differed in that the study of Haarman et al. was population-based.

The use of the ATN classification [4] can help us to better characterize all pathological features that can be found in patients with PM. It is interesting that none of the five most common combined categories had a tractional component of T1 or higher, which is understandable considering that in our sample, 89.4% of eyes did not have any tractional component. We also must consider that the T component refers to tractional damage to the macular area, but does not consider extramacular tractional damage and because of this, these extrafoveal features are missed in the ATN classification. Another limitation of this classification is that the neovascular dominion includes lacquer cracks, active CNV, and Fuch´s spots, but one patient may have more than one; however, only one of them may be detected. Nevertheless, this classification provides a very useful understanding of PM. The use of the IMI OCT classification [3] enables a complete evaluation of the patients with HM and PM without using any tools except OCT, and it is the only classification that includes DSM/RSM in the definitions of PM. OCT is the only tool that facilitates the diagnosis of most of the complications of HM. We believe that any patient with HM should undergo this examination regularly. Finally, as the definitions and classifications have changed throughout the past 20 years, it is difficult to compare results between different studies.

In our study, we looked for extrafoveal retinoschisis, in addition to the foveal retinoschisis already assessed with the ATN classification. In our evaluations, we found that inner plus outer retinoschisis was the most frequent presentation. Similar results were found in the study of Ruão et al. [23], who found extrafoveal retinoschisis in 23.9% of their patients' eyes. However, Xiao et al. reported that the most prevalent type of extrafoveal retinoschisis in their sample was the inner type [43], although they selected a sample of patients with a previous diagnosis of extrafoveal retinoschisis, which may explain the difference.

The prevalence of DSM in our sample was within the range previously published [44]. Interestingly, only one eye had subretinal fluid due to this condition, although it is the main recognized complication of DSM, whose prevalence has been reported to vary from 2% to 67% [44]. We also observed two eyes with RSM that was unrelated to inferior staphylomas, which was hypothesized to be an early sign of evolving DSM that is more frequently found in younger patients with HM [44].

Alterations in the optic nerve were common in our sample. Nearly half of the patients had circumpapillary atrophy, which extended toward the temporal side and involved the macular area in 23 eyes, whereas 40% of patients had a myopic crescent, unlike the results published by Haarman et al. [38], who reported a value of up to 80% of peripapillary atrophy in their sample, with a higher frequency in older patients, although they do not distinguish between myopic conus and circumpapillary atrophy. He et al. [45] identified peripapillary atrophy in 112 of 134 eyes and this was the most frequent sign observed in HM, whereas Fang et al. [42] reported a prevalence of 89.5%. All these figures along with our results indicate the high prevalence of this kind of lesion, which has already been reported. The evaluation of this sign is important because it is the most frequent sign of progression of PM and this area of peripapillary atrophy can extend toward the macula, as the previously mentioned authors found.

Macular pits, defined as focal excavations in atrophic areas [26,46,47], are viewed as focal depressions in the OCT scans, usually in areas of complete chorioretinal atrophy. In the fundus images, a greyish lesion inside the atrophic area is indicative of the presence of the pit. These lesions can be defined as hypofluorescence in fundus reflectance images of OCT (Figure 10). To our knowledge, no prevalence rates have been reported because only a small number of case series have been published. We found four eyes with a macular pit and two of them were accompanied by scleral dehiscence. In addition, six eyes had scleral dehiscence without a macular pit. All of them were found in atrophic areas. The cause of this kind of lesion remains unclear, although the uneven force of intraocular pressure in those areas of a debilitated ocular wall may affect its appearance [26].

Freund [48] first described ICC as pigmented retinal epithelium detachment in the peripapillary area. Toranzo et al. [49] later reported no pigmented retinal epithelium detachment and suggested its current name. ICC can be observed in structural OCT as a hyporeflectant space where the choroid should be. The frequency with which we observed this anomaly is similar to the one obtained by Shimada [50]m who reported a 4.6% prevalence rate in their sample. You et al. [51] reported a higher prevalence in the Beijing Eye Study in 15 of 89 subjects with HM with OCT images that showed ICC. In addition, Haarman et al. [38] reported similar prevalence levels of ICC in a Caucasian sample. These numbers indicated that ICC is not an uncommon alteration and wide-field SS-OCT is key to correctly detect and characterize it.

Forty-three percent of the patients' eyes had vessel folds, which is indicative of the rigidity of the vessel in contrast to the prevalent sign of retinal elongation in our study. Sayanagi et al. [52] also reported vascular folds in an HM sample, but that case series included only seven eyes.

We also identified PEV in 88.8% of eyes, a sign that some authors believe is a possible connection to CNV [53,54]. In fact, we did find an association between PEV and lacquer cracks, CNV, and Fuch´s spots in some eyes, but most eyes did not have any of these conditions or the PEVs were not in the same location. Since this finding is so frequent, it may also well be that colocalization of PEV and CNV occurs by chance.

We could not analyze the FAZ in all of the eyes due to segmentation errors, which made measurement difficult. When comparing our results with normal subjects, an increase in SPFAZ was observed across studies [55–59]. DPFAZ shows greater heterogeneity, with some studies showing smaller values [56,58,59], while others reported higher values [55,57]. These results indicate a change in the FAZ area of myopes compared to healthy subjects, which is probably caused by the elongation of the ocular layers. However, these comparisons should be considered carefully because the equipment and methodology vary greatly across studies. Table 3 shows an overview of the measurements of FAZ in different studies. The SPFAZ values are equal to the results published by Xiuyan et al. [30], although their sample consisted of moderate myopes, but the values were smaller than those reported by Lee et al. [31]. However, the DPFAZ area was slightly larger in our study than the one published by Lee et al. [31], but smaller than that reported by Xiuyan et al. [30].

We manually measured the retinal, choroidal, and scleral foveal thicknesses using the HD spotlight vertical line scan. Although seven eyes had to be eliminated because it was impossible to identify the fovea, we measured the fovea in most of the studied eyes. Our results indicate high dispersion, which may be explained by the different alterations that occur in myopic eyes, such as the different types of staphylomas, CNVs, DSMs, or the presence of macular atrophy that can affect the measurements. Global elongation results in thinning of the ocular layers [33–36,60]. This is evident when comparing the thicknesses of the HM eyes to those of healthy subjects [37]. Our results showed some variations compared to the published data. We found thinner mean retinal thicknesses compared to healthy adults, as expected [37]. However, our retinas were thicker compared to the results reported by Liu et al. [32] and Maruko et al. [35], but thinner than those reported by Xiuyan et al. [30]. Thus, it is possible to observe heterogeneity in the values obtained in the scientific literature. The results for choroidal and scleral thicknesses also showed thinner values compared to healthy eyes, with values that are nearly half of those published [37,61]. If we focused on studies about HM samples, high heterogeneity can also be detected. For choroidal thickness, Park et al. [33], Wong et al. [34], and Maruko et al. [35] reported smaller values than those obtained in our study. In contrast, Tan et al. [37] and Xiuyan et al. [30] reported higher values compared with the current study. Again, these differences may be explained by the heterogeneity of PM with different types of macular alterations that may affect the choroidal thickness. These differences also apply to the scleral thickness in that our results were higher than those of Park et al. [33], Wong et al. [34], Maruko et al. [35], and Hayashi et al. [36]. However, differences of up to 70 μm can be observed across studies that may be based on measurement methodologies, sample characteristics, or the type of OCT used.

We found that 12.5% of eyes had cilioretinal arteries in our sample, which is slightly lower than that reported by Zhu et al. [62], who found that 17.05% of their patients' eyes had a cilioretinal artery or the 14.5% reported by Meng [29]. The most common type of cilioretinal artery in the current study was a temporal ribbon, which is consistent with the results of Meng et al. [29] who used the same classification. The importance of this cilioretinal artery arises from the study of Zhu et al. [62], in that the results suggested that the presence of a cilioretinal artery may increase the macular vascular flow, resulting in better VA, which we could not verify with our data.

HM and PM are important causes of visual loss, but the existing literature on the associated causative pathologies is insufficient. Furthermore, studies have been conducted primarily in Asian countries. Thus, our results contribute to a better understanding of the frequency of observations of macular complications of HM and PM in a Caucasian sample. Likewise, it highlights the importance of novel equipment, such as SS-OCT, in the diagnosis of this pathology, as the PLEX® Elite 9000 OCT was the main diagnostic tool used in this study.

The main limitations of this study were the sample characteristics. We recruited patients with HM who sought consultation in an ophthalmic clinic. Thus, the frequency of observations that has been presented may be biased toward more severe pathology, in that patients with high myopes without symptoms may not seek ophthalmologic consultation. Nevertheless, we included the healthiest patients from the refractive unit to minimize this bias. Another limitation arises from the maximal length of the OCT spotlight scan used to diagnose staphyloma. Although 16 mm is long, it may be insufficient to detect all kinds of staphylomas, and optic nerve staphylomas may be more difficult to detect.

The current study was large and demonstrated the use of this tool to better assess the posterior pole in most patients with HM. We encourage clinicians to perform wide-field OCT in all patients with HM.

5. Conclusions

In this study, we presented the frequency of observations of lesions in the posterior pole using OCT in a HM Spanish Caucasian cohort, which may be important for epidemiologic purposes and for a better understanding of PM. The role of wide-field OCT as the main diagnostic tool to detect macular alterations in PM has been highlighted. SS-OCT is a novel tool that is more potent than previous generations of OCTs and can detect most major complications of PM in the posterior pole, such as retinoschisis or CNV, and less frequent alterations, such as macular pits or ICC. Most importantly, some pathologies, such as perforating scleral vessels, can only be identified with this new equipment; these vessels seem to more common than previously thought and they seem to be unrelated to CNV.

Author Contributions: R.M.C.-M. conceived the study, analyzed the data, revised the manuscript, interpreted, and validated the data, and ensured that questions related to the accuracy or integrity of any part of the work were appropriately investigated. P.A.-L. and M.A.C. collected the data. P.A.-L. also contributed to the writing of the paper and interpreted the data. I.F.-B. supervised the project and wrote the methodology. All authors have read and agreed to the published version of the manuscript.

Funding: This research received no external funding.

Institutional Review Board Statement: The study was conducted in accordance with the Declaration of Helsinki and approved by the Institutional Review Board (or Ethics Committee) of the Comité ético de investigación con medicamentos del área de salud de Valladolid Oeste (protocol code PI 21-2161 on 11 February 2021).

Informed Consent Statement: Written informed consent has been obtained from the patients to publish this paper.

Data Availability Statement: Authors can make their research data available, accessible, and usable if necessary.

Acknowledgments: The authors are grateful to M.J. Maldonado and Carolina Ossa Calderón that allowed the recruitment of patients from their clinics.

Conflicts of Interest: The authors declare no conflict of interest. Nevertheless, the University of Valladolid and the IOBA belong to the Advanced Retina Imaging (ARI) Network, with ZEISS PLEX Elite 9000 at its core, formed by expert leading clinicians and researchers around the world with scientists and developers at ZEISS to accelerate the development of innovations to benefit patients through an active exchange of ideas and findings. The aim of the ARI Network is to drive the development of new clinical applications and future OCT technologies (www.zeiss.com/arinetwork accessed on 23 February 2023).

References

1. Ohno-Matsui, K. Pathologic Myopia: *Asia-Pac. J. Ophthalmol.* **2016**, *5*, 415–423. [CrossRef]
2. Flitcroft, D.I.; He, M.; Jonas, J.B.; Jong, M.; Naidoo, K.; Ohno-Matsui, K.; Rahi, J.; Resnikoff, S.; Vitale, S.; Yannuzzi, L. IMI—Defining and Classifying Myopia: A Proposed Set of Standards for Clinical and Epidemiologic Studies. *Investig. Opthalmol. Vis. Sci.* **2019**, *60*, M20. [CrossRef] [PubMed]
3. Ohno-Matsui, K.; Wu, P.-C.; Yamashiro, K.; Vutipongsatorn, K.; Fang, Y.; Cheung, C.M.G.; Lai, T.Y.Y.; Ikuno, Y.; Cohen, S.Y.; Gaudric, A.; et al. IMI Pathologic Myopia. *Investig. Opthalmol. Vis. Sci.* **2021**, *62*, 5. [CrossRef] [PubMed]
4. Ruiz-Medrano, J.; Montero, J.A.; Flores-Moreno, I.; Arias, L.; García-Layana, A.; Ruiz-Moreno, J.M. Myopic maculopathy: Current status and proposal for a new classification and grading system (ATN). *Prog. Retin. Eye Res.* **2019**, *69*, 80–115. [CrossRef]
5. Spaide, R.F. Staphyloma. Part 1. In *Pathologic Myopia*; Springer: New York, NY, USA, 2013.
6. Curtin, B.J. The posterior staphyloma of pathologic myopia. *Trans. Am. Ophthalmol. Soc.* **1977**, *75*, 20.
7. Ohno-Matsui, K. Proposed Classification of Posterior Staphylomas Based on Analyses of Eye Shape by Three-Dimensional Magnetic Resonance Imaging and Wide-Field Fundus Imaging. *Ophthalmology* **2014**, *121*, 1798–1809. [CrossRef]
8. Németh, J.; Tapasztó, B.; Aclimandos, W.A.; Kestelyn, P.; Jonas, J.B.; De Faber, J.-T.H.N.; Januleviciene, I.; Grzybowsk, A.; Nagy, Z.Z.; Pärssinen, O. Update and guidance on management of myopia. European Society of Ophthalmology in cooperation with International Myopia Institute. *Eur. J. Ophthalmol.* **2021**, *31*, 853–883. [CrossRef]
9. Curtin, B.J.; Karlin, D.B. Axial length measurements and fundus changes of the myopic eye I. the posterior fundus. *Trans. Am. Ophthalmol. Soc.* **1970**, *68*, 23.
10. Avila, M.P.; Weiter, J.J.; Jalkh, A.E.; Trempe, C.L.; Pruett, R.C.; Schepens, C.L. Natural History of Choroidal Neovascularization in Degenerative Myopia. *Ophthalmology* **1984**, *91*, 1573–1581. [CrossRef]
11. Ohno-Matsui, K.; Kawasaki, R.; Jonas, J.B.; Cheung, C.M.G.; Saw, S.-M.; Verhoeven, V.J.M.; Klaver, C.C.W.; Moriyama, M.; Shinohara, K.; Kawasaki, Y.; et al. International Photographic Classification and Grading System for Myopic Maculopathy. *Am. J. Ophthalmol.* **2015**, *159*, 877–883.e7. [CrossRef]
12. Gohil, R.; Sivaprasad, S.; Han, L.T.; Mathew, R.; Kiousis, G.; Yang, Y. Myopic foveoschisis: A clinical review. *Eye* **2015**, *29*, 593–601. [CrossRef] [PubMed]
13. Xu, X.; Fang, Y.; Jonas, J.B.; Du, R.; Shinohara, K.; Tanaka, N.; Yokoi, T.; Onishi, Y.; Uramoto, K.; Kamoi, K.; et al. Ridge-shaped macula in young myopic patients and its differentiation from typical dome-sahped macula in elderly myopic patients. *Retina* **2020**, *40*, 225–232. [CrossRef] [PubMed]
14. Takano, M.; Kishi, S. Foveal retinoschisis and retinal detachment in severely myopic eyes with posterior staphyloma. *Am. J. Ophthalmol.* **1999**, *128*, 472–476. [CrossRef] [PubMed]
15. Ikuno, Y.; Jo, Y.; Hamasaki, T.; Tano, Y. Ocular Risk Factors for Choroidal Neovascularization in Pathologic Myopia. *Investig. Opthalmol. Vis. Sci.* **2010**, *51*, 3721. [CrossRef]
16. Leveziel, N.; Yu, Y.; Reynolds, R.; Tai, A.; Meng, W.; Caillaux, V.; Calvas, P.; Rosner, B.; Malecaze, F.; Souied, E.H.; et al. Genetic Factors for Choroidal Neovascularization Associated with High Myopia. *Investig. Opthalmol. Vis. Sci.* **2012**, *53*, 5004. [CrossRef]
17. Bruyère, E.; Miere, A.; Cohen, S.Y.; Martiano, D.; Sikorav, A.; Popeanga, A.; Semoun, O.; Querques, G.; Souied, E.H. Neovascularization secondary to high myopia imaged by optical coherence tomography angiography. *Retina* **2017**, *37*, 2095–2101. [CrossRef] [PubMed]
18. Miyata, M.; Ooto, S.; Hata, M.; Yamashiro, K.; Tamura, H.; Akagi-Kurashige, Y.; Nakanishi, H.; Ueda-Arakawa, N.; Takahashi, A.; Kuroda, Y.; et al. Detection of Myopic Choroidal Neovascularization Using Optical Coherence Tomography Angiography. *Am. J. Ophthalmol.* **2016**, *165*, 108–114. [CrossRef] [PubMed]
19. Zou, M.; Wang, S.; Chen, A.; Liu, Z.; Young, C.A.; Zhang, Y.; Jin, G.; Zheng, D. Prevalence of myopic macular degeneration worldwide: A systematic review and meta-analysis. *Br. J. Ophthalmol.* **2020**, *104*, 1748–1754. [CrossRef]
20. Hashemi, H.; Fotouhi, A.; Yekta, A.; Pakzad, R.; Ostadimoghaddam, H.; Khabazkhoob, M. Global and regional estimates of prevalence of refractive errors: Systematic review and meta-analysis. *J. Curr. Ophthalmol.* **2018**, *30*, 3–22. [CrossRef]

21. Sainz-Gómez, C.; Fernández-Robredo, P.; Salinas-Alamán, Á.; Montañés, J.M.; Berasategui, J.M.E.; Guillén-Grima, F.; Ruiz-Moreno, J.M.; Garcia-Layana, A. Prevalence and Causes of Bilateral Blindness and Visual Impairment among Institutionalized Elderly People in Pamplona, Spain. *Eur. J. Ophthalmol.* **2010**, *20*, 442–450. [CrossRef]
22. Coco-Martin, R.M.; Belani-Raju, M.; de la Fuente-Gomez, D.; Sanabria, M.R.; Fernández, I. Progression of myopic maculopathy in a Caucasian cohort of highly myopic patients with long follow-up: A multistate analysis. *Graefes Arch. Clin. Exp. Ophthalmol.* **2021**, *259*, 81–92. [CrossRef]
23. Ruão, M.; Andreu-Fenoll, M.; Dolz-Marco, R.; Gallego-Pinazo, R. Prevalence of Different Optical Coherence Tomography Findings in a Spanish Cohort With High Myopia. *J. Vitreoretin. Dis.* **2017**, *1*, 41–44. [CrossRef]
24. Lee, R.; Tham, Y.-C.; Cheung, C.Y.; Sidhartha, E.; Siantar, R.G.; Lim, S.-H.; Wong, T.Y.; Cheng, C.-Y. Factors affecting signal strength in spectral-domain optical coherence tomography. *Acta Ophthalmol.* **2018**, *96*, 54–58. [CrossRef] [PubMed]
25. Witmer, M.T.; Margo, C.E.; Drucker, M. Tilted Optic Disks. *Surv. Ophthalmol.* **2010**, *55*, 403–428. [CrossRef] [PubMed]
26. Ohno-Matsui, K.; Akiba, M.; Moriyama, M. Macular pits and scleral dehiscence in highly myopic eyes with macular chorioretinal atrophy. *Retin. Cases Brief Rep.* **2013**, *7*, 334–337. [CrossRef] [PubMed]
27. Meng, L.-H.; Yuan, M.-Z.; Zhao, X.-Y.; Chen, Y.-X. Macular Bruch's membrane defects and other myopic lesions in high myopia. *Int. J. Ophthalmol.* **2022**, *15*, 466–473. [CrossRef]
28. Faghihi, H.; Hajizadeh, F.; Riazi-Esfahani, M. Optical Coherence Tomographic Findings in Highly Myopic Eyes. *J. Ophthalmic Vis. Res.* **2010**, *5*, 110–121. [PubMed]
29. Meng, Y.; Wei, L.; Zhang, K.; He, W.; Lu, Y.; Zhu, X. Cilioretinal Arteries in Highly Myopic Eyes: A Photographic Classification System and Its Association With Myopic Macular Degeneration. *Front. Med.* **2020**, *7*, 595544. [CrossRef] [PubMed]
30. Xiuyan, Z.; Qingmei, T.; Qiuxin, W.; Tailiang, L.; Jing, X.; Guodong, T.; Ting, Y.; Shasha, L.; Xi, C.; Chenying, Q.; et al. Thickness, vessel density of retina and choroid on OCTA in young adults (18–24 years old). *Microvasc. Res.* **2021**, *136*, 104169. [CrossRef]
31. Lee, J.H.; Lee, M.W.; Baek, S.K.; Lee, Y.H. Repeatability of Manual Measurement of Foveal Avascular Zone Area in Optical Coherence Tomography Angiography Images in High Myopia. *Korean J. Ophthalmol.* **2020**, *34*, 113. [CrossRef]
32. Liu, X.; Shen, M.; Yuan, Y.; Huang, S.; Zhu, D.; Ma, Q.; Ye, X.; Lu, F. Macular Thickness Profiles of Intraretinal Layers in Myopia Evaluated by Ultrahigh-Resolution Optical Coherence Tomography. *Am. J. Ophthalmol.* **2015**, *160*, 53–61.e2. [CrossRef]
33. Park, U.C.; Lee, E.K.; Kim, B.H.; Oh, B.-L. Decreased choroidal and scleral thicknesses in highly myopic eyes with posterior staphyloma. *Sci. Rep.* **2021**, *11*, 7987. [CrossRef]
34. Wong, C.W.; Phua, V.; Lee, S.Y.; Wong, T.Y.; Cheung, C.M.G. Is Choroidal or Scleral Thickness Related to Myopic Macular Degeneration? *Investig. Opthalmol. Vis. Sci.* **2017**, *58*, 907. [CrossRef] [PubMed]
35. Maruko, I.; Iida, T.; Sugano, Y.; Oyamada, H.; Akiba, M.; Sekiryu, T. Morphologic Analysis in Pathologic Myopia Using High-Penetration Optical Coherence Tomography. *Investig. Opthalmol. Vis. Sci.* **2012**, *53*, 3834. [CrossRef] [PubMed]
36. Hayashi, M.; Ito, Y.; Takahashi, A.; Kawano, K.; Terasaki, H. Scleral thickness in highly myopic eyes measured by enhanced depth imaging optical coherence tomography. *Eye* **2013**, *27*, 410–417. [CrossRef] [PubMed]
37. Tan, C.S.H.; Cheong, K.X.; Lim, L.W.; Li, K.Z. Topographic variation of choroidal and retinal thicknesses at the macula in healthy adults. *Br. J. Ophthalmol.* **2014**, *98*, 339–344. [CrossRef]
38. Haarman, A.E.G.; Tedja, M.S.; Brussee, C.; Enthoven, C.A.; van Rijn, G.A.; Vingerling, J.R.; Keunen, J.E.E.; Boon, C.J.F.; Geerards, A.J.M.; Luyten, G.P.M.; et al. Prevalence of Myopic Macular Features in Dutch Individuals of European Ancestry With High Myopia. *JAMA Ophthalmol.* **2022**, *140*, 115. [CrossRef]
39. Shinohara, K.; Shimada, N.; Moriyama, M.; Yoshida, T.; Jonas, J.B.; Yoshimura, N.; Ohno-Matsui, K. Posterior Staphylomas in Pathologic Myopia Imaged by Widefield Optical Coherence Tomography. *Investig. Opthalmol. Vis. Sci.* **2017**, *58*, 3750. [CrossRef]
40. Frisina, R.; Baldi, A.; Cesana, B.M.; Semeraro, F.; Parolini, B. Morphological and clinical characteristics of myopic posterior staphyloma in Caucasians. *Graefes Arch. Clin. Exp. Ophthalmol.* **2016**, *254*, 2119–2129. [CrossRef]
41. Xu, X.; Fang, Y.; Uramoto, K.; Nagaoka, N.; Shinohara, K.; Yokoi, T.; Tanaka, N.; Ohno-Matsui, K. Clinical features of lacquer cracks in eyes with pathologic myopia. *Retina* **2019**, *39*, 1265–1277. [CrossRef]
42. Fang, Y.; Yokoi, T.; Nagaoka, N.; Shinohara, K.; Onishi, Y.; Ishida, T.; Yoshida, T.; Xu, X.; Jonas, J.B.; Ohno-Matsui, K. Progression of Myopic Maculopathy during 18-Year Follow-up. *Ophthalmology* **2018**, *125*, 863–877. [CrossRef]
43. Xiao, W.; Zhu, Z.; Odouard, C.; Xiao, O.; Guo, X.; He, M. Wide-Field En Face Swept-Source Optical Coherence Tomography Features of Extrafoveal Retinoschisis in Highly Myopic Eyes. *Investig. Opthalmol. Vis. Sci.* **2017**, *58*, 1037. [CrossRef] [PubMed]
44. Kumar, V.; Verma, S.; Azad, S.V.; Chawla, R.; Bhayana, A.A.; Surve, A.; Vohra, R.; Venkatesh, P. Dome-shaped macula—Review of literature. *Surv. Ophthalmol.* **2021**, *66*, 560–571. [CrossRef]
45. He, X.; Deng, J.; Xu, X.; Wang, J.; Cheng, T.; Zhang, B.; Zhao, H.; Luan, M.; Fan, Y.; Xiong, S.; et al. Design and Pilot data of the high myopia registration study: Shanghai Child and Adolescent Large-scale Eye Study (SCALE-HM). *Acta Ophthalmol.* **2021**, *99*, e489–e500. [CrossRef] [PubMed]
46. Fogel Levin, M.; Freund, K.B.; Gunnemann, F.; Greaves, G.; Sadda, S.; Sarraf, D. Myopic macular pits: A case series with multimodal imaging. *Can. J. Ophthalmol.* **2021**, S0008418221003483. [CrossRef] [PubMed]
47. Freitas-da-Costa, P.; Falcão, M.; Carneiro, Â. Infrared Reflectance Pattern of Macular Pits in Pathologic Myopia. *JAMA Ophthalmol.* **2015**, *133*, e1580. [CrossRef] [PubMed]
48. Freund, K.B. Peripapillary Detachment in Pathologic Myopia. *Arch. Ophthalmol.* **2003**, *121*, 197. [CrossRef]

49. Toranzo, J.; Cohen, S.Y.; Erginay, A.; Gaudric, A. Peripapillary Intrachoroidal Cavitation in Myopia. *Am. J. Ophthalmol.* **2005**, *140*, 731–732. [CrossRef]
50. Shimada, N. Characteristics of Peripapillary Detachment in Pathologic Myopia. *Arch. Ophthalmol.* **2006**, *124*, 46. [CrossRef]
51. You, Q.S.; Peng, X.Y.; Chen, C.X.; Xu, L.; Jonas, J.B. Peripapillary Intrachoroidal Cavitations. The Beijing Eye Study. *PLoS ONE* **2013**, *8*, e78743. [CrossRef]
52. Sayanagi, K.; Ikuno, Y.; Gomi, F.; Tano, Y. Retinal vascular microfolds in highly myopic eyes. *Am. J. Ophthalmol.* **2005**, *139*, 658–663. [CrossRef]
53. Ishida, T.; Watanabe, T.; Yokoi, T.; Shinohara, K.; Ohno-Matsui, K. Possible connection of short posterior ciliary arteries to choroidal neovascularisations in eyes with pathologic myopia. *Br. J. Ophthalmol.* **2019**, *103*, 457–462. [CrossRef] [PubMed]
54. Querques, G.; Corvi, F.; Balaratnasingam, C.; Casalino, G.; Parodi, M.B.; Introini, U.; Freund, K.B.; Bandello, F. Lacquer Cracks and Perforating Scleral Vessels in Pathologic Myopia: A Possible Causal Relationship. *Am. J. Ophthalmol.* **2015**, *160*, 759–766.e2. [CrossRef]
55. Falavarjani, K.; Shenazandi, H.; Naseri, D.; Anvari, P.; Kazemi, P.; Aghamohammadi, F.; Alissmail, F.; Alemzadeh, S. Foveal avascular zone and vessel density in healthy subjects: An optical coherence tomography angiography study. *J. Ophthalmic Vis. Res.* **2018**, *13*, 260. [CrossRef] [PubMed]
56. Noh, D.; Ryu, G.; Sagong, M. Analysis of Foveal Microvascular Structures Using Optical Coherence Tomography Angiography in Age-stratified Healthy Koreans. *J. Korean Ophthalmol. Soc.* **2017**, *58*, 1058. [CrossRef]
57. Iafe, N.A.; Phasukkijwatana, N.; Chen, X.; Sarraf, D. Retinal Capillary Density and Foveal Avascular Zone Area Are Age-Dependent: Quantitative Analysis Using Optical Coherence Tomography Angiography. *Investig. Opthalmol. Vis. Sci.* **2016**, *57*, 5780. [CrossRef] [PubMed]
58. Morales, D.; Wu, A.; Wu, L. The foveal avascular zone area in healthy eyes measured by ocular coherence tomography angiography using a full spectrum probabilistic algorithm. *Int. Ophthalmol.* **2021**, *41*, 2187–2196. [CrossRef]
59. Tan, C.S.; Lim, L.W.; Chow, V.S.; Chay, I.W.; Tan, S.; Cheong, K.X.; Tan, G.T.; Sadda, S.R. Optical Coherence Tomography Angiography Evaluation of the Parafoveal Vasculature and Its Relationship With Ocular Factors. *Investig. Opthalmol. Vis. Sci.* **2016**, *57*, OCT224. [CrossRef] [PubMed]
60. Jonas, J.B.; Wang, Y.X.; Dong, L.; Guo, Y.; Panda-Jonas, S. Advances in myopia research anatomical findings in highly myopic eyes. *Eye Vis.* **2020**, *7*, 45. [CrossRef]
61. Vurgese, S.; Panda-Jonas, S.; Jonas, J.B. Scleral Thickness in Human Eyes. *PLoS ONE* **2012**, *7*, e29692. [CrossRef] [PubMed]
62. Zhu, X.; Meng, J.; Wei, L.; Zhang, K.; He, W.; Lu, Y. Cilioretinal Arteries and Macular Vasculature in Highly Myopic Eyes. *Ophthalmol. Retina* **2020**, *4*, 965–972. [CrossRef] [PubMed]

Disclaimer/Publisher's Note: The statements, opinions and data contained in all publications are solely those of the individual author(s) and contributor(s) and not of MDPI and/or the editor(s). MDPI and/or the editor(s) disclaim responsibility for any injury to people or property resulting from any ideas, methods, instructions or products referred to in the content.

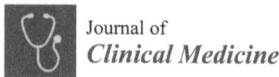

Article

The Short-Term Results of Autologous Platelet-Rich Plasma as an Adjuvant to Re-Intervention in the Treatment of Refractory Full-Thickness Macular Holes

Matilde Buzzi [1,*], Guglielmo Parisi [2], Paola Marolo [2], Francesco Gelormini [2], Mariantonia Ferrara [3], Raffaele Raimondi [4], Davide Allegrini [4], Tommaso Rossi [5], Michele Reibaldi [2] and Mario R. Romano [1,4,*]

1 Department of Biomedical Sciences, Humanitas University, 20090 Milan, Italy
2 Department of Surgical Sciences, Eye Clinic Section, University of Turin, 10124 Turin, Italy
3 Manchester Royal Eye Hospital, Manchester University Hospitals NHS Foundation Trust, Manchester M13 9WL, UK
4 Eye Unit, Department of Ophthalmology, Humanitas Gavazzeni-Castelli, 24125 Bergamo, Italy
5 IRCCS Fondazione Bietti ONLUS, 00198 Roma, Italy
* Correspondence: matilde.buzzi@humanitas.it (M.B.); mario.romano@hunimed.eu (M.R.R.)

Abstract: The purpose of this study was to investigate the short-term efficacy and safety of autologous platelet-rich plasma (a-PRP) as an adjuvant to revisional vitrectomy for refractory full-thickness macular holes (rFTMHs). We conducted a prospective, non-randomized interventional study including patients with rFTMH after a pars plana vitrectomy (PPV) with internal limiting membrane peeling and gas tamponade. We included 28 eyes from 27 patients with rFTMHs: 12 rFTMHs in highly myopic eyes (axial length greater than 26.5 mm or a refractive error greater than -6D or both); 12 large rFTMHs (minimum hole width > 400 µm); and 4 rFTMHs secondary to the optic disc pit. All patients underwent 25-G PPV with a-PRP, a median time of 3.5 ± 1.8 months after the primary repair. At the six-month follow-up, the overall rFTMH closure rate was 92.9%, distributed as follows: 11 out of 12 eyes (91.7%) in the highly myopic group, 11 out of 12 eyes (91.7%) in the large rFTMH group, and 4 out of 4 eyes (100%) in the optic disc pit group. Median best-corrected visual acuity significantly improved in all groups, in particular from 1.00 (interquartile range: 0.85 to 1.30) to 0.70 (0.40 to 0.85) LogMAR in the highly myopic group ($p = 0.016$), from 0.90 (0.70 to 1.49) to 0.40 (0.35 to 0.70) LogMAR in the large rFTMH group ($p = 0.005$), and from 0.90 (0.75 to 1.00) to 0.50 (0.28 to 0.65) LogMAR in the optic disc pit group. No intraoperative or postoperative complications were reported. In conclusion, a-PRP can be an effective adjuvant to PPV in the management of rFTMHs.

Keywords: autologous platelet-rich plasma; highly myopic full-thickness macular holes; optic disc pit maculopathy; pars plana vitrectomy; refractory full-thickness macular hole

Citation: Buzzi, M.; Parisi, G.; Marolo, P.; Gelormini, F.; Ferrara, M.; Raimondi, R.; Allegrini, D.; Rossi, T.; Reibaldi, M.; Romano, M.R. The Short-Term Results of Autologous Platelet-Rich Plasma as an Adjuvant to Re-Intervention in the Treatment of Refractory Full-Thickness Macular Holes. *J. Clin. Med.* **2023**, *12*, 2050. https://doi.org/10.3390/jcm12052050

Academic Editor: Alireza Karimi

Received: 31 January 2023
Revised: 24 February 2023
Accepted: 2 March 2023
Published: 4 March 2023

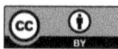

Copyright: © 2023 by the authors. Licensee MDPI, Basel, Switzerland. This article is an open access article distributed under the terms and conditions of the Creative Commons Attribution (CC BY) license (https://creativecommons.org/licenses/by/4.0/).

1. Introduction

Pars plana vitrectomy (PPV) with an internal limiting membrane (ILM) peeling and gas tamponade is the current gold standard for the primary repair of full-thickness macular holes (FTMHs), leading to an overall reported closure rate of 80–100% [1,2]. Moreover, the use of an inverted ILM flap has been demonstrated to further increase the primary anatomical success rate in large or highly myopic (HM) or both FTMHs, that are at a higher risk of a primary failure [3,4]. However, the FTMHs that fail to close in the first instance, so-called refractory FTMH (rFTMH), still represent a surgical challenge and have been associated with a lower closure rate in the case of secondary repair [5]. To optimize the outcomes of rFTMH repair, a variety of surgical techniques involving revisional PPV combined with additional maneuvers or adjuvant tissues or both, has been proposed, such as a repeated gas tamponade with or without the enlargement of the previous ILM peeling, the application of subretinal fluid, a retinal massage, placement of a micro drain, relaxation of the arcuate or radial retinotomies, transplantation of the ILM-free flaps, construction of an autologous or allogenic lens capsular flap, use of a human amniotic membrane plug or autologous neurosensory retinal flap, outpatient treatment of fluid or gas exchange alone or in combination with laser photocoagulation and macular buckling [5]. So far, there is no agreement on the best surgical approach for rFTMH [6].

The use of autologous platelet-rich plasma (a-PRP) has also been suggested as an effective adjuvant to revisional PPV for the repair of rFTMH [7–11], based on its potential beneficial effects on retinal pigment epithelium (RPE) cells and Müller cells, as well as a potential contributing mechanical effect on MH closure [5]. Indeed, the a-PRP, consisting of a portion of the plasma obtained by the centrifugation of the peripheral blood, is characterized by a platelet concentration and, thus, growth factors (GFs) content, significantly higher compared with that of the original sample [12]. These GFs have been shown to exert a modulating effect on tissue inflammation as well as a promoting effect on tissue repair and regeneration [12]. Concerning the eye, several GFs contained in platelets have been associated with the modulation and promotion of migration and growth of Müller cells, which have an established crucial role in the healing process of the macular hole [12–16]. In particular, it has been demonstrated that the incubation of rat Müller cells with platelet-derived GF (PDGF), fibroblast GF, epidermal GF or insulin-like GF 1, resulted in the enhancement of the proliferative and migratory activity of these cells [17]. These findings confirmed previous experimental studies demonstrating a stimulating effect on immortalized Müller cell migration and the proliferation of different platelet preparations in vitro [15]. Concerning RPE cells, there is experimental evidence of enhanced RPE cell migration and proliferation in response to incubation with human thrombocyte concentrate [18]. Furthermore, PDGF has been specifically involved in the promotion of the proliferative and migratory activity of human RPE cells [18]. Concerning the potential mechanical effect of a-PRP, it has been speculated that the platelets coagulum could act by sealing the macular hole and, thus, contribute to its closure [19]. The evidence of a hyperreflective plug overlying the hole has been reported the day after the surgery using both a-PRP [20] and plasma rich in growth factor [19].

In this light, it may be hypothesized that rFTMH at a high failure risk, such as large or highly myopic holes or both, might benefit from the use of a-PRP to further promote their closure. The purpose of our study was to evaluate the efficacy, in terms of both visual and anatomic outcomes, and the safety of a-PRP as an adjuvant to revisional PPV in rFTMHs.

2. Materials and Methods

We conducted a prospective, nonrandomized, interventional case series on patients affected by rFTMH and treated with PPV with a-PRP between January 2021 and June 2022. The study was conducted per the tenets of the Declaration of Helsinki, Institutional review board approval was obtained (Protocol Number 0041666) and all patients signed a written informed consent form after a detailed discussion regarding the procedure.

2.1. Inclusion and Exclusion Criteria

The inclusion criteria were the following:

- A previous PPV with ILM peeling and gas tamponade due to an idiopathic FTMH or myopic FTMH or optic disc pit maculopathy (ODPM), and
- adult patients (age > 18 years), and
- rFTMHs associated with high myopia (defined as eyes with an axial length greater than 26.5 mm or a refractive error greater than -6D or both), or
- large rFTMHs (minimum hole width > 400 μm, according to the (OCT)-based International Vitreomacular Traction Study Group (IVTS) classification [21]), or
- rFTMHs associated with ODPM.

The exclusion criteria included previously vitrectomized eyes at the time of the PPV for an FTMH repair (in case of idiopathic or highly myopic FTMH) or ODPM, any concomitant ocular or neurological condition that could affect the visual acuity, uncontrolled systemic conditions potentially leading to an unacceptable increased operative risk, as well as uncontrolled or untreated ocular pathologies, or both, that were likely to result in a significant increase in the risk of intraoperative or postoperative complications or both.

2.2. Surgical Procedure

All patients underwent surgery under local anesthesia. The surgeries were performed by three experienced vitreoretinal surgeons. The primary surgery consisted of a three-port, trans-conjunctival, sutureless 25-gauge PPV. If needed, posterior vitreous detachment (PVD) was induced and a core and peripheral vitrectomy were carried out. A blue dye was used to stain the ILM and a conventional ILM peeling of at least a two-disc diameter was performed. A foveal-sparing ILM peeling was performed in the case of an ODPM. After the indented search to rule out any undetected peripheral pathology to treat, a fluid-air exchange (FAX) was performed and followed by an air-gas exchange. In all phakic patients, a concomitant standard small-incision cataract surgery was performed. All the patients were requested to keep facedown positioning for 3 days postoperatively.

Concerning the revisional surgical procedure, to prepare the a-PRP, immediately before the surgery, the patient's peripheral venous blood was collected in a 10 mL tube with 1 mL of 3.2% sodium citrate, and centrifugated at 1600 revolutions per minute for 10 min. The PRP, identifiable as the middle of the 3 distinct visible layers (from the top; platelet-poor plasma, PRP, and red blood cells), was then collected in a sterile syringe.

The revisional PPV was performed using a 25-gauge PPV. The adequacy of the previous ILM peeling was checked after staining with a blue vital dye. None of the cases required an ILM peeling enlargement. The residual epiretinal traction, due to the initial foveal sparing, was removed from the eyes in the ODPM group. After FAX, 3 drops of aPRP were injected over the rFTMH and 12% perfluoropropane (C_3F_8) was used as tamponade. Finally, the patient was instructed to keep the supine position for 1 h, followed by the face-down position for 3 days.

2.3. Ophthalmic Evaluation

All of the patients were evaluated at a baseline, the day after the surgery and at a 1-, and 6-month follow-up (FU). At each FU, the patients underwent a complete ophthalmic examination, including a best-corrected visual acuity (BCVA) assessment, slit-lamp biomicroscopy, applanation tonometry, and dilated fundoscopy. In addition, spectral-domain optical coherence tomography (SD-OCT) of the macula was performed using the Heidelberg Spectralis SD-OCT (Heidelberg Engineering, Heidelberg, Germany) at the baseline and at the 1- and 6-month FU. A 30° × 25° posterior pole scan, 240 Sects., ART 20 was acquired for each patient and the crossline centered on the fovea was used to measure the hole diameter. According to the IVTS classification [21], the minimum hole width was manually drawing a line between the narrowest hole points at the level of the mid retina and parallel to the RPE, using the caliper function of the OCT device. According to the classification proposed by Rossi and coworkers [22], the MH closure pattern was classified as type 0 if the MH remained open with an exposed RPE, and type 1 in the case of MH closure with reconstitution of all of the retinal layers (1A), or with a residual defect of the external (1B) or internal (1C) retinal layers; as no autologous or heterologous tissue transplant was performed, the type 2 closure patter did not apply to this study. In addition, the presence of residual external limiting membrane (ELM) defects, ellipsoid zone (EZ) defects or fibrin-like hyperreflective (HR) tissue, or both, was documented. The closure pattern was classified as 1A if only the focal of the EZ and/or ELM were present.

2.4. Statistical Analysis

We carried out the statistical analysis using the IBM SPSS Statistics software (version 29; Armonk, NY, USA: IBM Corp.). As the visual acuity was measured in Snellen, the VA values were converted into logarithms of the minimal angle of resolution (logMAR) values for the statistical analysis. As previously performed in other studies, a logMAR value of 1.98, 2.28, 2.70, and 3.00 was considered equivalent to counting fingers, hand movements, perception of light, and no perception of light, respectively [23]. The BCVA values were expressed as a median and interquartile range. Before statistical analysis, the Shapiro-Wilk test was used to evaluate the continuous variables and, consequently, non-parametric statistical analyses were performed. The statistical significance of the differences between the median preoperative and postoperative BCVA was tested using the Wilcoxon signed-rank test for paired samples. The difference was considered statistically significant if the p-value < 0.05.

3. Results

A number of 28 eyes, from 27 patients with rFTMH, were included in the study. Specifically, 12 eyes (42.9%) were highly myopic (HM group), 12 eyes (42.9%) had a large rFTMH, and 4 eyes (14.3%) (L group) had rFTMHs associated with ODPM (ODPM group). All the patients completed the minimum follow-up of 6 months. The mean patient age was 61 ± 8.78 years. The demographic findings are resumed in Table 1. The mean baseline FTMH size (before primary surgery) was 385.5 ± 148.5 µm in the HM group and 567.6 ± 118.7 µm in the L group. All eyes in the OPDM group presented initially with subretinal and intraretinal fluid, involving both inner and outer retinal layers, and developed FTMH after a primary PPV and ILM peeling. The mean interval between the first and the second surgical procedure was 3.5 ± 1.8 months.

Table 1. The demographic and clinical findings.

	Overall	HM Group	L Group	ODPM Group
Age (mean, years)	61 ± 8.78	62.1 ± 6.6	65 ± 6.3	46 ± 4.5
Sex (% male)	42.8%	33.3%	41.7%	75%
Laterality (% right)	53.6%	66.7%	50%	25%

The mean macular hole size before the revisional PPV was 451.8 ± 162.4 µm in the whole cohort, and, specifically, 364 ± 147.7 µm in the HM group, 552.4 ± 145.4 µm in the L group, and 413.5 ± 79.9 µm in the ODPM group.

At the 6-month FU, hole closure was achieved in 26 out of 28 eyes (92.9%): 11 out of 12 eyes in the HM group (91.7%), 11 out of 12 eyes in the L group (91.7%) and 4 out of 4 eyes in the ODPM group (100%). The structural OCT outcomes at the 6-month FU are shown in Table 1. Complete reconstitution of all the retinal layers was detected in the majority of the rFTMHs as a type 1A closure pattern and was documented in 46.4% of the eyes, with the highest percentage in the ODPM group (75%). Residual EZ defects resulted to be more commonly detected than residual ELM defects, regardless of the initial type of rFTMH. Indeed, this trend was noted in all the groups, with the highest rate of residual EZ defect in the L group (Table 2). Larger FTMH showed a trend towards the residual EZ defect as the mean preoperative hole size was 465.4 ± 180.6 µm and 423.2 ± 119.3 µm in eyes with and without the residual postoperative EZ defect, respectively. Two representative cases are shown in Figures 1–3.

Table 2. The optical coherence tomography data at 6-month follow-up.

	Overall	Highly Myopic rFTMHs	Large rFTMHs	rFTMHs Associated with ODPM
Closure rate	26/28 (92.9%)	11/12 (91.7%)	11/12 (91.7%)	4/4 (100%)
Closure type 1A	13/28 (46.4%)	5/12 (41.7%)	5/12 (41.7%)	3/4 (75.0%)
Closure type 1B	2/28 (7.1%)	1/12 (8.3%)	0/12 (0%)	1/4 (25.0%)
Closure type 1C	11/28 (39.3%)	5/12 (41.7%)	6/12 (50.0%)	0/4 (0%)
Residual ELM defect	8/28 (25.6%)	6/12 (50.0%)	4/12 (33.3%)	1/4 (25%)
Residual EZ defect	21/28 (75.0%)	8/12 (66.7%)	11/12 (91.7%)	2/4 (50%)
Fibrin-like HR tissue	1/28 (3.6%)	1/12 (8.3%)	0/12 (0%)	0/4 (0%)

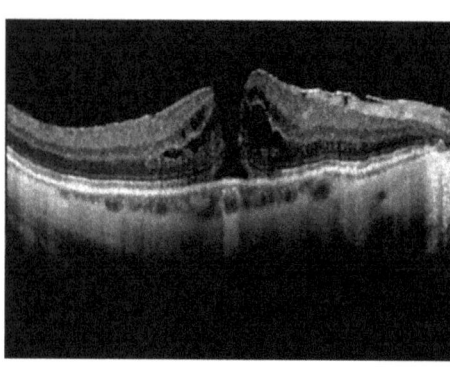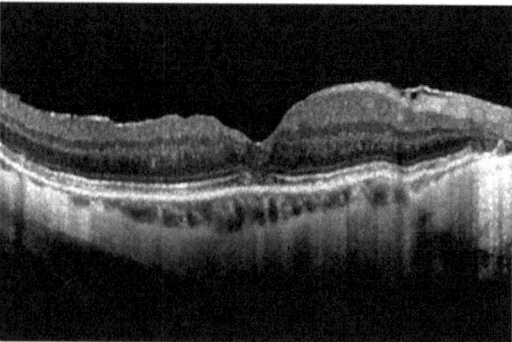

Figure 1. Case 1: A full-thickness refractory macular hole (rFTMH) of a highly myopic eye that did not close after a primary 25-G pars plana vitrectomy (PPV) with internal limiting membrane peeling (**left**). At 6 months after secondary PPV with autologous platelet-rich plasma and gas tamponade, complete closure of rFTMH is seen (**right**).

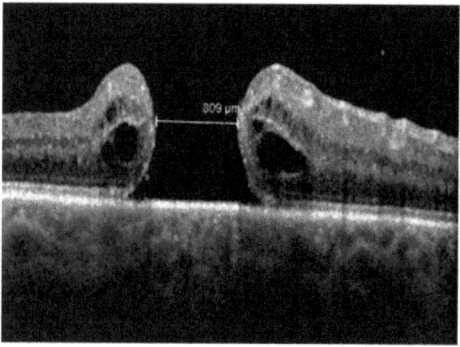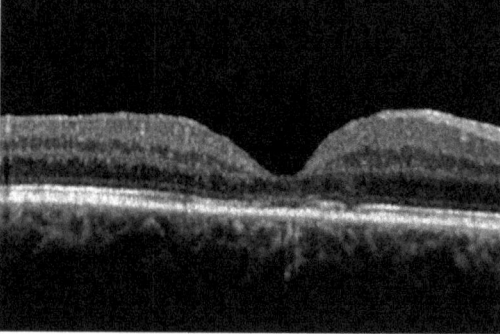

Figure 2. Case 2: A full-thickness refractory large macular hole (rFTMH) (minimum hole width 809 μm) that did not close after a primary 25-G pars plana vitrectomy (PPV) with internal limiting membrane peeling (**left**). At 6 months after secondary PPV with autologous platelet-rich plasma and gas tamponade, complete closure of rFTMH is seen (**right**).

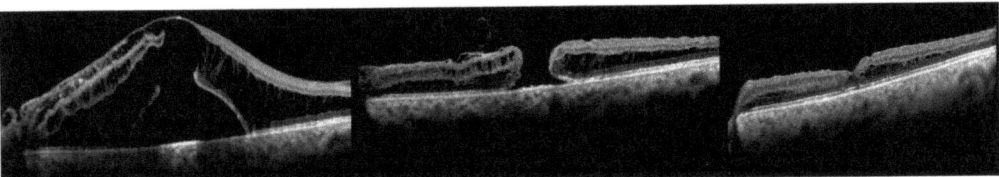

Figure 3. Case 3: An optic disc pit maculopathy with intraretinal fluid involving inner and outer retinal layers and subretinal fluid (**left**). A secondary full-thickness refractory macular hole after a primary 25-G pars plana vitrectomy (PPV) with internal limiting membrane peeling and foveal sparing (**middle**). The FTMH was closed at 3 months after the secondary PPV with autologous platelet-rich plasma and gas tamponade (**right**).

The median overall preoperative BCVA was 0.95 (0.75 to 1.15) LogMAR. In particular, the median preoperative BCVA was 1.00 (0.85 to 1.30) LogMAR in the highly myopic group, 0.90 (0.70 to 1.49) LogMAR in the large rFTMH group, and 0.90 (0.75 to 1.00) LogMAR in the optic disc pit group. At the final 6-month FU, a statistically significant improvement in BCVA was documented in both the whole cohort and each of the groups identified. In particular, the median BCVA improved from 0.95 (0.75 to 1.15) LogMAR to 0.50 (0.40 to 0.70) LogMAR in the whole cohort ($p < 0.001$), 1.00 (0.85 to 1.30) LogMAR to 0.70 (0.40 to 0.85) LogMAR in the highly myopic group ($p = 0.016$), and from 0.90 (0.70 to 1.49) LogMAR to 0.40 (0.35 to 0.70) LogMAR in the large rFTMH group ($p = 0.005$). The median BCVA improved from 0.90 (0.75 to 1.00) LogMAR to 0.50 (0.28 to 0.65) LogMAR in the ODPM group; however, the size of the sample was too small to be tested for statistical significance.

No intraoperative or postoperative complications were recorded.

ELM, external limiting membrane; EZ, ellipsoid zone; HR, hyperreflective; ODPM, optic disc pit maculopathy; rFTMHs, refractory full-thickness macular holes.

4. Discussion

Pars plana vitrectomy with ILM peeling and gas tamponade currently represents the established treatment of choice for the primary repair of idiopathic FTMH; in addition, the inverted ILM flap is gaining popularity for the primary repair of large or highly myopic FTMH, or both, as it has been associated with an increased closure rate in these types of FTMH, that are at higher risk of failure [1,24]. Unsuccessful closures of FTMH after primary surgical repair occurs in up to 10% of cases and there is currently no consensus on the best surgical management [5]. Performing a revisional PPV for rFTMH involves some specific challenges associated with the absence or limited availability of ILM in the macular area and a decreased rate of hole closure [25]. In addition, a higher risk of primary and secondary failure as well as poorer visual outcomes is known to be associated with large or highly myopic FTMH or both [5]. Refractory FTMHs associated with OPDM after the primary surgery can represent a surgical scenario similar to rFTMH after surgical repair for the idiopathic FTMH, as PPV and ILM peeling with or without an ILM inverted flap are gaining a growing popularity as the primary surgical approach in treating OPDM [26]. So far, various revisional surgical techniques have been proposed for the treatment of rFMTHs, but the strength of the evidence based on the available studies is limited by several important flaws, such as the predominance of retrospective studies, the absence of randomized controlled trials, the variety of methods used, and the surgical steps described [5]. Despite the above-mentioned limitations, the literature appears to support the combination of revisional PPV with the use of adjuvants aimed at the promotion and modulation of the intraretinal gliosis or the mechanical action of "scaffold" for the Müller cells or both [5].

In light of its high GF content, a-PRP has been long used to promote tissue regeneration or repair in different fields of medicine, including ophthalmology [12]. In this regard, PRP has been first and successfully used in the management of diseases of the ocular surface [27]. The application of a-PRP as an adjuvant in FTMH surgery has been supported by the experimental evidence of the stimulatory effect of platelet GFs on the migratory and proliferative activity of Müller cells, as well as RPE cell growth in vitro [11,13,17]. So far, the use of a-PRP has been associated with promising results in terms of the closure rate and visual gain in macular holes of different types, such as highly myopic FTMH [19], idiopathic large FTMH [28], rFTMH associated with Alport syndrome [20], FTMH associated with macular telangiectasia type 2 [29], lamellar macular holes [30], idiopathic rFTMH associated, or not associated, with high myopia [5]. However, it is worth noting that the strength of these findings is limited by the availability of only a few retrospective studies [5]. So far, only one randomized controlled trial compared the outcomes of PPV and ILM peeling with or without an intraoperative injection of autologous platelet concentrate (APC) in the eyes affected by recurrent FTMHs, highly myopic FTMHs, or large MHs [28]. Despite the inter-group difference in the closure rate not reaching statistical significance, the use of APC was associated with a trend towards a higher success rate compared with PPV and ILM peeling only, and so, it was suggested as a potential adjuvant in selected cases [28].

In this prospective study, we evaluated the efficacy and safety of a-PRP as an adjuvant to revisional PPV for rFTMHs at high risk of failure, such as large rFTMHs, highly myopic rFMTH, and rFTMHs associated with OPDM. Out of a total of 28 eyes included, a type 1 closure rate was achieved in 92.9% of cases (26 eyes), with one large and one highly myopic rFTMH that failed to close. These results are consistent with those of Figueroa et al. [19], who reported a successful hole closure in 10 of 11 highly myopic rFTMHs treated with revisional PPV and plasma rich in growth factors, a subtype of aPRP that need to be activated before the surgical use. The closure rate reported in the studies currently available on the use of a-PRP in rFTMH repair ranges from 60% to 85% [10,25,28,31,32]. The short median inter-surgery interval (3.5 ± 1.8 months) may have contributed to the high closure rate in our study, as a shorter time between the primary and secondary surgery may result in a higher anatomical success rate [11]. In addition, Degenhardt et al. [11] evaluated the outcomes of 103 eyes treated with revisional PPV and autologous platelet concentrate due to rFTMH and reported that there was a trend towards the correlation of greater axial length and a higher rate of anatomical failure. However, in this study, the closure rate was high (at 91.7%) in both the HM group and the L group, with only one hole that failed to close in each group. Finally, the use of a-PRP in revisional PPV has been associated with ILM peeling enlargement, if needed, and a different intraocular tamponade, including short-acting gas, long-acting gases and silicone oil [5]. In this regard, an additional strength of our study is the absence of the need for ILM peeling enlargement and the use of the same gas tamponade (C_3F_8) in all surgeries. Indeed, this ruled out the potential effect of the ILM peeling enlargement or different intraocular tamponade, or both, on the final closure rate.

In terms of the anatomical results, we also analyzed the restoration of EZ and ELM. It is known that ELM recovery is more common in the EZ recovery in eyes treated for FTMH [33]. The recovery of ELM and EZ has been previously correlated with better visual outcomes [34]. In our study, we observed a complete restoration of the ELM in the majority of the eyes (74.4%), whereas residual EZ defects were detected in 75% of the eyes at the 6-month FU. This finding appears consistent with the residual EZ damage in 76% and 81% of eyes treated for rFTMH previously reported by Purtskhvanidze et al. [10] and Degenhardt et al. [11], respectively. It has been speculated that the greater hole size may be correlated with a higher rate of residual EZ and ELM damage [19]; thus, the large size of the rFTMHs at the baseline may have contributed to the presence of residual EZ damage in our sample. Degenhardt et al. [11] also hypothesized that the EZ damage might be considered a potential complication of a-PRP. Nevertheless, as highlighted by the same authors [11], persistent damage of the EZ band is a known complication of the FTMH surgery itself and so far, there is no evidence supporting a specific role of a-PRP.

Another important structural complication potentially associated with the surgical repair of FTMH is the postoperative evidence of excessive intraretinal gliosis, which has been associated with worse reconstitutions of the ELM and EZ, as well as poorer visual outcomes due to a detrimental effect in retinal neuronal cells [35]. A potential beneficial effect of PRP in terms of the alleviation of the fibrotic reaction has been demonstrated in the rat model of dimethylnitrosamine-induced hepatic fibrosis [36]. This may support a modulating effect of platelet GFs in wound-healing processes, such as intraretinal gliosis. This potential beneficial effect of a-PRP might be also more important in eyes that may be at a higher risk of excessive intraretinal gliosis, such as highly myopic eyes. Consistent with this hypothesis, we detected HR fibrin-like tissue only in one highly myopic eye.

Concerning the functional results, we reported a significant improvement in BCVA from the baseline to the final FU visit, in all groups. The potential advantages of revisional PPV with aPRP compared to other revisional surgical techniques for rFTMHs, in terms of final VA and VA gain, have been recently highlighted. Indeed, in a recent retrospective multicentric study comparing several revisional surgical techniques for rFTMHs, revisional PPV and a-PRP were associated with the highest visual gain (a mean of 24 ETDRS letters gain, ranging from 12 to 38 letters) compared to revisional PPV with repeating gas tamponade, ILM-free flap, radial nerve fiber layer incisions, retinal massage, and the fitting of a micro drain [37]. In addition, a recent review comparing anatomical and functional outcomes of different surgical revisional techniques for treating rFTMHs concluded that revisional PPV with a-PRP represents one of the most efficient techniques available in light of the good anatomical and functional outcomes and the low level of complexity of surgical maneuvers [27]. In particular, Frisina et al. [38] confirmed the superiority of a-PRP in terms of the BCVA gain when compared with ILM-free flap transplantation and pointed out that the only surgical technique associated with BCVA gain greater than a-PRP was the use of a human amniotic membrane plug, that entails more invasive and challenging surgical maneuvers.

Finally, it is worth highlighting that additional advantages of a-PRP lie in its simplicity and safety. The collection and delivery protocol of a-PPR is minimally invasive, rapid, and repeatable. As briefly mentioned above, concerning the comparison with the use of a human amniotic membrane plug, this advantage of a-PRP is also more important if compared with the more complex surgical maneuvers of other validated revisional techniques, such as ILM-free flap transplantation, or the greater invasiveness, or both, for instance in the case of autologous retinal free flap transplantation. In addition, no intraoperative and postoperative complications were recorded. Although a theoretical risk of an increased risk of endophthalmitis and severe intraocular inflammation associated with the intraocular use of a-PRP has been raised in the past [9,39], this concern is not supported by any available evidence. Indeed, to the best of our knowledge, no case of postoperative endophthalmitis has ever been reported in eyes treated with PPV and different formulations of platelet concentrate. In addition, a recent retrospective case series that compared eyes with rFTMH treated with revisional PPV and heavy silicone oil versus revisional PPV with autologous platelets concentrate and SF_6, reported severe postoperative complications (namely endophthalmitis and retinal detachment associated with proliferative vitreoretinopathy) only in the former group, supporting the safety of a-PRP use [40]. A case has been described of temporary and self-resolved exudative retinal detachment during the second week after PPV with platelet concentrate and without ILM peeling [39]; in this case, the potential causative role of the platelet concentrate or the unusually high concentration of inflammatory mediators due to an unusual white cells/platelets breakdown in the concentrate, or both, has been speculated but no evidence supporting this hypothesis has been presented [39]. No other case of postoperative complications induced by severe intraocular inflammation has been reported in the literature, so far. Consistently, none of the patients included in this study experienced any infection or excessive intraocular inflammation.

We acknowledge that the small sample is a limitation of this study. However, we specifically focused on subgroups of rFTMH that are known to be at higher risk of failure and, differently to the currently available studies, we presented a study with a prospective design. In addition, future studies could analyze more detailed functional outcomes, such as metamorphopsia and retinal sensitivity. Finally, we did not compare the use of a-PRP in revisional PPV for rFTMH with alternative revisional techniques and we did not include a control group treated with revisional PPV and repeated gas tamponade alone. This analysis could be carried out in future larger prospective studies, ideally randomized.

In conclusion, revisional PPV with a-PRP can be an effective and safe treatment for rFTMHs, resulting in satisfactory visual and anatomical outcomes comparable with other surgical options and the advantage of a simple and reproducible procedure.

Author Contributions: Conceptualization, M.R.R. and M.R.; methodology, M.R.R., M.R., G.P., P.M. and F.G.; validation, M.R.R., M.R., G.P., P.M., F.G., M.F., T.R., R.R. and D.A.; formal analysis, M.B. and R.R.; resources, M.R., G.P., P.M., F.G. and M.F.; data curation, M.B., R.R., G.P., P.M. and F.G.; writing—original draft preparation, M.B. and R.R.; writing—review and editing, M.F. and D.A.; supervision, M.R.R., M.R. and T.R.; project administration, M.R.R. All authors have read and agreed to the published version of the manuscript.

Funding: This research received no external funding.

Institutional Review Board Statement: All procedures performed in studies involving human participants were in accordance with the ethical standards of the institutional and national research committee and with the 1964 Helsinki declaration and its later amendments or comparable ethical standards (Protocol Number 0041666).

Informed Consent Statement: Informed consent was obtained from all subjects involved in the study.

Data Availability Statement: The data that support the findings of this study are available from the corresponding author upon reasonable request.

Conflicts of Interest: The authors declare no conflict of interest.

References

1. Abdelkader, E.; Lois, N. Internal Limiting Membrane Peeling in Vitreo-Retinal Surgery. *Surv. Ophthalmol.* **2008**, *53*, 368–396. [CrossRef] [PubMed]
2. Ch'ng, S.W.; Patton, N.; Ahmed, M.; Ivanova, T.; Baumann, C.; Charles, S.; Jalil, A. The Manchester Large Macular Hole Study: Is It Time to Reclassify Large Macular Holes? *Am. J. Ophthalmol.* **2018**, *195*, 36–42. [CrossRef]
3. Chatziralli, I.; Machairoudia, G.; Kazantzis, D.; Theodossiadis, G.; Theodossiadis, P. Inverted Internal Limiting Membrane Flap Technique for Myopic Macular Hole: A Meta-Analysis. *Surv. Ophthalmol.* **2021**, *66*, 771–780. [CrossRef] [PubMed]
4. Chen, G.; Tzekov, R.; Jiang, F.; Mao, S.; Tong, Y.; Li, W. Inverted ILM Flap Technique versus Conventional ILM Peeling for Idiopathic Large Macular Holes: A Meta-Analysis of Randomized Controlled Trials. *PLoS ONE* **2020**, *15*, e0236431. [CrossRef]
5. Romano, M.R.; Rossi, T. Review Article Management of Refractory and Recurrent Macular Holes: A Comprehensive Review. *Surv. Ophthalmol.* **2022**, *67*, 908–931. [CrossRef] [PubMed]
6. Tam, A.L.C.; Yan, P.; Gan, N.Y.; Lam, W.C. The Current Surgical Management of Large, Recurrent, or Persistent Macular Holes. *Retina* **2018**, *38*, 1263–1275. [CrossRef] [PubMed]
7. Shpak, A.A.; Shkvorchenko, D.O.; Krupina, E.A. Surgical Treatment of Macular Holes with and without the Use of Autologous Platelet-Rich Plasma. *Int. Ophthalmol.* **2021**, *41*, 1043–1052. [CrossRef]
8. Figueroa, M.S.; Govetto, A.; Arriba-Palomero, P. de Short-Term Results of Platelet-Rich Plasma as Adjuvant to 23-G Vitrectomy in the Treatment of High Myopic Macular Holes. *Eur. J. Ophthalmol.* **2015**, *26*, 491–496. [CrossRef]
9. Cheung, C.M.G.; Munshi, V.; Mughal, S.; Mann, J.; Hero, M. Anatomical Success Rate of Macular Hole Surgery with Autologous Platelet without Internal-Limiting Membrane Peeling. *Eye* **2005**, *19*, 1191–1193. [CrossRef]
10. Purtskhvanidze, K.; Frühsorger, B.; Bartsch, S.; Hedderich, J.; Roider, J.; Treumer, F. Persistent Full-Thickness Idiopathic Macular Hole: Anatomical and Functional Outcome of Revitrectomy with Autologous Platelet Concentrate or Autologous Whole Blood. *Ophthalmologica* **2017**, *239*, 19–26. [CrossRef]
11. Degenhardt, V.; Busch, C.; Jochmann, C.; Meier, P.; Unterlauft, J.D.; Mößner, A.; Edel, E.; Tewari, R.; Wiedemann, P.; Rehak, M. Prognostic Factors in Patients with Persistent Full-Thickness Idiopathic Macular Holes Treated with Re-Vitrectomy with Autologous Platelet Concentrate. *Ophthalmologica* **2019**, *242*, 214–221. [CrossRef]
12. Alves, R.; Grimalt, R. A Review of Platelet-Rich Plasma: History, Biology, Mechanism of Action, and Classification. *Skin Appendage Disord.* **2018**, *4*, 18–24. [CrossRef]
13. Campochiaro, P.A.; Hackett, S.F.; Vinores, S.A.; Freund, J.; Csaky, C.; LaRochelle, W.; Henderer, J.; Johnson, M.; Rodriguez, I.R.; Friedman, Z.; et al. Platelet-Derived Growth Factor Is an Autocrine Growth Stimulator in Retinal Pigmented Epithelial Cells. *J. Cell Sci.* **1994**, *107*, 2459–2469. [CrossRef] [PubMed]

14. Zheng, C.; Zhu, Q.; Liu, X.; Huang, X.; He, C.; Jiang, L.; Quan, D.; Zhou, X.; Zhu, Z. Effect of Platelet-Rich Plasma (PRP) Concentration on Proliferation, Neurotrophic Function and Migration of Schwann Cells in Vitro. *J. Tissue Eng. Regen Med.* **2016**, *10*, 428–436. [CrossRef] [PubMed]
15. Burmeister, S.L.; Hartwig, D.; Astrid Limb, G.; Kremling, C.; Hoerauf, H.; Müller, M.; Geerling, G. Effect of Various Platelet Preparations on Retinal Müller Cells. *Investig. Ophthalmol. Vis. Sci.* **2009**, *50*, 4881–4886. [CrossRef]
16. Castelnovo, L.; Dosquet, C.; Gaudric, A.; Sahel, J.; Hicks, D. Human Platelet Suspension Stimulates Porcine Retinal Glial Proliferation and Migration in Vitro. *Investig. Ophthalmol. Vis. Sci.* **2000**, *41*, 601–609.
17. Wu, A.L.; Liu, Y.T.; da Chou, H.; Chuang, L.H.; Chen, K.J.; Chen, Y.P.; Liu, L.; Yeung, L.; Wang, N.K.; Hwang, Y.S.; et al. Role of Growth Factors and Internal Limiting Membrane Constituents in Müller Cell Migration. *Exp. Eye Res.* **2021**, *202*, 108352. [CrossRef] [PubMed]
18. Velhagen, K.H.; Druegg, A.; Rieck, P. Proliferation and Wound Healing of Retinal Pigment Epithelium Cells in Vitro. Effect of Human Thrombocyte Concentrate, Serum and PDGF. *Ophthalmologe* **1999**, *96*, 77–81. [CrossRef]
19. Figueroa, M.S.; Mora Cantallops, A.; Virgili, G.; Govetto, A. Long-Term Results of Autologous Plasma as Adjuvant to Pars Plana Vitrectomy in the Treatment of High Myopic Full-Thickness Macular Holes. *Eur. J. Ophthalmol.* **2021**, *31*, 2612–2620. [CrossRef]
20. D'Alterio, F.M.; Ferrara, M.; Bagnall, A.; Talks, K.L.; Hillier, R.J. Platelet-Rich Plasma and Macular Hole Surgery: A Clue to Their Mode of Action and the Influence of Anti-Platelet Agents. *Eur. J. Ophthalmol.* **2022**, 112067212210936. [CrossRef] [PubMed]
21. Duker, J.S.; Kaiser, P.K.; Binder, S.; de Smet, M.D.; Gaudric, A.; Reichel, E.; Sadda, S.R.; Sebag, J.; Spaide, R.F.; Stalmans, P. The International Vitreomacular Traction Study Group Classification of Vitreomacular Adhesion, Traction, and Macular Hole. *Ophthalmology* **2013**, *120*, 2611–2619. [CrossRef] [PubMed]
22. Rossi, T.; Bacherini, D.; Caporossi, T.; Telani, S.; Iannetta, D.; Rizzo, S.; Moysidis, S.N.; Koulisis, N.; Mahmoud, T.H.; Ripandelli, G. Macular Hole Closure Patterns: An Updated Classification. *Graefe's Arch. Clin. Exp. Ophthalmol.* **2020**, *258*, 2629–2638. [CrossRef]
23. Ferrara, M.; Mehta, A.; Qureshi, H.; Avery, P.; Yorston, D.; Laidlaw, D.A.; Williamson, T.H.; Steel, D.H.W.; Casswell, A.G.; Morris, A.H.C.; et al. Phenotype and Outcomes of Phakic Versus Pseudophakic Primary Rhegmatogenous Retinal Detachments: Cataract or Cataract Surgery Related? *Am. J. Ophthalmol.* **2021**, *222*, 318–327. [CrossRef]
24. Marques, R.E.; Sousa, D.C.; Leal, I.; Faria, M.Y.; Marques-Neves, C. Complete ILM Peeling versus Inverted Flap Technique for Macular Hole Surgery: A Meta-Analysis. *Ophthalmic. Surg. Lasers Imaging Retin.* **2020**, *51*, 187-A2. [CrossRef] [PubMed]
25. Hillenkamp, J.; Kraus, J.; Framme, C.; Jackson, T.L.; Roider, J.; Gabel, V.P.; Sachs, H.G. Retreatment of Full-Thickness Macular Hole: Predictive Value of Optical Coherence Tomography. *Br. J. Ophthalmol.* **2007**, *91*, 1445–1449. [CrossRef] [PubMed]
26. Babu, N.; Kohli, P.; Ramasamy, K. Comparison of Various Surgical Techniques for Optic Disc Pit Maculopathy: Vitrectomy with Internal Limiting Membrane (ILM) Peeling Alone versus Inverted ILM Flap "plug" versus Autologous Scleral "Plug". *Br. J. Ophthalmol.* **2020**, *104*, 1567–1573. [CrossRef] [PubMed]
27. Anitua, E.; de la Sen-Corcuera, B.; Orive, G.; Sánchez-Ávila, R.M.; Heredia, P.; Muruzabal, F.; Merayo-Lloves, J. Progress in the Use of Plasma Rich in Growth Factors in Ophthalmology: From Ocular Surface to Ocular Fundus. *Expert. Opin. Biol. Ther.* **2022**, *22*, 31–45. [CrossRef] [PubMed]
28. Kim, M.; Won, J.Y.; Choi, S.Y.; Kim, M.; Ra, H.; Jee, D.; Kwon, J.W.; Kang, K.D.; Roh, Y.J.; Park, Y.G.; et al. Therapeutic Efficacy of Autologous Platelet Concentrate Injection on Macular Holes with High Myopia, Large Macular Holes, or Recurrent Macular Holes: A Multicenter Randomized Controlled Trial. *J. Clin. Med.* **2021**, *10*, 2727. [CrossRef] [PubMed]
29. Rangel, C.M.; Blanco, N.A.; Pedraza-Concha, A.; Gomez, M.A.; Parra, M.M.; Arias, J.D. Plasma Rich in Growth Factors as Treatment for a Full-Thickness Macular Hole Due to Macular Telangiectasia Type 2. *Arch. Soc. Esp. Oftalmol.* **2022**, *97*, 219–223. [CrossRef]
30. Hagenau, F.; Luft, N.; Nobl, M.; Vogt, D.; Klaas, J.E.; Schworm, B.; Siedlecki, J.; Kreutzer, T.C.; Priglinger, S.G. Improving Morphological Outcome in Lamellar Macular Hole Surgery by Using Highly Concentrated Autologous Platelet-Rich Plasma. *Graefe's Arch. Clin. Exp. Ophthalmol.* **2022**, *260*, 1517–1524. [CrossRef]
31. Dimopoulos, S.; William, A.; Voykov, B.; Ziemssen, F.; Bartz-Schmidt, K.U.; Spitzer, M.S. Anatomical and Visual Outcomes of Autologous Thrombocyte Serum Concentrate in the Treatment of Persistent Full-Thickness Idiopathic Macular Hole after ILM Peeling with Brilliant Blue G and Membrane Blue Dual. *Acta Ophthalmol.* **2017**, *95*, e429–e430. [CrossRef]
32. Valldeperas, X.; Wong, D. Is It Worth Reoperating on Macular Holes? *Ophthalmology* **2008**, *115*, 158–163. [CrossRef]
33. Bodhankar, P.; Joshi, A.; Dronadula, M.; Patil, A. Postoperative Microstructural Re-Modelling and Functional Outcomes in Idiopathic Full Thickness Macular Hole. *Indian J. Ophthalmol.* **2022**, *70*, 2077. [CrossRef] [PubMed]
34. Bleidißel, N.; Friedrich, J.; Feucht, N.; Klaas, J.; Maier, M. Visual Improvement and Regeneration of Retinal Layers in Eyes with Small, Medium, and Large Idiopathic Full-Thickness Macular Holes Treated with the Inverted Internal Limiting Membrane Flap Technique over a Period of 12 Months. *Graefe's Arch. Clin. Exp. Ophthalmol.* **2022**, *260*, 3161–3171. [CrossRef] [PubMed]
35. Oh, J.; Yang, S.M.; Choi, Y.M.; Kim, S.W.; Huh, W. Glial Proliferation after Vitrectomy for a Macular Hole: A Spectral Domain Optical Coherence Tomography Study. *Graefe's Arch. Clin. Exp. Ophthalmol.* **2013**, *251*, 477–484. [CrossRef] [PubMed]
36. Salem, N.A.; Hamza, A.; Alnahdi, H.; Ayaz, N. Biochemical and Molecular Mechanisms of Platelet-Rich Plasma in Ameliorating Liver Fibrosis Induced by Dimethylnitrosurea. *Cell. Physiol. Biochem.* **2018**, *47*, 2331–2339. [CrossRef]
37. Maguire, M.J.; Steel, D.H.; Yorston, D.; Hind, J.; El-Faouri, M.; Jalil, A.; Tyagi, P.; Wickham, L.; Laidlaw, A.H. Outcome of Revision Procedures for Failed Primary Macular Hole Surgery. *Retina* **2021**, *41*, 1389–1395. [CrossRef]

38. Frisina, R.; Gius, I.; Tozzi, L.; Midena, E. Refractory Full Thickness Macular Hole: Current Surgical Management. *Eye* **2022**, *36*, 1344–1354. [CrossRef]
39. Gamulescu, M.A.; Roider, J.; Gabel, V.P. Exudative Retinal Detachment in Macular Hole Surgery Using Platelet Concentrates—A Case Report. *Graefe's Arch. Clin. Exp. Ophthalmol.* **2001**, *239*, 227–229. [CrossRef]
40. Schaub, F.; Gözlügöl, N.; von Goscinski, C.; Enders, P.; Heindl, L.M.; Dahlke, C. Outcome of Autologous Platelet Concentrate and Gas Tamponade Compared to Heavy Silicone Oil Tamponade in Persistent Macular Hole Surgery. *Eur. J. Ophthalmol.* **2021**, *31*, 664–672. [CrossRef]

Disclaimer/Publisher's Note: The statements, opinions and data contained in all publications are solely those of the individual author(s) and contributor(s) and not of MDPI and/or the editor(s). MDPI and/or the editor(s) disclaim responsibility for any injury to people or property resulting from any ideas, methods, instructions or products referred to in the content.

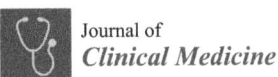

Journal of
Clinical Medicine

Article

Long-Term Effect of SARS-CoV-2 Infection on the Retinal and Choroidal Microvasculature

Magdalena Kal [1,2], Mateusz Winiarczyk [3,*], Dorota Zarębska-Michaluk [1,4], Dominik Odrobina [2,5], Elżbieta Cieśla [5], Bernadetta Płatkowska-Adamska [1,2], Michał Biskup [2], Paweł Pabjan [4,5], Stanisław Głuszek [1] and Jerzy Mackiewicz [3]

1. Collegium Medicum, Jan Kochanowski University of Kielce, 25-369 Kielce, Poland
2. Ophthalmic Clinic, The Voivodeship Hospital, 25-736 Kielce, Poland
3. Department of Vitreoretinal Surgery, Medical University of Lublin, 20-059 Lublin, Poland
4. Department of Infectious Disease, Provincial Hospital in Kielce, 25-736 Kielce, Poland
5. Institute of Medical Science, Jan Kochanowski University of Kielce, 25-369 Kielce, Poland
* Correspondence: mateuszwiniarczyk@umlub.pl

Abstract: The purpose of this study was to evaluate the persistent changes in microvascular parameters based on optical coherence tomography angiography (OCTA) in patients hospitalized due to COVID-19 bilateral pneumonia. The case-control prospective study was carried out among 49 patients with COVID-19 and 45 healthy age- and gender-matched 2 and 8 months after hospital discharge. We found a significantly decreased vessel density (VD) in superficial capillary plexus (SCP) in COVID-19 patients. Significantly decreased vessel density (VD) in the superficial capillary plexus (SCP), the deep capillary plexus (DCP), and choriocapillaris (CC), with significantly increased vessel density observed in the choriocapillaris in the foveal area (FCC). The foveal avascular zone in DCP (FAZd) was significantly increased in the COVID-19 group. We found differences between OCTA parameters according to gender. The foveal VD in SCP and DCP was significantly decreased in women compared to men. The FAZ area in SCP (FAZs) and superior VD in the choriocapillaris (SCC) were significantly increased in women. In conclusion, we noticed persistent changes in the ocular parameters of OCTA in COVID-19 patients. At the second follow-up visit, we observed a widened FAZ zone in SCP and decreased VD in some regions of the retina and choroid.

Keywords: COVID-19; SARS-CoV-2; optical coherence tomography angiography; vessel density; persistent microvascular changes

1. Introduction

The severe acute respiratory syndrome coronavirus 2 (SARS-CoV-2) spread worldwide in December 2019, causing the pandemic announced by World Health Organization (WHO) on 11 March 2020. This virus can cause a life-threatening infection associated with acute respiratory distress syndrome, a prothrombotic condition, cytokine storm, and multiorgan failure [1]. The SARS-CoV-2 virus binds via protein S to the ACE2 receptor present at high rates in the heart, lung, kidney, oleum, bladder epithelia Wells, and gastrointestinal system. This receptor is also present in the retina and choroid of the eye [2]. By damaging endothelial cells, this virus can lead to ischaemia, oedema, and hypercoagulability [3].

In our previous study, we used optical coherence tomography (OCT) to evaluate the retinal and choroidal microvasculature and neuroretinal structures in hospitalized patients with bilateral pneumonia due to SARS-CoV-2. We found a decreased vascular density (VD), enlarged foveal avascular zone (FAZ), thickened retinal nerve fibre layer (RNFL), and thinner ganglion cell layer (GCL) in foveal and parafoveal areas in COVID-19 patients compared to a cohort of age and sex-matched healthy controls [4]. Our results were consistent with those of other authors [5,6]. In the current study, we want to report the results of OCTA 6 months after the first study, in which persistent changes in some of its parameters are present. We decided to separate COVID-19 patients into two groups differentiating on gender due to the differences described in the literature in the course of the viral disease itself, the higher number of hospitalizations, and mortality among men due to COVID-19 [7]. The persisting symptoms such as fatigue and dyspnea, impaired pulmonary function [8,9], and chest image abnormalities due to SARS-CoV-2 infection were described [10]. These symptoms were more common in women than men, although there are no reports more than six months after follow-up [11–13].

2. Materials and Methods

2.1. Subjects

There was a double prospective study, controls in COVID-19 patients with bilateral pneumonia, who were hospitalized in the Department of Infectious Diseases of WSZ in Kielce during the pandemic spring wave caused by B.1.1.7 variant of SARS-CoV-2 from March to May 2021. The project was approved by the Bioethics Committee of Collegium Medicum of Jan Kochanowski University in Kielce (study code 54 approved on 1 July 2021).

As described in our previous paper, we excluded patients with eye and systemic diseases that could have affected the measurement outcomes, as previously described [4].

First, we examined 63 COVID-19 patients with bilateral pneumonia (120 eyes), 2 months after hospital discharge. Among this group we excluded 6 eyes: 2 eyes with hyperopia > 3 diopters, 1 eye with myopia > 3 diopters, 2 eyes after ocular trauma, and 1 eye after uveitis. After 6 months, we contacted these 62 patients and invited them to repeat the ocular examination; 49 patients (75 eyes) agreed to return. Among this group, we excluded the patients with these conditions and incomplete test results.

All patients signed the written informed consent to participate in the current study and underwent ophthalmological evaluation two and eight months after hospital discharge.

2.2. Characteristics of the Studied Group

The analyzed COVID-19 group consisted of 49 patients. In all, 31 men (63.27%) and 18 women (36.73%) with COVID-19 bilateral pneumonia participated in the analysis. A total of 75 eyes were included in the study group. The mean age of participants was 51.33 ± 1.45. The mean age of women was 55.1 ± 2.69, and men's was 49.6 ± 1.66 ($p = 0.075$). The mean (M) $\pm$ standard error of BMI M $\pm$ SEM was 28.56 (0.50) kg/m^2. There was no statistically significant difference in BMI between COVID-19 patients and the control group ($p = 0.051$).

The clinical diagnosis of COVID-19 was confirmed as previously described [4].

A total of 49 COVID-19 patients (75 eyes) underwent complete ophthalmic examination 8 months after hospital discharge. The visual acuity and reading vision were measured with a LogMAR scale. The intraocular pressure (IOP) measurement, a slit-lamp examination, OCT of the macula and optic nerve, and angio-OCT (OCTA) were performed. At the follow-up examination, the patients did not report any impairment of near or distant visual acuity or any visual complaints.

2.3. Characteristics of a Healthy Group

The control group included healthy patients who attended the ophthalmology department for a routine eye examination. This group consisted of 43 subjects ($n = 43$; eyes = 83) with a mean age of 47.76 ± 1.38. Written informed consent was obtained from all patients. Inclusion criteria for this group were as follows: age of 30–70 years, negative laboratory tests for SARS-CoV-2 infection (PCR from a nasopharyngeal swab), the absence of COVID-19 symptoms in the past or close contact with COVID-19 patients within the 14 days before the examination, and the absence of concomitant eye diseases. All patients had full distance and near vision of 6/6 in Snellen charts (0.0); the spherical equivalent was -0.67 (0.13), and the mean axial length was 23.35 (0.10) mm (Table 1).

Table 1. Ocular characteristics of COVID-19 patients at 0 months and 6 months.

Parameters	0 Month		6 Months		p
	$\bar{x}$ (SEM)	Me (IQR)	$\bar{x}$ (SEM)	Me (IQR)	
Visual acuity	6/6 (0.0)	6/6 (0.0)	6/6 (0.0)	6/6 (0.0)	0.593 [B]
Reading vision	6/6 (0.0)	6/6 (0.0)	6/6 (0.0)	6/6 (0.0)	0.285 [B]
Axial length	23.56 (0.10)	23.67 (1.1)	23.56 (0.10)	23.67 (1.1)	-
Intraocular pressure in mmHg (IOP)	16.66 (0.31)	16.85 (4.05)	16.42 (0.31)	16.40 (3.70)	0.504 [A]
Spherical equivalent (D)	0.19 (0.16)	0.0 (2.38)	0.20 (0.16)	0.0 (2.25)	0.673 [A]

[A]—t Student test; [B]—Wilcoxon rank test; D—diopters.

2.4. Optical Coherence Angiography Measurements

All scans were acquired with Swept Source DRI-OCT Triton SS-OCT Angio (Topcon Inc., Tokyo, Japan). OCTA protocols included the following parameters: 4.5 × 4.5 mm and 6 × 6 mm scanning protocols.

OCTA parameters evaluated were vessel density (VD) in the three different plexi: (superficial capillary plexus) SCP, deep capillary plexus (DCP), and choriocapillaris (CC) using the ETDRS grid subfields to define the areas of interest. The vessel density was measured in superior (S), inner nasal (N), inner inferior (I), and inner temporal (T) ETDRS subfields centered on the macula by fixation. Vessel density measurement was performed via the integrated software. The foveal avascular zone (FAZ) in the SCP and in the DCP was manually delineated by two independent graders, encompassing the central fovea, where no clear and demarcated vessels were seen on the OCTA. Scan quality over 65% was a threshold for eligibility for the study, as previously described [4].

2.5. Statistical Analysis

For quantitative traits, distributions were checked. The mean and standard error of the mean (SEM), median (Me), and interquartile range (IQR) were calculated separately for patients tested at 0 months, 6 months, and the control group separately. Student's t-tests for dependent samples and Wilcoxon's paired rank test were used to compare the variables for binary studies. For comparison of COVID-19 men and women in the 2 separate studies, and COVID-19 patients studied at months 0 and 6 versus the control group, the Student's t-test was used for independent samples and the Mann-Whitney, depending on their distribution. A statistical significance threshold of $p < 0.05$ was set. The analysis was performed with STATISTICA 13.3 statistical package, Polish version (STATSOFT, Krakow, Poland).

3. Results

3.1. OCT Angiography Outcomes

3.1.1. Case-Control Study (6 Months)

In the optical coherence tomography angiography (OCTA) analysis, a significantly decreased vessel density (VD) in superficial capillary plexus (SCP) was observed in COVID-19 patients at the 6-month examination compared to controls in the superior area (S SCP) (45.38 ± 0.40 vs. 48.23 ± 0.37, $p = 0.000$), nasal area (N SCP) (43.91 ± 0.27 vs. 44.99 ± 0.27, $p = 0.024$), inferior area (I SCP) (44.43 ± 0.40 vs. 47.30 ± 0.36, $p < 0.001$), temporal area (T SCP) (44.82 ± 0.23 vs. 46.44 ± 0.24, $p < 0.001$). The foveal avascular zone in SCP (FAZ s) was significantly increased in COVID-19 patients at the 6-month examination, compared to controls (328.95 ± 13.35 vs. 251.03 ± 12.10, $p < 0.001$).

The significantly decreased vessel density (VD) was also found in deep capillary plexus (DCP) in COVID-19 patients at the 6-month examination, compared to controls in foveal area (F DCP) (14.48 ± 0.55 vs. 16.93 ± 0.49, $p < 0.001$), superior area (S DCP) (47.31 ± 0.37 vs. 52.18 ± 0.40, $p < 0.001$), nasal area (N SCP) (45.62 ± 0.31 vs. 48.45 ± 0.32, $p < 0.001$), inferior area (I DCP) (45.83 ± 0.38 vs. 50.91 ± 0.40, $p < 0.001$), temporal area (T

DCP) (43.68 ± 0.28 vs. 47.20 ± 0.33, $p < 0.001$). The foveal avascular zone in DCP (FAZd) was significantly increased in COVID-19 patients at the 6-month examination, compared to controls (552.80 ± 23.74 vs. 235.05 ± 12.10, $p < 0.001$).

The significantly decreased vessel density (VD) was observed in the choriocapillaris (CC) in COVID-19 patients at the 6-month examination, compared to controls in the superior area (S CC) (52.07 ± 0.26 vs. 54.24 ± 0.28, $p < 0.001$), inferior area (I CC) (52.24 ± 0.25 vs. 54.26 ± 0.28, $p < 0.001$), temporal area (T CC) (52.99 ± 0.27 vs. 53.50 ± 0.50, $p < 0.001$) (Table 2).

Table 2. Comparison of foveal (F) and parafoveal parameters of OCTA (optical coherence tomography angiography) between COVID-19 patients (women and men) in the 6-month and control group: SCP—superficial capillary plexus, DCP—deep capillary plexus, CC—choriocapillaris, FAZ s—superficial foveal avascular zone, FAZ d—deep foveal avascular zone, F—foveal area, S—superior area, N—nasal area, I—inferior area, T—temporal area. Mean ± SEM (standard error of the mean) structural OCT values. Bold values denote statistical significance at the $p < 0.05$ level.

Variables	6th Month (n = 75 Eyes)		Control Group (n = 83 Eyes)		p
	$\bar{x}$ (SEM)	Me (IQR)	$\bar{x}$ (SEM)	Me (IQR)	
F SCP	19.93 (0.48)	19.86 (5.30)	20.70 (045)	21.14 (5.34)	0.239 [A]
F DCP	14.48 (0.55)	13.89 (6.11)	16.93 (0.49)	16.55 (6.92)	<0.001 [A]
F CCP	52.43 (0.34)	52.16 (2.97)	52.43 (0.47)	52.96 (6.38)	0.404 [B]
S SCP	45.38 (0.40)	46.26 (3.65)	48.23 (0.37)	48.19 (3.84)	0.000 [B]
S DCP	47.31 (0.37)	46.88 (3.41)	52.18 (0.40)	51.89 (4.63)	<0.001 [B]
S CCP	52.07 (0.26)	52.19 (3.59)	54.24 (0.28)	54.23 (2.44)	<0.001 [B]
N SCP	43.91 (0.27)	44.59 (2.70)	44.99 (0.27)	45.05 (3.57)	0.024 [B]
N DCP	45.62 (0.31)	45.60 (4.41)	48.45 (0.32)	47.91 (4.18)	<0.001 [A]
N CCP	52.79 (0.25)	52.75 (2.85)	53.22 (0.25)	53.32 (2.89)	0.148 [B]
I SCP	44.43 (0.40)	45.22 (5.06)	47.30 (0.36)	47.45 (5.13)	<0.001 [B]
I DCP	45.83 (0.38)	45.06 (4.02)	50.91 (0.40)	50.34 (4.39)	<0.001 [B]
I CCP	52.24 (0.25)	52.19 (3.10)	54.26 (0.28)	54.11 (2.45)	<0.001 [B]
T SCP	44.82 (0.23)	44.77 (2.06)	46.44 (0.24)	46.52 (3.29)	<0.001 [A]
T DCP	43.68 (0.28)	43.36 (3.30)	47.20 (0.33)	46.93 (4.39)	<0.001 [A]
T CCP	52.99 (0.27)	53.00 (2.65)	53.50 (0.50)	54.06 (2.43)	<0.001 [B]
FAZs (μm²)	328.95 (13.35)	329.59 (128.40)	251.03 (12.10)	243.07 (154.03)	<0.001 [A]
FAZd (μm²)	552.80 (23.74)	562.23 (325.06)	235.05 (12.10)	226.41 (157.03)	<0.001 [B]

[A]—t Student test; [B]—Wilcoxon rank test.

3.1.2. Prospective Cohort Study (0–6 Months)

In the optical coherence tomography angiography (OCTA) analysis, a significantly decreased vessel density (VD) in superficial capillary plexus (SCP) was observed in COVID-19 patients at the 6-month examination, compared to 0 month in the foveal area (F SCP) (19.93 ± 0.48 vs. 20.54 ± 0.51, $p = 0.006$), superior area (S SCP) (45.38 ± 0.40 vs. 48.44 ± 0.31, $p < 0.001$), nasal area (N SCP) (43.91 ± 0.27 vs. 44.92 ± 0.29, $p = 0.004$), inferior area (I SCP) (44.43 ± 0.40 vs. 47.29 ± 0.42, $p < 0.001$).

The significantly decreased vessel density (VD) was observed in deep capillary plexus (DCP) in COVID-19 patients at the 6-month examination, compared to 0 months in the foveal area (F DCP) (14.48 ± 0.55 vs. 17.11 ± 0.55, $p < 0.001$), superior area (S DCP) (47.31 ± 0.37 vs. 52.00 ± 0.35, $p < 0.001$), nasal area (N DCP) (45.62 ± 0.31 vs. 49.05 ± 0.34, $p < 0.001$), inferior area (I DCP) (45.83 ± 0.38 vs. 51.10 ± 0.48, $p < 0.001$).

The foveal avascular zone in DCP (FAZ d) was significantly increased in COVID-19 patients at the 6-month examination, compared to 0 months (552.80 ± 23.74 vs. 359.32 ± 16.92, $p < 0.001$).

The significantly decreased vessel density (VD) was observed in the choriocapillaris (CC) in COVID-19 patients at the 6-month examination, compared to 0 months in the superior area (S CC) (52.07 ± 54.07 ± 0.24, $p < 0.001$), nasal area (N CC) (52.79 ± 0.25 vs. 53.76 ± 0.26, $p = 0.003$), inferior area (I CC) (52.24 ± 0.25 vs. 54.13 ± 0.26, $p < 0.001$), temporal area (T CC) (52.99 ± 0.27 vs. 54.09 ± 0.20, $p < 0.001$).

The significantly increased vessel density (VD) was observed in the choriocapillaris (CC) in COVID-19 patients at the 6-month examination, compared to 0 months in the foveal area (FCC) (52.43 ± 0.34 vs. 51.34 ± 0.47, $p = 0.014$) (Table 3).

Table 3. Comparison of foveal (F) and parafoveal parameters of OCTA (optical coherence tomography angiography) between 0 months and the 6th month in all COVID-19 patients (women and men): SCP—superficial capillary plexus, DCP—deep capillary plexus, CC—choriocapillaris, FAZ s—superficial foveal avascular zone, FAZ d—deep foveal avascular zone, F—foveal area, S—superior area, N—nasal area, I—inferior area, T—temporal area. Mean ± SEM (standard error of the mean) structural OCT values. Bold values denote statistical significance at the $p < 0.05$ level.

Variables OCTA	0 Month (n = 75 Eyes)		6th Month (n = 75 Eyes)		p
	$\bar{x}$ (SEM)	Me (IQR)	$\bar{x}$ (SEM)	Me (IQR)	
F SCP	20.54 (0.51)	20.79 (4.97)	19.93 (0.48)	19.86 (5.30)	0.006 [A]
F DCP	17.11 (0.55)	16.92 (5.75)	14.48 (0.55)	13.89 (6.11)	<0.001 [A]
F CC	51.34 (0.47)	51.64 (4.91)	52.43 (0.34)	52.16 (2.97)	0.014 [B]
S SCP	48.44 (0.31)	48.58 (2.75)	45.38 (0.40)	46.26 (3.65)	<0.001 [B]
S DCP	52.00 (0.35)	52.04 (4.61)	47.31 (0.37)	46.88 (3.41)	<0.001 [A]
S CC	54.07 (0.24)	54.12 (2.43)	52.07 (0.26)	52.19 (3.59)	<0.001 [B]
N SCP	44.92 (0.29)	45.13 (3.95)	43.91 (0.27)	44.59 (2.70)	0.004 [A]
N DCP	49.05 (0.34)	48.51 (3.64)	45.62 (0.31)	45.60 (4.41)	<0.001 [B]
N CC	53.76 (0.26)	53.83 (2.67)	52.79 (0.25)	52.75 (2.85)	0.003 [A]
I SCP	47.29 (0.42)	48.01 (3.86)	44.43 (0.40)	45.22 (5.06)	<0.001 [B]
I DCP	51.10 (0.48)	51.14 (5.19)	45.83 (0.38)	45.06 (4.02)	<0.001 [B]
I CC	54.13 (0.26)	54.25 (3.37)	52.24 (0.25)	52.19 (3.10)	<0.001 [A]
T SCP	46.57 (0.24)	46.45 (3.16)	44.82 (0.23)	44.77 (2.06)	<0.001 [A]
T DCP	47.44 (0.31)	47.59 (3.88)	43.68 (0.28)	43.36 (3.30)	<0.001 [A]
T CC	54.09 (0.20)	53.94 (2.40)	52.99 (0.27)	53.00 (2.65)	<0.001 [A]
FAZs (µm²)	327.60 (12.64)	323.55 (128.40)	328.95 (13.35)	329.59 (128.40)	0.822 [A]
FAZd (µm²)	359.32 (16.29)	343.11 (155.06)	552.80 (23.74)	562.23 (325.06)	<0.001 [B]

[A]—t Student test; [B]—Wilcoxon rank test.

3.2. Gender Analysis

3.2.1. Gender Analysis at 0 Month

In OCTA analysis, the foveal VD in SCP was significantly decreased in women than in men (18.91 ± 0.85 vs. 21.62 ± 0.58, $p = 0.008$) at 0 months. The VD was significantly decreased in the temporal area in DCP in women than in men (46.55 ± 0.52 vs. 48.04 ± 0.36, $p = 0.018$).

The FAZ area in SCP (FAZs) was significantly increased in women than in men (367.86 ± 22.56 vs. 300.76 ± 13.53, $p = 0.008$) at 0 months (Table 4).

Table 4. Comparison of foveal (F) and parafoveal parameters of OCTA (optical coherence tomography angiography) parameters between women and men in COVID-19 patients in 0 month: SCP—superficial capillary plexus, DCP—deep capillary plexus, CC—choriocapillaris, FAZ s—superficial foveal avascular zone, FAZ d—deep foveal avascular zone, F—foveal area, S—superior area, N—nasal area, I—inferior area, T—temporal area. Mean ± SEM (standard error of the mean) structural OCT values. Bold values denote statistical significance at the $p < 0.05$ level.

Variables	Women—0 Month (n = 30 Eyes)		Men—0 Month (n = 45 Eyes)		p
	$\bar{x}$ (SEM)	Me (IQR)	$\bar{x}$ (SEM)	Me (IQR)	
F SCP	18.91 (0.85)	18.89 (3.75)	21.62 (0.58)	21.50 (4.04)	**0.008** [A]
F DCP	16.96 (0.83)	17.74 (5.00)	17.21 (0.74)	16.33 (5.65)	0.693 [B]
F CC	50.62 (0.83)	50.78 (5.48)	51.83 (0.55)	52.56 (3.74)	0.143 [B]
S SCP	49.11 (0.44)	49.41 (2.48)	47.99 (0.41)	48.44 (2.89)	0.071 [B]
S DCP	51.44 (0.66)	51.66 (5.27)	52.37 (0.39)	52.45 (4.00)	0.178 [A]
S CC	54.61 (0.44)	54.49 (2.19)	53.71 (0.26)	53.71 (1.84)	0.097 [B]
N SCP	45.38 (0.39)	45.79 (3.59)	44.62 (0.41)	44.70 (4.40)	0.221 [B]
N DCP	48.66 (0.62)	47.56 (4.43)	49.31 (0.39)	48.82 (2.68)	0.077 [B]
N CC	53.81 (0.38)	53.63 (2.17)	53.73 (0.35)	54.26 (3.00)	0.868 [A]
I SCP	48.31 (0.44)	48.46 (2.54)	46.61 (0.61)	47.62 (4.77)	0.083 [B]
I DCP	50.42 (0.68)	49.98 (3.18)	51.55 (0.66)	51.74 (5.23)	0.089 [B]
I CC	54.25 (0.39)	54.29 (3.73)	54.04 (0.35)	54.05 (3.05)	0.727 [A]
T SCP	46.93 (0.35)	46.64 (2.54)	46.33 (0.36)	46.22 (3.28)	0.258 [A]
T DCP	46.55 (0.52)	46.38 (3.68)	48.04 (0.36)	47.95 (3.46)	**0.018** [A]
T CC	54.14 (0.32)	53.81 (2.33)	54.06 (0.25)	53.98 (1.97)	0.847 [A]
FAZs (µm^2)	367.86 (22.56)	367.77 (114.43)	300.76 (13.53)	297.32 (101.35)	**0.008** [A]
FAZd (µm^2)	366.22 (24.63)	346.34 (115.90)	349.73 (21.80)	326.98 (161.64)	0.398 [B]

[A]—t Student test; [B]—Wilcoxon rank test.

3.2.2. Gender Analysis at the 6th Month

In OCTA analysis, the foveal VD in SCP was significantly decreased in women than in men (18.69 ± 0.88 vs. 20.75 ± 0.53, $p = 0.037$) at the 6th month. The VD was significantly decreased in the temporal area in DCP in women than in men (43.01 ± 0.46 vs. 44.13 ± 0.34, $p = 0.049$).

In OCTA analysis, the superior VD in CC (S CC) was significantly increased in women than in men (52.76 ± 0.45 vs. 51.61 ± 0.29, $p = 0.028$) at the 6th month.

The FAZ area in SCP (FAZs) was significantly increased in women than in men (379.17 ± 23.56 vs. 295.46 ± 13.86, $p = 0.002$) during the 6th month (Table 5).

Table 5. Comparison of foveal (F) and parafoveal parameters of OCTA (optical coherence tomography angiography) parameters between women and men in the 6th month in COVID-19 patients: SCP—superficial capillary plexus, DCP—deep capillary plexus, CC—choriocapillaris, FAZ s—superficial foveal avascular zone, FAZ d—deep foveal avascular zone, F—foveal area, S—superior area, N—nasal area, I—inferior area, T—temporal area. Mean ± SEM (standard error of the mean) structural OCT values. Bold values denote statistical significance at the $p < 0.05$ level.

Variables	Women—6th Month (n = 30 Eyes)		Men—6th Month (n = 45 Eyes)		p
	$\bar{x}$ (SEM)	Me (IQR)	$\bar{x}$ (SEM)	Me (IQR)	
F SCP	18.69 (0.88)	18.96 (5.29)	20.75 (0.53)	20.56 (4.46)	**0.037** [A]

Table 5. Cont.

Variables	Women—6th Month (n = 30 Eyes)		Men—6th Month (n = 45 Eyes)		p
	$\bar{x}$ (SEM)	Me (IQR)	$\bar{x}$ (SEM)	Me (IQR)	
F DCP	14.23 (0.92)	14.15 (6.25)	14.64 (0.70)	13.71 (5.61)	0.876 [B]
F CCP	51.91 (0.53)	51.69 (3.01)	52.78 (0.43)	52.55 (2.91)	0.209 [A]
S SCP	45.66 (0.63)	46.50 (3.62)	45.19 (0.52)	45.89 (3.49)	0.632 [B]
S DCP	47.31 (0.62)	47.26 (4.55)	47.31 (0.46)	46.39 (3.09)	0.885 [B]
S CCP	52.76 (0.45)	53.74 (3.45)	51.61 (0.29)	51.69 (2.40)	0.028 [A]
N SCP	44.50 (0.37)	44.87 (2.29)	43.51 (0.36)	43.87 (2.89)	0.055 [B]
N DCP	46.22 (0.42)	46.30 (3.50)	45.21 (0.43)	45.23 (4.56)	0.112 [A]
N CCP	52.59 (0.35)	52.55 (1.82)	52.92 (0.34)	53.30 (3.01)	0.523 [A]
I SCP	44.45 (0.59)	44.74 (3.51)	44.42 (0.54)	45.51 (5.35)	0.751 [B]
I DCP	45.46 (45.46)	44.72 (2.78)	46.08 (0.50)	45.193.87)	0.274 [B]
I CCP	52.67 (0.40)	52.38 (2.81)	51.95 (0.33)	52.02 (3.46)	0.914 [A]
T SCP	44.82 (0.28)	45.02 (1.72)	44.82 (0.35)	44.75 (2.38)	0.991 [A]
T DCP	43.01 (0.46)	43.26 (3.63)	44.13 (0.34)	43.65 (3.37)	0.049 [A]
T CCP	52.94 (0.38)	52.90 (2.76)	53.03 (0.38)	53.04 (2.75)	0.773 [B]
FAZs (μm^2)	379.17 (23.56)	381.50 (125.11)	295.46 (13.86)	289.75 (115.91)	0.002 [A]
FAZd (μm^2)	591.75 (40.67)	581.79 (302.26)	526.84 (28.54)	551.51 (301.16)	0.182 [A]

[A]—t Student test; [B]—Wilcoxon rank test.

4. Discussion

The current study aimed to evaluate and compare the short- and long-term changes in microvascular parameters based on optical coherence tomography angiography (OCTA) in COVID-19 patients hospitalized due to bilateral pneumonia caused by SARS-CoV-2.

The OCT is a non-invasive tool, which can successfully visualize the microvascular network of the retina and choroid in many ocular disorders and general diseases [14].

The results of our study were compared with the results of other researchers who evaluated the condition of the retina and choroid six months after the first examination, and, like them, we assessed whether the changes in the eye have a more severe course in women compared with men [15,16].

In our first study, we found decreased vessel density (VD) in the superficial capillary plexus (SCP), in the deep capillary plexus (DCP), and in the choriocapillaris (CC) in 63 COVID-19 patients, compared to a cohort of age and sex-matched healthy controls. The foveal avascular zone (FAZ) in SCP and in DCP were significantly increased in that study [4].

Six months later, we examined 49 of 63 hospitalized COVID-19 patients with bilateral pneumonia 8 months before and found a significantly decreased vessel density (VD) in superficial capillary plexus (SCP) in OCTA in COVID-19 patients at the 6-month examination, compared to controls in parafoveal areas and at the 6-month examination, compared to 0 months in foveal and parafoveal areas.

The foveal avascular zone in SCP (FAZ s) was significantly increased in COVID-19 patients at the 6-month examination, compared to controls.

We observed a significantly decreased vessel density (VD) in deep capillary plexus (DCP) in COVID-19 patients at the 6-month examination, compared to controls and compared to 0 months in foveal and parafoveal areas.

The foveal avascular zone in DCP (FAZ d) was significantly increased in COVID-19 patients at the 6-month examination, compared to controls and compared to 0 month.

The significantly decreased vessel density (VD) was observed in choriocapillaris (CC) in COVID-19 patients at the 6-month examination, compared to controls in parafoveal areas.

We found a significantly decreased vessel density (VD) in choriocapillaris (CC) in parafoveal areas and a significantly increased vessel density (VD) in foveal area of choriocapillaris (FCC) in COVID-19 patients at 6-month examination, compared to 0 month.

Changes in OCTA microvascular parameters described two months after hospitalization for SARS-CoV-2 infection are still present six months later. The similar findings may involve tissues that are embryologically and structurally similar to the retina, such as the brain. One study reports microstructural abnormalities and changes in cerebral blood flow three months after recovery from pneumonia in COVID-19 patients [17].

Many papers report persistent changes after SARS-CoV-2 infection, such as pulmonary dysfunction six months after the onset of symptoms, renal dysfunction, vascular dysfunction, and thromboembolic disease even one month after the illness [18,19].

SARS-CoV-2 can directly destroy endothelial cells by binding to angiotensin-converting enzyme 2 (ACE-2) [20,21]. This mechanism can develop coagulopathy leading to damage to the vessels in many human organs [22]. The retina and choroid are richly vascularized structures with the ACE2 receptor present, which is a choke point for the SARS-CoV-2 virus, so one might expect microangiopathy here. Many authors have described thrombotic-related findings in the retina, i.e., retinal haemorrhages, cotton wool balls, and dilated and tortuous retinal vessels in COVID-19 patients [23,24].

We compared parameters of OCTA between women and men at 0 months and at 6 months. Many studies have described persisting symptoms as more common in women, such as fatigue and dyspnea, impaired pulmonary function [8], and chest image abnormalities [10,13]. One may hypothesize that COVID-19 infection may lead to different sex-related complications.

The foveal VD in SCP was significantly decreased in women than in men at 0 months and 6 months. The VD was also significantly decreased in the temporal area in DCP in women than in men at 0 months and 6 months. The FAZ area in SCP (FAZs) was significantly increased in women than in men at 0 months and 6 months. The superior VD in the choriocapillaris (SCC) was significantly increased in women than in men at six months.

Some authors suggest a slower recovery process in women compared to men or even a gradual deterioration of ocular parameters based on the OCTA study in this group. This may suggest that women may have a higher risk of reduced VD in the months following COVID-19. Some researchers also report that women may be more predisposed to persistent neurological and psychological impairment, fatigue, post-activity polypnea, and alopecia [13,25].

Fernandez-de-las Penas C. et al. described that the number of post-COVID symptoms was significantly higher in women than in men ($p < 0.001$). Furthermore, he found that women were more predisposed to post-COVID symptomatology even eight months after hospital discharge [26]. Three multicenter studies reported that the female gender is a potential risk factor for the development of post-COVID symptoms, e.g., fatigue, dyspnea, or dermatological symptoms [27].

The issue of why the female sex is more predisposed to post-COVID symptoms is currently debated in the literature. First, there are biological differences in the expression of ACE2 I transmembrane protease serine 2 (TMPRSS2) receptors between males and females, and immunological differences; lower production of pro-inflammatory interleukin-6 (IL-6) due to viral infection in women [28,29]. Other factors that are considered in the more frequent development of post-COVID symptoms in women are more frequent hand washing, less exposure to infections, and higher psychological stress [30].

Many researchers have considered the effect of female hormones on the vascularization of the eyeball. Estrogen, progesterone, and testosterone are regulators of blood flow through the retina and choroid and are also key to regulating vascular tone in the body. Estrogen plays a protective role when there is a decrease in vascular resistance in the large vessels of the eye [28,29]. One study showed significantly greater choroidal blood flow in women under 40 compared to women over 55 men. Age was not significant for choroidal blood flow in men. Also, pulsatile ocular blood flow and pulse amplitude were significantly higher in pre-menopausal women compared to age-matched male and post-menopausal women not taking hormonal therapy [30]. Further sex-disaggregated studies evaluating retinal and choroidal blood circulation are needed.

Our study had several limitations. The separate groups of women and men consisted of too few individuals. An algorithm for the OCT examination is needed to assess which parameters of this examination may be highly helpful in assessing the ocular condition and general state of COVID-19 patients. The strength of our study was the highly selected group of patients hospitalized for SARS-CoV-2 infection and the strictly maintained time frame of the two follow-up examinations in this group.

5. Conclusions

A study that we performed twice in COVID-19 patients, two and six months after hospital discharge, showed a trend toward persistent decline in VD in retinal and choroidal vascular plexuses. Differences were observed between OCTA parameters between women and men to the disadvantage of the first group, such as reduced VD in SCP and in DCP and a widened FAZ zone in SCP. Further follow-up studies are needed in this group of patients stratified by sex to assess whether there are consequences in these ocular structures due to poor blood supply.

Author Contributions: Conceptualization, M.K.; methodology, M.K., M.W. and D.Z.-M.; software, D.O.; validation, E.C.; formal analysis, B.P.-A.; investigation, M.K. and M.W.; resources, M.K.; data curation, M.B.; writing—original draft preparation, M.K.; writing—review and editing, M.W., D.Z.-M. and B.P.-A.; visualization, D.Z.-M.; supervision, D.O., J.M. and S.G.; project administration, P.P., S.G. and J.M.; funding acquisition, M.K. All authors have read and agreed to the published version of the manuscript.

Funding: Project financed under the program of the Ministry of Education and Science called "Regional Initiative of Excellence" in the years 2019–2023, project no. 024/RID/2018/19. Amount of financing 1,199,900,000 PLN.

Institutional Review Board Statement: The study was conducted in accordance with the Declaration of Helsinki and approved by the Bioethics Committee of Collegium Medicum of Jan Kochanowski University in Kielce (study code 54 approved on 1 July 2021).

Informed Consent Statement: Informed consent was obtained from all subjects involved in the study.

Data Availability Statement: Not available.

Conflicts of Interest: The authors declare no conflict of interest.

References

1. Gu, S.X.; Tyagi, T.; Jain, K.; Gu, V.W.; Lee, S.H.; Hwa, J.M.; Kwan, J.M.; Krause, D.S.; Lee, A.I.; Halene, S.; et al. Thrombocytopathy and endotheliopathy: Crucial contributors to COVID-19 thromboinflammation. *Nat. Rev. Cardiol.* **2021**, *18*, 194–209. [CrossRef] [PubMed]
2. Holappa, M.; Vapaatalo, H.; Vaajanen, A. Many Faces of Renin-angiotensin System—Focus on Eye. *Open Ophthalmol. J.* **2017**, *11*, 122–142. [CrossRef] [PubMed]
3. Felsenstein, S.; Herbert, J.A.; McNamara, P.S.; Hedrich, C.M. COVID-19: Immunology and treatment options. *Clin. Immunol.* **2020**, *215*, 108448. [CrossRef]
4. Kal, M.; Winiarczyk, M.; Cieśla, E.; Płatkowska-Adamska, B.; Walczyk, A.; Biskup, M.; Pabjan, P.; Głuszek, S.; Odrobina, D.; Mackiewicz, J.; et al. Retinal Microvascular Changes in COVID-19 Bilateral Pneumonia Based on Optical Coherence Tomography Angiography. *J. Clin. Med.* **2022**, *11*, 3621. [CrossRef] [PubMed]
5. Huang, C.; Wang, Y.; Li, X.; Ren, L.; Zhao, J.; Hu, Y.; Zhang, L.; Fan, G.; Xu, J.; Gu, X.; et al. Clinical features of patients infected with 2019 novel coronavirus in Wuhan, China. *Lancet* **2020**, *395*, 497–506. [CrossRef] [PubMed]

6. Giannis, D.; Ziogas, I.A.; Gianni, P. Coagulation disorders in coronavirus infected patients: COVID-19, SARS-CoV-1, MERS-CoV and lessons from the past. *J. Clin. Virol.* **2020**, *127*, 104362. [CrossRef] [PubMed]
7. Magro, C.; Mulvey, J.J.; Berlin, D.; Nuovo, G.; Salvatore, S.; Harp, J.; Baxter-Stoltzfus, A.; Laurence, J. Complement associated microvascular injury and thrombosis in the pathogenesis of severe COVID-19 infection: A report of five cases. *Transl. Res.* **2020**, *220*, 1–13. [CrossRef]
8. Varga, Z.; Flammer, A.J.; Steiger, P.; Haberecker, M.; Andermatt, R.; Zinkernagel, A.S.; Mehra, M.R.; Schuepbach, R.A.; Ruschitzka, F.; Moch, H. Endothelial cell infection and endotheliitis in COVID-19. *Lancet* **2020**, *395*, 1417–1418. [CrossRef]
9. Bates, N.M.; Tian, J.; Smiddy, W.E.; Lee, W.-H.; Somfai, G.M.; Feuer, W.J.; Shiffman, J.C.; Kuriyan, A.E.; Gregori, N.Z.; Kostic, M.; et al. Relationship between the morphology of the foveal avascular zone, retinal structure, and macular circulation in patients with diabetes mellitus. *Sci. Rep.* **2018**, *8*, 5355. [CrossRef]
10. Invernizzi, A.; Torre, A.; Parrulli, S.; Zicarelli, F.; Schiuma, M.; Colombo, V.; Giacomelli, A.; Cigada, M.; Milazzo, L.; Ridolfo, A.; et al. Retinal findings in patients with COVID-19: Results from the SERPICO-19 study. *Eclinicalmedicine* **2020**, *27*, 100550. [CrossRef]
11. Virgo, J.; Mohamed, M. Paracentral acute middle maculopathy and acute macular neuroretinopathy following SARS-CoV-2 infection. *Eye* **2020**, *34*, 2352–2353. [CrossRef] [PubMed]
12. Cevik, M.; Kuppalli, K.; Kindrachuk, J.; Peiris, M. Virology, transmission, and pathogenesis of SARS-CoV-2. *BMJ* **2020**, *371*, m3862. [CrossRef]
13. Liu, C.; Ye, L.; Xia, R.; Zheng, X.; Yuan, C.; Wang, Z.; Lin, R.; Shi, D.; Gao, Y.; Yao, J.; et al. Chest Computed Tomography and Clinical Follow-Up of Discharged Patients with COVID-19 in Wenzhou City, Zhejiang, China. *Ann. Am. Thorac. Soc.* **2020**, *17*, 1231–1237. [CrossRef] [PubMed]
14. Torjesen, I. COVID-19: Middle aged women face greater risk of debilitating long term symptoms. *BMJ* **2021**, *372*, n829. [CrossRef] [PubMed]
15. Carfi, A.; Bernabei, R.; Landi, F.; for the Gemelli against COVID-19 Post-Acute Care Study Group. Persistent Symptoms in Patients after Acute COVID-19. *JAMA* **2020**, *324*, 603–605. [CrossRef] [PubMed]
16. Hryhorowicz, S.; Ustaszewski, A.; Kaczmarek-Ryś, M.; Lis, E.; Witt, M.; Pławski, A.; Ziętkiewicz, E. European context of the diversity and phylogenetic position of SARS-CoV-2 sequences from Polish COVID-19 patients. *J. Appl. Genet.* **2021**, *62*, 327–337. [CrossRef]
17. Bilbao-Malavé, V.; González-Zamora, J.; de Viteri, M.S.; de la Puente, M.; Gándara, E.; Casablanca-Piñera, A.; Boquera-Ventosa, C.; Zarranz-Ventura, J.; Landecho, M.; García-Layana, A. Persistent Retinal Microvascular Impairment in COVID-19 Bilateral Pneumonia at 6-Months Follow-Up Assessed by Optical Coherence Tomography Angiography. *Biomedicines* **2021**, *9*, 502. [CrossRef]
18. Turker, I.C.; Dogan, C.U.; Dirim, A.B.; Guven, D.; Kutucu, O.K. Evaluation of early and late COVID-19-induced vascular changes with OCTA. *Can. J. Ophthalmol.* **2022**, *57*, 236–241. [CrossRef]
19. Qin, Y.; Wu, J.; Chen, T.; Li, J.; Zhang, G.; Wu, D.; Zhou, Y.; Zheng, N.; Cai, A.; Ning, Q.; et al. Long-term microstructure and cerebral blood flow changes in patients recovered from COVID-19 without neurological manifestations. *J. Clin. Investig.* **2021**, *131*, e147329. [CrossRef]
20. Lam, M.H.-B.; Wing, Y.-K.; Yu, M.W.-M.; Leung, C.-M.; Ma, R.C.W.; Kong, A.P.S.; So, W.; Fong, S.Y.-Y.; Lam, S.-P. Mental Morbidities and Chronic Fatigue in Severe Acute Respiratory Syndrome Survivors: Long-term Follow-up. *Arch. Intern. Med.* **2009**, *169*, 2142–2147. [CrossRef] [PubMed]
21. Lee, M.-H.; Perl, D.P.; Nair, G.; Li, W.; Maric, D.; Murray, H.; Dodd, S.J.; Koretsky, A.P.; Watts, J.A.; Cheung, V.; et al. Microvascular Injury in the Brains of Patients with COVID-19. *N. Engl. J. Med.* **2021**, *384*, 481–483. [CrossRef]
22. Huang, C.; Huang, L.; Wang, Y.; Li, X.; Ren, L.; Gu, X.; Kang, L.; Guo, L.; Liu, M.; Zhou, X.; et al. 6-month consequences of COVID-19 in patients discharged from hospital: A cohort study. *Lancet* **2021**, *397*, 220–232. [CrossRef] [PubMed]
23. Fernández-De-Las-Peñas, C.; Martín-Guerrero, J.D.; Pellicer-Valero, J.; Navarro-Pardo, E.; Gómez-Mayordomo, V.; Cuadrado, M.L.; Arias-Navalón, J.A.; Cigarán-Méndez, M.; Hernández-Barrera, V.; Arendt-Nielsen, L. Female Sex Is a Risk Factor Associated with Long-Term Post-COVID Related-Symptoms but not with COVID-19 Symptoms: The LONG-COVID-EXP-CM Multicenter Study. *J. Clin. Med.* **2022**, *11*, 413. [CrossRef] [PubMed]
24. Sigfrid, L.; Drake, T.M.; Pauley, E.; Jesudason, E.C.; Olliaro, P.; Lim, W.S.; Gillesen, A.; Berry, C.; Lowe, D.J.; McPeake, J.; et al. Long Covid in adults discharged from UK hospitals after COVID-19: A prospective, multicentre cohort study using the ISARIC WHO Clinical Characterisation Protocol. *Lancet Reg. Health. Eur.* **2021**, *8*, 100186. [CrossRef]
25. Bwire, G.M. Coronavirus: Why Men are More Vulnerable to COVID-19 than Women? *SN Compr. Clin. Med.* **2020**, *2*, 874–876. [CrossRef] [PubMed]
26. Ortona, E.; Buonsenso, D.; Carfi, A.; Malorni, W. Long COVID: An estrogen-associated autoimmune disease? *Cell Death Discov.* **2021**, *7*, 77. [CrossRef]
27. Anca, P.S.; Toth, P.P.; Kempler, P.; Rizzo, M. Gender differences in the battle against COVID-19: Impact of genetics, comorbidities, inflammation and lifestyle on differences in outcomes. *Int. J. Clin. Pract.* **2021**, *75*, e13666. [CrossRef]
28. Schmidl, D.; Schmetterer, L.; Garhöfer, G.; Popa-Cherecheanu, A. Gender Differences in Ocular Blood Flow. *Curr. Eye Res.* **2015**, *40*, 201–212. [CrossRef]

29. Ustymowicz, A.; Mariak, Z.; Weigele, J.; Lyson, T.; Kochanowicz, J.; Krejza, J. Normal reference intervals and ranges of side-to-side and day-to-day variability of ocular blood flow Doppler parameters. *Ultrasound Med. Biol.* **2005**, *31*, 895–903. [CrossRef]
30. Kavroulaki, D.; Gugleta, K.; Kochkorov, A.; Katamay, R.; Flammer, J.; Orgul, S. Influence of gender and menopausal status on peripheral and choroidal circulation. *Acta Ophthalmol.* **2010**, *88*, 850–853. [CrossRef]

Disclaimer/Publisher's Note: The statements, opinions and data contained in all publications are solely those of the individual author(s) and contributor(s) and not of MDPI and/or the editor(s). MDPI and/or the editor(s) disclaim responsibility for any injury to people or property resulting from any ideas, methods, instructions or products referred to in the content.

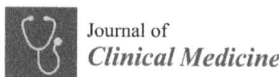

Review

Bruch's Membrane: A Key Consideration with Complement-Based Therapies for Age-Related Macular Degeneration

Sarah Hammadi [1,†], Nikolaos Tzoumas [1,2,†], Mariantonia Ferrara [3], Ingrid Porpino Meschede [4], Katharina Lo [4], Claire Harris [4,5], Majlinda Lako [1] and David H. Steel [1,2,*]

1. Biosciences Institute, Faculty of Medical Sciences, Newcastle University, Newcastle upon Tyne NE2 4HH, UK
2. Sunderland Eye Infirmary, Queen Alexandra Rd., Sunderland SR2 9H, UK
3. Manchester Royal Eye Hospital, Manchester M13 9WL, UK
4. Gyroscope Therapeutics Limited, a Novartis Company, Rolling Stock Yard, 6th Floor, 188 York Way, London N7 9AS, UK
5. Clinical and Translational Research Institute, Faculty of Medical Sciences, Newcastle University, Newcastle upon Tyne NE2 4HH, UK
* Correspondence: david.steel@ncl.ac.uk
† These authors contributed equally to this work.

Abstract: The complement system is crucial for immune surveillance, providing the body's first line of defence against pathogens. However, an imbalance in its regulators can lead to inappropriate overactivation, resulting in diseases such as age-related macular degeneration (AMD), a leading cause of irreversible blindness globally affecting around 200 million people. Complement activation in AMD is believed to begin in the choriocapillaris, but it also plays a critical role in the subretinal and retinal pigment epithelium (RPE) spaces. Bruch's membrane (BrM) acts as a barrier between the retina/RPE and choroid, hindering complement protein diffusion. This impediment increases with age and AMD, leading to compartmentalisation of complement activation. In this review, we comprehensively examine the structure and function of BrM, including its age-related changes visible through in vivo imaging, and the consequences of complement dysfunction on AMD pathogenesis. We also explore the potential and limitations of various delivery routes (systemic, intravitreal, subretinal, and suprachoroidal) for safe and effective delivery of conventional and gene therapy-based complement inhibitors to treat AMD. Further research is needed to understand the diffusion of complement proteins across BrM and optimise therapeutic delivery to the retina.

Keywords: Bruch's membrane; retinal pigment epithelium; choroid; age-related macular degeneration (AMD); complement system; complement therapies

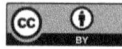

1. Introduction

Age-related macular degeneration (AMD) is a leading cause of irreversible sight loss, affecting around 200 million globally, including 25% of those over 60 in Europe [1,2]. It leads to reduced quality of life, increased anxiety and depression, and has a substantial economic impact upwards of GBP 1.6 billion per year in the UK [3]. With ageing populations, its personal and socioeconomic impact will continue to grow. AMD involves progressive degeneration of the macula, including drusen formation and tissue atrophy, leading to severe central visual loss in its late stages [4]. While intravitreal anti-vascular endothelial growth factor (VEGF) therapy has been successful in improving outcomes in neovascular AMD, the majority of cases (95%) are non-exudative and, until recently, have been without any available treatment options. Moreover, the current treatments for neovascular AMD are inadequate as they do not halt the underlying degeneration, which ultimately results in atrophy or scarring in a significant number of cases, with around one-third of patients still experiencing visual decline despite treatment [5]. New therapies are needed to address this issue.

AMD, a multifactorial eye disease involving hypoxia, inflammation, vascular insufficiency, oxidative stress, and chronic immune activation, remains a complex and challenging research area [6]. The complement system, with its crucial role in immune and homeostatic functions, is a major contributor to these processes and a focus of current research for effective treatments [7]. AMD first manifests in the retinal pigment epithelium (RPE) and choroid. Bruch's membrane, an elastin- and collagen-rich extracellular matrix situated between the retinal pigment epithelium and the choroid, has key structural and functional properties and acts as a molecular sieve to compartmentalise the retina from the systemic circulation. Systemic complement production, chiefly by hepatocytes, has well-known roles in homeostasis, but the effects of local complement production and action are less well recognised. Complement components are produced by several cell types within the retina. Müller cells produce most of the complement activators, retinal neurones factor I, while RPE cells express factor H and terminal complement components [8]. Thus, with the compartmentalisation afforded by BrM, this creates an environment discrete from many of the effects of systemic complement production. In vivo imaging of BrM and its surrounding area has seen significant progress in recent years, helping in early recognition of AMD. A detailed understanding of BrM properties is therefore crucial for both deciphering the pathogenesis of AMD and developing effective therapies.

This review covers the basics of BrM structure and function, its age-related changes visible on imaging, and its impact on complement dysfunction in AMD. We also discuss the potential and limitations of different delivery routes for effective and safe delivery of complement inhibition to the macula.

2. The Structure and Function of BrM

BrM is a 2–4 μm thin layer of extracellular matrix between the retina and choroid in the eye serving as a selectively permeable membrane between the RPE and choriocapillaris (CC). The RPE is a crucial monolayer of epithelial cells supporting the high metabolic activity of the neural retina through various key metabolic, transport, and immunoregulatory functions [9]. The CC, a 10 μm thick network of highly anastomosed and fenestrated capillaries, facilitates protein diffusion between the retina and choroid. The choroid, a vital vascular connective tissue, regulates blood flow and temperature and secretes growth factors to maintain eye homeostasis [10].

BrM is a continuous membrane posterior to the ora serrata, deficient only at the point of optic nerve insertion [11]. In 1971, Hogan described BrM as having five layers [12], which are described from inner to outer layers as follows:

- The RPE basement membrane is about 0.15 μm thick [13,14] and contains collagen IV α1–5, collagen V, heparan sulphate, chondroitin sulphate, laminins 1, 5, 10, and 11, and nindogen-1 [15–20].
- The inner collagenous layer (ICL) is about 1.4 μm thick containing crossed layers of collagen I, III, and V fibronectin, chondroitin sulphate, dermatan sulphate, apolipoprotein E (apoE), clusterin, heme, lipoproteins, and vitronectin [21–26].
- The central elastic layer (CEL) is about 0.8 μm thick, discontinuous in the macular region [27], and contains elastin fibres that are contiguous with the ICL and outer collagenous layer (OCL). The CEL is important for biomechanical properties, antiangiogenic barrier functions, and choroidal contractility [28].
- The OCL's thickness ranges from 1 to 5 μm [29] and contains collagen I, III, and V, fibronectin, fibulin-5, chondroitin sulphate, lipoproteins, dermatan sulphate, clusterin, and apoE [17,19,24,26,30–32].
- The choroidal endothelial cell (CEC) basement membrane is about 0.07 μm thick and contains collagen IV, α1, α2, V, and VI, heparan sulphate, laminin, endostatin, and chondroitin sulphate [15,19,20,33,34]. It is discontinuous due to the presence of choroidal inter-capillary pillars between CC lumens [28].

The exchange of nutrients, oxygen, minerals, and visual cycle by-products between the RPE and the CC is primarily regulated by BrM through passive diffusion. The permeability of BrM is largely determined by its structure and is mainly influenced by the molecular weight, size, and shape of the diffusing substance (Figure 1). While some complement proteins such as Factor H-like protein 1 (FHL-1), Factor D (FD), and C5a have been found to pass through BrM [35,36], it has been reported that C3a, despite its small molecular weight, is not able to do so. This observation may reflect the higher positive net charge of C3a at neutral pH [35], causing it to be trapped within the BrM, which is negatively charged due to the presence of glycosaminoglycans [35,37,38]. Post-translational modifications, such as N-linked glycosylation, may also impede diffusion of complement proteins such as Factor I (FI) through BrM, although these are not considered sufficient to explain the lack of diffusion of Factor H (FH) and Factor B (FB) [35,39]. Finally, solute transmission through BrM is determined by the hydrostatic pressure and the concentration gradient of molecules [14]. The CEL has the largest pore size and highest water diffusion [21], while the ICL has the smallest pore size and lowest water conductivity [21].

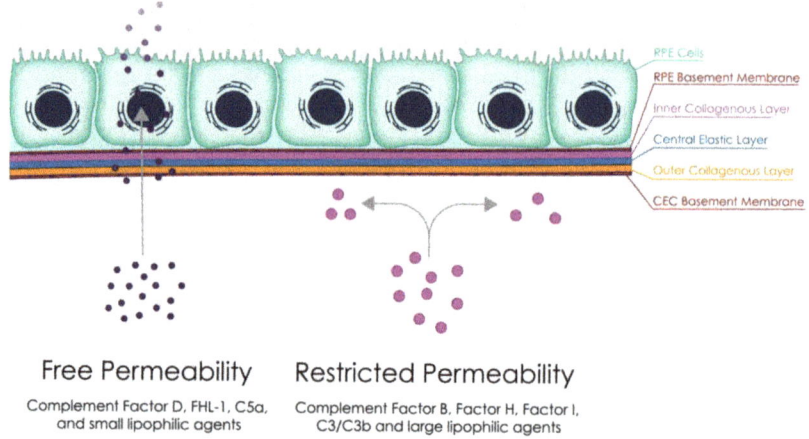

Figure 1. Complement diffusion through BrM. BrM has been shown to act as a barrier between the retina and choroid, allowing a limited number of complement proteins, such as FHL-1, factor D, and C5a, to diffuse through. This compartmentalisation may be exacerbated in ageing and disease, as lipid deposition in AMD has been shown to reduce FHL-1 diffusion. This could create two separate compartments for complement activation and regulation, namely the retinal and choroidal sides, with complement proteins remaining on their side of origin. Abbreviations: FHL-1, Factor H-like 1 protein; RPE, retinal pigment epithelium.

Additionally, BrM provides structural support to the RPE and has important transport functions. Its high elasticity, with an estimated modulus of 7 to 19 MPa [40], allows it to stretch and accommodate changes in intraocular pressure [28]. This is in stark contrast to the lower elasticity of the sclera, with a modulus of approximately 1.2 to 1.3 MPa [41], and the retina, which has an even lower modulus of 0.000208 MPa [42].

The BrM remodelling process involves three inactive forms of matrix metalloproteinases (MMPs) synthesised by the RPE, types 1, 2, and 9. These MMPs are important in BrM homeostasis and its physiological function [43]. The catalytic activity of MMPs is regulated by tissue inhibitors of MMPs (TIMPs). TIMP-1 and TIMP-2 are thought to move freely within the BrM, while TIMP-3 is thought to be bound to the RPE and CEC basement membrane [44].

3. Ageing Processes in BrM

BrM undergoes significant structural changes with ageing, particularly in terms of its permeability [28].

3.1. Anatomical Changes

BrM undergoes thickening with ageing [29,45–47], detectable using modern ophthalmic imaging (Figure 2). This phenomenon is likely due to the accumulation of lipids, including esterified cholesterol, fatty acids, and triglycerides [48,49], which reduces its permeability [50,51]. Changes in matrix molecules, such as an increase in MMPs 2 and 9 and their inhibitor TIMP-3, may also contribute to BrM thickening [43,52,53], as may advanced glycation end-products (AGEs) such as pentosides and carboxymethyllysine that cause inflammation via activation of AGE receptors on RPE and immune cells [54]. Changes in BrM laminin and proteoglycans, essential for its structural properties and RPE cell attachment, also occur with age [16]. RPE synthesises laminin 1 (α1ß1γ1), 5 (α3ß3γ2), and 10/11 (α5ß1/2γ1), allowing adhesion to BrM via integrin-mediated mechanisms [16]. However, heparan sulphate proteoglycans (HSPGs), key binders of the complement regulator Factor H (FH), have been shown to be reduced with age [55] and may lead to increased complement activation [56,57]. This may exacerbate the effect of the FH p.Y402H polymorphism (a major genetic risk factor for AMD) as it has been proposed that the variant protein binds less well to HSPGs than the wild-type protein [56,57].

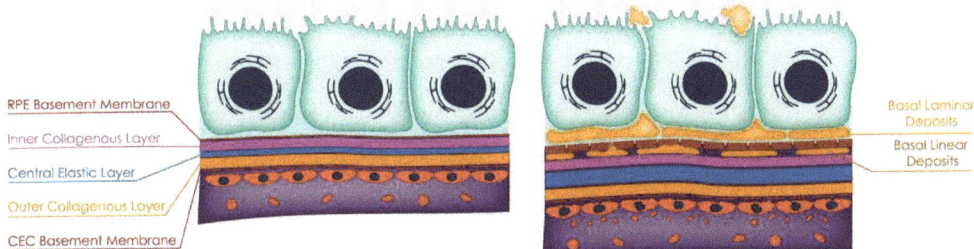

Figure 2. Age-related changes to BrM. With increasing age, BrM undergoes several alterations, including overall thickening due to increased deposition of collagen, lipids, TIMP-2, MMPs 2 and 9, calcium phosphate, and AGEs. Additionally, basal laminar and basal linear deposits are observed with age, and there is a reduction in heparan sulphate. These changes to BrM contribute to the pathogenesis of several retinal diseases, including age-related macular degeneration. Abbreviations: TIMP, tissue inhibitor of metalloproteinase; MMP, matrix metalloproteinase; AGEs, advanced glycation end-products; RPE, retinal pigment epithelium; CEC, choroidal endothelial cell.

3.2. Biomechanical Changes

Calcification with calcium phosphate deposition is also detected in the CEL with ageing [58], causing BrM to become stiffer. The elasticity of BrM has been shown to decrease linearly from as early as 21 years of age at a rate of approximately 1% per year [59], although this does not appear to be exaggerated in AMD [59].

3.3. Permeability Changes

The movement of water across BrM, as measured with Ussing chambers [60–63], decreases with age. The loss of water permeability is greatest in the ICL, particularly in the macular area as compared to the retinal periphery [62]. With age, there is also a reduction in the transport of protein molecules. One study observed an almost 100% reduction in the permeability of serum proteins across BrM from the first to the ninth decades of life (from 3.5×10^{-6} to 0.2×10^{-6} cm/s) [64]. The study further observed that in younger donors, BrM was permeable to serum proteins with molecular weights greater than 200 kDa, while in elderly donors, the threshold decreased to 100 kDa [64]. Nevertheless, these models may not fully capture the complexity of human physiology. For instance, recent research has indicated that some complement molecules with a molecular weight of less than 100 kDa cannot penetrate BrM, implying that there may be additional factors (such as sample preparation, pH, temperature, and osmolarity) that could influence the outcomes of such experiments.

Table 1 provides an overview of functional and anatomical changes in BrM associated with ageing, while Table 2 summarises the changes in the composition of each layer of BrM with age.

Table 1. Summary of functional and anatomical changes in BrM with age.

Functional Changes	Anatomical Changes
Decrease in elasticity Decrease in water permeability Decrease in protein permeability Decreased complement protein permeability	Accumulation of lipids, TIMP-3, MMP-2, MMP-9, calcium phosphate, and AGEs BrM thickening Reduced heparan sulphate Increased complement activation

Abbreviations: TIMP, tissue inhibitor of metalloproteinase; MMP, matrix metalloproteinase; AGEs, advanced glycation end-products; BrM, Bruch's membrane.

Table 2. Changes in the composition of each layer of BrM with age.

Layers	Composition	Changes with Age
RPE basement membrane	Chondroitin sulphate Collagen IV α1–5 Collagen V Heparan sulphate Laminins 1, 5, 10, and 11 Nidogen-1	BLamD accumulation
Inner collagenous layer	Apolipoprotein E Chondroitin sulphate Clusterin Collagen I, III, and V Dermatan sulphate Fibronectin Haem Lipoproteins Vitronectin	Lipoprotein deposition BLinD accumulation
Central elastic layer	Elastin	Elastin and calcium phosphate deposition

Table 2. Cont.

Layers	Composition	Changes with Age
Outer collagenous layer	Apolipoprotein E Chondroitin sulphate Clusterin Collagen I, III, and V Dermatan sulphate Fibronectin Fibulin-5 Lipoproteins	Lipoprotein deposition
Choroidal endothelial cell basement membrane	Chondroitin sulphate Collagen IV, α1, α2 Collagen V Collagen VI Endostatin Heparan sulphate Laminin	Unknown

Abbreviations: BLamD, basal laminar deposit; BLinD, basal linear deposit.

4. Overview of AMD

AMD classification has traditionally been based on anatomical changes observed through ophthalmic imaging, with early, intermediate, and advanced (or late) stages being distinguished. While early/intermediate forms have been associated with functional changes such as impaired dark adaptation, advanced AMD has been the primary focus of research due to most visual impairment being caused by this stage. Advanced AMD can be broadly classified into two clinical forms: neovascular AMD and geographic atrophy [45]. In neovascular (or exudative) AMD, subretinal neovascularisation develops below or above the RPE. These abnormal blood vessels often leak serous fluid or blood, resulting in macular oedema and/or haemorrhages that can lead to rapid visual loss. Repeated disruption of retinal architecture in this manner may also result in profound, irreversible vision loss. In geographic atrophy due to AMD, a zone of photoreceptor, RPE, and CC degeneration typically starts within the macula and expands to involve the fovea. It has recently been estimated that 16% of patients with bilateral geographic atrophy are registered severely sight impaired within an average of six years [4].

As the advanced subtypes of AMD are considered irreversible, it is important to understand the processes at early and intermediate stages of the disease to identify patients benefitting most from emerging therapies. Both advanced AMD subtypes are typically preceded by the accumulation of extracellular material in the BrM of the central retina. These are primarily termed drusen, focal deposits of proteins and neutral lipids such as esterified cholesterol, with apolipoproteins B and E located between the basal lamina of the RPE and the inner collagenous layer of BrM [65,66] (Figure 3). Of over 100 proteins identified in drusen, the commonest include vitronectin and clusterin (which both participate in the control of the lytic activity of complement), with TIMP-3, serum albumin, and crystallins [67] also identified—several of which have undergone oxidative protein modifications [68]. Two additional forms of BrM thickening are also observed in early disease, namely basal laminar deposits (BLamDs) and basal linear deposits (BLinDs), which are appreciable as diffuse thickening of the inner aspect of BrM on imaging. These are distinguished by their anatomical location: BLamDs are found above the RPE basement membrane, while BLinDs are located beneath this, adjacent to the BrM ICL. BLamDs also have characteristic staining patterns and may have a striated histological appearance due to long-spacing collagen [69,70]. These deposits have similar lipid and protein constituents to drusen [71] and are often confluent with them [70]. Collections of extracellular material in the subretinal space between the apical RPE and photoreceptors, known as subretinal drusenoid deposits or reticular pseudodrusen, have also been observed and are considered a high-risk phenotype for AMD progression [72].

4.1. Genetic Risk Factors

AMD is a complex disease resulting from the interplay of both genetic and environmental factors. Its strong genetic component, with an up to 10-fold increase in risk when a parent or sibling is affected, makes it one of the most heritable complex diseases [73,74]. Indeed, a large twin study has proposed heritability (additive genetic) estimates of 46% to 71% for AMD severity classification based on clinical examination and colour fundus photography [75]. The genetic basis of AMD has been widely studied through genome-wide association studies (GWASs). These studies identify various genetic variants associated with increased risks of developing AMD, including a common single nucleotide polymorphism (SNP) in the *CFH* gene (*CFH* p.Y402H) conferring an approximately two-fold higher risk of developing late-stage AMD per allele [76] and a common haplotype affecting the age-related maculopathy susceptibility 2 (*ARMS2*) and HtrA serine peptidase 1 (*HTRA1*) gene loci [77]. Subsequent GWASs have detected 52 independent and rare variants distributed across 34 loci that account for more than half of the condition's heritability [78]. These include many genes involved in the alternative pathway of complement activation (*CFH, CFI, CFB, C2, C3, C9*), as well as genes involved in cholesterol metabolism (*ABCA1, APOE, LIPC*), matrix remodelling (*TIMP3, COL8A1*), and other functions [78–80]. Both common and rare variants have been found to contribute to AMD risk, with rare variants in *CFI* associated with particularly high risk [81,82]. Further research is necessary to fully understand the role of these genetic variants in the development and progression of AMD.

4.2. Environmental Risk Factors

In addition to ageing, smoking is a significant environmental risk factor for AMD, with the odds ratio for current smokers compared to ex-smokers being estimated by one meta-analysis to be 1.78 (95% confidence intervals, 1.52–2.09) [73]. Smoking can increase inflammation and oxidative stress in the RPE, which can be further exacerbated by changes in the choriocapillaris such as abnormal blood vessel growth and vasoconstriction [83,84]. Large longitudinal studies have suggested that smokers remain at high risk of developing neovascular AMD up to 20 years after smoking cessation [85,86], although these analyses were not adjusted for socioeconomic status. The literature on possible associations of AMD with diet, sunlight exposure, and cardiovascular or metabolic disease is inconsistent, partly due to difficulties in quantifying or standardising these factors. Antioxidant vitamin and mineral supplementation may delay late AMD progression in some high-risk individuals, although this evidence is of low certainty [87].

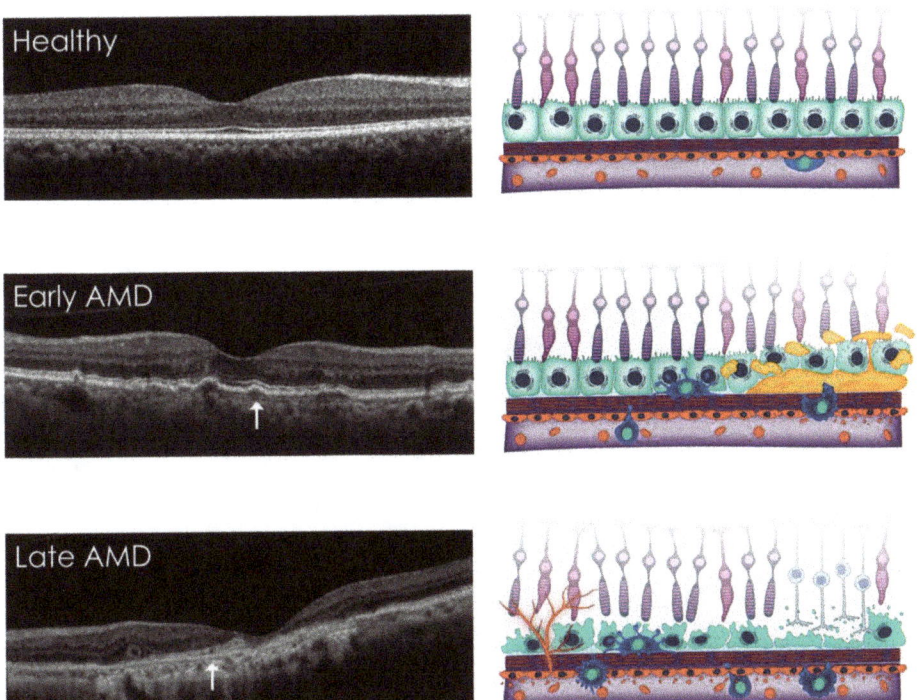

Figure 3. Pathological changes at the BrM interface in AMD. In healthy individuals (**top panels**), the retinal tissues are in a state of metabolic equilibrium. Early/intermediate AMD (**middle panels**) is characterised by the accumulation of extracellular deposits (illustrated in orange), such as soft drusen/BLinDs beneath the RPE and subretinal drusenoid deposits above it. These deposits mainly consist of lipoproteins of dietary and photoreceptor outer segment origin and are excreted by the RPE. They accumulate in the sub-RPE space and impede transit to the choroid due to ageing of the Bruch's membrane. The accumulation of these deposits is associated with underlying choriocapillaris vascular dropout and initiates an immune response that leads to the recruitment of inflammatory cells. These deposits increase the risk of advanced stages of AMD, including atrophy and neovascularisation (**bottom panels**). Notably, BrM is more visible in areas of RPE separation and choroidal neovascularisation (white arrows). Changes within the Bruch's membrane are not depicted in this figure. Open-source images used with permission [88]. Abbreviations: AMD, age-related macular degeneration; BLinDs, basal linear deposits; BrM, Bruch's membrane; RPE, retinal pigment epithelium.

5. Non-Invasive Imaging of BrM

Advances in ophthalmic imaging, particularly optical coherence tomography (OCT) and OCT-angiography, have improved visualisation of BrM in high resolution, allowing age-related changes and retinal pathologies such as AMD to be studied.

BrM, in conjunction with the RPE, is known as the RPE–BrM complex, identified as the fourth outer hyper-reflective band of the retina on commercially available spectral-domain or swept-source OCT devices [89]. In young adults, the interdigitation zone, RPE, BrM, and choriocapillaris can be distinguished; however, with age, their demarcation becomes less clear due to BrM thickening and BLamDs (Figure 4). Separation of the RPE and BrM due to choroidal neovascularisation (CNV), drusen, or RPE atrophy can sometimes be seen as a thin hyper-reflective line on OCT [90] (Figure 3). The increased thickness of the RPE–BrM complex with age may also correlate positively with quantitative autofluorescence [91]. As previously described, the BrM thickening is partly attributed to age-related accumulation of lipoprotein-related lipids that form basal linear deposits (BLinDs) and soft drusen. These deposits are not visible on OCT but may appear as scattered hypofluorescent spots on late-phase indocyanine green angiography [92].

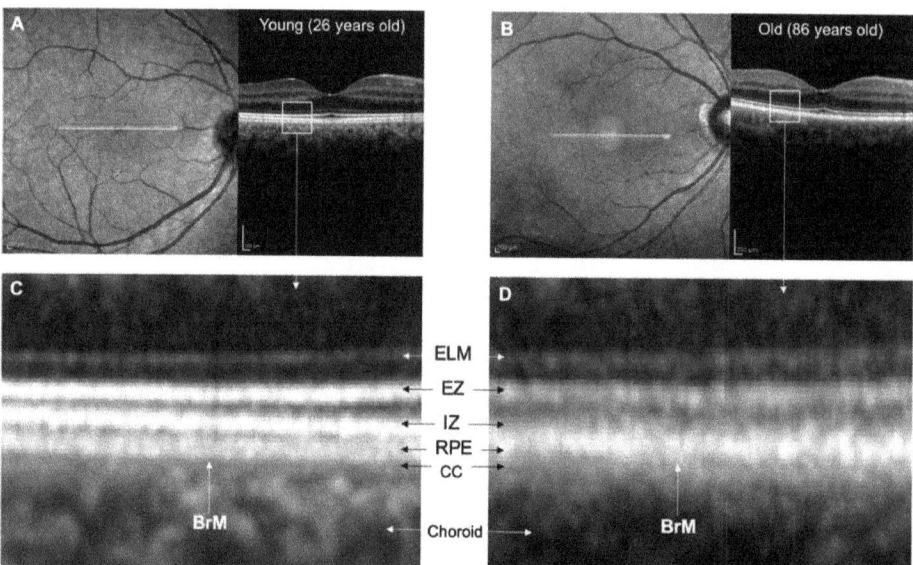

Figure 4. Comparison of OCT images of younger and older retinas. (**A**,**B**) show scanning laser ophthalmoscope fundal images and corresponding horizontal 15-degree OCT line scans of a 26-year-old female with a clear lens and an 86-year-old female who had undergone cataract surgery. The OCT images were averaged from 100 B-scans. (**C**,**D**) show high magnification views of the outer retina. In the 26-year-old individual, clear distinctions can be made between the IZ, RPE, BrM, and CC. However, in the 86-year-old individual, these structures are indistinct, and there is apparent thickening of BrM and thinning of the CC. Abbreviations: BrM, Bruch's membrane; CC, choriocapillaris; ELM, external limiting membrane; EZ, ellipsoid zone; IZ, interdigitation zone; OCT, optical coherence tomography; RPE; retinal pigment epithelium.

On OCT-angiography, BrM appears as a dark (hypoechoic), avascular band. In cases of type 1 and type 2 macular neovascularisation, OCT-angiography may show a signal crossing through the BrM [90]. However, it is important to note that projection artifacts can sometimes cause large retinal vessels to appear at the level of the BrM [90].

5.1. In Vivo Imaging of BrM in AMD

Eyes with early and/or intermediate AMD have a thicker RPE–BrM complex than healthy eyes according to global and/or low-density OCT spatial analysis [92,93]. The central macula shows the most significant thickening [94]. High-density OCT thickness analysis has shown that the central RPE–BrM complex is thicker in intermediate AMD than early AMD, likely due to the build-up of lipoprotein-related lipids [95]. The thickness of the RPE–BrM complex, outer plexiform, and outer nuclear layers decreases with increasing eccentricity from the foveal centre, which may relate to the loss of rod photoreceptors in AMD [95]. Recent data suggest that the thickening of the RPE–BrM complex in AMD eyes is mainly due to the accumulation of BLamDs and extracellular matrix material between the basal lamina and plasma membrane of the RPE, rather than accumulation within the RPE or BrM itself [69]. This can appear as a "double-layer sign" or splitting within the RPE–BrM complex on OCT [69], which is an emerging biomarker of neovascular AMD [96].

5.2. In Vivo Imaging of BrM in Inherited Retinal Degenerations (IRDs)

Thickening of BrM can also be seen in IRDs such as dominant drusen (DD), late-onset retinal degeneration (L-ORD), pseudoxanthoma elasticum, and Sorsby fundus dystrophy (SFD) [97]. OCT scans show a separation of the RPE and BrM, appearing as two distinct hyper-reflective bands in DD, L-ORD, and SFD, which has been suggested as a potential biomarker for these degenerative conditions [97]. The extent of separation of the RPE–BrM complex has been suggested to correspond with the degree of visual symptoms in DD and SFD [97]. This separation is thought to be caused by the accumulation of BLinDs and BLamDs between the elastic lamina of BrM and the visible apical RPE, where melanosomes are concentrated [97].

6. Overview of Complement

The complement system is a complex network of approximately 30 proteins that plays a vital role in the immune response. There are three main pathways: the classical pathway, the lectin pathway, and the alternative pathway (Figure 5). The complement system comprises both activating and controlling proteins that are found throughout the body in individual or complex forms. Complement represents a significant 15% of the globulin fraction of blood and is responsible for lytic activity against invading pathogens as part of the innate immune system [98]. However, recent evidence also indicates that complement has critical roles in adaptive immunity, cell senescence, and tissue remodelling [7]. Complement activation occurs through a process called "tick-over", in which the central component, C3, activates at a low level in plasma and initiates the alternative pathway (AP). This sets off a cascade of protein interactions that culminates in rapid inflammation and cell lysis via the formation of a pore on membranes of a bacterium or antibody-coated cell surface, known as the membrane attack complex (MAC) [7,99]. The primary impact of the MAC on nucleated cells is the induction of inflammation through multiple signalling pathways and activation of the NLRP3 inflammasome. Despite its potent pro-inflammatory properties, The MAC rarely leads to the lysis of nucleated cells due to the presence of ion pumps and endo/exocytotic mechanisms that prevent cellular damage [100]. These findings underscore the importance of the complement system in maintaining immune function and preventing disease.

The complement system's inability to distinguish self from non-self can lead to unintended consequences on healthy tissues in the vicinity of activation, resulting in local cell dysfunction, damage, or even death. While regulatory proteins normally coat our own cells and quickly inactivate activating proteins and complexes to control complement activation, even brief episodes of activation can contribute to disease progression over time.

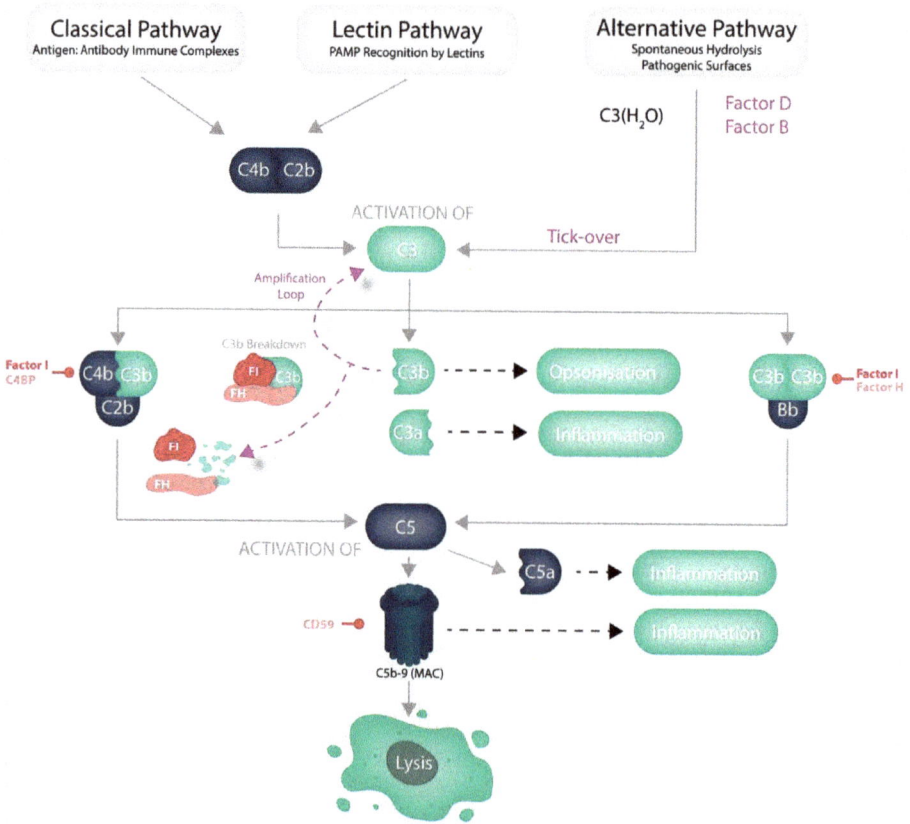

Figure 5. The pathways of the complement system. The complement system is a network of proteolytic pathways that work together to maintain the body's homeostasis. The alternative pathway is continuously activated through the hydrolysis of C3 to C3(H$_2$O) in a process known as "tick-over" and triggers the formation of C3 convertases (C4b:C2b, C3b:Bb (not shown)) and C5 convertases (C4b:C2b:C3b and C3b:Bb:C3b), leading to the production of anaphylatoxins, effector molecules, and the C5b-9 complex (MAC). Although it causes significant inflammation, cell lysis as a result of the MAC is a rare occurrence. Importantly, the production of C3b results in further C3 activation through the formation of the C3b:Bb convertase (also not shown) in a process known as the amplification loop. These pathways are regulated by various factors and cofactors that interact with complement components, activating enzymes, or each other. FH plays a critical role as a cofactor for FI by binding C3b and possessing cofactor/decay-accelerating activities that inhibit the alternative pathway amplification loop and initiate the breakdown pathway of C3b. Abbreviations: FH, Factor H; FI, Factor I; MAC, membrane attack complex; PAMP, pathogen-associated molecular pattern.

7. Complement Dysfunction in AMD

7.1. The Role of Complement in Choroidal Homeostasis

The relative importance of the RPE and CC in the development of AMD is a subject of ongoing debate, but it is clear that both tissues play a role [101,102]. Early in the disease process, there is a vascular loss of CC that corresponds to the presence of drusen [103]. In AMD and normal ageing, the accumulation of MAC on CC endothelium also increases in a process that is exacerbated by the presence of the *CFH* p.Y402H genotype [104–106].

This can result in the death of choroidal endothelial cells in culture [105–111]. Complement may play a constitutive role in the choroid and retina decades before the onset of AMD, as indicated in human tissue studies by higher MAC deposition [108,112], CD59 expression [113], and FH production relative to other retinal tissues. Thus, complement may have a significant impact on choroidal homeostasis through its effects on modulating macular neovascularisation and immune cell regulation.

7.2. The Role of Complement in RPE Function

Under normal conditions, RPE cells express complement proteins that facilitate the opsonisation and phagocytosis of photoreceptor outer segments and waste products of the visual cycle through a process known as autophagy [114,115]. This is supported by the presence of multiple complement components and regulators in drusen [67,114,116–118]. In fact, complement proteins C3 and Factor B (FB) have been found to be essential for drusen formation in mouse models of inherited retinal degeneration [119–121]. This model is triggered by inducing the missense p.R345W variant in the *EFEMP1* (EGF-containing fibulin-like extracellular matrix protein 1) gene, which encodes fibulin-3 involved in extracellular matrix development. This variant causes Doyne honeycomb retinal dystrophy in humans, which is characterised by early-onset macular and peripapillary drusen. In mice, this variant recreates many of the histological features of AMD, such as the accumulation of coalescing, electron-dense sub-RPE debris and general RPE and choroidal abnormalities, including degeneration, vacuolation, loss or disruption of RPE basal infoldings, choroidal atrophy, and focal thickening and invasion of cellular processes into BrM. Despite this, it is important to acknowledge the limitations of using murine models to study AMD, as has been explored elsewhere [122].

Under normal conditions, complement expression in the RPE and neural retina is generally low compared to the choroid [114], but this may increase under conditions of stress or stimulation. In ageing and AMD, there is increased expression of the complement protein C3 within RPE cells and on their basal membranes [114,123]. This is also seen in mice, where increased AP activation in the RPE/choroid has been identified [124]. Exosomes secreted by stressed RPE cells have also been found to be coated with complement components [125,126]. The role of this increased complement expression in the RPE is not yet clear, as it could either be protective or contribute to disease pathogenesis. To protect themselves from harmful complement activation, RPE cells secrete FH and express several regulators of the complement system, such as CD59 on their apical side [113,127,128] and CD46 (also known as membrane cofactor protein or MCP) on their basal side [113,129,130]. CD59 inhibits formation of the MAC, whereas FH and CD46 drive the breakdown of surface-bound C3b. In addition to its role in regulating the complement system, FH also binds to pro-inflammatory lipid peroxidation products on the surface of damaged RPE cells and controls inflammation in their vicinity [131].

7.3. Impact of Complement Overactivation on RPE Function and Viability

Reduced expression of FH and CD46 by RPE cells is observed in AMD, and this coincides with increased deposition of the MAC and cell lysis [132,133]. Dysfunctional FH, including the p.Y402H variant, can also lead to overactivation of the complement system, which can impair the essential functions of RPE cells, including autophagy, lysosomal function, and energy metabolism. This has been demonstrated in studies using RPE cells derived from patients with AMD with high-risk complement genotypes [134–137]. RPE cells with impaired lysosomal function are thought to be susceptible to MAC deposition due to their inability to adequately recycle and traffic complement inhibitors such as CD59 to the cell surface [138]. A lack of functional FH may also impair the clearance of lipid peroxidation products [131], leading to oxidative stress [139]. Oxidative stress, in turn, may downregulate the expression of complement regulators by RPE cells [113,127,140–142] through apoptotic shedding and exosomal release of CD46 and CD59 [143]. Furthermore, infiltrating subretinal macrophages in AMD may induce complement dysfunction in RPE cells [144]. These interactions can create a vicious cycle of complement activation, oxidative stress, and cellular dysfunction.

Complement-mediated dysfunction of the RPE may contribute to the development of AMD. As previously discussed, this has been implied in a variety of mouse models of inherited retinal degeneration, in which the presence of drusen-like deposits is dependent on complement for formation [119–121,145]. Complement activation leading to MAC deposition also has immunomodulatory effects on nucleated cells and stimulates the RPE to produce metalloproteinases and VEGF [146,147], which may drive macular neovascularisation, thus suggesting that complement overactivation may lead to both exudative and non-exudative AMD. In addition, our recent study of the UK Biobank, the largest repository of retinal imaging data to date, found that the common at-risk FH genotype (*CFH* p.Y402H) and different rare FI variants were associated with reduced RPE–BrM complex thickness in healthy participants, suggesting that complement overactivation may have a negative impact on the function and viability of RPE cells [81]. These effects may be more pronounced with advancing age or disease.

To protect against complement activation and cellular dysfunction, overexpression of secreted and membrane-bound complement regulatory proteins has been suggested as a therapeutic strategy [111,148–151].

7.4. Complement Dysfunction in Macular Neovascularisation

Several experiments using mouse models of laser-induced CNV have demonstrated that all complement pathways, particularly the alternative and terminal pathways, play a significant role in angiogenesis [150,152–163]. The alternative pathway is responsible for the majority of C5a and MAC formation [164], which suggests that the terminal pathway may be causative in CNV formation. Additionally, several studies have highlighted the potential role of the vascular endothelial growth factor (VEGF) pathway in mediating these effects. VEGF is an angiogenic protein that exerts its effects primarily through VEGF receptor 2 (VEGFR2). For example, sublytic levels of MAC have been shown to stimulate the release of growth factors from nucleated cells [99,100], including VEGF from RPE in cell culture studies [146,165]. In addition, the inhibition of CD46 by gene knockout in mouse models led to increased VEGF production in the retina and choroid, increased MAC deposition on these tissues, increased susceptibility to laser-induced CNV, and degenerative changes in retinal tissues resembling an AMD phenotype [166,167]. It is worth noting that the VEGF–complement interaction may also be reciprocal; VEGF inhibition has been shown to increase complement activation by decreasing FH expression in RPE and renal podocytes through VEGFR2- and PKC-α/CREB-dependent signalling [168].

The activation of complement can have varying effects depending on the stimulus or location in the body. For instance, the anaphylatoxins C3a and C5a have been found to enhance laser-induced CNV in some cases, but may have anti-angiogenic properties in mouse models of retinal hypoxia through the stimulation of mononuclear phagocytes to secrete soluble VEGF receptor 1 that inhibits VEGF [169,170]. There is also conflicting evidence on the role of FB, a serine protease involved in the alternative pathway of complement activation, in angiogenesis. Some studies have shown that FB has a pro-angiogenic effect mediated through increased VEGF and VEGFR2 expression by endothelial cells in mouse models of laser-induced CNV and retinal hypoxia [81,153,171]. MMP expression in choroidal endothelial cells has also been found to increase with MAC-dependent complement activation [172], suggesting that complement may promote angiogenesis through multiple pathways. In contrast, other research has shown that inhibiting FB in a mouse model of retinal hypoxia potentially leads to increased neovascularisation, as well as increased severity and duration of retinopathy, through a reduction in endothelial cell apoptosis and increased expression of CD55 [163], a regulator of complement. These findings suggest that complement may have complex and diverse roles in angiogenesis, and further research is needed to fully understand its mechanisms of action.

Understanding the complex interplay between complement and angiogenesis has significant implications for the development of effective and safe complement-based therapies. The balance of complement activation is crucial, as both underactivation and overactivation can have adverse effects. However, the effects of complete inhibition of complement in the eye remain unclear and require further exploration. For example, it is unclear why the development of macular neovascularisation is a possible emergent adverse event of intravitreally administered complement inhibitors for dry AMD and whether this is due to treatment modality (e.g., the PEGylation of agents such as pegcetacoplan and avacincaptad pegol) or target [173]. The complexity of this field is further compounded by limited evidence from case reports suggesting that intravitreal inhibition of VEGF may lead to disorders of complement overactivation in the kidneys [174]. Newer agents that target both complement and the VEGF pathways, such as Ranifitin (manufactured by *Apellis*, Waltham, MA, USA), may address these safety concerns. However, the role of VEGF secreted by the RPE in maintaining the choriocapillaris is still not fully understood [175]. Some studies have found a correlation between intravitreal anti-VEGF therapy for neovascular AMD and an increased risk of developing GA [176–179], but it is unclear if this is due to common advanced AMD processes or if VEGF inhibition leads to retinal cell damage related to complement. There is also debate over whether non-exudative macular neovascularisation can support photoreceptors and the RPE in GA [180–182]. Further research into the biological interactions between complement and VEGF will be important for guiding drug development and clinical trial design [183].

7.5. Immune Cell Regulation

Complement plays a vital role in directing the cellular immune response to diseases, largely explored in cancer and sepsis but also relevant for AMD [184].

A critical component in this area is the anaphylatoxin C5a, which plays multiple roles in immune regulation. While it has well-known pro-inflammatory functions mediated through its C5aR receptors and activation of the NLRP3 inflammasome (as previously reviewed [185,186]), it is also essential for the development and regulation of T-cell immunity [187–193]. C5a signalling generally leads to inflammation through the protection of CD4+ T-cells against apoptosis and the upregulation of pro-inflammatory cytokines such as IL-17 and IL-22 [187]. Furthermore, in the choriocapillaris, C5a upregulates the expression of leukocyte adhesion molecules on endothelial cells [109] and plays a key role in recruiting γδ T-cells [194], a specialised class of tissue-resident lymphocytes that rapidly expand in response to stress induced by pathogens or endogenous stimuli and initiate neutrophil recruitment, phagocyte activation, and granuloma formation [195].

It has also been shown that MAC recruits and activates leukocytes by coordinating inflammasome activation and endothelial cytokine signalling [196–200], which may initially preserve tissue function by rapidly suppressing danger; however, sustained production of reactive oxygen species, proteases, and inflammatory cytokines can contribute to dysfunction of retinal structures [6,201]. With increasing age, endothelial cells may become more sensitive to MAC injury due to higher cytoskeletal Rho kinase activity [202]. In a series of experiments, Calippe and colleagues showed somewhat surprisingly that FH prevents the clearance of subretinal mononuclear phagocytes through CD47-dependent mechanisms [203]. Interestingly, the common FH risk variant in AMD, *CFH* p.Y402H, resulted in even poorer microglial elimination [203]. These findings suggest that non-resolving subretinal inflammation due to complement may be exacerbated by genetic predispositions.

8. Local vs. Systemic Complement Production in AMD

The debate over the role of systemic versus local complement activation in AMD is highly relevant to drug design and delivery [204]. While most complement proteins are produced in the liver, others (such as C1q, C7, Factor D, and properdin) are produced at extrahepatic sites by various cells, including monocytes, macrophages, and glial and endothelial cells [7,204,205]. Local complement synthesis is regulated by cytokines and growth factors [206], and local biosynthesis is responsible for downstream complement effects in some tissues. Emerging evidence suggests that the effects of complement activation vary across tissues based on their structural properties, with some tissues being more susceptible to local activation and others being more prone to systemic activation. For example, in experimental mouse models, the renal tubular epithelium has been found to be more susceptible to donor kidney-derived C3, while the fenestrated capillaries of the renal glomerulus are more prone to systemic C3 activation [204,207]. This concept may be particularly relevant in the context of the kidney and eye, both of which have structural and developmental similarities [208] and are known to be susceptible to complement dysregulation [7,209]. These findings suggest that targeted complement inhibitors may be more effective in certain tissues at improving disease outcomes.

The BrM is believed to play a crucial role in partitioning complement activation into local or systemic pathways within the eye. As previously mentioned, its physical, electrostatic, and biochemical properties contribute to this function [14]. As noted previously in Section 2, BrM permeability declines with age [64]. Using donor eye tissue, Clark and colleagues found that certain complement proteins, such as C3/C3b, FH, FB, and FI, are unable to penetrate the BrM even at small quantities, while others, such as Factor D, Factor H-like protein 1 (FHL-1), and C5a, can cross the BrM but at reduced concentrations [35]. The fact that FHL-1 (49 kDa), a splice variant of the *CFH* gene, has better tissue penetration than the full-length, glycosylated FH protein (155 kDa) suggests that it may play a specialised role in controlling complement activation locally [35,36]. However, FHL-1 is not as effective at inhibiting AP overactivation as FH, as it has reduced binding to extracellular matrix proteins and cannot alter its conformation to conceal its catalytic domains when not bound to host structures [210]. Another clue that FHL-1 may have evolved specifically to control complement activation locally is that the genetic sequences consistent with FHL-1 expression are found in old world monkeys, but not in their new world ancestors [210]. Beyond FHL-1, it has also been shown that FI is found at significantly lower levels in the aqueous fluid of the eye compared to FI levels found in simultaneously sampled serum [211]. This finding provides further evidence for the concept that complement regulation in the eye is compartmentalised and distinct from systemic regulation. These results have important implications for the delivery of complement therapeutics across the BrM and should be considered in drug design and development.

There is evidence suggesting that levels of circulating complement activation products may be associated with the severity of AMD, although it is not yet clear whether this is a causal relationship or simply a result of ageing [212–217]. Systemic inflammation and endothelial dysfunction have been linked to reduced chorioretinal thickness [218], which may precede the development of AMD. Additionally, drusen, a hallmark of AMD containing systemic proteins, have been suggested to result from pathological transport of visual cycle by-products across the capillary wall or BrM [219]. However, patients with genetic abnormalities in the complement system tend to only develop overt disease in one organ (such as AMD, C3 glomerulopathy, or atypical haemolytic uraemic syndrome), even in the presence of rare, pathogenic variants or haploinsufficiency of FH and FI [81,220–223]. In a multicentre study of liver transplant patients, incident AMD was found to be associated with recipient, but not donor, *CFH* p.Y402H status, suggesting that systemic complement production by the liver may not contribute to retinal disease [224]. These findings suggest that the end-organ response to complement overactivation may be influenced by genetic determinants at a tissue level, which have yet to be fully mapped.

9. Complement as a Therapeutic Target

Despite facing numerous challenges in the past, such as a high plasma concentration, high daily turnover, and a volatile nature, the field of complement inhibition has made significant progress in recent years [225]. This is due in part to a better understanding of the genetic and functional roles of complement in various tissues, as well as improved structural information regarding the proteins involved. As a result, a number of complement inhibitors are currently in late-stage clinical trials for the treatment of AMD, with the first such agent (pegcetacoplan, manufactured by *Apellis*, Waltham, MA, USA) recently receiving approval from the U.S. Food and Drug Administration (FDA) for the treatment of GA [173]. Complement therapies can be delivered systemically or directly to the eye by intravitreal, subretinal, and suprachoroidal injections (Figure 6). These therapies are diverse in their design and delivery, though it remains to be seen which strategy will be most effective for ophthalmic indications. Given the potential for complement activation to contribute to the development of AMD and other conditions, inhibiting the alternative pathway of complement has garnered significant interest as a therapeutic strategy [226].

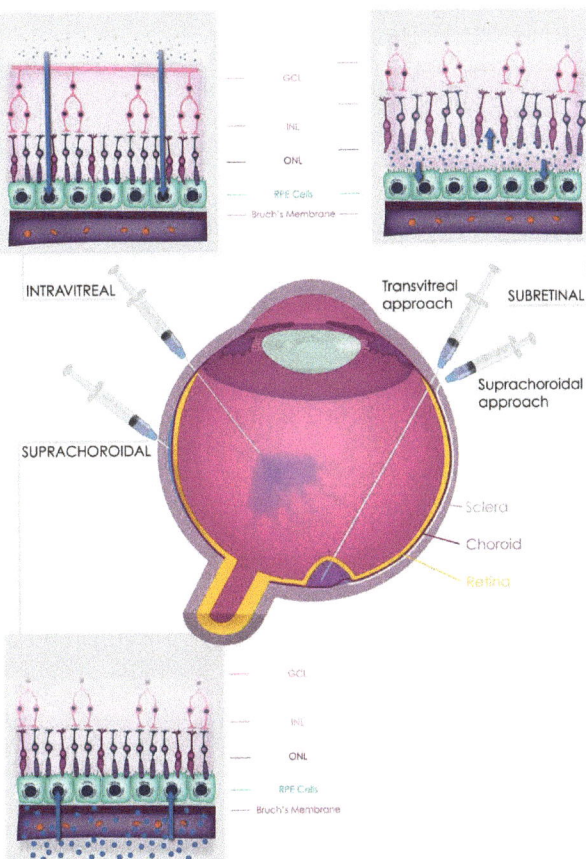

Figure 6. Different types of drug delivery route in the human eye. Intravitreal (IVT) injections are a common method of administering therapeutic agents to the eye. Other routes of administration, such as subretinal and suprachoroidal injections, are also being investigated. Subretinal agents may be administered transvitreally or by cannulation through the suprachoroidal space. Viral gene therapies targeting the retina vary in their vector distribution, retinal tropism, and transduction efficiency depending on the route of delivery used. While efficacy is a primary focus, safety is also a key consideration, as it relates to inflammation and iatrogenic complications. Abbreviations: GCL, ganglion cell layer; INL, inner nuclear layer; ONL, outer nuclear layer; RPE, retinal pigment epithelium.

9.1. Systemic Therapies

Systemic complement therapy, which involves delivering drugs orally, subcutaneously, or intravenously, is appealing due to its ease of administration. Additionally, the high blood flow in the choroid makes it possible for these therapies to quickly reach their target tissue [227]. However, as mentioned previously, although choroidal vessels are highly permeable, BrM is less so, making the diffusion of systemic therapies through it a challenge. The blood–retinal barrier (BRB)—comprising the tight junctional complexes between retinal capillary endothelial cells (inner BRB) and retinal pigment epithelial cells (outer BRB)—may also impede the diffusion of molecules from the systemic circulation to the retina. The inner BRB is only permeable to molecules with a small diameter or molecular weight (i.e., up to 2 nanometres or a few hundred daltons) [228], while the outer BRB is also highly selective, allowing hydrophilic and larger molecules to cross at a slower rate than their small, lipophilic counterparts [229]. However, as mentioned earlier, the relevance of diffusion chamber experiments to human health remains uncertain. Despite these challenges and limitations, it is possible that if complement-mediated choroidal dysfunction is a major contributor to AMD, saturating this tissue with systemic therapies may be sufficient to improve the disease.

While systemic administration of drugs has the potential to provide benefits in the treatment of posterior segment conditions, there is a lack of information about drug distribution in this area. Studies have simulated drug distribution from the plasma to the vitreous in rabbits [230], but it is unclear how these pharmacokinetics translate to humans and whether higher rates of systemic drug clearance may be a factor [228]. Other considerations for systemic administration include the effects of protein binding in the plasma on drug permeability, the potential for transcellular diffusion to bypass the tight junctions of the BRB and increase drug permeability [228], and the risk of systemic toxicity. Complement inhibition, in particular, has been associated with an increased risk of encapsulated bacterial infection and the loading of host cells with complement proteins upstream of the inhibited molecule [231,232], resulting in a need for vaccination and the exclusion of patients who are immunocompromised. Nevertheless, small molecule therapeutics such as the FDA-approved avacopan (an inhibitor of C5a Receptor 1, previously developed by *ChemoCentryx*, San Carlos, CA, USA, now by *Amgen*, Thousand Oaks, CA, USA) and iptacopan (also known as LNP023, an inhibitor of FB, developed by *Novartis*, Basel, Switzerland), which has recently achieved its Phase 3 outcomes, have shown that systemic complement inhibition can safely treat systemic conditions such as paroxysmal nocturnal haemoglobinuria [233,234]. Homing agents that bind to neoepitopes on complement proteins or stress-related antigens on apoptotic or necrotic cells may offer an additional way of restricting drug action to inflammation hotspots and reducing the risk of widespread systemic effects [225], though it is unclear how such a therapy would specifically target the eye.

To date, intravenous eculizumab (manufactured by *Alexion Pharmaceuticals*, New Haven, CT, USA), a monoclonal antibody against C5, is the only systemic complement inhibitor to have completed a randomised controlled trial in AMD, and it failed to show any significant benefits in terms of anatomy or function in a randomised controlled trial for GA [235]. Despite the limited duration of treatment (6 months) and small sample size with several methodological biases [173], its inability to demonstrate any clinical efficacy in terms of reducing GA progression or vision loss has raised questions about the usefulness of systemic complement inhibitors for AMD treatment. The results of Phase 2 clinical trials of several systemic agents are eagerly awaited and may provide more insight into the potential of systemic complement inhibitors for AMD [236]. These include IONIS-FB-LRx (developed by *Ionis Pharmaceuticals Inc.*, Carlsbad, CA, USA), a subcutaneous antisense oligonucleotide inhibitor of FB (NCT03815825, https://clinicaltrials.gov/ct2/show/NCT03815825), danicopan (formerly developed by *Achillion Pharmaceuticals*, CT, US, now by *AstraZeneca*, Cambridge, UK), an oral small molecule inhibitor of Factor D (NCT05019521, https://clinicaltrials.gov/ct2/show/NCT05019521), and iptacopan, the oral small molecule inhibitor of FB discussed above (NCT05230537, https://clinicaltrials.gov/ct2/show/NCT05230537). There are also many other systemic complement inhibitors in clinical development for other conditions [225].

9.2. Intravitreal Therapies

Intravitreal delivery of agents directly to the vitreous cavity of the eye is a commonly used approach for treating diseases of the central retina. This method has been particularly successful in the treatment of vascular retinal disorders such as neovascular AMD through the use of anti-VEGF agents. Intravitreal delivery is a relatively simple procedure that can be performed in an outpatient setting with minimal safety concerns [237]. Although achieving therapeutic levels with intravitreal formulations is challenging due to dilution in the vitreous and variable retinal penetration dictated by molecular characteristics, all of the complement inhibitors currently in late-stage clinical trials for AMD are being administered intravitreally, including pegcetacoplan, an anti-C3 agent, and avacincaptad pegol, an anti-C5 agent. In Phase 3 studies, these agents have shown anatomical benefits for the treatment of GA at one year, but it is still unknown whether they will meaningfully improve visual outcomes [173]. Furthermore, there are safety concerns regarding the induction of exudative AMD for both agents [173]. An interesting hypothesis relating to reduced C3 breakdown products on endothelial cell surfaces with a shift to a reparative proangiogenic macrophage phenotype has been proposed [238]. It is unclear whether this adverse event is related to class effects of complement inhibition or PEGylation, as discussed in Section 7.4, or other clinical factors such as the presence and activity of macular neovascularisation in the fellow eye of study participants. As such, longer-term studies following market authorisation will likely be needed to assess the real-world risks to patients. Pegcetacoplan has recently been granted FDA market authorisation for the treatment of GA due to its positive results in reducing GA progression for dosing up to 24 months. The submission of avacincaptad pegol to the FDA is anticipated to result in an outcome in Q3 2023. Both agents are still being evaluated by the European Medicines Agency (EMA).

Nevertheless, the frequent administration of these therapies (i.e., monthly or every other month) and the associated burden on healthcare systems and patients have led to a continued search for longer-acting treatments. One potential approach is the use of gene therapy to modulate complement expression in the retina over the long term. Gene therapy involves the delivery of nucleic acid cargo (such as DNA, mRNA, or small interfering RNA) using viral or non-viral vectors. In the retina, adeno-associated virus (AAV) vectors have shown promise as a gene therapy technology due to their effectiveness and ability to sustain gene expression for several years in certain IRDs [239–241]. While AMD is a complex genetic disease, advances in dual and triple AAV vectors with enhanced cargo capacity now allow for the delivery of larger genes [242], including anti-VEGF and complement regulatory molecules, which could potentially be used in gene therapy for AMD.

While intravitreal gene therapies have shown some efficacy in transducing inner retinal ganglion cells for the treatment of Leber hereditary optic neuropathy [243], transduction of photoreceptors in the outer retina has proven more challenging. The inner limiting membrane (ILM) and glial processes of the neural retina act as barriers to the diffusion of naturally occurring AAV serotypes in humans [244,245]. AAVs have a high affinity for extracellular matrix proteins such as heparan sulphate, which is found in both the ILM and BrM [244]. This affinity allows AAVs to home to the vitreoretinal interface and facilitates retinal transduction, though it also reduces their diffusion through the retina [246]. Transduction may be most effective at areas of thinner ILM, such as in the perivascular regions [247], resulting in variable effects across the retina. There have been attempts to manipulate the ILM to reduce the necessary viral load for effective transduction, including the use of proteases to digest the ILM [244,248,249], electric microcurrents [250], and non-penetrating AAV vectors to saturate heparan binding sites in the vitreous [251]. However, these techniques have not resulted in gene expression in the outer retina. Other experimental techniques, such as ILM peeling or vitrectomy [252,253], sub-ILM injection [254,255], and ILM photo-disruption with indocyanine green [256], have also been proposed, but their safety is uncertain.

One possible way to enhance outer retinal transduction through the ILM without further surgical intervention is to make amino acid substitutions in the viral capsid to reduce heparan affinity [246]. However, this approach may require higher vector concentrations to compensate for the long diffusion distance within the vitreous [247]. These higher doses may trigger a stronger immune response and increase titres of neutralising antibodies [257–259], which can spread through the blood and lymphatic tissues [260] and potentially lead to reduced transduction efficacy and a lack of transgene expression with repeated administration [261,262]. Additionally, triggering a systemic immune response against an AAV-based vector can result in unintended side effects such as transgene expression in lymphoid organs [263,264] or systemic complement activation [265,266]. The high prevalence and cross-reactivity of neutralising AAV antibodies [239] indicates that methods to mitigate anti-AAV immunity will be necessary before the safety and efficacy of high-dose intravitreal viral vector-based gene therapy can be fully evaluated [267]. Unfortunately, animal models may not always provide reliable data on this issue [268].

There is growing interest in the development of non-viral vectors, such as polymeric, liposomal, lipid, and inorganic vectors, due to concerns about the immunogenicity of viral vectors [269]. However, the anionic and composite properties of vitreal proteoglycans can also hinder the effectiveness of these agents [270]. Strategies such as PEGylation [271], charge modification [272], and coating with hyaluronate or chloroquine [273,274] have been shown to improve retinal transduction in animal models when administered intravitreally. However, more research is needed to fully understand the biological effects and potential adverse effects of delayed clearance of these approaches.

While there are numerous challenges to intravitreal gene therapy, transduction or transfection of the inner retina may be sufficient to treat AMD. Müller glia, which are the most abundant glial cells in the retina and play a multifaceted role in retinal homeostasis and response to injury, including potentially photoreceptor regeneration, may be a target for gene therapy [275,276]. Müller cells are also considered a major source of complement proteins in the inner retina [115,130,277]. However, it is unclear if Müller cell gliosis in advanced AMD could obstruct vector diffusion [278]. Early therapeutic intervention in the disease course may offer the greatest benefit [279], and there are several ongoing intravitreal gene therapy trials for advanced AMD [280], including JNJ-1887 (formerly AAVCAGsCD59), an intravitreal AAV-based vector expressing a soluble form of the MAC inhibitory protein CD59 that is being evaluated for the treatment of GA. In mice, JNJ-1887 has been shown to reduce laser-induced CNV formation beyond the site of vector delivery [150], indicating the potential superior coverage of intravitreal versus subretinal gene therapies. This investigational medicinal product has received Advanced Therapy Medicinal Product designation by the EMA and FDA fast track designation for dry AMD following positive Phase 1 safety signals announced in a recent press release (NCT03144999) (available online: https://www.jnj.com/janssen-announces-late-breaking-data-from-two-gene-therapy-programs-at-the-american-academy-of-ophthalmology-2022-annual-meeting (accessed on 2 April 2023)).

9.3. Subretinal Therapies

Subretinal administration is a method of delivering drugs to the retina that has been commonly used in IRD gene therapy trials [281]. In this approach, the subretinal space is approached transvitreally with a vitrectomy. The retina is then perforated via a fine retinotomy and surgically detached from the RPE through a subretinal injection, forming a transient subretinal "bleb" that lasts for less than 1–2 days [281]. This space has the advantage of being close to the target cell populations in the outer retina and having greater immune privilege compared to the vitreous [282]. Most AAV-based vector serotypes can be used to deliver genes to RPE and outer nuclear layer cells through the subretinal route [283], although transduction of other cell types may be variable [284]. Subretinal gene delivery has been shown to be more effective and have a faster onset than intravitreal delivery in animal models [260,285,286]. For example, subretinal, but not intravitreal, administration of a CR2–FH fusion protein has been shown to reverse smoking-induced RPE damage in a mouse model [286]. Subretinal delivery is also less likely to result in systemic exposure and, potentially, immunogenicity compared to intravitreal administration [260], and the effectiveness of subretinal gene therapy does not seem to be affected by the presence of neutralising antibodies in the host serum [287]. Ongoing phase 2 studies (NCT04437368 (https://clinicaltrials.gov/ct2/show/NCT04437368), NCT03846193 (https://clinicaltrials.gov/ct2/show/NCT03846193), NCT04566445 (https://clinicaltrials.gov/ct2/show/NCT04566445)) are exploring the potential of GT005 (developed by *Gyroscope Therapeutics Limited*, London, UK, a *Novartis* company), an investigational subretinal AAV-based vector expressing *CFI*, for the treatment of GA using two delivery methods (Figure 6).

Subretinal injections for viral gene therapy may trigger host immune responses [258,288–291], and the requirement for vitrectomy and transvitreal approaches can cause complications such as cataracts and retinal tear formation/detachment [292–294]. These issues may be partly addressed through the use of novel surgical delivery systems [295]. The subretinal space can be approached through the suprachoroidal space using a flexible conduit with transpupillary visualisation as it transits to the intended point of delivery. At this point, a microneedle is advanced into the subretinal space and the treatment delivered, avoiding the need for vitrectomy and its related complications. This method is being evaluated in the aforementioned GT005 trial using the Orbit™ Subretinal Delivery System (NCT03846193, https://clinicaltrials.gov/ct2/show/NCT03846193). One potential limitation is that it forms a BrM perforation point, which in AMD eyes in particular could theoretically increase the risk of macular neovascularisation if positioned posteriorly near the fovea, although this has not been observed to date. Utilisation of more anterior delivery avoids this and would be appropriate for secreted protein gene therapy as with FI.

Increased activation of glial responses and chronic choroidal inflammation following subretinal, but not intravitreal, AAV vector administration has additionally been reported in primates [257]. Dose-dependent immune responses have also been observed, with high doses potentially leading to persistent inflammation and clinically significant vision loss in patients receiving high-dose AAV2 vector-based subretinal *RPE65* therapy [296]. Systemic steroids are often used to mitigate this phenomenon, but the long-term effects of this approach on the retina are unclear [281]. Moreover, subfoveal viral gene therapy has been associated with various adverse effects, such as RPE alterations, retinal thinning, foveal morphological changes, vision loss, and the variable duration of clinical effects [281,294,296–298]. ROCK inhibitors may improve synaptic remodelling and ameliorate these negative effects in the future [299]. Finally, the limited lateral diffusion of subretinal agents may not fully suppress complement activation in distal retinal sites [282]. Overall, while subretinal viral gene therapy has a favourable safety profile [300], it is important to carefully consider the potential risks and limitations of the procedure.

Although non-viral vectors have been explored for subretinal administration, they have generally been associated with toxicity and lower transduction levels compared to viral vectors [301]. Additionally, the viscosity of these formulations may limit their ability to adequately cover the subretinal area [302]. This highlights the importance of carefully considering the choice of vector for subretinal gene therapy.

9.4. Suprachoroidal Therapies

The suprachoroidal route for drug delivery, initially proposed 20 years ago, has gained increasing attention as a potential alternative to traditional subretinal and intravitreal routes [303]. This approach involves injecting a small amount of agent into the suprachoroidal space, a potential space consisting of tightly packed connective tissue between the choroid and sclera that extends from the supraciliary space at the front of the eye to the optic nerve at the back. It is bound anteriorly by the scleral spur and posteriorly by the optic nerve and posterior ciliary arteries [304]. Its structural continuity and small volume are important for understanding the potential of the suprachoroidal space as a drug delivery route, which allows for rapid dissemination of a small amount of agent around most of the eye [305]. For example, bevacizumab (149 kDa) has been shown to effectively diffuse into the choroid, RPE, and photoreceptors through this route [306]. Furthermore, the suprachoroidal route offers faster diffusion for smaller, lipophilic agents [307] and, as an ab externo approach, avoids the intraocular complications associated with intravitreal and subretinal administration [308]. Overall, the suprachoroidal route represents a promising option for delivering drugs to the outer retina.

Co-localisation with a polymer may improve particle durability and spread [309]. Nevertheless, particle clearance may be less a concern for gene vector-based therapies delivered via the suprachoroidal route. For example, suprachoroidal injection of an AAV-based vector in large animals achieved a wider distribution of outer retinal transduction than subretinal therapy [310–312] and lower systemic distribution and inflammation than the intravitreal route [310,312]. These experiments suggest that the suprachoroidal route is less immunogenic than the intravitreal space but more immunogenic than the subretinal space. It is possible that the exposure of these agents to the resident macrophages and lymphatic lacunae of the choroid may enhance their antigen presentation systemically, which could lead to subretinal immune cell infiltration and the neutralization of antibody production in nonhuman primates and rats [310,312].

Despite the preclinical concerns surrounding suprachoroidal viral gene therapy, the Phase 2 study of RGX-314 (developed by *REGENXBIO*, Rockville, MD, USA, in partnership with *AbbVie*, North Chicago, IL, USA; NCT04514653, https://clinicaltrials.gov/ct2/show/NCT04514653) has recently shown positive interim results (available online: https://regenxbio.gcs-web.com/news-releases/news-release-details/regenxbio-announces-additional-positive-interim-data-trials-rgx (accessed on 2 April 2023)). RGX-314 is an investigational suprachoroidal AAV-based vector that expresses an anti-VEGF antibody fragment and is being developed for the treatment of exudative AMD. These interim results indicate efficacy and limited intraocular inflammation, despite the use of a non-native protein and administration in patients who are neutralising antibody-positive without prophylactic steroid use.

Non-viral-based vectors are also currently being actively explored as alternative suprachoroidally administered therapeutics [313]. BrM may also pose a barrier to the diffusion of therapies to the retina due to its dense proteoglycan content that can sequester viral-based vectors and electrostatically repel non-viral formulations. A small molecule Factor D inhibitor (A01017, formerly developed by *Achillion Pharmaceuticals*, now by *AstraZeneca*) showed promising results in a preclinical study with biological efficacy up to three months after suprachoroidal administration in rabbits, though further studies have not been made publicly available [314]. It is unclear whether this drug was biosimilar to the orally administered danicopan currently in development.

10. Conclusions

The ability to visualise changes associated with age and retinal pathologies, including AMD, using high-resolution ophthalmic imaging techniques such as OCT and OCT-angiography has facilitated the study of BrM as a critical component in AMD pathogenesis. The results of the first Phase 3 trials using intravitreal complement inhibitors have brought exciting and promising advancements in the treatment of this disease that affects millions of people. Further research is needed to fully understand the transit of complement proteins and vectors across BrM and the RPE to achieve effective therapeutic delivery of inhibitors and regulators, which will be crucial in targeting complement activation that occurs on both sides of BrM.

Author Contributions: S.H.: writing—original draft preparation; N.T.: writing—original draft preparation; M.F.: writing—original draft preparation; C.H.: writing—review and editing; M.L.: writing—review and editing; I.P.M.: writing—review and editing; K.L.: writing—review and editing; D.H.S.: writing—conceptualisation and original draft preparation. All authors have read and agreed to the published version of the manuscript.

Funding: Sarah Hammadi is supported by Newcastle University and Gyroscope Therapeutics, a Novartis company; Nikolaos Tzoumas is supported by an NIHR Academic Clinical Fellowship (ACF-2021-01-008); Majlinda Lako is supported by Retina UK (#GR602 and #GR601) and Macular Society UK; Claire Harris received research grant support from companies developing complement therapeutics; David H Steel has research funding from Gyroscope Therapeutics (a Novartis company) (relevant to work under consideration), Alcon, Boehringer Ingelheim, Bayer, DORC, and Roche.

Institutional Review Board Statement: Not applicable.

Informed Consent Statement: Not applicable.

Data Availability Statement: Not applicable.

Conflicts of Interest: Nikolaos Tzoumas, Majlinda Lako, and Mariantonia Ferrara have no disclosures. Sarah Hammadi is supported by funding from Gyroscope Therapeutics, a Novartis company. Claire Harris is an employee of Gyroscope Therapeutics, a Novartis company. Claire Harris recent (last three years) consultant or Advisory Board member for Gyroscope Therapeutics, Q32 Bio Inc, Biocryst Pharmaceuticals, Chinook Therapeutics. Receipt of research funding frim Ra Pharmaceuticals. Ingrid Porpino Meschede and Katharina Lo are employees of Gyroscope Therapeutics, a Novartis Company. David Steel provides consultancy for Gyroscope Therapeutics (a Novartis company) (relevant to work under consideration), Apellis (relevant to work under consideration), Alcon, BVI, Roche, and Novo Nordisk.

References

1. Wong, W.L.; Su, X.; Li, X.; Cheung, C.M.; Klein, R.; Cheng, C.Y.; Wong, T.Y. Global prevalence of age-related macular degeneration and disease burden projection for 2020 and 2040: A systematic review and meta-analysis. *Lancet Glob. Health* **2014**, *2*, e106–e116. [CrossRef] [PubMed]
2. Li, J.Q.; Welchowski, T.; Schmid, M.; Mauschitz, M.M.; Holz, F.G.; Finger, R.P. Prevalence and incidence of age-related macular degeneration in Europe: A systematic review and meta-analysis. *Br. J. Ophthalmol.* **2020**, *104*, 1077–1084. [CrossRef]
3. Minassian, D.; Reidy, A. Future Sight Loss UK (2): An Epidemiological and Economic Model for Sight Loss in the Decade 2010–2020. 2009. Available online: https://media.rnib.org.uk/documents/FSUK_Report_2_0.doc (accessed on 2 April 2023).
4. Chakravarthy, U.; Bailey, C.C.; Johnston, R.L.; McKibbin, M.; Khan, R.S.; Mahmood, S.; Downey, L.; Dhingra, N.; Brand, C.; Brittain, C.J.; et al. Characterizing Disease Burden and Progression of Geographic Atrophy Secondary to Age-Related Macular Degeneration. *Ophthalmology* **2018**, *125*, 842–849. [CrossRef]
5. Rofagha, S.; Bhisitkul, R.B.; Boyer, D.S.; Sadda, S.R.; Zhang, K.; Group, S.-U.S. Seven-year outcomes in ranibizumab-treated patients in ANCHOR, MARINA, and HORIZON: A multicenter cohort study (SEVEN-UP). *Ophthalmology* **2013**, *120*, 2292–2299. [CrossRef]
6. Guillonneau, X.; Eandi, C.M.; Paques, M.; Sahel, J.A.; Sapieha, P.; Sennlaub, F. On phagocytes and macular degeneration. *Prog. Retin. Eye Res.* **2017**, *61*, 98–128. [CrossRef] [PubMed]
7. Tzoumas, N.; Hallam, D.; Harris, C.L.; Lako, M.; Kavanagh, D.; Steel, D.H.W. Revisiting the role of factor H in age-related macular degeneration: Insights from complement-mediated renal disease and rare genetic variants. *Surv. Ophthalmol.* **2021**, *66*, 378–401. [CrossRef] [PubMed]
8. Pauly, D.; Agarwal, D.; Dana, N.; Schafer, N.; Biber, J.; Wunderlich, K.A.; Jabri, Y.; Straub, T.; Zhang, N.R.; Gautam, A.K.; et al. Cell-Type-Specific Complement Expression in the Healthy and Diseased Retina. *Cell. Rep.* **2019**, *29*, 2835–2848.E4. [CrossRef]
9. Lakkaraju, A.; Umapathy, A.; Tan, L.X.; Daniele, L.; Philp, N.J.; Boesze-Battaglia, K.; Williams, D.S. The cell biology of the retinal pigment epithelium. *Prog. Retin. Eye Res.* **2020**, *78*, 100846. [CrossRef] [PubMed]
10. Nickla, D.L.; Wallman, J. The multifunctional choroid. *Prog. Retin. Eye Res.* **2010**, *29*, 144–168. [CrossRef]
11. Edwards, M.; Lutty, G.A. Bruch's Membrane and the Choroid in Age-Related Macular Degeneration. *Adv. Exp. Med. Biol.* **2021**, *1256*, 89–119. [CrossRef]
12. Hogan, M.J.; Alvarado, A.J.; Weddell, J.E. *Histology of the Human. Eye: An. Atlas and Textbook*; Saunders: Philadelphia, PA, USA, 1971.
13. Guymer, R.; Luthert, P.; Bird, A. Changes in Bruch's membrane and related structures with age. *Prog. Retin. Eye Res.* **1999**, *18*, 59–90. [CrossRef] [PubMed]
14. Booij, J.C.; Baas, D.C.; Beisekeeva, J.; Gorgels, T.G.; Bergen, A.A. The dynamic nature of Bruch's membrane. *Prog. Retin. Eye Res.* **2010**, *29*, 1–18. [CrossRef] [PubMed]

15. Chen, L.; Miyamura, N.; Ninomiya, Y.; Handa, J.T. Distribution of the collagen IV isoforms in human Bruch's membrane. *Br. J. Ophthalmol.* **2003**, *87*, 212–215. [CrossRef]
16. Aisenbrey, S.; Zhang, M.; Bacher, D.; Yee, J.; Brunken, W.J.; Hunter, D.D. Retinal pigment epithelial cells synthesize laminins, including laminin 5, and adhere to them through alpha3- and alpha6-containing integrins. *Investig. Ophthalmol. Vis. Sci.* **2006**, *47*, 5537–5544. [CrossRef] [PubMed]
17. Call, T.W.; Hollyfield, J.G. Sulfated proteoglycans in Bruch's membrane of the human eye: Localization and characterization using cupromeronic blue. *Exp. Eye Res.* **1990**, *51*, 451–462. [CrossRef]
18. Beattie, J.R.; Pawlak, A.M.; Boulton, M.E.; Zhang, J.; Monnier, V.M.; McGarvey, J.J.; Stitt, A.W. Multiplex analysis of age-related protein and lipid modifications in human Bruch's membrane. *FASEB J.* **2010**, *24*, 4816–4824. [CrossRef] [PubMed]
19. Das, A.; Frank, R.N.; Zhang, N.L.; Turczyn, T.J. Ultrastructural localization of extracellular matrix components in human retinal vessels and Bruch's membrane. *Arch. Ophthalmol.* **1990**, *108*, 421–429. [CrossRef]
20. Lin, W.L.; Essner, E.; McCarthy, K.J.; Couchman, J.R. Ultrastructural immunocytochemical localization of chondroitin sulfate proteoglycan in Bruch's membrane of the rat. *Investig. Ophthalmol. Vis. Sci.* **1992**, *33*, 2072–2075.
21. Marmor, M.F.; Wolfensberger, T.J. *The Retinal Pigment Epithelium*; Oxford University Press: New York, NY, USA, 1998.
22. Ruberti, J.W.; Curcio, C.A.; Millican, C.L.; Menco, B.P.; Huang, J.D.; Johnson, M. Quick-freeze/deep-etch visualization of age-related lipid accumulation in Bruch's membrane. *Investig. Ophthalmol. Vis. Sci.* **2003**, *44*, 1753–1759. [CrossRef] [PubMed]
23. Hageman, G.S.; Mullins, R.F.; Russell, S.R.; Johnson, L.V.; Anderson, D.H. Vitronectin is a constituent of ocular drusen and the vitronectin gene is expressed in human retinal pigmented epithelial cells. *FASEB J.* **1999**, *13*, 477–484. [CrossRef]
24. Anderson, D.H.; Ozaki, S.; Nealon, M.; Neitz, J.; Mullins, R.F.; Hageman, G.S.; Johnson, L.V. Local cellular sources of apolipoprotein E in the human retina and retinal pigmented epithelium: Implications for the process of drusen formation. *Am. J. Ophthalmol.* **2001**, *131*, 767–781. [CrossRef] [PubMed]
25. Tezel, T.H.; Geng, L.; Lato, E.B.; Schaal, S.; Liu, Y.; Dean, D.; Klein, J.B.; Kaplan, H.J. Synthesis and secretion of hemoglobin by retinal pigment epithelium. *Investig. Ophthalmol. Vis. Sci.* **2009**, *50*, 1911–1919. [CrossRef]
26. Sakaguchi, H.; Miyagi, M.; Shadrach, K.G.; Rayborn, M.E.; Crabb, J.W.; Hollyfield, J.G. Clusterin is present in drusen in age-related macular degeneration. *Exp. Eye Res.* **2002**, *74*, 547–549. [CrossRef]
27. Chong, N.H.; Keonin, J.; Luthert, P.J.; Frennesson, C.I.; Weingeist, D.M.; Wolf, R.L.; Mullins, R.F.; Hageman, G.S. Decreased thickness and integrity of the macular elastic layer of Bruch's membrane correspond to the distribution of lesions associated with age-related macular degeneration. *Am. J. Pathol.* **2005**, *166*, 241–251. [CrossRef]
28. Johnson, M.; Curcio, C.A. *Structure, Function, and Pathology of Bruch's Membrane*; Elsevier: Amsterdam, The Netherlands, 2012; Volume 1.
29. Newsome, D.A.; Huh, W.; Green, W.R. Bruch's membrane age-related changes vary by region. *Curr. Eye Res.* **1987**, *6*, 1211–1221. [CrossRef]
30. Huang, J.D.; Presley, J.B.; Chimento, M.F.; Curcio, C.A.; Johnson, M. Age-related changes in human macular Bruch's membrane as seen by quick-freeze/deep-etch. *Exp. Eye Res.* **2007**, *85*, 202–218. [CrossRef] [PubMed]
31. Wang, L.; Li, C.M.; Rudolf, M.; Belyaeva, O.V.; Chung, B.H.; Messinger, J.D.; Kedishvili, N.Y.; Curcio, C.A. Lipoprotein particles of intraocular origin in human Bruch membrane: An unusual lipid profile. *Investig. Ophthalmol. Vis. Sci.* **2009**, *50*, 870–877. [CrossRef]
32. Mullins, R.F.; Olvera, M.A.; Clark, A.F.; Stone, E.M. Fibulin-5 distribution in human eyes: Relevance to age-related macular degeneration. *Exp. Eye Res.* **2007**, *84*, 378–380. [CrossRef]
33. Bhutto, I.A.; Kim, S.Y.; McLeod, D.S.; Merges, C.; Fukai, N.; Olsen, B.R.; Lutty, G.A. Localization of collagen XVIII and the endostatin portion of collagen XVIII in aged human control eyes and eyes with age-related macular degeneration. *Investig. Ophthalmol. Vis. Sci.* **2004**, *45*, 1544–1552. [CrossRef]
34. Yamada, Y.; Tian, J.; Yang, Y.; Cutler, R.G.; Wu, T.; Telljohann, R.S.; Mattson, M.P.; Handa, J.T. Oxidized low density lipoproteins induce a pathologic response by retinal pigmented epithelial cells. *J. Neurochem.* **2008**, *105*, 1187–1197. [CrossRef] [PubMed]
35. Clark, S.J.; McHarg, S.; Tilakaratna, V.; Brace, N.; Bishop, P.N. Bruch's Membrane Compartmentalizes Complement Regulation in the Eye with Implications for Therapeutic Design in Age-Related Macular Degeneration. *Front. Immunol.* **2017**, *8*, 1778. [CrossRef]
36. Clark, S.J.; Schmidt, C.Q.; White, A.M.; Hakobyan, S.; Morgan, B.P.; Bishop, P.N. Identification of factor H-like protein 1 as the predominant complement regulator in Bruch's membrane: Implications for age-related macular degeneration. *J. Immunol.* **2014**, *193*, 4962–4970. [CrossRef] [PubMed]
37. Langford-Smith, A.; Day, A.J.; Bishop, P.N.; Clark, S.J. Complementing the Sugar Code: Role of GAGs and Sialic Acid in Complement Regulation. *Front. Immunol.* **2015**, *6*, 25. [CrossRef] [PubMed]
38. Clark, S.J.; Bishop, P.N.; Day, A.J. The proteoglycan glycomatrix: A sugar microenvironment essential for complement regulation. *Front. Immunol.* **2013**, *4*, 412. [CrossRef]
39. Tsiftsoglou, S.A.; Arnold, J.N.; Roversi, P.; Crispin, M.D.; Radcliffe, C.; Lea, S.M.; Dwek, R.A.; Rudd, P.M.; Sim, R.B. Human complement factor I glycosylation: Structural and functional characterisation of the N-linked oligosaccharides. *Biochim. Biophys. Acta* **2006**, *1764*, 1757–1766. [CrossRef]
40. Chan, W.H.; Hussain, A.A.; Marshall, J. Youngs Modulus of Bruchs Membrane: Implications for AMD. *Investig. Ophthalmol. Vis. Sci.* **2007**, *48*, 2187.

41. Friberg, T.R.; Lace, J.W. A comparison of the elastic properties of human choroid and sclera. *Exp. Eye Res.* **1988**, *47*, 429–436. [CrossRef]
42. Jones, I.L.; Warner, M.; Stevens, J.D. Mathematical modelling of the elastic properties of retina: A determination of Young's modulus. *Eye* **1992**, *6 Pt 6*, 556–559. [CrossRef]
43. Guo, L.; Hussain, A.A.; Limb, G.A.; Marshall, J. Age-dependent variation in metalloproteinase activity of isolated human Bruch's membrane and choroid. *Invest. Ophthalmol. Vis. Sci.* **1999**, *40*, 2676–2682.
44. Vranka, J.A.; Johnson, E.; Zhu, X.; Shepardson, A.; Alexander, J.P.; Bradley, J.M.; Wirtz, M.K.; Weleber, R.G.; Klein, M.L.; Acott, T.S. Discrete expression and distribution pattern of TIMP-3 in the human retina and choroid. *Curr. Eye Res.* **1997**, *16*, 102–110. [CrossRef]
45. Sarks, S.H. Ageing and degeneration in the macular region: A clinico-pathological study. *Br. J. Ophthalmol.* **1976**, *60*, 324–341. [CrossRef] [PubMed]
46. Okubo, A.; Rosa, R.H., Jr.; Bunce, C.V.; Alexander, R.A.; Fan, J.T.; Bird, A.C.; Luthert, P.J. The relationships of age changes in retinal pigment epithelium and Bruch's membrane. *Investig. Ophthalmol. Vis. Sci.* **1999**, *40*, 443–449.
47. Ramrattan, R.S.; van der Schaft, T.L.; Mooy, C.M.; de Bruijn, W.C.; Mulder, P.G.; de Jong, P.T. Morphometric analysis of Bruch's membrane, the choriocapillaris, and the choroid in aging. *Investig. Ophthalmol. Vis. Sci.* **1994**, *35*, 2857–2864.
48. Pauleikhoff, D.; Wojteki, S.; Muller, D.; Bornfeld, N.; Heiligenhaus, A. Adhesive properties of basal membranes of Bruch's membrane. Immunohistochemical studies of age-dependent changes in adhesive molecules and lipid deposits. *Ophthalmologe* **2000**, *97*, 243–250. [CrossRef] [PubMed]
49. Haimovici, R.; Gantz, D.L.; Rumelt, S.; Freddo, T.F.; Small, D.M. The lipid composition of drusen, Bruch's membrane, and sclera by hot stage polarizing light microscopy. *Investig. Ophthalmol. Vis. Sci.* **2001**, *42*, 1592–1599.
50. Bird, A.C.; Marshall, J. Retinal pigment epithelial detachments in the elderly. *Trans. Ophthalmol. Soc. UK* **1986**, *105 Pt 6*, 674–682.
51. Hussain, A.A.; Rowe, L.; Marshall, J. Age-related alterations in the diffusional transport of amino acids across the human Bruch's-choroid complex. *J. Opt. Soc. Am. A Opt. Image Sci. Vis.* **2002**, *19*, 166–172. [CrossRef]
52. Kamei, M.; Hollyfield, J.G. TIMP-3 in Bruch's membrane: Changes during aging and in age-related macular degeneration. *Investig. Ophthalmol. Vis. Sci.* **1999**, *40*, 2367–2375.
53. Handa, J.T.; Verzijl, N.; Matsunaga, H.; Aotaki-Keen, A.; Lutty, G.A.; te Koppele, J.M.; Miyata, T.; Hjelmeland, L.M. Increase in the advanced glycation end product pentosidine in Bruch's membrane with age. *Investig. Ophthalmol. Vis. Sci.* **1999**, *40*, 775–779.
54. Pietkiewicz, J.; Seweryn, E.; Bartys, A.; Gamian, A. Receptors for advanced glycation end products and their physiological and clinical significance. *Postepy Hig. Med. Dosw.* **2008**, *62*, 511–523.
55. Keenan, T.D.; Pickford, C.E.; Holley, R.J.; Clark, S.J.; Lin, W.; Dowsey, A.W.; Merry, C.L.; Day, A.J.; Bishop, P.N. Age-dependent changes in heparan sulfate in human Bruch's membrane: Implications for age-related macular degeneration. *Investig. Ophthalmol. Vis. Sci.* **2014**, *55*, 5370–5379. [CrossRef] [PubMed]
56. Clark, S.J.; Higman, V.A.; Mulloy, B.; Perkins, S.J.; Lea, S.M.; Sim, R.B.; Day, A.J. His-384 allotypic variant of factor H associated with age-related macular degeneration has different heparin binding properties from the non-disease-associated form. *J. Biol. Chem.* **2006**, *281*, 24713–24720. [CrossRef] [PubMed]
57. Prosser, B.E.; Johnson, S.; Roversi, P.; Herbert, A.P.; Blaum, B.S.; Tyrrell, J.; Jowitt, T.A.; Clark, S.J.; Tarelli, E.; Uhrin, D.; et al. Structural basis for complement factor H linked age-related macular degeneration. *J. Exp. Med.* **2007**, *204*, 2277–2283. [CrossRef]
58. Davis, W.L.; Jones, R.G.; Hagler, H.K. An electron microscopic histochemical and analytical X-ray microprobe study of calcification in Bruch's membrane from human eyes. *J. Histochem. Cytochem.* **1981**, *29*, 601–608. [CrossRef] [PubMed]
59. Ugarte, M.; Hussain, A.A.; Marshall, J. An experimental study of the elastic properties of the human Bruch's membrane-choroid complex: Relevance to ageing. *Br. J. Ophthalmol.* **2006**, *90*, 621–626. [CrossRef]
60. Moore, D.J.; Hussain, A.A.; Marshall, J. Age-related variation in the hydraulic conductivity of Bruch's membrane. *Investig. Ophthalmol. Vis. Sci.* **1995**, *36*, 1290–1297.
61. Starita, C.; Hussain, A.A.; Pagliarini, S.; Marshall, J. Hydrodynamics of ageing Bruch's membrane: Implications for macular disease. *Exp. Eye Res.* **1996**, *62*, 565–572. [CrossRef]
62. Starita, C.; Hussain, A.A.; Patmore, A.; Marshall, J. Localization of the site of major resistance to fluid transport in Bruch's membrane. *Investig. Ophthalmol. Vis. Sci.* **1997**, *38*, 762–767.
63. Hillenkamp, J.; Hussain, A.A.; Jackson, T.L.; Cunningham, J.R.; Marshall, J. The influence of path length and matrix components on ageing characteristics of transport between the choroid and the outer retina. *Investig. Ophthalmol. Vis. Sci.* **2004**, *45*, 1493–1498. [CrossRef]
64. Moore, D.J.; Clover, G.M. The effect of age on the macromolecular permeability of human Bruch's membrane. *Investig. Ophthalmol. Vis. Sci.* **2001**, *42*, 2970–2975.
65. Green, W.R.; Enger, C. Age-related macular degeneration histopathologic studies. The 1992 Lorenz E. Zimmerman Lecture. *Ophthalmology* **1993**, *100*, 1519–1535. [CrossRef]
66. Curcio, C.A.; Presley, J.B.; Millican, C.L.; Medeiros, N.E. Basal deposits and drusen in eyes with age-related maculopathy: Evidence for solid lipid particles. *Exp. Eye Res.* **2005**, *80*, 761–775. [CrossRef] [PubMed]
67. Crabb, J.W.; Miyagi, M.; Gu, X.; Shadrach, K.; West, K.A.; Sakaguchi, H.; Kamei, M.; Hasan, A.; Yan, L.; Rayborn, M.E.; et al. Drusen proteome analysis: An approach to the etiology of age-related macular degeneration. *Proc. Natl. Acad. Sci. USA* **2002**, *99*, 14682–14687. [CrossRef]

68. Mitchell, P.; Liew, G.; Gopinath, B.; Wong, T.Y. Age-related macular degeneration. *Lancet* **2018**, *392*, 1147–1159. [CrossRef]
69. Sura, A.A.; Chen, L.; Messinger, J.D.; Swain, T.A.; McGwin, G., Jr.; Freund, K.B.; Curcio, C.A. Measuring the Contributions of Basal Laminar Deposit and Bruch's Membrane in Age-Related Macular Degeneration. *Investig. Ophthalmol. Vis. Sci.* **2020**, *61*, 19. [CrossRef]
70. Sarks, S.; Cherepanoff, S.; Killingsworth, M.; Sarks, J. Relationship of Basal laminar deposit and membranous debris to the clinical presentation of early age-related macular degeneration. *Investig. Ophthalmol. Vis. Sci.* **2007**, *48*, 968–977. [CrossRef]
71. Penfold, P.L.; Madigan, M.C.; Gillies, M.C.; Provis, J.M. Immunological and aetiological aspects of macular degeneration. *Prog. Retin. Eye Res.* **2001**, *20*, 385–414. [CrossRef] [PubMed]
72. Spaide, R.F.; Ooto, S.; Curcio, C.A. Subretinal drusenoid deposits AKA pseudodrusen. *Surv. Ophthalmol.* **2018**, *63*, 782–815. [CrossRef]
73. Chakravarthy, U.; Wong, T.Y.; Fletcher, A.; Piault, E.; Evans, C.; Zlateva, G.; Buggage, R.; Pleil, A.; Mitchell, P. Clinical risk factors for age-related macular degeneration: A systematic review and meta-analysis. *BMC Ophthalmol.* **2010**, *10*, 31. [CrossRef]
74. Shahid, H.; Khan, J.C.; Cipriani, V.; Sepp, T.; Matharu, B.K.; Bunce, C.; Harding, S.P.; Clayton, D.G.; Moore, A.T.; Yates, J.R.; et al. Age-related macular degeneration: The importance of family history as a risk factor. *Br. J. Ophthalmol.* **2012**, *96*, 427–431. [CrossRef] [PubMed]
75. Seddon, J.M.; Cote, J.; Page, W.F.; Aggen, S.H.; Neale, M.C. The US twin study of age-related macular degeneration: Relative roles of genetic and environmental influences. *Arch. Ophthalmol.* **2005**, *123*, 321–327. [CrossRef] [PubMed]
76. Klein, R.J.; Zeiss, C.; Chew, E.Y.; Tsai, J.Y.; Sackler, R.S.; Haynes, C.; Henning, A.K.; SanGiovanni, J.P.; Mane, S.M.; Mayne, S.T.; et al. Complement factor H polymorphism in age-related macular degeneration. *Science* **2005**, *308*, 385–389. [CrossRef]
77. Iyengar, S.K.; Song, D.; Klein, B.E.; Klein, R.; Schick, J.H.; Humphrey, J.; Millard, C.; Liptak, R.; Russo, K.; Jun, G.; et al. Dissection of genomewide-scan data in extended families reveals a major locus and oligogenic susceptibility for age-related macular degeneration. *Am. J. Hum. Genet.* **2004**, *74*, 20–39. [CrossRef]
78. Fritsche, L.G.; Igl, W.; Bailey, J.N.; Grassmann, F.; Sengupta, S.; Bragg-Gresham, J.L.; Burdon, K.P.; Hebbring, S.J.; Wen, C.; Gorski, M.; et al. A large genome-wide association study of age-related macular degeneration highlights contributions of rare and common variants. *Nat. Genet.* **2016**, *48*, 134–143. [CrossRef] [PubMed]
79. Winkler, T.W.; Grassmann, F.; Brandl, C.; Kiel, C.; Gunther, F.; Strunz, T.; Weidner, L.; Zimmermann, M.E.; Korb, C.A.; Poplawski, A.; et al. Genome-wide association meta-analysis for early age-related macular degeneration highlights novel loci and insights for advanced disease. *BMC Med. Genom.* **2020**, *13*, 120. [CrossRef]
80. de Breuk, A.; Acar, I.E.; Kersten, E.; Schijvenaars, M.; Colijn, J.M.; Haer-Wigman, L.; Bakker, B.; de Jong, S.; Meester-Smoor, M.A.; Verzijden, T.; et al. Development of a Genotype Assay for Age-Related Macular Degeneration: The EYE-RISK Consortium. *Ophthalmology* **2021**, *128*, 1604–1617. [CrossRef]
81. Tzoumas, N.; Kavanagh, D.; Cordell, H.J.; Lotery, A.J.; Patel, P.J.; Steel, D.H. Rare complement factor I variants associated with reduced macular thickness and age-related macular degeneration in the UK Biobank. *Hum. Mol. Genet.* **2022**, *31*, 2678–2692. [CrossRef]
82. Khan, A.H.; Sutton, J.; Cree, A.J.; Khandhadia, S.; De Salvo, G.; Tobin, J.; Prakash, P.; Arora, R.; Amoaku, W.; Charbel Issa, P.; et al. Prevalence and phenotype associations of complement factor I mutations in geographic atrophy. *Hum. Mutat.* **2021**, *42*, 1139–1152. [CrossRef] [PubMed]
83. Roth, F.; Bindewald, A.; Holz, F.G. Keypathophysiologic pathways in age-related macular disease. *Graefes Arch. Clin. Exp. Ophthalmol.* **2004**, *242*, 710–716. [CrossRef] [PubMed]
84. Age-Related Eye Disease Study Research, G. Risk factors associated with age-related macular degeneration. A case-control study in the age-related eye disease study: Age-Related Eye Disease Study Report Number 3. *Ophthalmology* **2000**, *107*, 2224–2232. [CrossRef]
85. Vingerling, J.R.; Hofman, A.; Grobbee, D.E.; de Jong, P.T. Age-related macular degeneration and smoking. The Rotterdam Study. *Arch. Ophthalmol.* **1996**, *114*, 1193–1196. [CrossRef] [PubMed]
86. Delcourt, C.; Diaz, J.L.; Ponton-Sanchez, A.; Papoz, L. Smoking and age-related macular degeneration. The POLA Study. Pathologies Oculaires Liees a l'Age. *Arch. Ophthalmol.* **1998**, *116*, 1031–1035. [CrossRef] [PubMed]
87. Evans, J.R.; Lawrenson, J.G. Antioxidant vitamin and mineral supplements for slowing the progression of age-related macular degeneration. *Cochrane Database Syst. Rev.* **2017**, *7*, CD000254. [CrossRef]
88. Gholami, P.; Lakshminarayanan, V. Optical Coherence Tomography Image Retinal Database. Available online: https://www.openicpsr.org/openicpsr/project/108503/version/V1/view (accessed on 2 April 2023).
89. Staurenghi, G.; Sadda, S.; Chakravarthy, U.; Spaide, R.F.; International Nomenclature for Optical Coherence Tomography (IN•OCT) Panel. Proposed lexicon for anatomic landmarks in normal posterior segment spectral-domain optical coherence tomography: The IN*OCT consensus. *Ophthalmology* **2014**, *121*, 1572–1578. [CrossRef] [PubMed]
90. Schottenhamml, J.; Moult, E.M.; Ploner, S.B.; Chen, S.; Novais, E.; Husvogt, L.; Duker, J.S.; Waheed, N.K.; Fujimoto, J.G.; Maier, A.K. OCT-OCTA segmentation: Combining structural and blood flow information to segment Bruch's membrane. *Biomed. Opt. Express* **2021**, *12*, 84–99. [CrossRef]
91. Cozzi, M.; Viola, F.; Belotti, M.; Cigada, M.; Cherepanoff, S.; Staurenghi, G.; Invernizzi, A. The In Vivo Correlation between Retinal Pigment Epithelium Thickness and Quantitative Fundus Autofluorescence in a White Population. *Ophthalmol. Retin.* **2021**, *5*, 365–373. [CrossRef]

92. Chen, L.; Yang, P.; Curcio, C.A. Visualizing lipid behind the retina in aging and age-related macular degeneration, via indocyanine green angiography (ASHS-LIA). *Eye* **2022**, *36*, 1735–1746. [CrossRef]
93. Lamin, A.; Oakley, J.D.; Dubis, A.M.; Russakoff, D.B.; Sivaprasad, S. Changes in volume of various retinal layers over time in early and intermediate age-related macular degeneration. *Eye* **2019**, *33*, 428–434. [CrossRef]
94. Trinh, M.; Khou, V.; Kalloniatis, M.; Nivison-Smith, L. Location-Specific Thickness Patterns in Intermediate Age-Related Macular Degeneration Reveals Anatomical Differences in Multiple Retinal Layers. *Investig. Ophthalmol. Vis. Sci.* **2021**, *62*, 13. [CrossRef]
95. Trinh, M.; Kalloniatis, M.; Alonso-Caneiro, D.; Nivison-Smith, L. High-Density Optical Coherence Tomography Analysis Provides Insights Into Early/Intermediate Age-Related Macular Degeneration Retinal Layer Changes. *Investig. Ophthalmol. Vis. Sci.* **2022**, *63*, 36. [CrossRef]
96. Wykoff, C.C.; Rosenfeld, P.J.; Waheed, N.K.; Singh, R.P.; Ronca, N.; Slakter, J.S.; Staurenghi, G.; Mones, J.; Baumal, C.R.; Saroj, N.; et al. Characterizing New-Onset Exudation in the Randomized Phase 2 FILLY Trial of Complement Inhibitor Pegcetacoplan for Geographic Atrophy. *Ophthalmology* **2021**, *128*, 1325–1336. [CrossRef] [PubMed]
97. Khan, K.N.; Borooah, S.; Lando, L.; Dans, K.; Mahroo, O.A.; Meshi, A.; Kalitzeos, A.; Agorogiannis, G.; Moghimi, S.; Freeman, W.R.; et al. Quantifying the Separation Between the Retinal Pigment Epithelium and Bruch's Membrane using Optical Coherence Tomography in Patients with Inherited Macular Degeneration. *Transl. Vis. Sci. Technol.* **2020**, *9*, 26. [CrossRef] [PubMed]
98. Walport, M.J. Complement first of two parts. *N. Engl. J. Med.* **2001**, *344*, 1058–1066. [CrossRef] [PubMed]
99. Morgan, B.P.; Walters, D.; Serna, M.; Bubeck, D. Terminal complexes of the complement system: New structural insights and their relevance to function. *Immunol. Rev.* **2016**, *274*, 141–151. [CrossRef]
100. Morgan, B.P. The membrane attack complex as an inflammatory trigger. *Immunobiology* **2016**, *221*, 747–751. [CrossRef]
101. Fields, M.A.; Del Priore, L.V.; Adelman, R.A.; Rizzolo, L.J. Interactions of the choroid, Bruch's membrane, retinal pigment epithelium, and neurosensory retina collaborate to form the outer blood-retinal-barrier. *Prog. Retin. Eye Res.* **2020**, *76*, 100803. [CrossRef]
102. Lejoyeux, R.; Benillouche, J.; Ong, J.; Errera, M.-H.; Rossi, E.A.; Singh, S.R.; Dansingani, K.K.; da Silva, S.; Sinha, D.; Sahel, J.-A.; et al. Choriocapillaris: Fundamentals and advancements. *Prog. Retin. Eye Res.* **2022**, *87*, 100997. [CrossRef]
103. Mullins, R.F.; Johnson, M.N.; Faidley, E.A.; Skeie, J.M.; Huang, J. Choriocapillaris vascular dropout related to density of drusen in human eyes with early age-related macular degeneration. *Investig. Ophthalmol. Vis. Sci.* **2011**, *52*, 1606–1612. [CrossRef]
104. Gerl, V.B.; Bohl, J.r.; Pitz, S.; Stoffelns, B.; Pfeiffer, N.; Bhakdi, S. Extensive deposits of complement C3d and C5b-9 in the choriocapillaris of eyes of patients with diabetic retinopathy. *Investig. Ophthalmol. Vis. Sci.* **2002**, *43*, 1104–1108.
105. Hageman, G.S.; Anderson, D.H.; Johnson, L.V.; Hancock, L.S.; Taiber, A.J.; Hardisty, L.I.; Hageman, J.L.; Stockman, H.A.; Borchardt, J.D.; Gehrs, K.M. A common haplotype in the complement regulatory gene factor H (HF1/CFH) predisposes individuals to age-related macular degeneration. *Proc. Natl. Acad. Sci. USA* **2005**, *102*, 7227–7232. [CrossRef]
106. Seth, A.; Cui, J.; To, E.; Kwee, M.; Matsubara, J. Complement-associated deposits in the human retina. *Investig. Ophthalmol. Vis. Sci.* **2008**, *49*, 743–750. [CrossRef] [PubMed]
107. Mullins, R.F.; Dewald, A.D.; Streb, L.M.; Wang, K.; Kuehn, M.H.; Stone, E.M. Elevated membrane attack complex in human choroid with high risk complement factor H genotypes. *Exp. Eye Res.* **2011**, *93*, 565–567. [CrossRef] [PubMed]
108. Mullins, R.F.; Schoo, D.P.; Sohn, E.H.; Flamme-Wiese, M.J.; Workamelahu, G.; Johnston, R.M.; Wang, K.; Tucker, B.A.; Stone, E.M. The membrane attack complex in aging human choriocapillaris: Relationship to macular degeneration and choroidal thinning. *Am. J. Pathol.* **2014**, *184*, 3142–3153. [CrossRef] [PubMed]
109. Skeie, J.M.; Fingert, J.H.; Russell, S.R.; Stone, E.M.; Mullins, R.F. Complement component C5a activates ICAM-1 expression on human choroidal endothelial cells. *Investig. Ophthalmol. Vis. Sci.* **2010**, *51*, 5336–5342. [CrossRef]
110. Chirco, K.R.; Tucker, B.A.; Stone, E.M.; Mullins, R.F. Selective accumulation of the complement membrane attack complex in aging choriocapillaris. *Exp. Eye Res.* **2016**, *146*, 393–397. [CrossRef]
111. Mulfaul, K.; Mullin, N.K.; Giacalone, J.C.; Voigt, A.P.; R DeVore, M.; Stone, E.M.; Tucker, B.A.; Mullins, R.F. Local factor H production by human choroidal endothelial cells mitigates complement deposition: Implications for macular degeneration. *J. Pathol.* **2022**, *257*, 29–38. [CrossRef]
112. Whitmore, S.S.; Sohn, E.H.; Chirco, K.R.; Drack, A.V.; Stone, E.M.; Tucker, B.A.; Mullins, R.F. Complement activation and choriocapillaris loss in early AMD: Implications for pathophysiology and therapy. *Prog. Retin. Eye Res.* **2015**, *45*, 1–29. [CrossRef]
113. Ebrahimi, K.B.; Fijalkowski, N.; Cano, M.; Handa, J.T. Decreased membrane complement regulators in the retinal pigmented epithelium contributes to age-related macular degeneration. *J. Pathol.* **2013**, *229*, 729–742. [CrossRef]
114. Anderson, D.H.; Radeke, M.J.; Gallo, N.B.; Chapin, E.A.; Johnson, P.T.; Curletti, C.R.; Hancox, L.S.; Hu, J.; Ebright, J.N.; Malek, G.; et al. The pivotal role of the complement system in aging and age-related macular degeneration: Hypothesis re-visited. *Prog. Retin. Eye Res.* **2010**, *29*, 95–112. [CrossRef]
115. Menon, M.; Mohammadi, S.; Davila-Velderrain, J.; Goods, B.A.; Cadwell, T.D.; Xing, Y.; Stemmer-Rachamimov, A.; Shalek, A.K.; Love, J.C.; Kellis, M.; et al. Single-cell transcriptomic atlas of the human retina identifies cell types associated with age-related macular degeneration. *Nat. Commun.* **2019**, *10*, 4902. [CrossRef]
116. Hageman, G.S.; Luthert, P.J.; Victor Chong, N.H.; Johnson, L.V.; Anderson, D.H.; Mullins, R.F. An integrated hypothesis that considers drusen as biomarkers of immune-mediated processes at the RPE-Bruch's membrane interface in aging and age-related macular degeneration. *Prog. Retin. Eye Res.* **2001**, *20*, 705–732. [CrossRef]

117. Baudouin, C.; Peyman, G.A.; Fredj-Reygrobellet, D.; Gordon, W.C.; Lapalus, P.; Gastaud, P.; Bazan, N.G. Immunohistological study of subretinal membranes in age-related macular degeneration. *Jpn. J. Ophthalmol.* **1992**, *36*, 443–451. [PubMed]
118. Johnson, L.V.; Leitner, W.P.; Rivest, A.J.; Staples, M.K.; Radeke, M.J.; Anderson, D.H. The Alzheimer's A beta -peptide is deposited at sites of complement activation in pathologic deposits associated with aging and age-related macular degeneration. *Proc. Natl. Acad. Sci. USA* **2002**, *99*, 11830–11835. [CrossRef] [PubMed]
119. Fernandez-Godino, R.; Garland, D.L.; Pierce, E.A. A local complement response by RPE causes early-stage macular degeneration. *Hum. Mol. Gen.* **2015**, *24*, 5555–5569. [CrossRef] [PubMed]
120. Garland, D.L.; Pierce, E.A.; Fernandez-Godino, R. Complement C5 is not critical for the formation of sub-RPE deposits in Efemp1 mutant mice. *Sci. Rep.* **2021**, *11*, 10416. [CrossRef]
121. Crowley, M.A.; Garland, D.L.; Sellner, H.; Banks, A.; Fan, L.; Rejtar, T.; Buchanan, N.; Delgado, O.; Xu, Y.Y.; Jose, S.; et al. Complement factor B is critical for sub-RPE deposit accumulation in a model of Doyne honeycomb retinal dystrophy with features of age-related macular degeneration. *Hum. Mol. Gen.* **2023**, *32*, 204–217. [CrossRef]
122. Ramkumar, H.L.; Zhang, J.; Chan, C.C. Retinal ultrastructure of murine models of dry age-related macular degeneration (AMD). *Prog. Retin. Eye Res.* **2010**, *29*, 169–190. [CrossRef]
123. Chen, M.; Muckersie, E.; Robertson, M.; Forrester, J.V.; Xu, H. Up-regulation of complement factor B in retinal pigment epithelial cells is accompanied by complement activation in the aged retina. *Exp. Eye Res.* **2008**, *87*, 543–550. [CrossRef]
124. Chen, M.; Liu, B.; Lukas, T.J.; Neufeld, A.H. The aged retinal pigment epithelium/choroid: A potential substratum for the pathogenesis of age-related macular degeneration. *PLoS ONE* **2008**, *3*, e2339. [CrossRef]
125. Wang, A.L.; Lukas, T.J.; Yuan, M.; Du, N.; Tso, M.O.; Neufeld, A.H. Autophagy and exosomes in the aged retinal pigment epithelium: Possible relevance to drusen formation and age-related macular degeneration. *PLoS ONE* **2009**, *4*, e4160. [CrossRef]
126. Wang, A.L.; Lukas, T.J.; Yuan, M.; Du, N.; Tso, M.O.; Neufeld, A.H. Autophagy, exosomes and drusen formation in age-related macular degeneration. *Autophagy* **2009**, *5*, 563–564. [CrossRef] [PubMed]
127. Chen, M.; Forrester, J.V.; Xu, H. Synthesis of complement factor H by retinal pigment epithelial cells is down-regulated by oxidized photoreceptor outer segments. *Exp. Eye Res.* **2007**, *84*, 635–645. [CrossRef]
128. Kim, Y.H.; He, S.; Kase, S.; Kitamura, M.; Ryan, S.J.; Hinton, D.R. Regulated secretion of complement factor H by RPE and its role in RPE migration. *Graefes Arch. Clin. Exp. Ophthalmol.* **2009**, *247*, 651–659. [CrossRef] [PubMed]
129. McLaughlin, B.J.; Fan, W.; Zheng, J.J.; Cai, H.; Del Priore, L.V.; Bora, N.S.; Kaplan, H.J. Novel role for a complement regulatory protein (CD46) in retinal pigment epithelial adhesion. *Investig. Ophthalmol. Vis. Sci.* **2003**, *44*, 3669–3674. [CrossRef] [PubMed]
130. Vogt, S.D.; Barnum, S.R.; Curcio, C.A.; Read, R.W. Distribution of complement anaphylatoxin receptors and membrane-bound regulators in normal human retina. *Exp. Eye Res.* **2006**, *83*, 834–840. [CrossRef]
131. Weismann, D.; Hartvigsen, K.; Lauer, N.; Bennett, K.L.; Scholl, H.P.N.; Issa, P.C.; Cano, M.; Brandstätter, H.; Tsimikas, S.; Skerka, C.; et al. Complement factor H binds malondialdehyde epitopes and protects from oxidative stress. *Nature* **2011**, *478*, 76–81. [CrossRef] [PubMed]
132. Bhutto, I.A.; Baba, T.; Merges, C.; Juriasinghani, V.; McLeod, D.S.; Lutty, G.A. C-reactive protein and complement factor H in aged human eyes and eyes with age-related macular degeneration. *Br. J. Ophthalmol.* **2011**, *95*, 1323–1330. [CrossRef]
133. Vogt, S.D.; Curcio, C.A.; Wang, L.; Li, C.-M.; McGwin, G., Jr.; Medeiros, N.E.; Philp, N.J.; Kimble, J.A.; Read, R.W. Retinal pigment epithelial expression of complement regulator CD46 is altered early in the course of geographic atrophy. *Exp. Eye Res.* **2011**, *93*, 413–423. [CrossRef]
134. Cerniauskas, E.; Kurzawa-Akanbi, M.; Xie, L.; Hallam, D.; Moya-Molina, M.; White, K.; Steel, D.; Doherty, M.; Whitfield, P.; Al-Aama, J.; et al. Complement modulation reverses pathology in Y402H-retinal pigment epithelium cell model of age-related macular degeneration by restoring lysosomal function. *Stem Cells Transl. Med.* **2020**, *9*, 1585–1603. [CrossRef]
135. Ebeling, M.C.; Geng, Z.; Kapphahn, R.J.; Roehrich, H.; Montezuma, S.R.; Dutton, J.R.; Ferrington, D.A. Impaired Mitochondrial Function in iPSC-Retinal Pigment Epithelium with the Complement Factor H Polymorphism for Age-Related Macular Degeneration. *Cells* **2021**, *10*, 789. [CrossRef]
136. Hallam, D.; Collin, J.; Bojic, S.; Chichagova, V.; Buskin, A.; Xu, Y.; Lafage, L.; Otten, E.G.; Anyfantis, G.; Mellough, C.; et al. An Induced Pluripotent Stem Cell Patient Specific Model of Complement Factor H (Y402H) Polymorphism Displays Characteristic Features of Age-Related Macular Degeneration and Indicates a Beneficial Role for UV Light Exposure. *Stem Cells* **2017**, *35*, 2305–2320. [CrossRef] [PubMed]
137. Ferrington, D.A.; Kapphahn, R.J.; Leary, M.M.; Atilano, S.R.; Terluk, M.R.; Karunadharma, P.; Chen, G.K.-J.; Ratnapriya, R.; Swaroop, A.; Montezuma, S.R.; et al. Increased retinal mtDNA damage in the CFH variant associated with age-related macular degeneration. *Exp. Eye Res.* **2016**, *145*, 269–277. [CrossRef]
138. Tan, L.X.; Toops, K.A.; Lakkaraju, A. Protective responses to sublytic complement in the retinal pigment epithelium. *Proc. Natl. Acad. Sci. USA* **2016**, *113*, 8789–8794. [CrossRef] [PubMed]
139. Armento, A.; Honisch, S.; Panagiotakopoulou, V.; Sonntag, I.; Jacob, A.; Bolz, S.; Kilger, E.; Deleidi, M.; Clark, S.; Ueffing, M. Loss of Complement Factor H impairs antioxidant capacity and energy metabolism of human RPE cells. *Sci. Rep.* **2020**, *10*, 10320. [CrossRef]
140. Thurman, J.M.; Renner, B.; Kunchithapautham, K.; Ferreira, V.P.; Pangburn, M.K.; Ablonczy, Z.; Tomlinson, S.; Holers, V.M.; Rohrer, B. Oxidative stress renders retinal pigment epithelial cells susceptible to complement-mediated injury. *J. Biol. Chem.* **2009**, *284*, 16939–16947. [CrossRef]

141. Wu, Z.; Lauer, T.W.; Sick, A.; Hackett, S.F.; Campochiaro, P.A. Oxidative stress modulates complement factor H expression in retinal pigmented epithelial cells by acetylation of FOXO3. *J. Biol. Chem.* **2007**, *282*, 22414–22425. [CrossRef] [PubMed]
142. Yang, P.; Baciu, P.; Kerrigan, B.C.P.; Etheridge, M.; Sung, E.; Toimil, B.A.; Berchuck, J.E.; Jaffe, G.J. Retinal Pigment Epithelial Cell Death by the Alternative Complement Cascade: Role of Membrane Regulatory Proteins, Calcium, PKC, and Oxidative Stress. *Investig. Ophthalmol. Vis. Sci.* **2014**, *55*, 3012–3021. [CrossRef]
143. Ebrahimi, K.B.; Fijalkowski, N.; Cano, M.; Handa, J.T. Oxidized low-density-lipoprotein-induced injury in retinal pigment epithelium alters expression of the membrane complement regulatory factors CD46 and CD59 through exosomal and apoptotic bleb release. *Adv. Exp. Med. Biol.* **2014**, *801*, 259–265. [PubMed]
144. Luo, C.; Zhao, J.; Madden, A.; Chen, M.; Xu, H. Complement expression in retinal pigment epithelial cells is modulated by activated macrophages. *Exp. Eye Res.* **2013**, *112*, 93–101. [CrossRef] [PubMed]
145. Toomey, C.B.; Kelly, U.; Saban, D.R.; Bowes Rickman, C. Regulation of age-related macular degeneration-like pathology by complement factor H. *Proc. Natl. Acad. Sci. USA* **2015**, *112*, E3040–E3049. [CrossRef]
146. Lueck, K.; Wasmuth, S.; Williams, J.; Hughes, T.R.; Morgan, B.P.; Lommatzsch, A.; Greenwood, J.; Moss, S.E.; Pauleikhoff, D. Sub-lytic C5b-9 induces functional changes in retinal pigment epithelial cells consistent with age-related macular degeneration. *Eye* **2011**, *25*, 1074–1082. [CrossRef] [PubMed]
147. Bandyopadhyay, M.; Rohrer, B. Matrix metalloproteinase activity creates pro-angiogenic environment in primary human retinal pigment epithelial cells exposed to complement. *Investig. Ophthalmol. Vis. Sci.* **2012**, *53*, 1953–1961. [CrossRef]
148. Sweigard, J.H.; Cashman, S.M.; Kumar-Singh, R. Adenovirus-mediated delivery of CD46 attenuates the alternative complement pathway on RPE: Implications for age-related macular degeneration. *Gene Ther.* **2011**, *18*, 613–621. [CrossRef] [PubMed]
149. Leaderer, D.; Cashman, S.M.; Kumar-Singh, R. Adeno-associated virus mediated delivery of an engineered protein that combines the complement inhibitory properties of CD46, CD55 and CD59. *J. Gene Med.* **2015**, *17*, 101–115. [CrossRef]
150. Cashman, S.M.; Ramo, K.; Kumar-Singh, R. A non membrane-targeted human soluble CD59 attenuates choroidal neovascularization in a model of age related macular degeneration. *PLoS ONE* **2011**, *6*, e19078. [CrossRef] [PubMed]
151. Ahmad, A.; Mandwie, M.; Dreismann, A.K.; Smyth, C.M.; Doyle, H.; Malik, T.H.; Pickering, M.C.; Lachmann, P.J.; Alexander, I.E.; Logan, G.J. Adeno-Associated Virus Vector Gene Delivery Elevates Factor I Levels and Downregulates the Complement Alternative Pathway In Vivo. *Hum. Gene Ther.* **2021**, *32*, 1370–1381. [CrossRef]
152. Schnabolk, G.; Coughlin, B.; Joseph, K.; Kunchithapautham, K.; Bandyopadhyay, M.; O'Quinn, E.C.; Nowling, T.; Rohrer, B. Local production of the alternative pathway complement component factor B is sufficient to promote laser-induced choroidal neovascularization. *Investig. Ophthalmol. Vis. Sci.* **2015**, *56*, 1850–1863. [CrossRef]
153. Rohrer, B.; Coughlin, B.; Kunchithapautham, K.; Long, Q.; Tomlinson, S.; Takahashi, K.; Holers, V.M. The alternative pathway is required, but not alone sufficient, for retinal pathology in mouse laser-induced choroidal neovascularization. *Mol. Immunol.* **2011**, *48*, e1–e8. [CrossRef] [PubMed]
154. Bora, N.S.; Kaliappan, S.; Jha, P.; Xu, Q.; Sohn, J.H.; Dhaulakhandi, D.B.; Kaplan, H.J.; Bora, P.S. Complement activation via alternative pathway is critical in the development of laser-induced choroidal neovascularization: Role of factor B and factor H. *J. Immunol.* **2006**, *177*, 1872–1878. [CrossRef]
155. Bora, P.S.; Sohn, J.H.; Cruz, J.M.; Jha, P.; Nishihori, H.; Wang, Y.; Kaliappan, S.; Kaplan, H.J.; Bora, N.S. Role of complement and complement membrane attack complex in laser-induced choroidal neovascularization. *J. Immunol.* **2005**, *174*, 491–497. [CrossRef]
156. Nozaki, M.; Raisler, B.J.; Sakurai, E.; Sarma, J.V.; Barnum, S.R.; Lambris, J.D.; Chen, Y.; Zhang, K.; Ambati, B.K.; Baffi, J.Z.; et al. Drusen complement components C3a and C5a promote choroidal neovascularization. *Proc. Natl. Acad. Sci. USA* **2006**, *103*, 2328–2333. [CrossRef] [PubMed]
157. Ramo, K.; Cashman, S.M.; Kumar-Singh, R. Evaluation of adenovirus-delivered human CD59 as a potential therapy for AMD in a model of human membrane attack complex formation on murine RPE. *Investig. Ophthalmol. Vis. Sci.* **2008**, *49*, 4126–4136. [CrossRef]
158. Gandhi, J.; Cashman, S.M.; Kumar-Singh, R. Soluble CD59 expressed from an adenovirus in vivo is a potent inhibitor of complement deposition on murine liver vascular endothelium. *PLoS ONE* **2011**, *6*, e21621. [CrossRef] [PubMed]
159. Bora, N.S.; Jha, P.; Lyzogubov, V.V.; Kaliappan, S.; Liu, J.; Tytarenko, R.G.; Fraser, D.A.; Morgan, B.P.; Bora, P.S. Recombinant membrane-targeted form of CD59 inhibits the growth of choroidal neovascular complex in mice. *J. Biol. Chem.* **2010**, *285*, 33826–33833. [CrossRef] [PubMed]
160. Rohrer, B.; Long, Q.; Coughlin, B.; Wilson, R.B.; Huang, Y.; Qiao, F.; Tang, P.H.; Kunchithapautham, K.; Gilkeson, G.S.; Tomlinson, S. A targeted inhibitor of the alternative complement pathway reduces angiogenesis in a mouse model of age-related macular degeneration. *Investig. Ophthalmol. Vis. Sci.* **2009**, *50*, 3056–3064. [CrossRef]
161. Birke, K.; Lipo, E.; Birke, M.T.; Kumar-Singh, R. Topical application of PPADS inhibits complement activation and choroidal neovascularization in a model of age-related macular degeneration. *PLoS ONE* **2013**, *8*, e76766. [CrossRef]
162. Bora, N.S.; Kaliappan, S.; Jha, P.; Xu, Q.; Sivasankar, B.; Harris, C.L.; Morgan, B.P.; Bora, P.S. CD59, a complement regulatory protein, controls choroidal neovascularization in a mouse model of wet-type age-related macular degeneration. *J. Immunol.* **2007**, *178*, 1783–1790. [CrossRef]
163. Sweigard, J.H.; Yanai, R.; Gaissert, P.; Saint-Geniez, M.; Kataoka, K.; Thanos, A.; Stahl, G.L.; Lambris, J.D.; Connor, K.M. The alternative complement pathway regulates pathological angiogenesis in the retina. *FASEB J.* **2014**, *28*, 3171–3182. [CrossRef]

164. Harboe, M.; Ulvund, G.; Vien, L.; Fung, M.; Mollnes, T.E. The quantitative role of alternative pathway amplification in classical pathway induced terminal complement activation. *Clin. Exp. Immunol.* **2004**, *138*, 439–446. [CrossRef]
165. Kunchithapautham, K.; Rohrer, B. Sublytic membrane-attack-complex (MAC) activation alters regulated rather than constitutive vascular endothelial growth factor (VEGF) secretion in retinal pigment epithelium monolayers. *J. Biol. Chem.* **2011**, *286*, 23717–23724. [CrossRef]
166. Lyzogubov, V.; Wu, X.; Jha, P.; Tytarenko, R.; Triebwasser, M.; Kolar, G.; Bertram, P.; Bora, P.S.; Atkinson, J.P.; Bora, N.S. Complement Regulatory Protein CD46 Protects against Choroidal Neovascularization in Mice. *Am. J. Pathol.* **2014**, *184*, 2537–2548. [CrossRef] [PubMed]
167. Lyzogubov, V.V.; Bora, P.S.; Wu, X.; Horn, L.E.; de Roque, R.; Rudolf, X.V.; Atkinson, J.P.; Bora, N.S. The Complement Regulatory Protein CD46 Deficient Mouse Spontaneously Develops Dry-Type Age-Related Macular Degeneration–Like Phenotype. *Am. J. Pathol.* **2016**, *186*, 2088–2104. [CrossRef] [PubMed]
168. Keir, L.S.; Firth, R.; Aponik, L.; Feitelberg, D.; Sakimoto, S.; Aguilar, E.; Welsh, G.I.; Richards, A.; Usui, Y.; Satchell, S.C. VEGF regulates local inhibitory complement proteins in the eye and kidney. *J. Clin. Investig.* **2017**, *127*, 199–214. [CrossRef] [PubMed]
169. Kahr, W.H. Complement halts angiogenesis gone wild. *Blood* **2010**, *116*, 4393–4394. [CrossRef]
170. Langer, H.F.; Chung, K.J.; Orlova, V.V.; Choi, E.Y.; Kaul, S.; Kruhlak, M.J.; Alatsatianos, M.; DeAngelis, R.A.; Roche, P.A.; Magotti, P.; et al. Complement-mediated inhibition of neovascularization reveals a point of convergence between innate immunity and angiogenesis. *Blood* **2010**, *116*, 4395–4403. [CrossRef]
171. Murray, H.; Qiu, B.; Ho, S.Y.; Wang, X. Complement Factor B Mediates Ocular Angiogenesis through Regulating the VEGF Signaling Pathway. *Int. J. Mol. Sci.* **2021**, *22*, 9580. [CrossRef]
172. Zeng, S.; Whitmore, S.S.; Sohn, E.H.; Riker, M.J.; Wiley, L.A.; Scheetz, T.E.; Stone, E.M.; Tucker, B.A.; Mullins, R.F. Molecular response of chorioretinal endothelial cells to complement injury: Implications for macular degeneration. *J. Pathol.* **2016**, *238*, 446–456. [CrossRef]
173. Tzoumas, N.R.G.; Williams, M.A.; Steel, D.H. Complement inhibitors for age-related macular degeneration. *Cochrane Database Syst. Rev.* **2023**; in press. [CrossRef]
174. Hanna, R.M.; Barsoum, M.; Arman, F.; Selamet, U.; Hasnain, H.; Kurtz, I. Nephrotoxicity induced by intravitreal vascular endothelial growth factor inhibitors: Emerging evidence. *Kidney Int.* **2019**, *96*, 572–580. [CrossRef]
175. Saint-Geniez, M.; Kurihara, T.; Sekiyama, E.; Maldonado, A.E.; D'Amore, P.A. An essential role for RPE-derived soluble VEGF in the maintenance of the choriocapillaris. *Proc. Natl. Acad. Sci. USA* **2009**, *106*, 18751–18756. [CrossRef]
176. Grunwald, J.E.; Daniel, E.; Huang, J.; Ying, G.-s.; Maguire, M.G.; Toth, C.A.; Jaffe, G.J.; Fine, S.L.; Blodi, B.; Klein, M.L.; et al. Risk of Geographic Atrophy in the Comparison of Age-related Macular Degeneration Treatments Trials. *Ophthalmology* **2014**, *121*, 150–161. [CrossRef]
177. Young, M.; Chui, L.; Fallah, N.; Or, C.; Merkur, A.B.; Kirker, A.W.; Albiani, D.A.; Forooghian, F. Exacerbation of choroidal and retinal pigment epithelial atrophy after anti-vascular endothelial growth factor treatment in neovascular age-related macular degeneration. *Retina* **2014**, *34*, 1308–1315. [CrossRef]
178. Xu, L.; Mrejen, S.; Jung, J.J.; Gallego-Pinazo, R.; Thompson, D.; Marsiglia, M.; Freund, K.B. Geographic atrophy in patients receiving anti-vascular endothelial growth factor for neovascular age-related macular degeneration. *Retina* **2015**, *35*, 176–186. [CrossRef] [PubMed]
179. Rosenfeld, P.J.; Shapiro, H.; Tuomi, L.; Webster, M.; Elledge, J.; Blodi, B. Characteristics of Patients Losing Vision after 2 Years of Monthly Dosing in the Phase III Ranibizumab Clinical Trials. *Ophthalmology* **2011**, *118*, 523–530. [CrossRef]
180. Pfau, M.; Möller, P.T.; Künzel, S.H.; von der Emde, L.; Lindner, M.; Thiele, S.; Dysli, C.; Nadal, J.; Schmid, M.; Schmitz-Valckenberg, S.; et al. Type 1 Choroidal Neovascularization Is Associated with Reduced Localized Progression of Atrophy in Age-Related Macular Degeneration. *Ophthalmol. Retin.* **2020**, *4*, 238–248. [CrossRef] [PubMed]
181. Capuano, V.; Miere, A.; Querques, L.; Sacconi, R.; Carnevali, A.; Amoroso, F.; Bandello, F.; Souied, E.H.; Querques, G. Treatment-naïve quiescent choroidal neovascularization in geographic atrophy secondary to nonexudative age-related macular degeneration. *Am. J. Ophthalmol.* **2017**, *182*, 45–55. [CrossRef]
182. Heiferman, M.J.; Fawzi, A.A. Progression of subclinical choroidal neovascularization in age-related macular degeneration. *PLoS ONE* **2019**, *14*, e0217805. [CrossRef]
183. Apte, R.S.; Chen, D.S.; Ferrara, N. VEGF in Signaling and Disease: Beyond Discovery and Development. *Cell* **2019**, *176*, 1248–1264. [CrossRef] [PubMed]
184. Roumenina, L.T.; Daugan, M.V.; Petitprez, F.; Sautès-Fridman, C.; Fridman, W.H. Context-dependent roles of complement in cancer. *Nat. Rev. Cancer* **2019**, *19*, 698–715. [CrossRef]
185. Wood, A.J.T.; Vassallo, A.; Summers, C.; Chilvers, E.R.; Conway-Morris, A. C5a anaphylatoxin and its role in critical illness-induced organ dysfunction. *Eur. J. Clin. Investig.* **2018**, *48*, e13028. [CrossRef]
186. Triantafilou, M.; Hughes, T.R.; Morgan, B.P.; Triantafilou, K. Complementing the inflammasome. *Immunology* **2016**, *147*, 152–164. [CrossRef] [PubMed]
187. Strainic, M.G.; Liu, J.; Huang, D.; An, F.; Lalli, P.N.; Muqim, N.; Shapiro, V.S.; Dubyak, G.R.; Heeger, P.S.; Medof, M.E. Locally produced complement fragments C5a and C3a provide both costimulatory and survival signals to naive CD4+ T cells. *Immunity* **2008**, *28*, 425–435. [CrossRef]

188. Peng, Q.; Li, K.; Wang, N.; Li, Q.; Asgari, E.; Lu, B.; Woodruff, T.M.; Sacks, S.H.; Zhou, W. Dendritic cell function in allostimulation is modulated by C5aR signaling. *J. Immunol.* **2009**, *183*, 6058–6068. [CrossRef] [PubMed]
189. Piao, C.; Zhang, W.-M.; Li, T.-T.; Zhang, C.-c.; Qiu, S.; Liu, Y.; Liu, S.; Jin, M.; Jia, L.-X.; Song, W.-C. Complement 5a stimulates macrophage polarization and contributes to tumor metastases of colon cancer. *Exp. Cell. Res.* **2018**, *366*, 127–138. [CrossRef]
190. Han, G.; Geng, S.; Li, Y.; Chen, G.; Wang, R.; Li, X.; Ma, Y.; Shen, B.; Li, Y. γδT-cell function in sepsis is modulated by C5a receptor signalling. *Immunology* **2011**, *133*, 340–349. [CrossRef]
191. Zaal, A.; Lissenberg-Thunnissen, S.N.; van Schijndel, G.; Wouters, D.; van Ham, S.M.; ten Brinke, A. Crosstalk between Toll like receptors and C5a receptor in human monocyte derived DCs suppress inflammatory cytokine production. *Immunobiology* **2013**, *218*, 175–180. [CrossRef]
192. Li, K.; Fazekasova, H.; Wang, N.; Peng, Q.; Sacks, S.H.; Lombardi, G.; Zhou, W. Functional modulation of human monocytes derived DCs by anaphylatoxins C3a and C5a. *Immunobiology* **2012**, *217*, 65–73. [CrossRef]
193. Li, X.X.; Clark, R.J.; Woodruff, T.M. C5aR2 Activation Broadly Modulates the Signaling and Function of Primary Human Macrophages. *J. Immunol.* **2020**, *205*, 1102–1112. [CrossRef] [PubMed]
194. Coughlin, B.; Schnabolk, G.; Joseph, K.; Raikwar, H.; Kunchithapautham, K.; Johnson, K.; Moore, K.; Wang, Y.; Rohrer, B. Connecting the innate and adaptive immune responses in mouse choroidal neovascularization via the anaphylatoxin C5a and γδT-cells. *Sci. Rep.* **2016**, *6*, 23794. [CrossRef]
195. Ribot, J.C.; Lopes, N.; Silva-Santos, B. γδ T cells in tissue physiology and surveillance. *Nat. Rev. Immunol.* **2021**, *21*, 221–232. [CrossRef]
196. Jane-Wit, D.; Manes, T.D.; Yi, T.; Qin, L.; Clark, P.; Kirkiles-Smith, N.C.; Abrahimi, P.; Devalliere, J.; Moeckel, G.; Kulkarni, S. Alloantibody and complement promote T cell–mediated cardiac allograft vasculopathy through noncanonical nuclear factor-κB signaling in endothelial cells. *Circulation* **2013**, *128*, 2504–2516. [CrossRef]
197. Xie, C.B.; Qin, L.; Li, G.; Fang, C.; Kirkiles-Smith, N.C.; Tellides, G.; Pober, J.S.; Jane-Wit, D. Complement membrane attack complexes assemble NLRP3 inflammasomes triggering IL-1 activation of IFN-γ–primed human endothelium. *Circ. Res.* **2019**, *124*, 1747–1759. [CrossRef]
198. Kilgore, K.S.; Schmid, E.; Shanley, T.P.; Flory, C.M.; Maheswari, V.; Tramontini, N.L.; Cohen, H.; Ward, P.A.; Friedl, H.P.; Warren, J.S. Sublytic concentrations of the membrane attack complex of complement induce endothelial interleukin-8 and monocyte chemoattractant protein-1 through nuclear factor-kappa B activation. *Am. J. Pathol.* **1997**, *150*, 2019. [PubMed]
199. Brunn, G.J.; Saadi, S.; Platt, J.L. Differential regulation of endothelial cell activation by complement and interleukin 1α. *Circ. Res.* **2006**, *98*, 793–800. [CrossRef]
200. Saadi, S.; Holzknecht, R.A.; Patte, C.P.; Platt, J.L. Endothelial cell activation by pore-forming structures: Pivotal role for interleukin-1α. *Circulation* **2000**, *101*, 1867–1873. [CrossRef]
201. Copland, D.A.; Theodoropoulou, S.; Liu, J.; Dick, A.D. A Perspective of AMD Through the Eyes of Immunology. *Investig. Ophthalmol. Vis. Sci.* **2018**, *59*, AMD83–AMD92. [CrossRef] [PubMed]
202. Cabrera, A.P.; Bhaskaran, A.; Xu, J.; Yang, X.; Scott, H.A.; Mohideen, U.; Ghosh, K. Senescence Increases Choroidal Endothelial Stiffness and Susceptibility to Complement Injury: Implications for Choriocapillaris Loss in AMD. *Investig. Ophthalmol. Vis. Sci.* **2016**, *57*, 5910–5918. [CrossRef] [PubMed]
203. Calippe, B.; Augustin, S.; Beguier, F.; Charles-Messance, H.; Poupel, L.; Conart, J.-B.; Hu, S.J.; Lavalette, S.; Fauvet, A.; Rayes, J.; et al. Complement Factor H Inhibits CD47-Mediated Resolution of Inflammation. *Immunity* **2017**, *46*, 261–272. [CrossRef]
204. Li, K.; Sacks, S.H.; Zhou, W. The relative importance of local and systemic complement production in ischaemia, transplantation and other pathologies. *Mol. Immunol.* **2007**, *44*, 3866–3874. [CrossRef]
205. Kouser, L.; Abdul-Aziz, M.; Nayak, A.; Stover, C.M.; Sim, R.B.; Kishore, U. Properdin and factor h: Opposing players on the alternative complement pathway "see-saw". *Front. Immunol.* **2013**, *4*, 93. [CrossRef]
206. Laufer, J.; Katz, Y.; Passwell, J.H. Extrahepatic synthesis of complement proteins in inflammation. *Mol. Immunol.* **2001**, *38*, 221–229. [CrossRef]
207. Sheerin, N.S.; Abe, K.; Risley, P.; Sacks, S.H. Accumulation of immune complexes in glomerular disease is independent of locally synthesized c3. *J. Am. Soc. Nephrol.* **2006**, *17*, 686–696. [CrossRef] [PubMed]
208. Wong, C.W.; Wong, T.; Cheng, C.-Y.; Sabanayagam, C. Kidney and eye diseases: Common risk factors, etiological mechanisms, and pathways. *Kidney Int.* **2014**, *85*, 1290–1302. [CrossRef] [PubMed]
209. Duvall-Young, J.; MacDonald, M.K.; McKechnie, N.M. Fundus changes in (type II) mesangiocapillary glomerulonephritis simulating drusen: A histopathological report. *Br. J. Ophthalmol.* **1989**, *73*, 297–302. [CrossRef]
210. Dopler, A.; Guntau, L.; Harder, M.J.; Palmer, A.; Höchsmann, B.; Schrezenmeier, H.; Simmet, T.; Huber-Lang, M.; Schmidt, C.Q. Self versus nonself discrimination by the soluble complement regulators factor H and FHL-1. *J. Immunol.* **2019**, *202*, 2082–2094. [CrossRef] [PubMed]
211. Hallam, T.M.; Marchbank, K.J.; Harris, C.L.; Osmond, C.; Shuttleworth, V.G.; Griffiths, H.; Cree, A.J.; Kavanagh, D.; Lotery, A.J. Rare genetic variants in complement factor I lead to low FI plasma levels resulting in increased risk of age-related macular degeneration. *Investig. Ophthalmol. Vis. Sci.* **2020**, *61*, 18. [CrossRef]
212. Reynolds, R.; Hartnett, M.E.; Atkinson, J.P.; Giclas, P.C.; Rosner, B.; Seddon, J.M. Plasma complement components and activation fragments: Associations with age-related macular degeneration genotypes and phenotypes. *Investig. Ophthalmol. Vis. Sci.* **2009**, *50*, 5818–5827. [CrossRef]

213. Scholl, H.P.; Issa, P.C.; Walier, M.; Janzer, S.; Pollok-Kopp, B.; Börncke, F.; Fritsche, L.G.; Chong, N.V.; Fimmers, R.; Wienker, T. Systemic complement activation in age-related macular degeneration. *PLoS ONE* **2008**, *3*, e2593. [CrossRef]
214. Lin, J.B.; Serghiou, S.; Miller, J.W.; Vavvas, D.G. Systemic Complement Activation Profiles in Nonexudative Age-Related Macular Degeneration: A Systematic Review. *Ophthalmol. Sci.* **2022**, *2*, 100118. [CrossRef]
215. Heesterbeek, T.J.; Lechanteur, Y.T.; Lorés-Motta, L.; Schick, T.; Daha, M.R.; Altay, L.; Liakopoulos, S.; Smailhodzic, D.; den Hollander, A.I.; Hoyng, C.B. Complement activation levels are related to disease stage in AMD. *Investig. Ophthalmol. Vis. Sci.* **2020**, *61*, 18. [CrossRef]
216. Lorés-Motta, L.; Paun, C.C.; Corominas, J.; Pauper, M.; Geerlings, M.J.; Altay, L.; Schick, T.; Daha, M.R.; Fauser, S.; Hoyng, C.B. Genome-wide association study reveals variants in CFH and CFHR4 associated with systemic complement activation: Implications in age-related macular degeneration. *Ophthalmology* **2018**, *125*, 1064–1074. [CrossRef] [PubMed]
217. Lynch, A.M.; Mandava, N.; Patnaik, J.L.; Frazer-Abel, A.A.; Wagner, B.D.; Palestine, A.G.; Mathias, M.T.; Siringo, F.S.; Cathcart, J.N.; Holers, V.M. Systemic activation of the complement system in patients with advanced age-related macular degeneration. *Eur. J. Ophthalmol.* **2020**, *30*, 1061–1068. [CrossRef]
218. Balmforth, C.; van Bragt, J.J.; Ruijs, T.; Cameron, J.R.; Kimmitt, R.; Moorhouse, R.; Czopek, A.; Hu, M.K.; Gallacher, P.J.; Dear, J.W. Chorioretinal thinning in chronic kidney disease links to inflammation and endothelial dysfunction. *JCI insight* **2016**, *1*, e89173. [CrossRef] [PubMed]
219. Bergen, A.A.; Arya, S.; Koster, C.; Pilgrim, M.G.; Wiatrek-Moumoulidis, D.; van der Spek, P.J.; Hauck, S.M.; Boon, C.J.; Emri, E.; Stewart, A.J. On the origin of proteins in human drusen: The meet, greet and stick hypothesis. *Prog. Retin. Eye Res.* **2019**, *70*, 55–84. [CrossRef] [PubMed]
220. Kavanagh, D.; Yu, Y.; Schramm, E.C.; Triebwasser, M.; Wagner, E.K.; Raychaudhuri, S.; Daly, M.J.; Atkinson, J.P.; Seddon, J.M. Rare genetic variants in the CFI gene are associated with advanced age-related macular degeneration and commonly result in reduced serum factor I levels. *Hum. Mol. Genet.* **2015**, *24*, 3861–3870. [CrossRef]
221. Wong, E.K.S.; Kavanagh, D. Diseases of complement dysregulation-an overview. *Semin. Immunopathol.* **2018**, *40*, 49–64. [CrossRef]
222. Raychaudhuri, S.; Iartchouk, O.; Chin, K.; Tan, P.L.; Tai, A.K.; Ripke, S.; Gowrisankar, S.; Vemuri, S.; Montgomery, K.; Yu, Y.; et al. A rare penetrant mutation in CFH confers high risk of age-related macular degeneration. *Nat. Genet.* **2011**, *43*, 1232–1236. [CrossRef] [PubMed]
223. Recalde, S.; Tortajada, A.; Subias, M.; Anter, J.; Blasco, M.; Maranta, R.; Coco, R.; Pinto, S.; Noris, M.; Garcia-Layana, A.; et al. Molecular Basis of Factor H R1210C Association with Ocular and Renal Diseases. *J. Am. Soc. Nephrol.* **2016**, *27*, 1305–1311. [CrossRef] [PubMed]
224. Khandhadia, S.; Hakobyan, S.; Heng, L.Z.; Gibson, J.; Adams, D.H.; Alexander, G.J.; Gibson, J.M.; Martin, K.R.; Menon, G.; Nash, K.; et al. Age-related Macular Degeneration and Modification of Systemic Complement Factor H Production Through Liver Transplantation. *Ophthalmology* **2013**, *120*, 1612–1618. [CrossRef]
225. Harris, C.L. Expanding horizons in complement drug discovery: Challenges and emerging strategies. *Semin. Immunopathol.* **2018**, *40*, 125–140. [CrossRef]
226. Mastellos, D.C.; Ricklin, D.; Lambris, J.D. Clinical promise of next-generation complement therapeutics. *Nat. Rev. Drug. Discov.* **2019**, *18*, 707–729. [CrossRef]
227. Bill, A.; Sperber, G.O. Control of retinal and choroidal blood flow. *Eye* **1990**, *4*, 319–325. [CrossRef] [PubMed]
228. del Amo, E.M.; Rimpelä, A.-K.; Heikkinen, E.; Kari, O.K.; Ramsay, E.; Lajunen, T.; Schmitt, M.; Pelkonen, L.; Bhattacharya, M.; Richardson, D.; et al. Pharmacokinetic aspects of retinal drug delivery. *Prog. Retin. Eye Res.* **2017**, *57*, 134–185. [CrossRef]
229. Pitkänen, L.; Ranta, V.-P.; Moilanen, H.; Urtti, A. Permeability of Retinal Pigment Epithelium: Effects of Permeant Molecular Weight and Lipophilicity. *Investig. Ophthalmol. Vis. Sci.* **2005**, *46*, 641–646. [CrossRef] [PubMed]
230. Vellonen, K.-S.; Soini, E.-M.; del Amo, E.M.; Urtti, A. Prediction of Ocular Drug Distribution from Systemic Blood Circulation. *Mol. Pharm.* **2016**, *13*, 2906–2911. [CrossRef] [PubMed]
231. Hillmen, P.; Szer, J.; Weitz, I.; Röth, A.; Höchsmann, B.; Panse, J.; Usuki, K.; Griffin, M.; Kiladjian, J.-J.; de Castro, C. Pegcetacoplan versus eculizumab in paroxysmal nocturnal hemoglobinuria. *N. Engl. J. Med.* **2021**, *384*, 1028–1037. [CrossRef]
232. McKinley, C.E.; Richards, S.J.; Munir, T.; Griffin, M.; Mitchell, L.D.; Arnold, L.; Riley, K.; Copeland, N.; Newton, D.J.; Hill, A. Extravascular hemolysis due to C3-loading in patients with PNH treated with eculizumab: Defining the clinical syndrome. *Blood* **2017**, *130*, 3471.
233. Jayne, D.R.W.; Merkel, P.A.; Schall, T.J.; Bekker, P.; Group, A.S. Avacopan for the Treatment of ANCA-Associated Vasculitis. *N. Engl. J. Med.* **2021**, *384*, 599–609. [CrossRef]
234. Risitano, A.M.; Roth, A.; Soret, J.; Frieri, C.; de Fontbrune, F.S.; Marano, L.; Alashkar, F.; Benajiba, L.; Marotta, S.; Rozenberg, I.; et al. Addition of iptacopan, an oral factor B inhibitor, to eculizumab in patients with paroxysmal nocturnal haemoglobinuria and active haemolysis: An open-label, single-arm, phase 2, proof-of-concept trial. *Lancet Haematol.* **2021**, *8*, e344–e354. [CrossRef]
235. Yehoshua, Z.; Alexandre de Amorim Garcia Filho, C.; Nunes, R.P.; Gregori, G.; Penha, F.M.; Moshfeghi, A.A.; Zhang, K.; Sadda, S.; Feuer, W.; Rosenfeld, P.J. Systemic Complement Inhibition with Eculizumab for Geographic Atrophy in Age-Related Macular Degeneration: The COMPLETE Study. *Ophthalmology* **2014**, *121*, 693–701. [CrossRef]
236. Boyer, D.D.; Ko, Y.-P.; Podos, S.D.; Cartwright, M.E.; Gao, X.; Wiles, J.A.; Huang, M. Danicopan, an Oral Complement Factor D Inhibitor, Exhibits High and Sustained Exposure in Ocular Tissues in Preclinical Studies. *Transl. Vis. Sci. Technol.* **2022**, *11*, 37. [CrossRef] [PubMed]

237. Sampat, K.M.; Garg, S.J. Complications of intravitreal injections. *Curr. Opin. Ophthalmol.* **2010**, *21*, 178–183. [CrossRef] [PubMed]
238. Liao, D.S.; Grossi, F.V.; El Mehdi, D.; Gerber, M.R.; Brown, D.M.; Heier, J.S.; Wykoff, C.C.; Singerman, L.J.; Abraham, P.; Grassmann, F.; et al. Complement C3 Inhibitor Pegcetacoplan for Geographic Atrophy Secondary to Age-Related Macular Degeneration: A Randomized Phase 2 Trial. *Ophthalmology* **2020**, *127*, 186–195. [CrossRef] [PubMed]
239. Verdera, H.C.; Kuranda, K.; Mingozzi, F. AAV Vector Immunogenicity in Humans: A Long Journey to Successful Gene Transfer. *Mol. Ther.* **2020**, *28*, 723–746. [CrossRef]
240. Van Craenenbroeck, K.; Vanhoenacker, P.; Haegeman, G. Episomal vectors for gene expression in mammalian cells. *Eur. J. Biochem.* **2000**, *267*, 5665–5678. [CrossRef]
241. Leroy, B.P.; Fischer, M.D.; Flannery, J.G.; MacLaren, R.E.; Dalkara, D.; Scholl, H.P.N.; Chung, D.C.; Spera, C.; Viriato, D.; Banhazi, J. Gene therapy for inherited retinal disease: Long-term durability of effect. *Ophthalmic Res.* **2022**, *66*, 179–196. [CrossRef]
242. Trapani, I.; Colella, P.; Sommella, A.; Iodice, C.; Cesi, G.; de Simone, S.; Marrocco, E.; Rossi, S.; Giunti, M.; Palfi, A.; et al. Effective delivery of large genes to the retina by dual AAV vectors. *EMBO Mol. Med.* **2014**, *6*, 194–211. [CrossRef]
243. Newman, N.J.; Yu-Wai-Man, P.; Carelli, V.; Moster, M.L.; Biousse, V.; Vignal-Clermont, C.; Sergott, R.C.; Klopstock, T.; Sadun, A.A.; Barboni, P.; et al. Efficacy and Safety of Intravitreal Gene Therapy for Leber Hereditary Optic Neuropathy Treated within 6 Months of Disease Onset. *Ophthalmology* **2021**, *128*, 649–660. [CrossRef]
244. Dalkara, D.; Kolstad, K.D.; Caporale, N.; Visel, M.; Klimczak, R.R.; Schaffer, D.V.; Flannery, J.G. Inner limiting membrane barriers to AAV-mediated retinal transduction from the vitreous. *Mol. Ther.* **2009**, *17*, 2096–2102. [CrossRef]
245. Hellstrom, M.; Ruitenberg, M.J.; Pollett, M.A.; Ehlert, E.M.; Twisk, J.; Verhaagen, J.; Harvey, A.R. Cellular tropism and transduction properties of seven adeno-associated viral vector serotypes in adult retina after intravitreal injection. *Gene Ther.* **2009**, *16*, 521–532. [CrossRef]
246. Dalkara, D.; Byrne, L.C.; Klimczak, R.R.; Visel, M.; Yin, L.; Merigan, W.H.; Flannery, J.G.; Schaffer, D.V. In vivo-directed evolution of a new adeno-associated virus for therapeutic outer retinal gene delivery from the vitreous. *Sci. Transl. Med.* **2013**, *5*, 189ra176. [CrossRef]
247. Ross, M.; Ofri, R. The future of retinal gene therapy: Evolving from subretinal to intravitreal vector delivery. *Neural Regen. Res.* **2021**, *16*, 1751–1759. [PubMed]
248. Boye, S.L.; Bennett, A.; Scalabrino, M.L.; McCullough, K.T.; Van Vliet, K.; Choudhury, S.; Ruan, Q.; Peterson, J.; Agbandje-McKenna, M.; Boye, S.E. Impact of Heparan Sulfate Binding on Transduction of Retina by Recombinant Adeno-Associated Virus Vectors. *J. Virol.* **2016**, *90*, 4215–4231. [CrossRef] [PubMed]
249. Woodard, K.T.; Liang, K.J.; Bennett, W.C.; Samulski, R.J. Heparan Sulfate Binding Promotes Accumulation of Intravitreally Delivered Adeno-associated Viral Vectors at the Retina for Enhanced Transduction but Weakly Influences Tropism. *J. Virol.* **2016**, *90*, 9878–9888. [CrossRef] [PubMed]
250. Song, H.; Zeng, Y.; Sardar Pasha, S.P.B.; Bush, R.A.; Vijayasarathy, C.; Qian, H.; Wei, L.; Wiley, H.E.; Wu, Z.; Sieving, P.A. Trans-Ocular Electric Current In Vivo Enhances AAV-Mediated Retinal Transduction in Large Animal Eye After Intravitreal Vector Administration. *Transl. Vis. Sci. Technol.* **2020**, *9*, 28. [CrossRef]
251. Ross, M.; Obolensky, A.; Averbukh, E.; Ezra-Elia, R.; Yamin, E.; Honig, H.; Dvir, H.; Rosov, A.; Hauswirth, W.W.; Gootwine, E. Evaluation of photoreceptor transduction efficacy of capsid-modified adeno-associated viral vectors following intravitreal and subretinal delivery in sheep. *Hum. Gene Ther.* **2020**, *31*, 719–729. [CrossRef]
252. Teo, K.Y.C.; Lee, S.Y.; Barathi, A.V.; Tun, S.B.B.; Tan, L.; Constable, I.J. Surgical removal of internal limiting membrane and layering of AAV vector on the retina under air enhances gene transfection in a nonhuman primate. *Investig. Ophthalmol. Vis. Sci.* **2018**, *59*, 3574–3583. [CrossRef]
253. Takahashi, K.; Igarashi, T.; Miyake, K.; Kobayashi, M.; Yaguchi, C.; Iijima, O.; Yamazaki, Y.; Katakai, Y.; Miyake, N.; Kameya, S. Improved intravitreal AAV-mediated inner retinal gene transduction after surgical internal limiting membrane peeling in cynomolgus monkeys. *Mol. Ther.* **2017**, *25*, 296–302. [CrossRef]
254. Boye, S.E.; Alexander, J.J.; Witherspoon, C.D.; Boye, S.L.; Peterson, J.J.; Clark, M.E.; Sandefer, K.J.; Girkin, C.A.; Hauswirth, W.W.; Gamlin, P.D. Highly Efficient Delivery of Adeno-Associated Viral Vectors to the Primate Retina. *Hum. Gene Ther.* **2016**, *27*, 580–597. [CrossRef]
255. Gamlin, P.D.; Alexander, J.J.; Boye, S.L.; Witherspoon, C.D.; Boye, S.E. SubILM injection of AAV for gene delivery to the retina. In *Adeno-Associated Virus Vectors. Methods in Molecular Biology*; Humana Press: New York, NY, USA, 2019; pp. 249–262.
256. Peynshaert, K.; Vanluchene, H.; De Clerck, K.; Minnaert, A.-K.; Verhoeven, M.; Gouspillou, N.; Bostan, N.; Hisatomi, T.; Accou, G.; Sauvage, F.; et al. ICG-mediated photodisruption of the inner limiting membrane enhances retinal drug delivery. *J. Control. Release* **2022**, *349*, 315–326. [CrossRef] [PubMed]
257. Ramachandran, P.S.; Lee, V.; Wei, Z.; Song, J.Y.; Casal, G.; Cronin, T.; Willett, K.; Huckfeldt, R.; Morgan, J.I.; Aleman, T.S.; et al. Evaluation of Dose and Safety of AAV7m8 and AAV8BP2 in the Non-Human Primate Retina. *Hum. Gene Ther.* **2017**, *28*, 154–167. [CrossRef]
258. Reichel, F.F.; Dauletbekov, D.L.; Klein, R.; Peters, T.; Ochakovski, G.A.; Seitz, I.P.; Wilhelm, B.; Ueffing, M.; Biel, M.; Wissinger, B.; et al. AAV8 Can Induce Innate and Adaptive Immune Response in the Primate Eye. *Mol. Ther.* **2017**, *25*, 2648–2660. [CrossRef] [PubMed]

259. Reichel, F.F.; Peters, T.; Wilhelm, B.; Biel, M.; Ueffing, M.; Wissinger, B.; Bartz-Schmidt, K.U.; Klein, R.; Michalakis, S.; Fischer, M.D.; et al. Humoral Immune Response After Intravitreal But Not After Subretinal AAV8 in Primates and Patients. *Investig. Ophthalmol. Vis. Sci.* **2018**, *59*, 1910–1915. [CrossRef] [PubMed]
260. Seitz, I.P.; Michalakis, S.; Wilhelm, B.; Reichel, F.F.; Ochakovski, G.A.; Zrenner, E.; Ueffing, M.; Biel, M.; Wissinger, B.; Bartz-Schmidt, K.U.; et al. Superior Retinal Gene Transfer and Biodistribution Profile of Subretinal Versus Intravitreal Delivery of AAV8 in Nonhuman Primates. *Investig. Ophthalmol. Vis. Sci.* **2017**, *58*, 5792–5801. [CrossRef] [PubMed]
261. Li, Q.; Miller, R.; Han, P.-Y.; Pang, J.; Dinculescu, A.; Chiodo, V.; Hauswirth, W.W. Intraocular route of AAV2 vector administration defines humoral immune response and therapeutic potential. *Mol. Vis.* **2008**, *14*, 1760–1769.
262. Kotterman, M.A.; Yin, L.; Strazzeri, J.M.; Flannery, J.G.; Merigan, W.H.; Schaffer, D.V. Antibody neutralization poses a barrier to intravitreal adeno-associated viral vector gene delivery to non-human primates. *Gene Ther.* **2015**, *22*, 116–126. [CrossRef]
263. Fitzpatrick, Z.; Leborgne, C.; Barbon, E.; Masat, E.; Ronzitti, G.; van Wittenberghe, L.; Vignaud, A.; Collaud, F.; Charles, S.; Sola, M.S. Influence of pre-existing anti-capsid neutralizing and binding antibodies on AAV vector transduction. *Mol. Ther. Methods Clin. Dev.* **2018**, *9*, 119–129. [CrossRef] [PubMed]
264. Wang, L.; Calcedo, R.; Wang, H.; Bell, P.; Grant, R.; Vandenberghe, L.H.; Sanmiguel, J.; Morizono, H.; Batshaw, M.L.; Wilson, J.M. The pleiotropic effects of natural AAV infections on liver-directed gene transfer in macaques. *Mol. Ther.* **2010**, *18*, 126–134. [CrossRef]
265. Zaiss, A.K.; Cotter, M.J.; White, L.R.; Clark, S.A.; Wong, N.C.W.; Holers, V.M.; Bartlett, J.S.; Muruve, D.A. Complement Is an Essential Component of the Immune Response to Adeno-Associated Virus Vectors. *J. Virol.* **2008**, *82*, 2727–2740. [CrossRef]
266. Denard, J.; Marolleau, B.; Jenny, C.; Rao, T.N.; Fehling, H.J.; Voit, T.; Svinartchouk, F. C-reactive protein (CRP) is essential for efficient systemic transduction of recombinant adeno-associated virus vector 1 (rAAV-1) and rAAV-6 in mice. *J. Virol.* **2013**, *87*, 10784–10791. [CrossRef]
267. Chan, Y.K.; Wang, S.K.; Chu, C.J.; Copland, D.A.; Letizia, A.J.; Costa Verdera, H.; Chiang, J.J.; Sethi, M.; Wang, M.K.; Neidermyer, W.J., Jr.; et al. Engineering adeno-associated viral vectors to evade innate immune and inflammatory responses. *Sci. Transl. Med.* **2021**, *13*, eabd3438. [CrossRef]
268. Short, B.G. Safety evaluation of ocular drug delivery formulations: Techniques and practical considerations. *Toxicol. Pathol.* **2008**, *36*, 49–62. [CrossRef] [PubMed]
269. Yin, H.; Kanasty, R.L.; Eltoukhy, A.A.; Vegas, A.J.; Dorkin, J.R.; Anderson, D.G. Non-viral vectors for gene-based therapy. *Nat. Rev. Genet.* **2014**, *15*, 541–555. [CrossRef] [PubMed]
270. Rowe-Rendleman, C.L.; Durazo, S.A.; Kompella, U.B.; Rittenhouse, K.D.; Di Polo, A.; Weiner, A.L.; Grossniklaus, H.E.; Naash, M.I.; Lewin, A.S.; Horsager, A.; et al. Drug and Gene Delivery to the Back of the Eye: From Bench to Bedside. *Investig. Ophthalmol. Vis. Sci.* **2014**, *55*, 2714–2730. [CrossRef] [PubMed]
271. Peeters, L.; Sanders, N.N.; Braeckmans, K.; Boussery, K.; Van de Voorde, J.; De Smedt, S.C.; Demeester, J. Vitreous: A Barrier to Nonviral Ocular Gene Therapy. *Investig. Ophthalmol. Vis. Sci.* **2005**, *46*, 3553–3561. [CrossRef]
272. Kim, H.; Robinson, S.B.; Csaky, K.G. Investigating the movement of intravitreal human serum albumin nanoparticles in the vitreous and retina. *Pharm. Res.* **2009**, *26*, 329–337. [CrossRef] [PubMed]
273. Huang, D.; Chen, Y.-S.; Green, C.R.; Rupenthal, I.D. Hyaluronic acid coated albumin nanoparticles for targeted peptide delivery in the treatment of retinal ischaemia. *Biomaterials* **2018**, *168*, 10–23. [CrossRef]
274. Mashal, M.; Attia, N.; Martínez-Navarrete, G.; Soto-Sánchez, C.; Fernández, E.; Grijalvo, S.; Eritja, R.; Puras, G.; Pedraz, J.L. Gene delivery to the rat retina by non-viral vectors based on chloroquine-containing cationic niosomes. *J. Control. Release* **2019**, *304*, 181–190. [CrossRef] [PubMed]
275. Yao, K.; Qiu, S.; Wang, Y.V.; Park, S.J.; Mohns, E.J.; Mehta, B.; Liu, X.; Chang, B.; Zenisek, D.; Crair, M.C. Restoration of vision after de novo genesis of rod photoreceptors in mammalian retinas. *Nature* **2018**, *560*, 484–488. [CrossRef]
276. Devoldere, J.; Peynshaert, K.; De Smedt, S.C.; Remaut, K. Müller cells as a target for retinal therapy. *Drug. Discov.* **2019**, *24*, 1483–1498. [CrossRef]
277. de Jong, S.; Gagliardi, G.; Garanto, A.; de Breuk, A.; Lechanteur, Y.T.E.; Katti, S.; van den Heuvel, L.P.; Volokhina, E.B.; den Hollander, A.I. Implications of genetic variation in the complement system in age-related macular degeneration. *Prog. Retin. Eye Res.* **2021**, *84*, 100952. [CrossRef] [PubMed]
278. Li, M.; Huisingh, C.; Messinger, J.; Dolz-Marco, R.; Ferrara, D.; Freund, K.B.; Curcio, C.A. Histology of geographic atrophy secondary to age-related macular degeneration: A multilayer approach. *Retina* **2018**, *38*, 1937. [CrossRef] [PubMed]
279. Scholl, H.P. Complement Inhibition in Age-Related Macular Degeneration—Treat Early! *JAMA Ophthalmol.* **2022**, *140*, 250–251. [CrossRef]
280. Thomas, C.N.; Sim, D.A.; Lee, W.H.; Alfahad, N.; Dick, A.D.; Denniston, A.K.; Hill, L.J. Emerging therapies and their delivery for treating age-related macular degeneration. *Br. J. Pharmacol.* **2022**, *179*, 1908–1937. [CrossRef]
281. Garafalo, A.V.; Cideciyan, A.V.; Héon, E.; Sheplock, R.; Pearson, A.; WeiYang Yu, C.; Sumaroka, A.; Aguirre, G.D.; Jacobson, S.G. Progress in treating inherited retinal diseases: Early subretinal gene therapy clinical trials and candidates for future initiatives. *Prog. Retin. Eye Res.* **2020**, *77*, 100827. [CrossRef]
282. Trapani, I.; Auricchio, A. Seeing the Light after 25 Years of Retinal Gene Therapy. *Trends Mol. Med.* **2018**, *24*, 669–681. [CrossRef]

283. Jüttner, J.; Szabo, A.; Gross-Scherf, B.; Morikawa, R.K.; Rompani, S.B.; Hantz, P.; Szikra, T.; Esposti, F.; Cowan, C.S.; Bharioke, A.; et al. Targeting neuronal and glial cell types with synthetic promoter AAVs in mice, non-human primates and humans. *Nat. Neurosci.* **2019**, *22*, 1345–1356. [CrossRef]
284. Vandenberghe, L.H.; Auricchio, A. Novel adeno-associated viral vectors for retinal gene therapy. *Gene Ther.* **2012**, *19*, 162–168. [CrossRef]
285. Mowat, F.M.; Gornik, K.R.; Dinculescu, A.; Boye, S.L.; Hauswirth, W.W.; Petersen-Jones, S.M.; Bartoe, J.T. Tyrosine capsid-mutant AAV vectors for gene delivery to the canine retina from a subretinal or intravitreal approach. *Gene Ther.* **2014**, *21*, 96–105. [CrossRef]
286. Annamalai, B.; Parsons, N.; Nicholson, C.; Obert, E.; Jones, B.; Rohrer, B. Subretinal Rather Than Intravitreal Adeno-Associated Virus-Mediated Delivery of a Complement Alternative Pathway Inhibitor Is Effective in a Mouse Model of RPE Damage. *Investig. Ophthalmol. Vis. Sci.* **2021**, *62*, 11. [CrossRef]
287. Amado, D.; Mingozzi, F.; Hui, D.; Bennicelli, J.L.; Wei, Z.; Chen, Y.; Bote, E.; Grant, R.L.; Golden, J.A.; Narfstrom, K. Safety and efficacy of subretinal readministration of a viral vector in large animals to treat congenital blindness. *Sci. Transl. Med.* **2010**, *2*, 21ra16. [CrossRef]
288. Ye, G.J.; Budzynski, E.; Sonnentag, P.; Nork, T.M.; Miller, P.E.; Sharma, A.K.; Ver Hoeve, J.N.; Smith, L.M.; Arndt, T.; Calcedo, R.; et al. Safety and Biodistribution Evaluation in Cynomolgus Macaques of rAAV2tYF-PR1.7-hCNGB3, a Recombinant AAV Vector for Treatment of Achromatopsia. *Hum. Gene Ther. Clin. Dev.* **2016**, *27*, 37–48. [CrossRef] [PubMed]
289. Vandenberghe, L.H.; Bell, P.; Maguire, A.M.; Cearley, C.N.; Xiao, R.; Calcedo, R.; Wang, L.; Castle, M.J.; Maguire, A.C.; Grant, R.; et al. Dosage thresholds for AAV2 and AAV8 photoreceptor gene therapy in monkey. *Sci. Transl. Med.* **2011**, *3*, 88ra54. [CrossRef] [PubMed]
290. Khabou, H.; Cordeau, C.; Pacot, L.; Fisson, S.; Dalkara, D. Dosage Thresholds and Influence of Transgene Cassette in Adeno-Associated Virus-Related Toxicity. *Hum. Gene Ther.* **2018**, *29*, 1235–1241. [CrossRef]
291. MacLachlan, T.K.; Milton, M.N.; Turner, O.; Tukov, F.; Choi, V.W.; Penraat, J.; Delmotte, M.H.; Michaut, L.; Jaffee, B.D.; Bigelow, C.E. Nonclinical Safety Evaluation of scAAV8-RLBP1 for Treatment of RLBP1 Retinitis Pigmentosa. *Mol. Ther. Methods Clin. Dev.* **2018**, *8*, 105–120. [CrossRef] [PubMed]
292. Treatment of Leber Congenital Amaurosis Due to RPE65 Mutations by Ocular Subretinal Injection of Adeno-Associated Virus Gene Vector: Short-Term Results of a Phase I Trial. *Hum. Gene Ther.* **2008**, *19*, 979–990. [CrossRef] [PubMed]
293. Maguire, A.M.; Simonelli, F.; Pierce, E.A.; Pugh, E.N., Jr.; Mingozzi, F.; Bennicelli, J.; Banfi, S.; Marshall, K.A.; Testa, F.; Surace, E.M. Safety and efficacy of gene transfer for Leber's congenital amaurosis. *N. Engl. J. Med.* **2008**, *358*, 2240–2248. [CrossRef]
294. Jacobson, S.G.; Cideciyan, A.V.; Ratnakaram, R.; Heon, E.; Schwartz, S.B.; Roman, A.J.; Peden, M.C.; Aleman, T.S.; Boye, S.L.; Sumaroka, A.; et al. Gene therapy for leber congenital amaurosis caused by RPE65 mutations: Safety and efficacy in 15 children and adults followed up to 3 years. *Arch. Ophthalmol.* **2012**, *130*, 9–24. [CrossRef]
295. Sastry, A.; Li, J.D.; Raynor, W.; Viehland, C.; Song, Z.; Xu, L.; Farsiu, S.; Izatt, J.A.; Toth, C.A.; Vajzovic, L. Microscope-Integrated OCT-Guided Volumetric Measurements of Subretinal Blebs Created by a Suprachoroidal Approach. *Transl. Vis. Sci. Technol.* **2021**, *10*, 24. [CrossRef]
296. Bainbridge, J.W.; Mehat, M.S.; Sundaram, V.; Robbie, S.J.; Barker, S.E.; Ripamonti, C.; Georgiadis, A.; Mowat, F.M.; Beattie, S.G.; Gardner, P.J. Long-term effect of gene therapy on Leber's congenital amaurosis. *N. Engl. J. Med.* **2015**, *372*, 1887–1897. [CrossRef]
297. Xue, K.; Groppe, M.; Salvetti, A.P.; MacLaren, R.E. Technique of retinal gene therapy: Delivery of viral vector into the subretinal space. *Eye* **2017**, *31*, 1308–1316. [CrossRef]
298. Gardiner, K.L.; Cideciyan, A.V.; Swider, M.; Dufour, V.L.; Sumaroka, A.; Komáromy, A.M.; Hauswirth, W.W.; Iwabe, S.; Jacobson, S.G.; Beltran, W.A. Long-term structural outcomes of late-stage RPE65 gene therapy. *Mol. Ther.* **2020**, *28*, 266–278. [CrossRef]
299. Halász, É.; Townes-Anderson, E.; Zarbin, M.A. Improving outcomes in retinal detachment: The potential role of rho-kinase inhibitors. *Curr. Opin. Ophthalmol.* **2020**, *31*, 192–198. [CrossRef]
300. MacLaren, R.E.; Groppe, M.; Barnard, A.R.; Cottriall, C.L.; Tolmachova, T.; Seymour, L.; Clark, K.R.; During, M.J.; Cremers, F.P.; Black, G.C.; et al. Retinal gene therapy in patients with choroideremia: Initial findings from a phase 1/2 clinical trial. *Lancet* **2014**, *383*, 1129–1137. [CrossRef]
301. Adijanto, J.; Naash, M.I. Nanoparticle-based technologies for retinal gene therapy. *Eur. J. Pharm. Biopharm.* **2015**, *95*, 353–367. [CrossRef]
302. Botto, C.; Rucli, M.; Tekinsoy, M.D.; Pulman, J.; Sahel, J.-A.; Dalkara, D. Early and late stage gene therapy interventions for inherited retinal degenerations. *Prog. Retin. Eye Res.* **2022**, *86*, 100975. [CrossRef]
303. Einmahl, S.; Savoldelli, M.; D'Hermies, F.o.; Tabatabay, C.; Gurny, R.; Behar-Cohen, F. Evaluation of a novel biomaterial in the suprachoroidal space of the rabbit eye. *Investig. Ophthalmol. Vis. Sci.* **2002**, *43*, 1533–1539.
304. Chiang, B.; Kim, Y.C.; Edelhauser, H.F.; Prausnitz, M.R. Circumferential flow of particles in the suprachoroidal space is impeded by the posterior ciliary arteries. *Exp. Eye Res.* **2016**, *145*, 424–431. [CrossRef]
305. Patel, S.R.; Lin, A.S.; Edelhauser, H.F.; Prausnitz, M.R. Suprachoroidal drug delivery to the back of the eye using hollow microneedles. *Pharm. Res.* **2011**, *28*, 166–176. [CrossRef]
306. Olsen, T.W.; Feng, X.; Wabner, K.; Csaky, K.; Pambuccian, S.; Cameron, J.D. Pharmacokinetics of pars plana intravitreal injections versus microcannula suprachoroidal injections of bevacizumab in a porcine model. *Investig. Ophthalmol. Vis. Sci.* **2011**, *52*, 4749–4756. [CrossRef]

307. Rai, U.D.J.P.; Young, S.A.; Thrimawithana, T.R.; Abdelkader, H.; Alani, A.W.G.; Pierscionek, B.; Alany, R.G. The suprachoroidal pathway: A new drug delivery route to the back of the eye. *Drug. Discov.* **2015**, *20*, 491–495. [CrossRef]
308. Peden, M.C.; Min, J.; Meyers, C.; Lukowski, Z.; Li, Q.; Boye, S.L.; Levine, M.; Hauswirth, W.W.; Ratnakaram, R.; Dawson, W. Ab-externo AAV-mediated gene delivery to the suprachoroidal space using a 250 micron flexible microcatheter. *PLoS ONE* **2011**, *6*, e17140. [CrossRef]
309. Chiang, B.; Venugopal, N.; Edelhauser, H.F.; Prausnitz, M.R. Distribution of particles, small molecules and polymeric formulation excipients in the suprachoroidal space after microneedle injection. *Exp. Eye Res.* **2016**, *153*, 101–109. [CrossRef]
310. Chung, S.H.; Mollhoff, I.N.; Mishra, A.; Sin, T.-N.; Ngo, T.; Ciulla, T.; Sieving, P.; Thomasy, S.M.; Yiu, G. Host immune responses after suprachoroidal delivery of AAV8 in nonhuman primate eyes. *Hum. Gene Ther.* **2021**, *32*, 682–693. [CrossRef]
311. Ding, K.; Shen, J.; Hafiz, Z.; Hackett, S.F.; e Silva, R.L.; Khan, M.; Lorenc, V.E.; Chen, D.; Chadha, R.; Zhang, M. AAV8-vectored suprachoroidal gene transfer produces widespread ocular transgene expression. *J. Clin. Investig.* **2019**, *129*, 4901–4911. [CrossRef]
312. Yiu, G.; Chung, S.H.; Mollhoff, I.N.; Nguyen, U.T.; Thomasy, S.M.; Yoo, J.; Taraborelli, D.; Noronha, G. Suprachoroidal and Subretinal Injections of AAV Using Transscleral Microneedles for Retinal Gene Delivery in Nonhuman Primates. *Mol. Ther. Methods Clin. Dev.* **2020**, *16*, 179–191. [CrossRef]
313. Kansara, V.; Muya, L.; Wan, C.-r.; Ciulla, T.A. Suprachoroidal delivery of viral and nonviral gene therapy for retinal diseases. *J. Ocul. Pharmacol. Ther.* **2020**, *36*, 384–392. [CrossRef]
314. Hancock, S.E.; Phadke, A.; Kansara, V.; Boyer, D.; Rivera, J.; Marlor, C.; Podos, S.; Wiles, J.; McElheny, R.; Ciulla, T.A.; et al. Ocular Pharmacokinetics and Safety of Suprachoroidal A01017, Small Molecule Complement Inhibitor, Injectable Suspension in Rabbits. *Investig. Ophthalmol. Vis. Sci.* **2020**, *61*, 3694.

Disclaimer/Publisher's Note: The statements, opinions and data contained in all publications are solely those of the individual author(s) and contributor(s) and not of MDPI and/or the editor(s). MDPI and/or the editor(s) disclaim responsibility for any injury to people or property resulting from any ideas, methods, instructions or products referred to in the content.

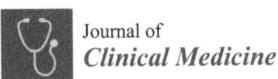

Review

Intraoperative OCT for Lamellar Corneal Surgery: A User Guide

Antonio Moramarco [1,2,*], Natalie di Geronimo [1,2], Matteo Airaldi [3,4], Lorenzo Gardini [1,2], Francesco Semeraro [3,4], Danilo Iannetta [1,2], Vito Romano [3,4] and Luigi Fontana [1,2]

[1] Ophthalmology Unit, Department of Medical and Surgical Sciences (DIMEC), Alma Mater Studiorum—University of Bologna, 40126 Bologna, Italy
[2] Ophthalmology Unit, IRCCS Azienda Ospedaliero-Universitaria di Bologna, 40126 Bologna, Italy
[3] Eye Unit, ASST Spedali Civili di Brescia, Piazzale Spedali Civili, 1, 25123 Brescia, Italy
[4] Eye Unit, Department of Medical and Surgical Specialties, Radiological Sciences and Public Health, University of Brescia, Viale Europa 15, 25123 Brescia, Italy
* Correspondence: moramarco.antonio@libero.it

Abstract: Intraoperative OCT is an innovative and promising technology which allows anterior and posterior segment ocular surgeons to obtain a near-histologic cross-sectional and tomographic image of the tissues. Intraoperative OCT has several applications in ocular surgery which are particularly interesting in the context of corneal transplantation. Indeed, iOCT images provide a direct and meticulous visualization of the anatomy, which could guide surgical decisions. In particular, during both big-bubble and manual DALK, the visualization of the relationship between the corneal layers and instruments allows the surgeon to obtain a more desirable depth of the trephination, thus achieving more type 1 bubbles, better regularity of the plane, and a reduced risk of DM perforation. During EK procedures, iOCT supplies information about proper descemetorhexis, graft orientation, and interface quality in order to optimize the postoperative adhesion and reduce the need for re-bubbling. Finally, mushroom PK, a challenging technique for many surgeons, can be aided through the use of iOCT since it guides the correct apposition of the lamellae and their centration. The technology of iOCT is still evolving: a larger field of view could allow for the visualization of all surgical fields, and automated tracking and iOCT autofocusing guarantee the continued centration of the image.

Keywords: anterior segment imaging; artificial intelligence; multimodal imaging; ophthalmic imaging; optical coherence tomography; DALK; corneal transplantation; endothelial keratoplasty; mushroom PK

1. Intraoperative OCT: Technology and Characteristics

Anterior segment OCT (AS-OCT) was described for the first time in 1994 by Izatt et al. as an essential tool for the clinical diagnosis and follow up of many corneal pathologies [1]. Thanks to its high level of resolution, AS-OCT provides a near-histologic cross-sectional and tomographic image of the tissues, allowing for the detailed evaluation of clinical conditions, and is able to impact medical and surgical decisions. The introduction of this technology into the operating room was a natural consequence considering its several potential applications during both anterior and posterior segment surgery. Indeed, intraoperative OCT (iOCT) provides immediate feedback on the tissues' anatomic configuration and could potentially directly guide surgical manipulations.

Standard OCT systems were unsuitable for a surgical setting due to their large dimensions and the traditional sitting position required for image acquisition, which was not practical for supine patients. The introduction of portable OCT systems allowed for the introduction of this tool into the operating room. The first two iOCT systems developed were the Bioptigen EnVisu (Bioptigen, Research Triangle Park, NC/Leica, Wetzlar, Germany) and the Optovue iVue (Optovue, Fremont, CA, USA) [2–7]. These systems were available in different configurations such as handheld, externally mounted, and microscope-mounted. Handheld imagine acquisition, although characterized by excellent image quality, is limited by potential motion artifacts, which could delay image capture and affect the quality of the resulting frames. In order to surpass these limitations, microscope-mounted systems were developed. These systems provided better stability; moreover, foot-pedal control of the microscope allowed for control of the probe location, with enhanced image reproducibility [8,9].

A major advance was achieved with the introduction of microscope-integrated OCT (MIOCT), which could finally enable the acquisition of real-time intraoperative OCT sections and the visualization of the instrument–tissue interaction [10,11]. Two of the currently most diffuse systems are the Zeiss OPMI LUMERA 700 (Carl Zeiss Meditec, Inc., Oberkochen, Germany) and the Leica Proveo 8 (Leica Microsystems, Wetzlar, Germany). Similar to the microscope-mounted systems, an MIOCT can be controlled by a foot pedal; furthermore, a heads-up display provides a combined visualization of the surgical field and the OCT data stream.

At first, iOCT was employed in vitreoretinal surgery, focusing on macular hole [8,12,13], vitreomacular traction [14,15], epiretinal membrane [16,17], and retinal detachment surgery [18,19]. More recently, it has been applied to glaucoma surgery [20], implantable collamer lens (ICL) implantation [21], cataract surgery [22], and corneal transplantation [23,24]. Concerning corneal surgery, its application is mainly related to lamellar surgery, both anterior and endothelial. Indeed, iOCT allows for a better visualization of the corneal layers, an evaluation of the instrument's depth during anterior lamellar surgery, and confirmation of the complete adhesion of the lamella during endothelial surgery.

In this narrative review, we describe the application of iOCT during different types of corneal lamellar surgery and provide a useful and complete guide for both novice and expert corneal surgeons.

2. Intraoperative OCT Applications for Lamellar Corneal Surgery

Guiding Big-Bubble Deep Anterior Lamellar Keratoplasty (BB-DALK)

Deep anterior lamellar keratoplasty (DALK) is the gold standard for the treatment of diseases of the anterior cornea, such as corneal ectasia, anterior stromal leucomas, and stromal dystrophies. In terms of improved visual acuity, DALK is associated with better outcomes than penetrating keratoplasty thanks to lower incidences of post-operative astigmatism and rejection [25,26]. Moreover, this technique does not require an open-sky approach, thus limiting possible risks and complications associated with the surgery [27,28].

There are several applications of iOCT, aimed mostly at avoiding the conversion to PK. First, it allows for the assessment of the corneal and anterior segment architecture, thus determining corneal thickness and regularity, and for the detection of the presence of anomalies such as Descemet's membrane (DM) rupture or peripheral anterior synechiae. The definition of corneal anatomy aids in making decisions about the depth of trephination, which can be identified by a vertical hyperreflective band along the anterior stroma in the peripheral cornea, where the cut was made. In their study, Santorum et al. suggested an intended stromal bed of 150 μm within the posterior corneal surface, measured with the built-in caliper tool of the intraoperative OCT software (InVivoVue, IVV 2.18, Lumivero. Denver, CO, USA) [29]. However, in all their eyes, they needed to further extend the groove after the first trephination in order to obtain the desirable depth. Usually, we establish the depth of trephination based on the full thickness measured on the iOCT. The aim is to leave a residual stromal thickness of about 100 μm and thus reach the pre-Descemetic plane. The PIONEER study detected an incidence of further dissection after the initial trephination in 55.6% of cases, determined by an evaluation made by the surgeon in light of an iOCT scan [9].

In BB-DALK surgery, the second step is the insertion of a cannula or needle into the stroma to create an air bubble. iOCT allows for the real-time visualization of the instrument, which can aid in guiding the insertion to the desirable depth and in the right direction. However, the visualization of the layers under the cannula can be masked by the hyperreflectivity of the instrument itself, hampering the correct assessment of the thickness of the tissue. In order to obtain the measurement of the residual stromal tissue, it is possible to remove the cannula and then, by acquiring a longitudinal iOCT scan, observe the presence of a stromal pocket, which is visible as an hyperreflective line along the posterior stroma [30]. Alternatively, even if the cannula is not removed from the scleral pocket, a transversal iOCT scan across the width of the instrument can still allow for the visualization of a hyperreflective line extending laterally to the shadow of the cannula, similar to a "seagull wing" appearance (Figure 1). Once this line is identified, the measurement of the residual stromal bed can be performed with the caliper, which is usually integrated into the iOCT's software, using the "seagull wing" as a reference.

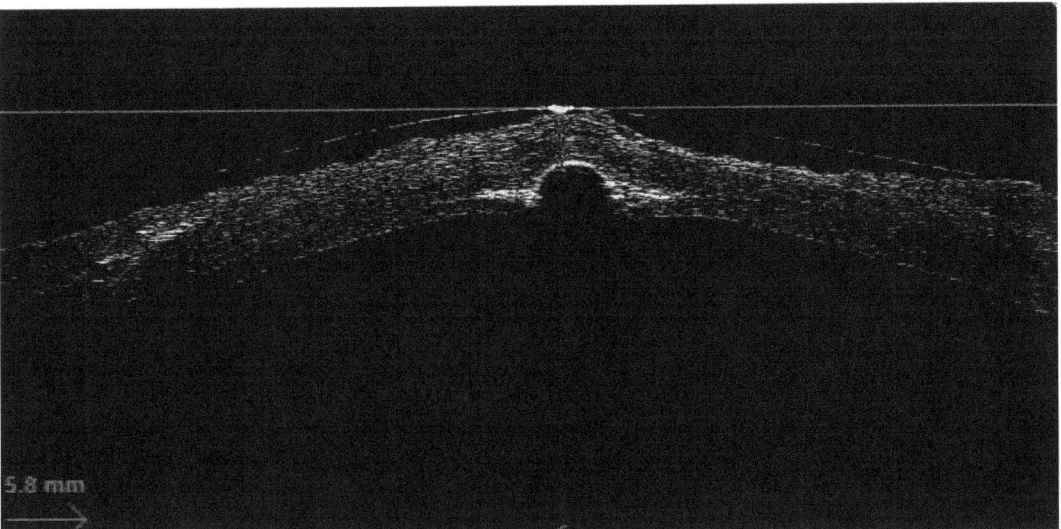

Figure 1. Seagull wing sign.

The proper identification of the residual stromal thickness under the cannula is useful for predicting the probability of achieving the big bubble. In 2013, Scorcia and colleagues observed how the distance between the cannula tip and the DM was significantly smaller (90.4 ± 27.7 µm) in cases in which a big bubble was achieved than in a group of unsuccessful surgeries (136.7 ± 24.2 µm) [31]. Indeed, corneal surgeons routinely employing iOCT could corroborate their evaluation of stromal depth with actual real-time thickness measurements, deciding whether a repositioning of the cannula to a deeper stromal plane is advisable and weighing the higher chances of achieving a big bubble with the increased risk of perforation.

The next step is the creation of the big bubble itself is to obtain a cleavage plan of the posterior stroma. The successful formation of the bubble is visualized on iOCT scans by observing the separation between the corneal stroma and DM, visible as a clear space between the internal concave surface and the external convex surface [32]. iOCT is capable of detecting sub-clinical big bubbles that are indistinguishable to the human eye in 40% of cases [33]. Moreover, iOCT could theoretically help to differentiate a type 1-BB from a type 2-BB by measuring the posterior wall of the bubble, which is made by pre-Descemetic stroma (the so-called Dua's layer) and DM in type 1 and by DM only in type 2. The posterior wall of type 2 bubbles should therefore be thinner than the type 1 wall, even though this difference is in the order of a few microns and modern iOCT has not yet attained an image resolution capable of consistently differentiating the two bubbles [34]. In cases of formation of small air bubbles distributed over the whole stroma, iOCT helps in identifying each bubble, allowing the surgeon to puncture them with a sharp instrument (e.g., a 15-degree blade) to create a bigger cavity, thus rescuing the surgery and proceeding with the stromal dissection without the need of a conversion to PK [35] (Figure 2).

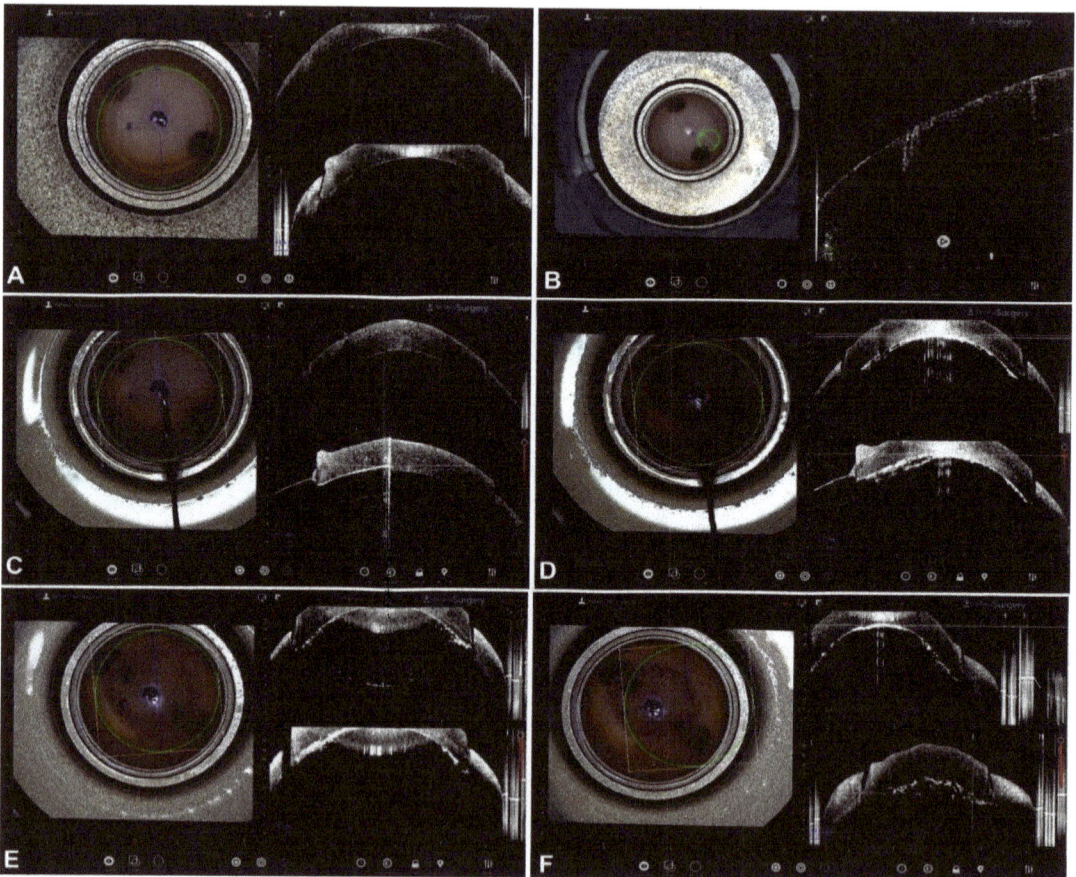

Figure 2. BB-DALK. (**A**) Stromal trephination. (**B**) Detail of the vertical hyperreflective band along the anterior stroma. (**C**) Insertion of the cannula. (**D**) Injection of air and bubble formation. (**E**) Bubble profile. (**F**) Detail of bubble and trephination.

3. Guiding Manual Stromal Dissection DALK

Although BB-DALK is the preferred technique for performing anterior lamellar keratoplasty, there are few situations in which a bubble cannot be achieved or is associated with a high risk of perforation. Specifically, in cases in which corneal opacities do not allow for the visualization of the depth of the stromal involvement, or cases in which the bubble could easily provoke DM ruptures (e.g., radial keratotomies), the majority of corneal surgeons prefer to perform manual stromal dissection.

Intraoperative OCT could be helpful during the multiple surgical steps of DALK by stromal dissection. Firstly, iOCT permits the determination of the depth of the opacity and therefore the type of ALK to perform. Variations in corneal thickness at different points may be visualized in irregular or ectatic corneas, helping surgeons decide on a safe depth of initial trephination [7]. In other words, iOCT guides decision making with respect to the depth of trephination and prompts further eventual dissection.

iOCT is especially useful because it allows the surgeon to better control the incision depth and assess the uniformity of the dissection plane to optimize visual outcomes, especially when coaxial microscopy does not offer an excellent evaluation of the depth of a corneal incision [34,36]. In addition, iOCT could be very useful in assessing the residual stroma during dissection. Regarding the BB technique, the aim is to reach the pre-Descemetic plane, which guarantees a combination of good visual outcomes and a low risk of Descemet perforation. Hence, the optimal stromal bed should have a thickness of no more than 100 µm [24,33].

Moreover, the use of OCT enables surgeons to attempt manual dissection in the case of an emphysematous opaque cornea after a failed big bubble attempt: the opaque bubble layer hampers visualization during subsequent dissection; thus, iOCT can help surgeons perform a safe manual dissection and minimize the risk of DM perforation [37].

During manual stromal dissection in particular, sharp instruments inserted too deeply into the stroma can cause a DM rupture. In these cases, iOCT can detect the location of the rupture and guide further dissection. When a DM rupture is present, it can be advantageous to inject air into the anterior chamber to keep it formed. However, in cases of narrow iridocorneal angles, the air can be misdirected into the posterior chamber, causing an iris protrusion, which can be readily detected by the iOCT [38].

Once the proper plan is achieved, it is possible to proceed with the graft placement. In this step, iOCT might be useful in detecting residual interface fluid, allowing the surgeon to evacuate it by applying moderate massage on the corneal surface, leading to a reduced risk of a double anterior chamber in the postoperative period. After lamellar dissection, iOCT aids in the assessment of graft thickness, graft–host apposition, and interface regularity, as well as in the evaluation of any residual stromal pathology or disparities in the graft–host sizing [35].

Finally, iOCT can aid in the management of post-DALK Descemet's membrane detachment (DMD) by determining the localization of maximal DMD, managing an iOCT-assisted injection of isoexpansile gas SF6 (BVI Medical, Waltham, USA) into the anterior chamber, guiding the location for venting incisions to drain the interface fluid, and confirming the apposition of the grafts [39].

4. Guiding Ultra-Thin Descemet Stripping Automated Endothelial Keratoplasy

Descemet Stripping automated endothelial keratoplasty (DSAEK) is one of the leading procedures for the management of corneal endothelial dysfunction [40]. Compared to PK, DSAEK has faster recovery times and better final visual and contrast acuity with less surgically induced astigmatism and fewer higher-order aberrations [41,42]. Graft rejection is also much more frequent in PK compared to DSAEK [43]. Some intra- and postoperative challenges specific to endothelial keratoplasty exist, such as graft visualization, graft apposition and dislocation, and interface complications [9]. However, iOCT can aid the corneal surgeon during every step of the DSAEK procedure, addressing each of these challenges [44].

During graft preparation, either one or two consecutive passes of a microkeratome blade allow for the creation of a very thin lenticule in a procedure known as UltraThin-DSAEK (UT-DSAEK), which has become the standard modern approach to DSAEK [40,45,46]. In cases in which this preparation is carried out in the operating room rather than at the eye bank, iOCT allows the surgeon to easily check the residual stromal thickness, the smoothness of the cut, and the regularity of the UT-DSAEK lenticule [47–51] (Figure 3).

The iOCT can also be useful for visualizing the DM during descemetorhexis, as well as for locating DM residues and guiding their removal under direct visualization, even in cases of poor visibility due to corneal edema or scarring [9,52–54]. With the help of iOCT,

DSAEK can be successful in patients affected by a clinically opaque cornea, which would otherwise be treated with a penetrating keratoplasty [52].

One of the most significant contributions of iOCT comes at perhaps the most crucial step of DSAEK: the apposition of the DSAEK lenticule to the recipient stroma. The assessment of the graft attachment and the evaluation of the residual interface fluid between the graft and the recipient stroma are readily available to the surgeon using iOCT. The routinary use of iOCT could, for instance, supersede the use of venting incisions, which have been developed to preemptively drain any potential residual fluid in the graft–stroma interface. Under direct iOCT visualization, residual fluid can be expressed out of the interface through focal manipulation and sweeping of the cornea [44,53,55]. Residual fluid is associated with early graft nonadherence and can result in textural interface opacities due to delayed gap closure, precipitated solutes, the retention of a viscoelastic substance, or lamellar irregularities caused by delayed adhesion or uneven matching of lamellar fibrils [56,57].

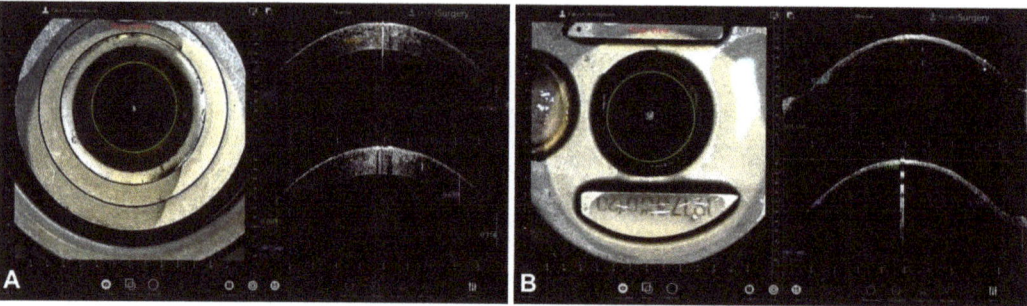

Figure 3. DSAEK preparation (**A**) Pre-cut thickness. (**B**) Post-cut thickness.

The iOCT can also aid in positioning the graft in cases of uneven posterior corneal surfaces, such as in cases of a previous penetrating keratoplasty in which the posterior lip of the trephination margin could hamper the successful attachment of a DSAEK graft. If a focal irregularity of the posterior corneal surface is detected, the graft can be recentered far from the irregular area [44].

Finally, iOCT's role could be even more prominent in times in which nanothin (<50 μm) DSAEK is gaining popularity: in complex eyes at a higher risk for rejection and graft detachment, nanothin DSAEK offers comparable results to Descemet membrane endothelial keratoplasty (DMEK) with lower rates of complication, and its results are enhanced by the use of iOCT for correct positioning and orientation [58,59] (Figure 4).

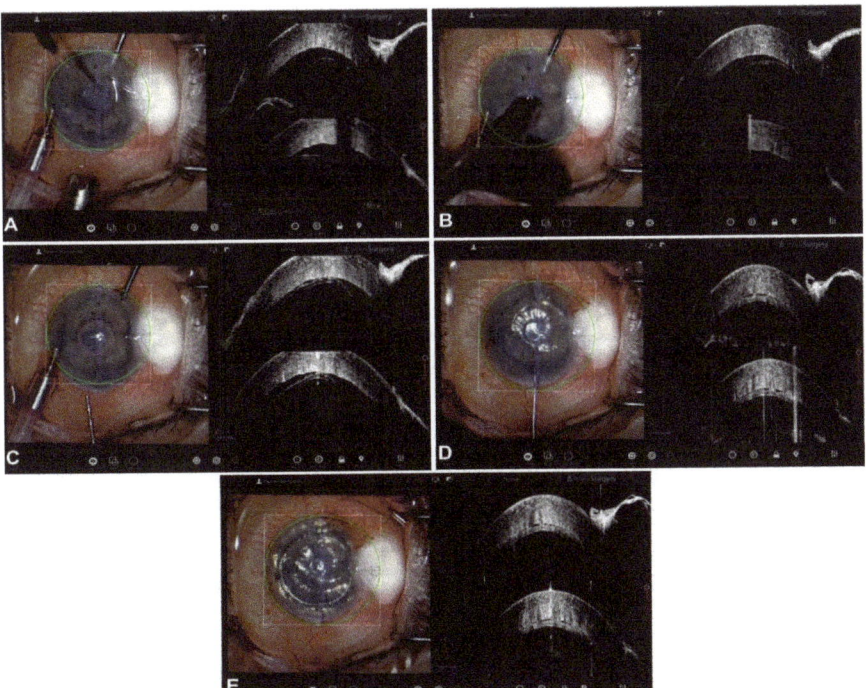

Figure 4. DSAEK. (**A**) Pull-through insertion. (**B**) Deployment. (**C**) Partial AC filling. (**D**) Interface fluid. (**E**) Apposition and AC filling.

5. Guiding Descemet Membrane Endothelial Keratoplasty

Although it is steadily gaining popularity, Descemet membrane endothelial keratoplasty (DMEK) is still considered to be a difficult technique characterized by a steep learning curve [60–62]. iOCT can facilitate the procedure, helping the expert and the novice surgeon alike [44,63–66].

One of the most useful applications of iOCT in DMEK surgery is the possibility of confirming the correct orientation of the graft in real time, with the endothelial side facing the anterior chamber [37,63,65–68]. The graft can be delivered with the endothelium folded either outwards, which represents its natural scrolled configuration, or inwards. In the inwards configuration, the membrane is folded in the opposite way to its natural scrolling tendency but it requires minimal time for unfolding inside the eye since it is perceived as an unnatural conformation [69–71]. In either cases, the unfolding of the graft can be monitored with iOCT even in cases of cloudy corneas, and the correct orientation can be confirmed [64]. As strategies to mark the tissue can result in endothelial damage or are inherently subtractive of endothelial cells, the possibility of checking the orientation of the graft indirectly could improve the long-term survival of the transplant [61,72,73].

At present, the orientation must be confirmed qualitatively by the surgeon based on the rolling and unfolding properties of the graft, as shown by iOCT [65]. However, the semi-automated or automated classification of graft orientation will most likely be integrated with iOCT: in 2013, Steven and colleagues correlated the intraoperative scrolling properties of DMEK grafts with donor age by mathematically describing the average curvature of the grafts, based on an image analysis of iOCT frames [63]. Building on this concept of curvature in relation to orientation of the graft, the deep learning segmentation of DMEK grafts has been applied to individual iOCT frames to automatically recognize the free-floating graft, compute its local curvature, and predict its orientation, with results comparable to a cornea specialist [68,74].

As in DSAEK surgery, iOCT during DMEK can be helpful not only to check the configuration and orientation of the graft but also to visualize areas of synechiae, remnants of Descemet membrane, the presence of fluid or folds at the graft–stromal interface, and to center the graft [63,64,75,76]. Finally, iOCT can also help in the preparation of the graft as well as in teaching novice surgeons. In fact, iOCT has been used to quantitatively assess the quality of donor corneas and pre-stripped grafts and to monitor each step of the stripping procedure [47,48]. Likewise, wet labs equipped with microscope-integrated iOCT allow expert surgeons to monitor the progression of their pupils and correct them accordingly [77]. (Figure 5).

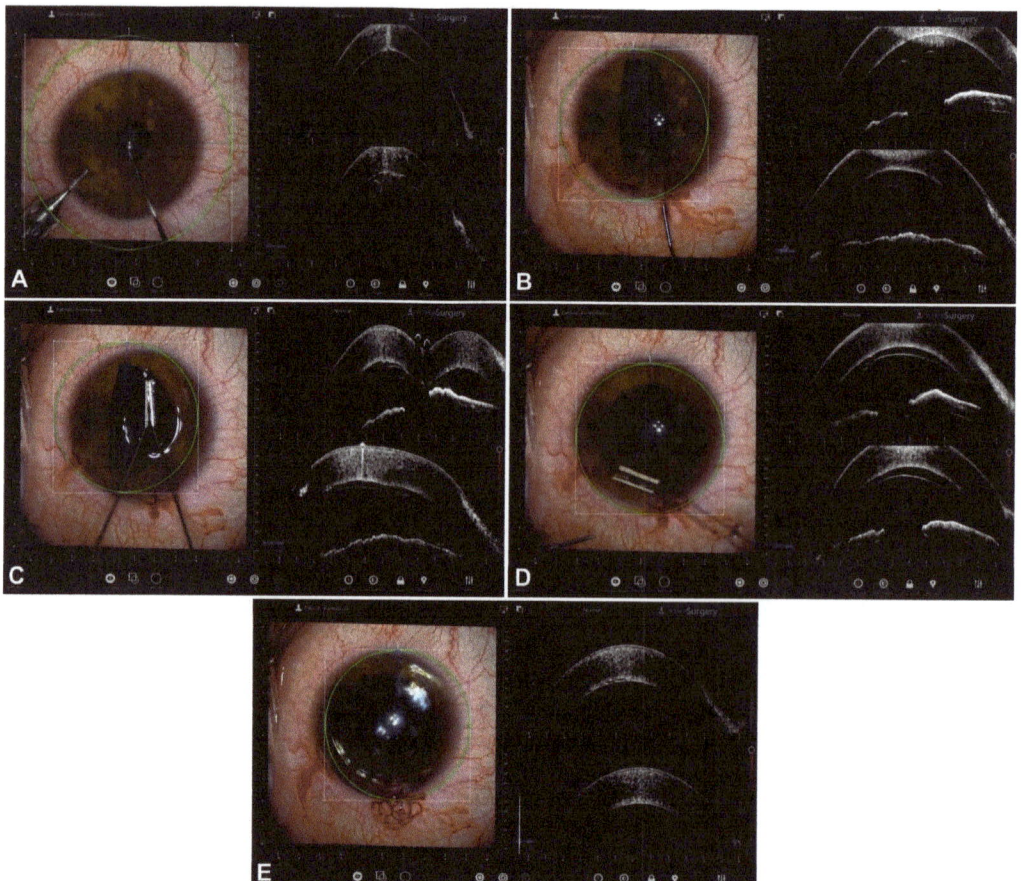

Figure 5. DMEK. (**A**) Deschemetorexhis. (**B**) Graft scroll. (**C**) Dirisamer maneuver. (**D**) Graft orientation and interface fluid. (**E**) AC filling.

6. Guiding Mushroom Penetrating Keratoplasty

The idea of asymmetrically shaping grafts in order to take advantage of the specific features of each layer of the cornea is not new [26,78,79]. The term "mushroom PK" was created in the 1950s, and its purpose is to minimize the replacement of the recipient's healthy endothelium while maintaining a large diameter of the superficial, refractive part of the graft [78,80]. This combines the benefits of lower incidences of induced astigmatism and rapid postoperative healing while minimizing endothelial cell loss and the risk of immunologic rejection and graft failure [80–83].

A variety of technique for preparing mushroom grafts have been described, from manual trephination to femtosecond-laser-assisted mushroom PK [82,84]. In 2005, Busin and colleagues created a two-piece mushroom PK by splitting the donor cornea in two with the help of a microkeratome and then punching the anterior and posterior lamellae to different sizes [80,81,85].

Although no publication in the literature thus far has focused on the use of iOCT in mushroom PK, its unique ability to examine the profile of asymmetric cuts and their relationship with the recipient tissue in real time can surely be of great help to the surgeon. In Figure 6, various steps of an iOCT-guided mushroom PK surgery are displayed. It is immediately obvious how iOCT can contribute and improve this complex surgery by visualizing the relationship between the graft layers and host tissue, allowing the surgeon to check for the correct positioning of the transplant.

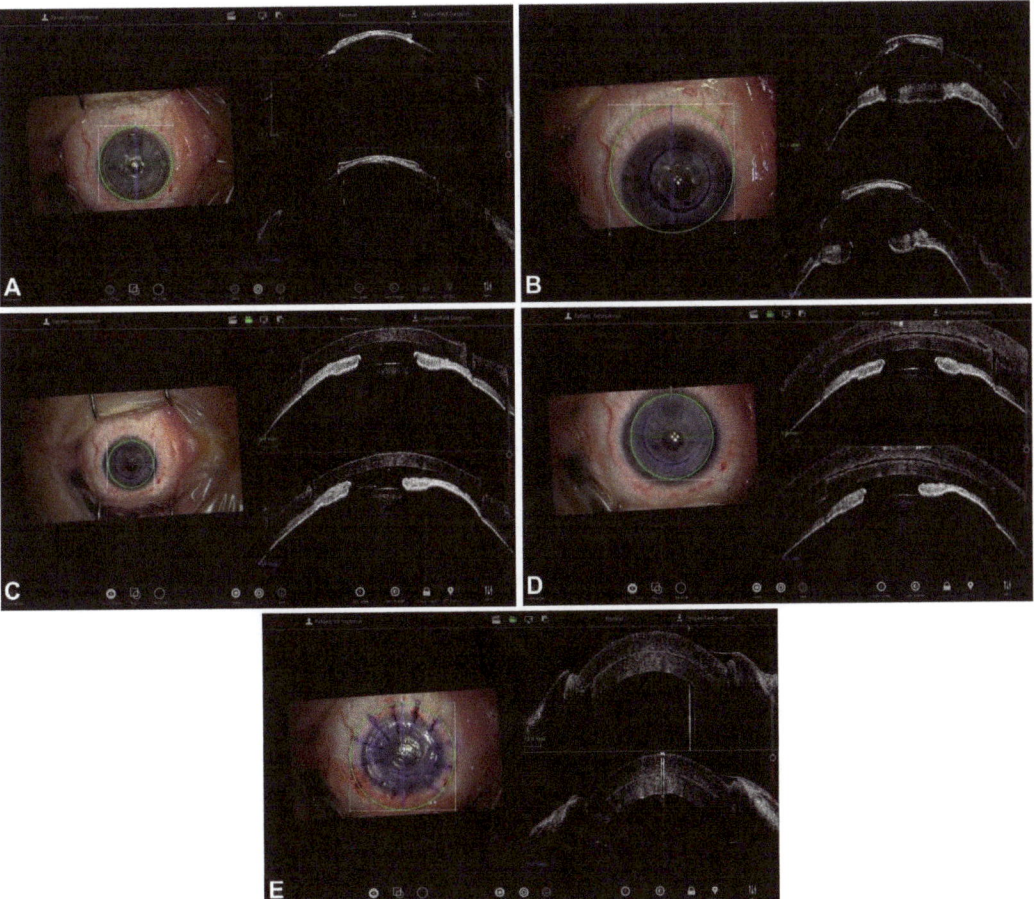

Figure 6. Mushroom PK. (**A**) Dissection. (**B**) Trephination. (**C**) Internal lamella placement. (**D**) External lamella placement. (**E**) Interface.

Mushroom PK is only one of the possible asymmetric graft configurations; the most well-known other configurations are the top-hat, the anvil, and the zig-zag configurations.

Each exploits the benefits of their particular shape and is tailored to the need of the individual diseased recipient corneas [86,87]. Asymmetric configurations, and in particular mushroom PK, are particularly suited to cases of thin, one-sided recipient corneas such as in very peripheral ectasias [82]. In fact, mushroom PK allows the surgeon to address the mismatch in thickness between the graft and the host by leaving behind a non-visually significant step between the two posterior surfaces while guaranteeing a continuous and smooth interface at the anterior refractive surface [75,82]. iOCT can clearly aid the surgeon in the positioning of mismatching surfaces in mushroom PK. Another possibility in mushroom PK that can greatly benefit from real-time positioning thanks to iOCT is the differential centration of the anterior and posterior lamellae, with the former usually being centered on the corneoscleral limbus and the latter on the visual axis, as described by Busin in 2005 [85].

7. Future Developments

To date, the most important limiting factor of a wider adoption of iOCTs is the entry cost of the device. The use of OCT in the operating room has transitioned from handheld OCTs to microscope-mounted OCTs and finally to microscope-integrated iOCTs, which have largely superseded earlier devices. This means that the entry cost for a state-of-the-art iOCT also includes, in more cases than not, the purchase of an integrated microscope.

The DISCOVER and PIONEER studies provided solid evidence of the utility of iOCT in modern eye surgery, but no large clinical randomized trial has definitely proven the superiority of iOCT to microscopy alone [9,11].

It is reasonable to think that with the increased adoption of these devices, their cost will also be mitigated [44]. The wider diffusion of this technology would allow its application in even more types of eye surgery, such as refractive surgery, and in the SMILE technique first of all. Indeed, the iOCT's aid permits the better visualization of the stromal lenticule and confirms the absence of cap–lenticule adhesion [88].

Furthermore, iOCTs are still evolving devices and, in addition to decreasing costs, their technical specifications are also expected to improve. Available iOCT devices currently employ a central wavelength of 840–860 nm and are capable of axial resolutions between 2.5 and 5 μm in the order of high-resolution posterior segment OCT [89]. However, their lateral resolution and A-Scan rate, arguably more relevant to corneal lamellar surgery, are currently working at 15–30 μm and 10–36 kHz, respectively. As a result of the latter, the acquisition of volume scans takes several seconds to complete and is not feasible during active surgical steps. Instead, continuous, high-resolution, single-line B-scans are usually employed to track the action [90]. On the other hand, increasing the lateral resolution could improve the visualization of finer details of the corneal anatomy and pathology [90].

Further developments of iOCT would also include even larger fields of view than what is currently available (up to 16–30 mm, depending on the device), which could allow the surgeon to easily monitor the entire surgical field, from the center of the cornea to the periphery of the anterior chamber, in one glimpse. Moreover, improvement of the automated tracking of surgical instruments and iOCT autofocusing on the corneal structure of interest, which may escape the field of view during surgical movements, are warranted [91].

Finally, with the goal of creating an all-in-one platform, microscope-integrated iOCT could be augmented with automated image analysis, providing useful insights on what is happening in the surgical field in real time, such as the analysis of graft orientation [68], or with the concurrently developing 3D imaging and robotically assisted surgery [92].

Author Contributions: Conceptualization, M.A.; Methodology, A.M.; formal analysis, D.I.; investigation, L.G.; data curation, N.d.G. and M.A.; writing—original draft, A.M., N.d.G., M.A., L.G. and V.R.; writing—review & editing, L.F.; visualization, V.R.; supervision, A.M., F.S., V.R. and L.F.; project administration, D.I. and V.R. All authors have read and agreed to the published version of the manuscript.

Funding: This research received no external funding.

Institutional Review Board Statement: Not applicable.

Informed Consent Statement: Not applicable.

Data Availability Statement: No new data were created or analyzed in this study. Data sharing is not applicable to this article.

Conflicts of Interest: The authors declare no conflict of interest.

References

1. Izatt, J.A.; Hee, M.R.; Swanson, E.A.; Lin, C.P.; Huang, D.; Schuman, J.S.; Puliafito, C.A.; Fujimoto, J.G. Micrometer-Scale Resolution Imaging of the Anterior Eye In Vivo with Optical Coherence Tomography. *Arch. Ophthalmol.* **1994**, *112*, 1584–1589. [CrossRef] [PubMed]
2. Mallipatna, A.; Vinekar, A.; Jayadev, C.; Dabir, S.; Sivakumar, M.; Krishnan, N.; Mehta, P.; Berendschot, T.; Yadav, N.K. The use of handheld spectral domain optical coherence tomography in pediatric ophthalmology practice: Our experience of 975 infants and children. *Indian J. Ophthalmol.* **2015**, *63*, 586–593. [CrossRef] [PubMed]
3. Ang, M.; Dubis, A.M.; Wilkins, M.R. Descemet Membrane Endothelial Keratoplasty: Intraoperative and Postoperative Imaging Spectral-Domain Optical Coherence Tomography. *Case Rep. Ophthalmol. Med.* **2015**, *2015*, 506251. [CrossRef] [PubMed]
4. Branchini, L.A.; Gurley, K.; Duker, J.S.; Reichel, E. Use of Handheld Intraoperative Spectral-Domain Optical Coherence Tomography in a Variety of Vitreoretinal Diseases. *Ophthalmic Surg. Lasers Imaging Retin.* **2016**, *47*, 49–54. [CrossRef] [PubMed]
5. Khademi, M.R.; Riazi-Esfahani, M.; Mazloumi, M.; Khodabandeh, A.; Riazi-Esfahani, H. Macular surgery using intraoperative spectral domain optical coherence tomography. *J. Ophthalmic Vis. Res.* **2015**, *10*, 309–315. [CrossRef] [PubMed]
6. Mendez, N.; Nayak, N.V.; Kolomeyer, A.M.; Szirth, B.C.; Khouri, A.S. Feasibility of Spectral Domain Optical Coherence Tomography Acquisition Using a Handheld Versus Conventional Tabletop Unit. *J. Diabetes Sci. Technol.* **2015**, *10*, 277–281. [CrossRef] [PubMed]
7. De Benito-Llopis, L.; Mehta, J.S.; Angunawela, R.I.; Ang, M.; Tan, D.T. Intraoperative Anterior Segment Optical Coherence Tomography: A Novel Assessment Tool during Deep Anterior Lamellar Keratoplasty. *Am. J. Ophthalmol.* **2013**, *157*, 334–341.e3. [CrossRef] [PubMed]
8. Ray, R.; Barañano, D.E.; Fortun, J.A.; Schwent, B.J.; Cribbs, B.E.; Bergstrom, C.S.; Hubbard, G.B.; Srivastava, S.K. Intraoperative Microscope-Mounted Spectral Domain Optical Coherence Tomography for Evaluation of Retinal Anatomy during Macular Surgery. *Ophthalmology* **2011**, *118*, 2212–2217. [CrossRef]
9. Ehlers, J.P.; Dupps, W.J.; Kaiser, P.K.; Goshe, J.; Singh, R.P.; Petkovsek, D.; Srivastava, S.K. The Prospective Intraoperative and Perioperative Ophthalmic ImagiNg with Optical CoherEncE TomogRaphy (PIONEER) Study: 2-Year Results. *Am. J. Ophthalmol.* **2014**, *158*, 999–1007.e1. [CrossRef]
10. Ehlers, J.P. Intraoperative optical coherence tomography: Past, present, and future. *Eye* **2015**, *30*, 193–201. [CrossRef]
11. Ehlers, J.P.; Modi, Y.S.; Pecen, P.E.; Goshe, J.; Dupps, W.J.; Rachitskaya, A.; Sharma, S.; Yuan, A.; Singh, R.; Kaiser, P.K.; et al. The DISCOVER Study 3-Year Results: Feasibility and Usefulness of Microscope-Integrated Intraoperative OCT during Ophthalmic Surgery. *Ophthalmology* **2018**, *125*, 1014–1027. [CrossRef]
12. Yee, P.; Sevgi, D.D.; Abraham, J.; Srivastava, S.K.; Le, T.K.; Uchida, A.; Figueiredo, N.; Rachitskaya, A.V.; Sharma, S.; Reese, J.; et al. iOCT-assisted macular hole surgery: Outcomes and utility from the DISCOVER study. *Br. J. Ophthalmol.* **2020**, *105*, 403–409. [CrossRef] [PubMed]
13. Wykoff, C.C.; Berrocal, A.M.; Schefler, A.C.; Uhlhorn, S.R.; Ruggeri, M.; Hess, D. Intraoperative OCT of a Full-Thickness Macular Hole Before and After Internal Limiting Membrane Peeling. *Ophthalmic Surg. Lasers Imaging Retin.* **2010**, *41*, 7–11. [CrossRef] [PubMed]
14. Huang, H.J.; Sevgi, D.D.; Srivastava, S.K.; Reese, J.; Ehlers, J.P. Vitreomacular Traction Surgery from the DISCOVER Study: Intraoperative OCT Utility, Ellipsoid Zone Dynamics, and Outcomes. *Ophthalmic Surg. Lasers Imaging Retin.* **2021**, *52*, 544–550. [CrossRef]
15. Falkner-Radler, C.I.; Glittenberg, C.; Gabriel, M.; Binder, S. Intrasurgical microscopeintegrated spectral domain optical coherence Tomography-Assisted membrane peeling. *Retina* **2015**, *35*, 2100–2106. [CrossRef] [PubMed]
16. Bruyère, E.; Philippakis, E.; Dupas, B.; Nguyen-Kim, P.; Tadayoni, R.; Couturier, A. Benefit of intraoperative optical coherence tomography for vitreomacular surgery in highly myopic eyes. *Retina* **2018**, *38*, 2035–2044. [CrossRef]
17. Ehlers, J.P.; Khan, M.; Petkovsek, D.; Stiegel, L.; Kaiser, P.K.; Singh, R.P.; Reese, J.L.; Srivastava, S.K. Outcomes of Intraoperative OCT–Assisted Epiretinal Membrane Surgery from the PIONEER Study. *Ophthalmol. Retin.* **2018**, *2*, 263–267. [CrossRef] [PubMed]
18. Abraham, J.R.; Srivastava, S.K.; Le, T.K.; Sharma, S.; Rachitskaya, A.; Reese, J.L.; Ehlers, J.P. Intraoperative OCT-Assisted Retinal Detachment Repair in the DISCOVER Study: Impact and Outcomes. *Ophthalmol. Retin.* **2020**, *4*, 378–383. [CrossRef]
19. Abraham, J.; Srivastava, S.K.; Reese, J.L.; Ehlers, J.P. Intraoperative OCT Features and Postoperative Ellipsoid Mapping in Primary Macula-Involving Retinal Detachments from the PIONEER Study. *Ophthalmol. Retin.* **2018**, *3*, 252–257. [CrossRef]
20. Heindl, L.M.; Siebelmann, S.; Dietlein, T.; Hüttmann, G.; Lankenau, E.; Cursiefen, C.; Steven, P. Future Prospects: Assessment of Intraoperative Optical Coherence Tomography in *Ab Interno* Glaucoma Surgery. *Curr. Eye Res.* **2014**, *40*, 1288–1291. [CrossRef]

21. Zaldivar, R.; Zaldivar, R.; Adamek, P.; Cerviño, A. Intraoperative adjustment of implantable collamer lens vault by lens rotation aided by intraoperative OCT. *J. Cataract. Refract. Surg.* **2022**, *48*, 999–1003. [CrossRef] [PubMed]
22. Toro, M.D.; Milan, S.; Tognetto, D.; Rejdak, R.; Costagliola, C.; Zweifel, S.A.; Posarelli, C.; Figus, M.; Rejdak, M.; Avitabile, T.; et al. Intraoperative Anterior Segment Optical Coherence Tomography in the Management of Cataract Surgery: State of the Art. *J. Clin. Med.* **2022**, *11*, 3867. [CrossRef] [PubMed]
23. Carlà, M.M.; Boselli, F.; Giannuzzi, F.; Gambini, G.; Caporossi, T.; De Vico, U.; Mosca, L.; Guccione, L.; Baldascino, A.; Rizzo, C.; et al. An Overview of Intraoperative OCT-Assisted Lamellar Corneal Transplants: A Game Changer? *Diagnostics* **2022**, *12*, 727. [CrossRef] [PubMed]
24. Eguchi, H.; Hotta, F.; Kusaka, S.; Shimomura, Y. Intraoperative Optical Coherence Tomography Imaging in Corneal Surgery: A Literature Review and Proposal of Novel Applications. *J. Ophthalmol.* **2020**, *2020*, 1–10. [CrossRef] [PubMed]
25. Gadhvi, K.A.; Romano, V.; Cueto, L.F.-V.; Aiello, F.; Day, A.C.; Allan, B.D. Deep Anterior Lamellar Keratoplasty for Keratoconus: Multisurgeon Results. *Am. J. Ophthalmol.* **2019**, *201*, 54–62. [CrossRef]
26. Gadhvi, K.A.; Romano, V.; Cueto, L.F.-V.; Aiello, F.; Day, A.C.; Gore, D.M.; Allan, B.D. Femtosecond Laser–Assisted Deep Anterior Lamellar Keratoplasty for Keratoconus: Multi-surgeon Results. *Am. J. Ophthalmol.* **2020**, *220*, 191–202. [CrossRef]
27. Han, D.C.; Mehta, J.S.; Por, Y.M.; Htoon, H.M.; Tan, D.T. Comparison of Outcomes of Lamellar Keratoplasty and Penetrating Keratoplasty in Keratoconus. *Am. J. Ophthalmol.* **2009**, *148*, 744–751.e1. [CrossRef]
28. Riss, S.; Heindl, L.M.; Bachmann, B.O.; Kruse, F.E.; Cursiefen, C. Pentacam-Based Big Bubble Deep Anterior Lamellar Keratoplasty in Patients with Keratoconus. *Cornea* **2012**, *31*, 627–632. [CrossRef]
29. Santorum, P.; Yu, A.C.; Bertelli, E.; Busin, M. Microscope-Integrated Intraoperative Optical Coherence Tomography–Guided Big-Bubble Deep Anterior Lamellar Keratoplasty. *Cornea* **2021**, *41*, 125–129. [CrossRef]
30. Titiyal, J.S.; Kaur, M.; Nair, S.; Sharma, N. Intraoperative optical coherence tomography in anterior segment surgery. *Surv. Ophthalmol.* **2020**, *66*, 308–326. [CrossRef]
31. Scorcia, V.; Busin, M.; Lucisano, A.; Beltz, J.; Carta, A.; Scorcia, G. Anterior Segment Optical Coherence Tomography–Guided Big-Bubble Technique. *Ophthalmology* **2013**, *120*, 471–476. [CrossRef] [PubMed]
32. Myerscough, J.; Friehmann, A.; Busin, M.; Goor, D. Successful Visualization of a Big Bubble during Deep Anterior Lamellar Keratoplasty using Intraoperative OCT. *Ophthalmology* **2019**, *126*, 1062. [CrossRef] [PubMed]
33. Ehlers, J.P.; Goshe, J.; Dupps, W.; Kaiser, P.; Singh, R.P.; Gans, R.; Eisengart, J.; Srivastava, S.K. Determination of Feasibility and Utility of Microscope-Integrated Optical Coherence Tomography During Ophthalmic Surgery: The DISCOVER Study RESCAN Results. *JAMA Ophthalmol.* **2015**, *133*, 1124–1132. [CrossRef] [PubMed]
34. Altaan, S.L.; Termote, K.; Elalfy, M.S.; Hogan, E.; Werkmeister, R.; Schmetterer, L.; Holland, S.; Dua, H.S. Optical coherence tomography characteristics of different types of big bubbles seen in deep anterior lamellar keratoplasty by the big bubble technique. *Eye* **2016**, *30*, 1509–1516. [CrossRef] [PubMed]
35. Steven, P.; Le Blanc, C.; Lankenau, E.; Krug, M.; Oelckers, S.; Heindl, L.M.; Gehlsen, U.; Huettmann, G.; Cursiefen, C. Optimising deep anterior lamellar keratoplasty (DALK) using intraoperative online optical coherence tomography (iOCT). *Br. J. Ophthalmol.* **2014**, *98*, 900–904. [CrossRef] [PubMed]
36. Au, J.; Goshe, J.; Dupps, W.J.; Srivastava, S.K.; Ehlers, J.P. Intraoperative Optical Coherence Tomography for Enhanced Depth Visualization in Deep Anterior Lamellar Keratoplasty from the PIONEER Study. *Cornea* **2015**, *34*, 1039–1043. [CrossRef]
37. Muijzer, M.B.; Schellekens, P.A.; Beckers, H.J.M.; de Boer, J.H.; Imhof, S.M.; Wisse, R.P.L. Clinical applications for intraoperative optical coherence tomography: A systematic review. *Eye* **2021**, *36*, 379–391. [CrossRef]
38. Eguchi, H.; Kusaka, S.; Arimura-Koike, E.; Tachibana, K.; Tsujioka, D.; Fukuda, M.; Shimomura, Y. Intraoperative optical coherence tomography (RESCAN®700) for detecting iris incarceration and iridocorneal adhesion during keratoplasty. *Int. Ophthalmol.* **2016**, *37*, 761–765. [CrossRef] [PubMed]
39. Sharma, N.; Aron, N.; Kakkar, P.; Titiyal, J.S. Continuous intraoperative OCT guided management of post-deep anterior lamellar keratoplasty descemet's membrane detachment. *Saudi J. Ophthalmol.* **2016**, *30*, 133–136. [CrossRef]
40. Busin, M.; Albè, E. Does thickness matter: Ultrathin Descemet stripping automated endothelial keratoplasty. *Curr. Opin. Ophthalmol.* **2014**, *25*, 312–318. [CrossRef] [PubMed]
41. Bahar, I.; Kaiserman, I.; Levinger, E.; Sansanayudh, W.; Slomovic, A.R.; Rootman, D.S. Retrospective Contralateral Study Comparing Descemet Stripping Automated Endothelial Keratoplasty with Penetrating Keratoplasty. *Cornea* **2009**, *28*, 485–488. [CrossRef]
42. Fenech, M.T.; Coco, G.; Pagano, L.; Gadhvi, K.A.; Titley, M.; Levis, H.J.; Parekh, M.; Kaye, S.B.; Romano, V. Thinning rate over 24 months in ultrathin DSAEK. *Eye* **2022**, *37*, 655–659. [CrossRef]
43. Romano, V.; Parekh, M.; Virgili, G.; Coco, G.; Leon, P.; Islein, K.; Ponzin, D.; Ferrari, S.; Fasolo, A.; Yu, A.C.; et al. Gender Matching Did Not Affect 2-year Rejection or Failure Rates Following DSAEK for Fuchs Endothelial Corneal Dystrophy. *Am. J. Ophthalmol.* **2021**, *235*, 204–210. [CrossRef] [PubMed]
44. Price, F.W. Intraoperative Optical Coherence Tomography: Game-Changing Technology. *Cornea* **2020**, *40*, 675–678. [CrossRef] [PubMed]
45. Romano, V.; Steger, B.; Myneni, J.; Batterbury, M.; Willoughby, C.E.; Kaye, S.B. Preparation of ultrathin grafts for Descemet-stripping endothelial keratoplasty with a single microkeratome pass. *J. Cataract. Refract. Surg.* **2017**, *43*, 12–15. [CrossRef] [PubMed]

46. Romano, V.; Pagano, L.; Gadhvi, K.A.; Coco, G.; Titley, M.; Fenech, M.T.; Ferrari, S.; Levis, H.J.; Parekh, M.; Kaye, S. Clinical outcomes of pre-loaded ultra-thin DSAEK and pre-loaded DMEK. *BMJ Open Ophthalmol.* **2020**, *5*, e000546. [CrossRef] [PubMed]
47. Kobayashi, A.; Yokogawa, H.; Mori, N.; Sugiyama, K. Visualization of precut DSAEK and pre-stripped DMEK donor corneas by intraoperative optical coherence tomography using the RESCAN 700. *BMC Ophthalmol.* **2016**, *16*, 135. [CrossRef]
48. Agarwal, R.; Shakarwal, C.; Sharma, N.; Titiyal, J. Intraoperative optical coherence tomography-guided donor corneal tissue assessment and preparation. *Indian J. Ophthalmol.* **2022**, *70*, 3496. [CrossRef]
49. Ruzza, A.; Parekh, M.; Avoni, L.; Wojcik, G.; Ferrari, S.; Desneux, L.; Ponzin, D.; Levis, H.J.; Romano, V. Ultra-thin DSAEK using an innovative artificial anterior chamber pressuriser: A proof-of-concept study. *Graefe's Arch. Clin. Exp. Ophthalmol.* **2021**, *259*, 1871–1877. [CrossRef]
50. Pagano, L.; Gadhvi, K.A.; Parekh, M.; Coco, G.; Levis, H.J.; Ponzin, D.; Ferrari, S.; Virgili, G.; Kaye, S.B.; Edwards, R.T.; et al. Cost analysis of eye bank versus surgeon prepared endothelial grafts. *BMC Health Serv. Res.* **2021**, *21*, 801. [CrossRef]
51. Romano, V.; Tey, A.; Hill, N.M.E.; Ahmad, S.; Britten, C.; Batterbury, M.; Willoughby, C.; Kaye, S.B. Influence of graft size on graft survival following Descemet stripping automated endothelial keratoplasty. *Br. J. Ophthalmol.* **2015**, *99*, 784–788. [CrossRef] [PubMed]
52. Pasricha, N.D.; Shieh, C.; Carrasco-Zevallos, O.; Keller, B.; Izatt, J.A.; Toth, C.A.; Kuo, A.N. Real-Time Microscope-Integrated OCT to Improve Visualization in DSAEK for Advanced Bullous Keratopathy. *Cornea* **2015**, *34*, 1606–1610. [CrossRef] [PubMed]
53. Steverink, J.G.; Wisse, R.P.L. Intraoperative optical coherence tomography in descemet stripping automated endothelial keratoplasty: Pilot experiences. *Int. Ophthalmol.* **2016**, *37*, 939–944. [CrossRef] [PubMed]
54. Shazly, T.A.; To, L.K.; Conner, I.P.; Espandar, L. Intraoperative Optical Coherence Tomography-Assisted Descemet Stripping Automated Endothelial Keratoplasty for Anterior Chamber Fibrous Ingrowth. *Cornea* **2017**, *36*, 757–758. [CrossRef] [PubMed]
55. Nowinska, A.; Wylegala, E.; Wroblewska-Czajka, E.; Janiszewska, D. Donor disc attachment assessment with intraoperative spectral optical coherence tomography during descemet stripping automated endothelial keratoplasty. *Indian J. Ophthalmol.* **2013**, *61*, 511–513. [CrossRef] [PubMed]
56. Juthani, V.V.; Goshe, J.M.; Srivastava, S.K.; Ehlers, J.P. Association Between Transient Interface Fluid on Intraoperative OCT and Textural Interface Opacity After DSAEK Surgery in the PIONEER Study. *Cornea* **2014**, *33*, 887–892. [CrossRef]
57. Hallahan, K.M.; Cost, B.; Goshe, J.M.; Dupps, W.J.; Srivastava, S.K.; Ehlers, J.P. Intraoperative Interface Fluid Dynamics and Clinical Outcomes for Intraoperative Optical Coherence Tomography–Assisted Descemet Stripping Automated Endothelial Keratoplasty From the PIONEER Study. *Am. J. Ophthalmol.* **2016**, *173*, 16–22. [CrossRef]
58. Yokogawa, H.; Kobayashi, A.; Mori, N.; Nishino, T.; Nozaki, H.; Sugiyama, K. Intraoperative optical coherence tomography-guided nanothin Descemet stripping automated endothelial keratoplasty in a patient with a remarkably thickened cornea. *Am. J. Ophthalmol. Case Rep.* **2022**, *25*, 101414. [CrossRef]
59. Kurji, K.H.; Cheung, A.Y.; Eslani, M.; Rolfes, E.J.; Chachare, D.Y.; Auteri, N.J.; Nordlund, M.L.; Holland, E.J. Comparison of Visual Acuity Outcomes Between Nanothin Descemet Stripping Automated Endothelial Keratoplasty and Descemet Membrane Endothelial Keratoplasty. *Cornea* **2018**, *37*, 1226–1231. [CrossRef]
60. Parekh, M.M.; Ruzza, A.B.; Romano, V.; Favaro, E.B.; Baruzzo, M.B.; Salvalaio, G.R.; Grassetto, A.M.; Ferrari, S.; Ponzin, D. Descemet Membrane Endothelial Keratoplasty Learning Curve for Graft Preparation in an Eye Bank Using 645 Donor Corneas. *Cornea* **2018**, *37*, 767–771. [CrossRef]
61. Moramarco, A.; Romano, V.; Modugno, R.L.; Coco, G.; Viola, P.; Fontana, L.M. Yogurt Technique for Descemet Membrane Endothelial Keratoplasty Graft Preparation: Early Clinical Outcomes. *Cornea* **2022**, *42*, 27–31. [CrossRef] [PubMed]
62. Borroni, D.; de Lossada, C.R.; Parekh, M.; Gadhvi, K.; Bonzano, C.; Romano, V.; Levis, H.J.; Tzamalis, A.; Steger, B.; Rechichi, M.; et al. Tips, Tricks, and Guides in Descemet Membrane Endothelial Keratoplasty Learning Curve. *J. Ophthalmol.* **2021**, *2021*, 1819454. [CrossRef] [PubMed]
63. Steven, P.; Le Blanc, C.; Velten, K.; Lankenau, E.; Krug, M.; Oelckers, S.; Heindl, L.M.; Gehlsen, U.; Hüttmann, G.; Cursiefen, C. Optimizing Descemet Membrane Endothelial Keratoplasty Using Intraoperative Optical Coherence Tomography. *JAMA Ophthalmol.* **2013**, *131*, 1135–1142. [CrossRef] [PubMed]
64. Sharma, N.; Sahay, P.; Maharana, P.K.; Kumar, S.; Ahsan, S.; Titiyal, J.S. Microscope Integrated Intraoperative Optical Coherence Tomography-Guided DMEK in Corneas with Poor Visualization. *Clin. Ophthalmol.* **2020**, *14*, 643–651. [CrossRef] [PubMed]
65. Patel, A.S.; Goshe, J.M.; Srivastava, S.K.; Ehlers, J.P. Intraoperative Optical Coherence Tomography–Assisted Descemet Membrane Endothelial Keratoplasty in the DISCOVER Study: First 100 Cases. *Am. J. Ophthalmol.* **2019**, *210*, 167–173. [CrossRef]
66. Muijzer, M.B.; Soeters, N.; Godefrooij, D.A.; van Luijk, C.M.; Wisse, R.P.L. Intraoperative Optical Coherence Tomography–Assisted Descemet Membrane Endothelial Keratoplasty: Toward More Efficient, Safer Surgery. *Cornea* **2020**, *39*, 674–679. [CrossRef] [PubMed]
67. Cost, B.; Goshe, J.M.; Srivastava, S.; Ehlers, J.P. Intraoperative Optical Coherence Tomography–Assisted Descemet Membrane Endothelial Keratoplasty in the DISCOVER Study. *Am. J. Ophthalmol.* **2015**, *160*, 430–437. [CrossRef] [PubMed]
68. Muijzer, M.B.; Heslinga, F.G.; Couwenberg, F.; Noordmans, H.-J.; Oahalou, A.; Pluim, J.P.W.; Veta, M.; Wisse, R.P.L. Automatic evaluation of graft orientation during Descemet membrane endothelial keratoplasty using intraoperative OCT. *Biomed. Opt. Express* **2022**, *13*, 2683. [CrossRef] [PubMed]

69. Yu, A.C.; Myerscough, J.; Spena, R.; Fusco, F.; Socea, S.; Furiosi, L.; De Rosa, L.; Bovone, C.; Busin, M. Three-Year Outcomes of Tri-Folded Endothelium-In Descemet Membrane Endothelial Keratoplasty with Pull-Through Technique. *Am. J. Ophthalmol.* **2020**, *219*, 121–131. [CrossRef]
70. Price, M.; Lisek, M.; Kelley, M.; Feng, M.T.; Price, F.W. Endothelium-in Versus Endothelium-out Insertion with Descemet Membrane Endothelial Keratoplasty. *Cornea* **2018**, *37*, 1098–1101. [CrossRef]
71. Parekh, M.; Ruzza, A.; Ferrari, S.; Ahmad, S.; Kaye, S.; Ponzin, D.; Romano, V. Endothelium-in versus endothelium-out for Descemet membrane endothelial keratoplasty graft preparation and implantation. *Acta Ophthalmol.* **2016**, *95*, 194–198. [CrossRef] [PubMed]
72. Romano, V.; Parekh, M.; Ruzza, A.; Willoughby, C.; Ferrari, S.; Ponzin, D.; Kaye, S.B.; Levis, H.J. Comparison of preservation and transportation protocols for preloaded Descemet membrane endothelial keratoplasty. *Br. J. Ophthalmol.* **2017**, *102*, 549–555. [CrossRef] [PubMed]
73. Tzamalis, A.; Vinciguerra, R.; Romano, V.; Arbabi, E.; Borroni, D.; Wojcik, G.; Ferrari, S.; Ziakas, N.; Kaye, S. The "Yogurt" Technique for Descemet Membrane Endothelial Keratoplasty Graft Preparation: A Novel Quick and Safe Method for Both Inexperienced and Senior Surgeons. *Cornea* **2020**, *39*, 1190–1195. [CrossRef] [PubMed]
74. Menassa, N.; Pagano, L.; Gadhvi, K.A.; Coco, G.; Kaye, S.B.; Levis, H.J.; Romano, V. Free-Floating DMEK in the Host Anterior Chamber: Surgical Management. *Cornea* **2020**, *39*, 1453–1456. [CrossRef] [PubMed]
75. Lang, S.J.; Heinzelmann, S.; Böhringer, D.; Reinhard, T.; Maier, P. Indications for intraoperative anterior segment optical coherence tomography in corneal surgery. *Int. Ophthalmol.* **2020**, *40*, 2617–2625. [CrossRef] [PubMed]
76. Saad, A.; Guilbert, E.; Grise-Dulac, A.; Sabatier, P.; Gatinel, D. Intraoperative OCT-Assisted DMEK: 14 Consecutive Cases. *Cornea* **2015**, *34*, 802–807. [CrossRef] [PubMed]
77. Famery, N.; Abdelmassih, Y.; El-Khoury, S.; Guindolet, D.; Cochereau, I.; Gabison, E.E. Artificial chamber and 3D printed iris: A new wet lab model for teaching Descemet's membrane endothelial keratoplasty. *Acta Ophthalmol.* **2018**, *97*, e179–e183. [CrossRef] [PubMed]
78. Franceschetti, A. The Different Techniques of Corneal Grafting and Their Indications. *Am. J. Ophthalmol.* **1955**, *39*, 61–66. [CrossRef] [PubMed]
79. Stocker, F.W. A new Technique for Corneal Mushroom Grafts. *Am. J. Ophthalmol.* **1959**, *48*, 27–30. [CrossRef]
80. Busin, M.; Madi, S.; Scorcia, V.; Santorum, P.; Nahum, Y. A Two-Piece Microkeratome-Assisted Mushroom Keratoplasty Improves the Outcomes and Survival of Grafts Performed in Eyes with Diseased Stroma and Healthy Endothelium (An American Ophthalmological Society Thesis). *Am. J. Ophthalmol.* **2015**, *113*, T1.
81. Yu, A.C.; Spena, R.; Fusco, F.; Dondi, R.; Myerscough, J.; Fabbri, F.; Bovone, C.; Busin, M. Long-Term Outcomes of Two-Piece Mushroom Keratoplasty for Traumatic Corneal Scars. *Am. J. Ophthalmol.* **2021**, *236*, 20–31. [CrossRef] [PubMed]
82. Saelens, I.E.Y.; Bartels, M.C.; Van Rij, G. Manual trephination of mushroom keratoplasty in advanced keratoconus. *Cornea* **2008**, *27*, 650–655. [CrossRef]
83. Scorcia, V.; Busin, M. Survival of Mushroom Keratoplasty Performed in Corneas with Postinfectious Vascularized Scars. *Am. J. Ophthalmol.* **2012**, *153*, 44–50.e1. [CrossRef] [PubMed]
84. Levinger, E.; Trivizki, O.; Levinger, S.; Kremer, I. Outcome of "Mushroom" Pattern Femtosecond Laser–Assisted Keratoplasty Versus Conventional Penetrating Keratoplasty in Patients with Keratoconus. *Cornea* **2014**, *33*, 481–485. [CrossRef]
85. Busin, M.; Arffa, R.C. Microkeratome-assisted Mushroom Keratoplasty with Minimal Endothelial Replacement. *Am. J. Ophthalmol.* **2005**, *140*, 138–140. [CrossRef] [PubMed]
86. Canovetti, A.; Rossi, F.; Rossi, M.; Menabuoni, L.; Malandrini, A.; Pini, R.; Ferrara, P. Anvil-profiled penetrating keratoplasty: Load resistance evaluation. *Biomech. Model. Mechanobiol.* **2018**, *18*, 319–325. [CrossRef]
87. Lee, H.P.; Zhuang, H. Biomechanical study on the edge shapes for penetrating keratoplasty. *Comput. Methods Biomech. Biomed. Eng.* **2012**, *15*, 1071–1079. [CrossRef]
88. Urkude, J.; Titiyal, J.S.; Sharma, N. Intraoperative Optical Coherence Tomography–Guided Management of Cap–Lenticule Adhesion During SMILE. *J. Refract. Surg.* **2017**, *33*, 783–786. [CrossRef] [PubMed]
89. Spaide, R.F.; Lally, D.R. High Resolution Spectral Domain Optical Coherence Tomography of Multiple Evanescent White Dot Syndrome. *Retin. Cases Brief Rep.* **2021**. [CrossRef]
90. Carrasco-Zevallos, O.M.; Viehland, C.; Keller, B.; Draelos, M.; Kuo, A.N.; Toth, C.A.; Izatt, J.A. Review of intraoperative optical coherence tomography: Technology and applications [Invited]. *Biomed. Opt. Express* **2017**, *8*, 1607–1637. [CrossRef] [PubMed]
91. Hahn, P.; Carrasco-Zevallos, O.; Cunefare, D.; Migacz, J.; Farsiu, S.; Izatt, J.A.; Toth, C.A. Intrasurgical Human Retinal Imaging with Manual Instrument Tracking Using a Microscope-Integrated Spectral-Domain Optical Coherence Tomography Device. *Transl. Vis. Sci. Technol.* **2015**, *4*, 1. [CrossRef] [PubMed]
92. Chen, C.-W.; Francone, A.A.; Gerber, M.J.; Lee, Y.-H.; Govetto, A.; Tsao, T.-C.; Hubschman, J.-P. Semiautomated optical coherence tomography-guided robotic surgery for porcine lens removal. *J. Cataract. Refract. Surg.* **2019**, *45*, 1665–1669. [CrossRef] [PubMed]

Disclaimer/Publisher's Note: The statements, opinions and data contained in all publications are solely those of the individual author(s) and contributor(s) and not of MDPI and/or the editor(s). MDPI and/or the editor(s) disclaim responsibility for any injury to people or property resulting from any ideas, methods, instructions or products referred to in the content.

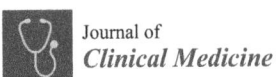

Article

Long-Term Safety and Efficacy of Pars Plana Vitrectomy for Uveitis: Experience of a Tertiary Referral Centre in the United Kingdom

Muhannd El Faouri [1,2], Naseer Ally [1], Myrta Lippera [1], Siddharth Subramani [3], George Moussa [1], Tsveta Ivanova [1], Niall Patton [1], Felipe Dhawahir-Scala [1], Carlos Rocha-de-Lossada [4,5,6,7], Mariantonia Ferrara [1,8] and Assad Jalil [1,*]

1. Manchester Royal Eye Hospital, Oxford Road, Manchester M13 9WL, UK; muhannad_fa3ouri@hotmail.com (M.E.F.); george.moussa@nhs.net (G.M.); tsveta.ivanova@mft.nhs.uk (T.I.); niall.patton@mft.nhs.uk (N.P.); mariantonia.ferrara@gmail.com (M.F.)
2. Faculty of Medicine, The Hashemite University, P.O. Box 330127, Zarqa 13133, Jordan
3. Khoo Teck Puat Hospital, Singapore 768828, Singapore
4. Qvision, Opththalmology Department, VITHAS Almería Hospital, 04120 Almería, Spain
5. Ophthalmology Department, VITHAS Málaga, 29016 Málaga, Spain
6. Regional Universityu Hospital of Malaga, Plaza del Hospital Civil, 29010 Málaga, Spain
7. Surgery Department, University of Sevilla, 41009 Seville, Spain
8. School of Medicine, University of Málaga, 29016 Málaga, Spain
* Correspondence: assad.jalil@mft.nhs.uk

Abstract: Aim: To evaluate the effectiveness of pars plana vitrectomy (PPV) without macular intervention on uveitis eyes with persistent vitreous inflammation/opacities in terms of visual acuity (VA), intraocular inflammation and macular profile. Methods: We carried out a single-center retrospective study of patients with uveitic eyes that underwent PPV without intervention on the macula due to persistent vitreous inflammation/opacities. The primary outcome measures were best-corrected visual acuity (BCVA), intraocular inflammation and macular profile at 3, 12 and 24 months after surgery. Results: Twenty-seven eyes of twenty-six patients were analyzed. Overall, 77.8% had an improvement of VA (55% by 0.3 LogMAR or more); 62.5% of patients had no intraocular inflammation, and the number of patients on systemic steroids and second-line immunosuppressives was reduced by 26% at 12 months; 87.5% of patients had resolution of macular oedema at 12 months. Conclusion: PPV for persistent vitreous inflammation/opacities is safe and effective, showing beneficial outcomes in terms of improvement of BCVA and the reduction in inflammation.

Keywords: intraocular inflammation; pars plana vitrectomy; uveitis; vitreous debris; visual acuity; vitreous opacities

1. Introduction

Uveitis is a heterogenous group of pathological conditions characterized by intraocular inflammation and is associated with a wide variety of etiologies [1]. Both adults and, less commonly, pediatric patients can be affected by uveitis, and the consequences of a protracted or recurrent inflammation can be severe, potentially leading to significant visual impairment [2–4]. In particular, uveitis can cause vision loss in up to 20% of eyes, with chronic macular oedema being the main reason for a moderate level of vision loss, and macular scarring being the most common cause of irreversible severe vision loss [3]. Pars plana vitrectomy (PPV) currently represents one of the treatment options, and it is increasingly used to treat uveitis for diagnostic and/or therapeutic purposes [1]. Indeed, there can be multiple indications for performing PPV to treat uveitic eyes. First, large amounts of vitreous material can be obtained for microbiological and histopathological analyses to help identify the etiology in cases of atypical clinical presentation or history, inconclusive laboratory or radiologic testing or persistent inflammation or appropriate immunosuppression [5]. Second, PPV has a primary role in the management of posterior segment complications associated with uveitis, including vitreous hemorrhage, epiretinal membrane (ERM), full-thickness macular holes, retinal detachment (RD) and cyclitic membranes causing hypotony [6,7]. In addition, although its exact role as an anti-inflammatory therapy for uveitis remains uncertain, PPV has shown to be effective in improving visual acuity, intraocular inflammation and macular oedema and causing a reduction in immunosuppressive medications [8]. It has been speculated that the therapeutic effect of PPV may be due to the removal of inflammatory cells, cytokines and immune complexes from the vitreous body [8]. However, to date, therapeutic PPV has not been integrated in the routine management of uveitis, mainly due to the lack of specific indications and concerns regarding the potential complications of PPV in eyes with active inflammation and the stability of long-term outcomes [9,10].

In light of this background, the aim of our study was to evaluate the long-term safety and efficacy of PPV given to patients with uveitic eyes in terms of the control of intraocular inflammation, visual acuity and the macular profile. Specifically, in order to better assess the role of the PPV itself and exclude the potential bias associated with additional surgical maneuvers, such as ERM peeling, we focused on eyes where persistent vitreous involvement was the only indication for surgery, and no macular intervention was performed.

2. Materials and Methods

We conducted a retrospective, single-center, non-randomized interventional study of consecutive patients affected by uveitis with persistent vitreous inflammation/opacities who underwent PPV without intervention on their macula at the Manchester Royal Eye Hospital. The study was registered with the clinical audit department, and the research adhered to the tenets of the Declaration of Helsinki. Approved patient consent was obtained before all procedures and all surgeries were performed prior to the study design.

2.1. Participants and Data Collection

Data were identified and collected from the surgical database of the vitreoretinal unit and were anonymized for the analysis. We included eyes treated with PPV due to persistent vitreous inflammation/opacities associated with uveitis and a minimum follow-up (FU) of 24 months. Diagnosis of uveitis etiology was based on the patients' history, clinical examination and investigations such as blood tests, chest radiographs and vitreous sampling (if performed) at the time of vitrectomy. The exclusion criteria were: (i) having undergone a surgical procedure on the macula (peeling of the ERM and/or internal limiting membrane); (ii) having a reason for being treated with PPV other than persistent vitreous inflammation/opacities, such as ERM, retinal detachment, a full-thickness macular hole and dislocated intraocular lens (IOL); (iii) having eyes where the vitreous sample was diagnostic for a non-inflammatory disease, specifically vitreoretinal lymphoma; (iv) patients with an incomplete FU.

Data collection included the patients' demographics, the type of uveitis, indication for PPV, surgical details, therapeutic regimen and preoperative clinical findings and 3, 12 and 24 months after the surgery. At each follow-up, the ophthalmic examination included an assessment of best-corrected visual acuity (BCVA) expressed as a logarithm of the minimal angle of resolution (LogMAR) and intraocular pressure (IOP), a slit lamp examination, a dilated fundus examination and optical coherence tomography (OCT) of the macula. Uveitis activity was defined based on anterior chamber (AC) and graded by applying the SUN criteria [11], and vitreous inflammation was graded according to Nussenblatt's method [12]. In particular, uveitis activity was defined as "mild", "moderate" or "severe" if AC and/or vitreous inflammation values were $\leq +1$, $+2$ or $+3$, and $+4$, respectively. The presence of cystoid macular edema (CME) and central retinal thickness were recorded by analyzing macular OCT scans. The therapeutic regimen was defined as being given: (i) no medication, (ii) a topical steroid (TS), (iii) an oral steroid (OS), (iv) conventional or biologic Disease Modifying Anti-Rheumatic Drugs (DMARDs) or (v) a combination of them.

2.2. Surgical Procedure

All surgical procedures were performed by a consultant surgeon or a vitreoretinal fellow under local anesthesia. Three-port standard PPV (23, 25 or 27 gauge) was carried out using the Stellaris vitrectomy system (Bausch and Lomb, St. Louis, MO, USA) or Constellation vitrectomy system (Alcon Laboratories, Inc, Fort Worth, TX, USA). Combined cataract surgery with intraocular lens implantation was performed if lens' opacity was detected preoperatively. Posterior vitreous detachment was induced, if it was needed, and core vitrectomy and peripheral vitreous shaving were performed. A vitreous sample was sent to the histopathological department for analysis. After the peripheral retinal check to look for retinal breaks, air or gas was used as an intraocular tamponade. All patients were given topical steroids, cycloplegia and antibiotics postoperatively. The topical steroid dose and, if necessary, oral steroid therapy was adjusted perioperatively to control inflammation.

2.3. Statistical Analysis

All data were analyzed using Stata 16.1 (Statacorp, College Station Texas, USA). Means (standard deviation, SD) were used to represent demographic data that had a normal distribution, and medians (Interquartile ranges) were used for skewed data. Crude analysis of paired skewed data was carried out using the Wilcoxon sign rank test. Due to the retrospective nature of the study and the presence of missing data at some time points, multiple imputation using chained equations was used to account for the missing data. As this study was a longitudinal analysis of the four main outcomes at four consecutive time periods, multi-level mixed effects models were used to account for the covariance of the data at each time point. Specifically, BCVA and CRT were assessed using mixed effects linear regression models. Uveitis activity and the presence of CME were assessed using a mixed effects ordinal logistic regression and mixed effects logistic regression models, respectively. All three FU visits were compared to the baseline. Other independent variables of clinical importance were added to generate the final multivariate models. Graphs of means were generated for time series data, with 95% confidence intervals represented. A p-value of <0.05 was regarded as significant.

3. Results

A total of 27 eyes of 26 patients met the inclusion criteria and underwent PPV for persistent uveitis-related vitreous inflammation/opacities and were included in the analysis. The baseline characteristics are presented in Table 1. The mean (SD) age at the time of vitrectomy was 45.8 (18.7) years, with the range being from 8 to 86 years. Eight eyes underwent combined phaco-PPV, whereas the remaining ones were treated with vitrectomy only. Six eyes underwent cataract surgery during the FU period analyzed. In terms of ocular co-pathologies potentially affecting the visual outcomes at the final FU, we documented cases of CME (two eyes), ERM (two eyes), CME and ERM (two eyes), a macular scar (one eye) and a cataract (one eye) (Figures 1 and 2). In addition, out of 27 eye, 6 eyes underwent glaucoma surgery during the FU (3 were treated with trabeculectomy and 3 was treated with glaucoma drainage implantation).

Overall, the crude change in BCVA was significant across all the follow-ups. The median (interquartile range, IQR) BCVA significantly improved from the preoperative value of 0.7 (0.50–1.00) logMAR to 0.30 (0.20–0.50) logMAR at the 3-month follow-up ($p < 0.001$), 0.30 (0.14–0.60) logMAR at the 12-month FU ($p = 0.005$) and 0.40 (0.10–0.60) logMAR at the 24-month FU ($p = 0.003$). Of the sample analyzed, 77.8% ($n = 21$) experienced improvement in BCVA, 11.1 % ($n = 3$) remained stable and 11.1.% ($n = 3$) worsened. The change in visual acuity outcomes over the study period are presented in Table 2 below. Univariate analysis showed that compared to the baseline, the visual acuity of patients improved by 0.45, 0.43 and 0.36 at 3, 12 and 24 months, respectively. The most significant improvement occurred in the period after the vitrectomy, and it slowly tapered off as the study period elapsed. Age and the presence of CME were also significant predictors. Every decade increase in age resulted in a 0.07 logMAR deterioration in visual acuity over two years. The presence of CME resulted in a 0.41 logMAR decrease in visual acuity if it was present over the entire study period. The pattern of visual recovery was maintained in the multivariate analysis, with patients improving by 0.43, 0.37 and 0.29 logMAR, respectively, over the three FU visits. Age, however, did not retain significance in the multivariate model, but the presence of CME did. The type of uveitis based on anatomical classification appears to have had an impact on the functional results, with intermediate uveitis showing a postoperative value of 0.35 logMAR, which is a better BCVA than that of posterior uveitis ($p = 0.01$). No significant difference was found when intermediate and panuveitis cases were compared, although there was a trend towards better results in the former group ($p = 0.097$). The combination of cataract surgery and PPV was significantly associated with postoperative BCVA as per univariate analysis ($p = 0.014$), but this association lost significance in the multivariate analysis ($p = 0.21$). Figure 3 below is a time series plot of the mean visual acuity with a 95% confidence interval at the baseline and each of the follow-up visits.

Table 1. Baseline characteristics of study patients and eyes that underwent vitrectomy.

Baseline Characteristic	
Age (years) mean (SD)	45.8 (18.7)
Sex, male n (%)	16 (59.3)
Lens status—n (%)	Phakic without cataract—11 (40.8)
	Phakic with cataract—8 (29.6)
	Pseudophakic—8 (29.6)
Uveitis etiology—n (%)	Idiopathic—4 (14.8)
	Sarcoidosis—9 (33)
	Toxoplasma—5 (18.5)
	Tuberculosis—1 (3.7)
	Fuchs Uveitis Syndrome—6 (22.2)
	Varicella-zoster virus—primary/active—1 (3.7)
	Toxocara—1 (3.7)
SUN classification—n (%)	Intermediate—9 (33)
	Posterior—9 (33)
	Panuveitis—9 (33)
Primary indication for vitrectomy—n (%)	Clearance of inflammatory debris—20 (74.1)
	Clearance of Hemorrhagic debris—3 (11.1)
	Cytological sampling—4 (14.8)

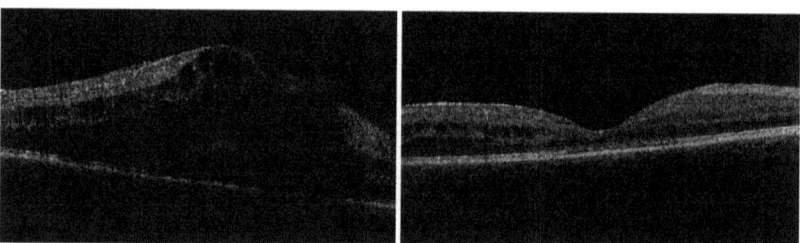

Figure 1. Case 1: Eye with vitritis and cystoid macular edema at the baseline (**left**); at 24-month, cystoid macular edema significantly improved, with persistence of small intraretinal cysts temporally involving the outer and inner nuclear layers (**right**).

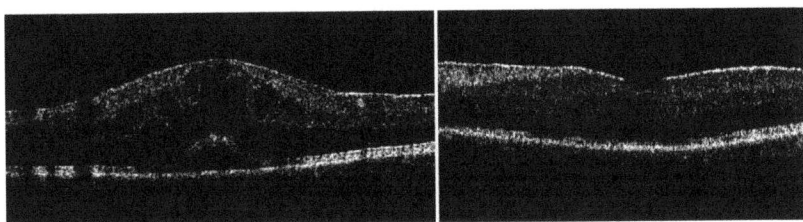

Figure 2. Case 2: Eye with vitritis and cystoid macular edema at the baseline (**left**); at 24-month, resolved cystoid macular edema and epiretinal membrane with preserved retinal layers (**right**).

Table 2. Multi-level mixed effects linear regression model of visual acuity outcome.

Variable	Change in LogMAR Visual Acuity Compared to Baseline	95% CI	p Value
Univariate			
3-month visit	−0.45	−0.76–−0.13	0.006
12-month visit	−0.43	−0.75–−0.11	0.008
24-month visit	−0.36	−0.69–−0.04	0.027
Age (Decade)	0.07	0.001–0.013	0.027
CME	0.41	0.15–0.68	0.002
Posterior compared to Intermediate	0.56	0.29–0.84	<0.001
Panuveitis compared to Intermediate	0.15	−0.13–0.42	0.29
Baseline Pseudophakic compared to phakic	−0.23	−0.51–0.04	0.098
Combined phacovitrectomy	0.32	0.07–0.58	0.014
Multivariate			
3-month visit	−0.46	−0.74–−0.18	0.002
12-month visit	−0.39	−0.67–−0.11	0.007
24-month visist	−0.30	−0.59–−0.013	0.041
Age (Decade)	0.04	−0.002–0.011	0.17
CME	0.36	0.11–0.62	0.005
Posterior compared to Intermediate	0.35	0.08–0.61	0.01
Panuveitis compared to Intermediate	0.21	−0.04–0.45	0.097
Baseline pseudophakic compared to phakic *	−0.21	−0.45–0.04	0.093
Combined phacovitrectomy *	0.16	−0.09–0.40	0.21

* Baseline lens status and combined phacovitrectomy were assessed separately in the multivariate models. Final reported coefficients were based on visit, CMO and diagnosis data.

The crude analysis of uveitis activity revealed that at the baseline, 7.4% ($n = 2$), 48.1% ($n = 13$), 37.0% ($n = 10$) and 7.4% ($n = 2$) patients had no activity and mild, moderate and severe activity, respectively. This improved to 44.4% ($n = 12$), 44.4% ($n = 12$), 3.7% ($n = 1$) and 3.7% ($n = 1$) with no activity and mild, moderate and severe activity at 3 months, respectively ($p = 0.003$). At the 12-month FU, the proportions of patients with no activity and mild, moderate and severe activity were 51.9% ($n = 14$), 40.7% ($n = 11$), 3.7% ($n = 1$) and 0%, respectively ($p < 0.001$). At the 24-month FU, the proportions of patients with no activity and mild, moderate and severe activity were 48.1% ($n = 13$), 40.7% ($n = 11$), 3.7% ($n = 1$) and 0%, respectively ($p = 0.002$). Table 3 below shows the change in uveitis activity at each of the follow-up visits compared to that of the baseline. The multivariate model shows a highly significant temporal relationship with uveitis grading, which decreased by 1.97, 2.28 and 2.19 at 3, 12 and 24 months, respectively (Table 4). Age was not a significant predictor of uveitis activity. Uveitis type was associated with the uveitis activity, with intermediate uveitis showing better response than panuveitis did ($p = 0.002$), but not posterior uveitis ($p = 0.834$). Figure 4 below shows the uveitis activity at each FU visit. As expected, due to the changes in uveitis activity, the therapeutic regimen was different at different FU visits.

The therapeutic regimes at each FU are detailed in Table 3. In particular, at the baseline, 12 patients were on oral steroids, which was compared to 4 at the final FU.

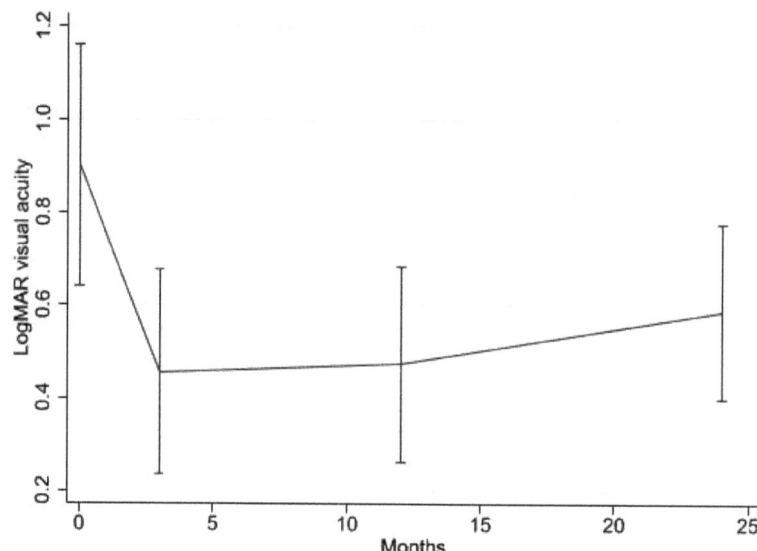

Figure 3. Time series plot of visual acuity recovery after pars plana vitrectomy in eyes of uveitic patients.

Table 3. Therapeutic regimen during the follow-up.

Therapeutic Regimen	Baseline Eyes, n (%)	3 m FU Eyes, n (%)	12 m FU Eyes, n (%)	24 m FU Eyes, n (%)
None	7 (25.9)	2 (7.4)	5 (18.5)	6 (22.2)
TS	8 (29.6)	19 (70.4)	15 (55.6)	15 (55.6)
OS	2 (7.4)	0 (0)	0 (0)	0 (0)
TS + OS	7 (25.9)	4 (14.8)	5 (18.5)	2 (7.4)
TS + DMARD	0	1 (3.7)	1 (3.7)	1 (3.7)
TS + OS + DMARD	3 (11.1)	1 (3.7)	1 (3.7)	2 (7.4)

Table 4. Multi-level mixed effects ordered logistic regression model of uveitis activity.

Variable	Change in Uveitis Activity Compared to that of the Baseline	95% CI	p Value
3-month visit	−2.14	−3.3−−1.00	<0.001
12-month visit	−2.50	−3.66−−1.33	<0.001
24-month visit	−2.34	−3.5−−1.16	<0.001
Age	0.005	−0.02−−0.03	0.625
Posterior compared to Intermediate	−0.11	−1.14−0.92	0.834
Panuveitis compared to Intermediate	1.53	0.56−2.51	0.002

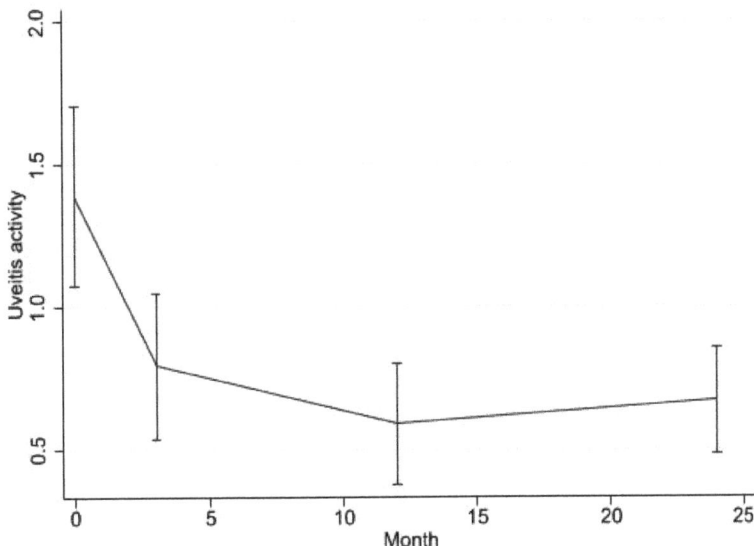

Figure 4. Change in uveitis activity at each follow-up visit in post-vitrectomized eyes.

The mean CRT values at the baseline, 3, 12 and 24 months were 360 (147.1), 339 (77.9), 284 (41.9) and 245 (30.4), respectively. Table 5 below shows a non-significant change over time in CRT. There is, however, a trend towards significance with each follow-up visit, with the upper limit of the 95% confidence interval at 24 months being only 5.9 µm thicker than the baseline measurement is, while the lower limit is 119.7 µm thinner than the baseline measurement is. CME was a significant predictor of CRT, with patients with CME having a 78.5 µm thicker CRTs over the study period. Figure 5 illustrates the CRTs at the baseline and each follow-up visit.

Table 5. Multilevel mixed effects linear regression model.

Variable	Change in Central Retinal Thickness Compared to that of the Baseline	95% CI	p Value
3-month visit	−7.8	−71.2–55.6	0.809
12-month visit	−34.4	−101.5–32.6	0.312
24-month visit	−56.9	−119.7–5.9	0.076
Age	−0.15	−1.7−−1.4	0.847
CME	78.5	26.0–131.0	0.003

We also specifically focused on the presence or absence of CME. At the baseline, 3, 12 and 24 months, 25.9% ($n = 7$), 14.8% ($n = 4$), 11.1% ($n = 3$), and 11.1% ($n = 3$) of patients had CME. The odds of developing CME over the study period did not significantly change when it was compared to that of the baseline as shown in Table 6 below.

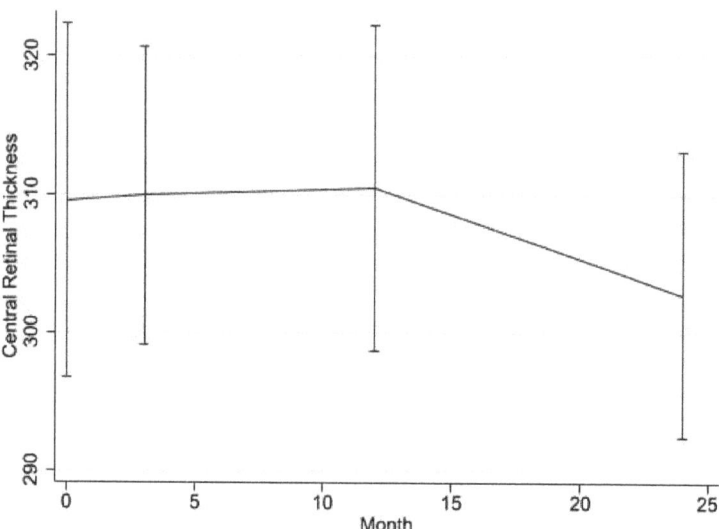

Figure 5. Time series plot of CRTs at baseline and each follow-up visit.

Table 6. Multi-level mixed effects logistic regression model.

Variable	Odds Ratio of CME Compared to Baseline	95% CI	p Value
3-month visit	0.66	0.2–2.9	0.576
12-month visit	0.51	0.1–2.5	0.404
24-month visit	0.50	0.98–2.5	0.394
Age	0.99	0.96–1.03	0.834
CME	1.03	0.07–3.06	0.993

4. Discussion

This study evaluated the long-term safety and efficacy of PPV for therapeutic and/or diagnostic purposes via persistent vitreous involvement in uveitic eyes, focusing on the postoperative control of intraocular inflammation, visual acuity and the macular profile. The rationale for including these patients relies on the attempt to selectively assess the potential effect of PPV itself and avoid confounding factors, in particular, concomitant pathologies. Indeed, the therapeutic role of PPV in uveitis has been variously reported as being beneficial for treating several diseases of the posterior segment affecting uveitic eyes, such as ERM, retinal detachment and persistent CME [6,7]. Our study demonstrated a beneficial effect of PPV in terms of BCVA, uveitis activity and the macular profile.

The improvement in visual acuity after the vitrectomy of uveitic eyes has been variously reported over recent decades [1,10]. Becker et al. reported 44 case series published between 1981 and 2005 and documented an improvement in vision in 708 eyes (68%) [8]. Shin et al. [9] analyzed the 12-month outcomes after PPV among patients with intermediate uveitis and reported a VA improvement in 69.7% of eyes, with mean preoperative BCVA improving from 0.81 (0.64) logMAR to 0.41 (0.50) logMAR postoperatively. Branson et al. [13] reviewed 11 studies reporting variable visual outcomes of PPV for macular pathology in uveitis, but this may be due to the masking of chronic permanent macular damage due to ERM or macular holes. Indeed, positive functional outcomes were further supported by a recent review reporting that the postoperative visual acuity improved in 69% of the eyes included, whereas no change and worsening were documented in 18% and 13%, respectively [10]. Our results appear to be consistent with previous studies, as the BCVA significantly improved at each FU visit. Interestingly, we report, for the first time, that although the BCVA improvement remained significant at 24-month FU, there was a significant trend towards a worsening of visual acuity with time. This finding may be explained by the presence of concomitant/subsequent ocular pathologies, such as glaucoma, ERM, cataract or posterior capsule opacification.

The functional improvement of eyes with uveitis after PPV has been also associated with the reportedly improved intraocular inflammation [9,14–20]. The effect of PPV on the inflammation status of eyes with uveitis has been evaluated in several previous studies, and the clearance of active inflammatory mediators from the vitreous cavity has been advocated as the main factor responsible for the decreased uveitis activity. However, other factors may contribute to the positive impact of PPV on intraocular inflammation, such as the increased clearance of inflammatory cells and the enhanced penetration of drugs used to control inflammation in vitrectomized eyes, as well as changes in the intraocular gradients of oxygen [21]. Conversely, in our study that included uveitis with different etiologies and anatomical location, most of previous studies focused on a specific type of uveitis. Shin et al. [9] studied the long-term implications of PPV performed in cases of complications, such as ERM, tractional retinal detachment and vitreous opacity, in 66 eyes with intermediate uveitis. The study demonstrated that in eyes treated with PPV, there was a decrease in the frequency of uveitis attacks, a reduction in the need for further therapy such as peri- or intraocular steroid injections or systemic medications, and an improvement in visual acuity during the 12-month follow up, which was independent of the degree of preoperative inflammation. Giuliari et al. [18] showed that PPV is safe and effective for the management of chronic pediatric uveitis and is associated with the reduction in systemic anti-inflammatory medications. Interestingly, Quinones et al. [22] performed a small randomized trial of 18 eyes, reporting more the improved control of intermediate uveitis after PPV compared with that of immunomodulatory therapy. Similar to our study, Scott et al. [15] included 41 eyes with intermediate cases, posterior cases or panuveitis treated with PPV, reporting an overall improvement in inflammation and visual acuity at the 12-month FU. Despite the better control of inflammation, the use of oral steroids and DMARDs remained unchanged in this cohort [15]. Takayama et al. [20] compared 38 eyes with granulomatous uveitis and 17 eyes with non-granulomatous uveitis treated with PPV and showed improvement in visual acuity and inflammation status 6 months after PPV. However, in the latter series, there was no analysis of the immunosuppressive and corticosteroid therapy [20]. Consistent with previous reports, we found a positive effect of PPV in terms of uveitis activity, which was significantly reduced at each FU analyzed. In terms of therapeutic regimen, we followed a step-wise approach, increasing the treatment from topical to oral steroids to determine the minimum amount of second-line immunosuppressives needed to achieve adequate control of intraocular inflammation. In addition, preoperative steroid and immunosuppressive therapy was avoided if PPV was performed for diagnostic purposes in order to improve the diagnostic yield. Improved inflammation control was also confirmed by the reduced proportion of patients requiring oral steroids 12 and 24 months after PPV. It is important to note that the control of inflammation without the need to use oral steroids is the main aim in the management of uveitis due to the potential steroid side effects, especially among children.

Our study also supported the safety of PPV in uveitic eyes. Indeed, we reported a limited number of intraoperative and postoperative complications. In this regard, the dramatic advances of vitrectomy machines over the last two decades, resulting in a less invasive and more efficient procedure [23–25], have been advocated as a significant contributing factor to the wide use of PPV, even for eyes with uveitis.

The improved control of inflammation post-PPV may contribute to the reported beneficial effect on CRT and CME. Macular edema is defined as the thickening of the retina in the macula caused by a breakdown in the blood–retinal barrier (BRB) with an accumulation of extracellular fluid in the intra or sub-retinal area [26]. The uveitic ME can range from 20% to 70% and can occur as a complication in anterior, intermediate or posterior uveitis. It is frequently observed in chronic and intermediate or posterior uveitis and panuveitis [27,28]. Macular oedema is the major cause of visual loss in uveitis, causing a visual acuity of 20/60 or less in approximately 40% of eyes [26,27,29]. Macular edema can occur in uveitis with different patterns: cystoid ME, in up to 80% of the cases, diffuse ME and serous retinal detachment [28]. The pathogenesis of ME in uveitis is multi-factorial, and although mechanical vitreomacular interactions and membrane formation on the macular surface can play a role, persistent subclinical or chronic inflammation is a key factor in the process [26]. Indeed, inflammation causes retinal pigment epithelial pump dysfunction and the consequent breakdown of the blood–retina barrier with the leakage of fluid in the retinal tissue [26,28]. The accumulation of inflammatory cytokines in the vitreous, which acts as a depot, could also be partly responsible for the macular oedema [8,30]. Therefore, performing PPV to remove the vitreous can theoretically eliminate the accumulation of inflammatory mediators close to the macula and help resolve or reduce the mechanical vitreomacular interactions [8]. In our study, only seven patients had preoperative macular oedemas. Considering that macular oedemas are a common complication of uveitis [28], the occurrence of macular oedemas in our study is limited. One of the factors could be due to under-reporting and obscuration of the macula from significant vitreous debris in the patients. Furthermore, we excluded all PPV with surgical maneuvers performed on the macula, including internal limiting membrane peeling, which has been proposed as a therapeutic option when the persistent CME is the main indication for PPV [31–33]. In addition, the impact of ILM peeling in severe CME of different etiologies is still controversial [32–34]. Although PPV was not specifically used in any of our cases to treat a macular oedema, we reported the resolution of macular edemas in four of seven patients (57%). This is better than reports elsewhere with rates with a range of 40–60% [8,14,15,31,35,36]. The true percentage of improvement, and hence, the protective effect on the macula may potentially be greater if it is assumed that more patients may have had an undiagnosed macular oedema prior to PPV due to hazy media. In addition, we found a trend towards the reduction in CRT during the entire FU, further supporting the long-term beneficial effect of PPV on the macular profile. These results, along with the risk of irreversible macular damage associated with undiagnosed chronic CME, might encourage early PPV in uveitic eyes with persistent vitreous inflammation/opacities. In addition, the removal of inflammatory debris with the secondary reduction of the macular oedema following PPV may allow the safe tapering of immunosuppressive medications.

We acknowledge that this study has several limitations. Firstly, the retrospective design will inherently lead to case selection bias. Moreover, due to the small sample size, we did not subgroup the uveitis conditions based on etiology, as this would have made the group sizes very small and provided inconclusive results. However, it should be highlighted that uveitis is not a common condition, and the application of strict inclusion and exclusion criteria allowed us to present a more homogeneous sample and exclude potential biases associated with specific surgical maneuvers (e.g., ERM peeling) or other main surgical indications (e.g., RD).

In conclusion, we report one of the largest studies on uveitic vitrectomies looking at both the control of inflammation and the use of immunosuppressive medications at 24 months following the surgery for all types of uveitis irrespective of the cause. Our results have shown that PPV, even without macular intervention for uveitis, leads to an overall improvement in VA, macular oedema and intraocular inflammation. Furthermore, there is an overall reduction in the use of combination medical therapy to control intraocular inflammation. The development of a well-designed randomized controlled trial for PPV in improving outcomes for uveitis will be useful, but it remains a challenge to conduct this type of study due to the heterogenous causes of uveitis.

Author Contributions: Conceptualization, A.J. and S.S.; methodology, M.F., N.A., G.M. and M.L.; validation, A.J., T.I., N.P., F.D.-S. and C.R.-d.-L.; formal analysis, N.A.; resources, M.L., G.M. and M.F.; writing—original draft preparation, S.S., M.F., M.L., N.A. and C.R.-d.-L.; writing—review and editing, A.J., T.I. and M.E.F.; supervision, N.A., F.D.-S. and M.E.F.; project administration, A.J. All authors have read and agreed to the published version of the manuscript.

Funding: This research received no external funding.

Institutional Review Board Statement: All procedures performed in studies involving human participants were in accordance with the ethical standards of the institutional and national research committee and with the 1964 Helsinki declaration and its later amendments or comparable ethical standards.

Informed Consent Statement: Patient consent was waived due to the retrospective nature of this study, and due to the subjects' anonymity and minimal risk to patients.

Data Availability Statement: The data that support the findings of this study are available from the corresponding author upon reasonable request.

Conflicts of Interest: The authors declare no conflict of interest.

References

1. Hung, J.H.; Rao, N.A.; Chiu, W.C.; Sheu, S.J. Vitreoretinal surgery in the management of infectious and non-infectious uveitis—A narrative review. *Graefe's Arch. Clin. Exp. Ophthalmol.* **2023**, *261*, 913–923. [CrossRef] [PubMed]
2. Ferrara, M.; Eggenschwiler, L.; Stephenson, A.; Montieth, A.; Nakhoul, N.; Araùjo-Miranda, R.; Foster, C.S. The Challenge of Pediatric Uveitis: Tertiary Referral Center Experience in the United States. *Ocul. Immunol. Inflamm.* **2019**, *27*, 410–417. [CrossRef]
3. Tomkins-Netzer, O.; Talat, L.; Bar, A.; Lula, A.; Taylor, S.R.; Joshi, L.; Lightman, S. Long-term clinical outcome and causes of vision loss in patients with uveitis. *Ophthalmology* **2014**, *121*, 2387–2392. [CrossRef]
4. Miserocchi, E.; Fogliato, G.; Modorati, G.; Bandello, F. Review on the worldwide epidemiology of uveitis. *Eur. J. Ophthalmol.* **2013**, *23*, 705–717. [CrossRef] [PubMed]
5. Jeroudi, A.; Yeh, S. Diagnostic vitrectomy for infectious uveitis. *Int. Ophthalmol. Clin.* **2014**, *54*, 173–197. [CrossRef] [PubMed]
6. Tanawade, R.G.; Tsierkezou, L.; Bindra, M.S.; Patton, N.A.; Jones, N.P. Visual outcomes of pars plana vitrectomy with epiretinal membrane peel in patients with uveitis. *Retina* **2015**, *35*, 736–741. [CrossRef] [PubMed]
7. Cristescu, I.-E.; Ivanova, T.; Moussa, G.; Ferrara, M.; Patton, N.; Dhawahir-Scala, F.; Ch'ng, S.W.; Mitra, A.; Tyagi, A.K.; Lett, K.S.; et al. Functional and Anatomical Outcomes of Pars Plana Vitrectomy for Epiretinal Membrane in Patients with Uveitis. *Diagnostics* **2022**, *12*, 3044. [CrossRef]
8. Becker, M.; Davis, J. Vitrectomy in the treatment of uveitis. *Am. J. Ophthalmol.* **2005**, *140*, 1096–1105. [CrossRef]
9. Shin, Y.U.; Shin, J.Y.; Ma, D.J.; Cho, H.; Yu, H.G. Preoperative Inflammatory Control and Surgical Outcome of Vitrectomy in Intermediate Uveitis. *J. Ophthalmol.* **2017**, *2017*, 5946240. [CrossRef]
10. Vithalani, N.M.; Basu, S. Therapeutic Vitrectomy in the Management of Uveitis: Opportunities and Challenges. *Semin. Ophthalmol.* **2022**, *37*, 820–829. [CrossRef]
11. Jabs, D.A.; Nussenblatt, R.B.; Rosenbaum, J.T. Standardization of Uveitis Nomenclature (SUN) Working Group. Standardization of uveitis nomenclature for reporting clinical data. Results of the First International Workshop. *Am. J. Ophthalmol.* **2005**, *140*, 509–516. [PubMed]
12. Nussenblatt, R.B.; Palestine, A.G.; Chan, C.C.; Roberge, F. Standardization of vitreal inflammatory activity in intermediate and posterior uveitis. *Ophthalmology* **1985**, *92*, 467–471. [CrossRef]
13. Branson, S.V.; McClafferty, B.R.; Kurup, S.K. Vitrectomy for Epiretinal Membranes and Macular Holes in Uveitis Patients. *J. Ocul. Pharmacol. Ther.* **2017**, *33*, 298–303. [CrossRef] [PubMed]
14. Heiligenhaus, A.; Bornfeld, N.; Wessing, A. Long-term results of pars plana vitrectomy in the management of intermediate uveitis. *Curr. Opin. Ophthalmol.* **1996**, *7*, 77–79. [CrossRef]
15. Scott, R.A.; Haynes, R.J.; Orr, G.M.; Cooling, R.J.; Pavésio, C.E.; Charteris, D.G. Vitreous surgery in the management of chronic endogenous posterior uveitis. *Eye* **2003**, *17*, 221–227. [CrossRef]
16. Eckardt, C.; Bacskulin, A. Vitrectomy in intermediate uveitis. *Dev. Ophthalmol.* **1992**, *23*, 232–238. [PubMed]
17. Dev, S.; Mieler, W.F.; Pulido, J.S.; Mittra, R.A. Visual outcomes after pars plana vitrectomy for epiretinal membranes associated with pars planitis. *Ophthalmology* **1999**, *106*, 1086–1090. [CrossRef] [PubMed]
18. Giuliari, G.P.; Chang, P.Y.; Thakuria, P.; Hinkle, D.M.; Foster, C.S. Pars plana vitrectomy in the management of paediatric uveitis: The Massachusetts Eye Research and Surgery Institution experience. *Eye* **2010**, *24*, 7–13. [CrossRef]
19. Verbraeken, H. Therapeutic pars plana vitrectomy for chronic uveitis: A retrospective study of the long-term results. *Graefe's Arch. Clin. Exp. Ophthalmol.* **1996**, *234*, 288–293. [CrossRef]
20. Takayama, K.; Tanaka, A.; Ishikawa, S.; Mochizuki, M.; Takeuchi, M. Comparison between Outcomes of Vitrectomy in Granulomatous and Nongranulomatous Uveitis. *Ophthalmologica* **2016**, *235*, 18–25. [CrossRef]

21. Svozilkova, P.; Heissigerova, J.; Brichova, M.; Kalvodova, B.; Dvorak, J.; Rihova, E. The role of pars plana vitrectomy in the diagnosis and treatment of uveitis. *Eur. J. Ophthalmol.* **2011**, *21*, 89–97. [CrossRef] [PubMed]
22. Quinones, K.; Choi, J.Y.; Yilmaz, T.; Kafkala, C.; Letko, E.; Foster, C.S. Pars plana vitrectomy versus immunomodulatory therapy for intermediate uveitis: A prospective, randomized pilot study. *Ocul. Immunol. Inflamm.* **2010**, *18*, 411–417. [CrossRef]
23. Romano, M.R.; Stocchino, A.; Ferrara, M.; Lagazzo, A.; Repetto, R. Fluidics of Single and Double Blade Guillotine Vitrectomy Probes in Balanced Salt Solution and Artificial Vitreous. *Transl. Vis. Sci. Technol.* **2018**, *7*, 19. [CrossRef]
24. Bansal, R.; Dogra, M.; Chawla, R.; Kumar, A. Pars plana vitrectomy in uveitis in the era of microincision vitreous surgery. *Indian J. Ophthalmol.* **2020**, *68*, 1844–1851. [CrossRef] [PubMed]
25. Lin, X.; Apple, D.; Hu, J.; Tewari, A. Advancements of vitreoretinal surgical machines. *Curr. Opin. Ophthalmol.* **2017**, *28*, 242–245. [CrossRef] [PubMed]
26. Fardeau, C.; Champion, E.; Massamba, N.; LeHoang, P. Uveitic macular edema. *Eye* **2016**, *30*, 1277–1292. [CrossRef]
27. Lardenoye, C.W.T.A.; van Kooij, B.; Rothova, A. Impact of macular edema on visual acuity in uveitis. *Ophthalmology* **2006**, *113*, 1446–1449. [CrossRef]
28. Accorinti, M.; Okada, A.A.; Smith, J.R.; Gilardi, M. Epidemiology of Macular Edema in Uveitis. *Ocul. Immunol. Inflamm.* **2019**, *27*, 169–180. [CrossRef]
29. Rothova, A.; Suttorp-van Schulten, M.S.; Frits Treffers, W.; Kijlstra, A. Causes and frequency of blindness in patients with intraocular inflammatory disease. *Br. J. Ophthalmol.* **1996**, *80*, 332–336. [CrossRef]
30. Algvere, P.; Alanko, H.; Dickhoff, K.; Lähde, Y.; Saari, K.M. Pars plana vitrectomy in the management of intraocular inflammation. *Acta Ophthalmol.* **1981**, *59*, 727–736. [CrossRef]
31. Radetzky, S.; Walter, P.; Fauser, S.; Koizumi, K.; Kirchhof, B.; Joussen, A.M. Visual outcome of patients with macular edema after pars plana vitrectomy and indocyanine green-assisted peeling of the internal limiting membrane. *Graefe's Arch. Clin. Exp. Ophthalmol.* **2004**, *242*, 273–278. [CrossRef]
32. Cho, M.; D'Amico, D.J. Transconjunctival 25-gauge pars plana vitrectomy and internal limiting membrane peeling for chronic macular edema. *Clin. Ophthalmol.* **2012**, *6*, 981–989. [CrossRef] [PubMed]
33. Schaal, S.; Tezel, T.H.; Kaplan, H.J. Surgical intervention in refractory CME–role of posterior hyaloid separation and internal limiting membrane peeling. *Ocul. Immunol. Inflamm.* **2008**, *16*, 209–210. [CrossRef] [PubMed]
34. Romano, M.R.; Allegrini, D.; Della Guardia, C.; Schiemer, S.; Baronissi, I.; Ferrara, M.; Cennamo, G. Vitreous and intraretinal macular changes in diabetic macular edema with and without tractional components. *Graefe's Arch. Clin. Exp. Ophthalmol.* **2019**, *257*, 1–8. [CrossRef]
35. Dugel, P.U.; Rao, N.A.; Ozler, S.; Liggett, P.E.; Smith, R.E. Pars plana vitrectomy for intraocular inflammation-related cystoid macular edema unresponsive to corticosteroids. A preliminary study. *Ophthalmology* **1992**, *99*, 1535–1541. [CrossRef] [PubMed]
36. Kiryu, J.; Kita, M.; Tanabe, T.; Yamashiro, K.; Miyamoto, N.; Ieki, Y. Pars plana vitrectomy for cystoid macular edema secondary to sarcoid uveitis. *Ophthalmology* **2001**, *108*, 1140–1144. [CrossRef]

Disclaimer/Publisher's Note: The statements, opinions and data contained in all publications are solely those of the individual author(s) and contributor(s) and not of MDPI and/or the editor(s). MDPI and/or the editor(s) disclaim responsibility for any injury to people or property resulting from any ideas, methods, instructions or products referred to in the content.

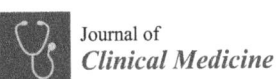

Journal of
Clinical Medicine

Review

Deceptive Tricks in Artificial Intelligence: Adversarial Attacks in Ophthalmology

Agnieszka M. Zbrzezny [1,2,*] and Andrzej E. Grzybowski [3,*]

1. Faculty of Mathematics and Computer Science, University of Warmia and Mazury, 10-710 Olsztyn, Poland
2. Faculty of Design, SWPS University of Social Sciences and Humanities, Chodakowska 19/31, 03-815 Warsaw, Poland
3. Institute for Research in Ophthalmology, Foundation for Ophthalmology Development, 60-836 Poznan, Poland
* Correspondence: agnieszka.zbrzezny@matman.uwm.edu.pl (A.M.Z.); ae.grzybowski@gmail.com (A.E.G.)

Abstract: The artificial intelligence (AI) systems used for diagnosing ophthalmic diseases have significantly progressed in recent years. The diagnosis of difficult eye conditions, such as cataracts, diabetic retinopathy, age-related macular degeneration, glaucoma, and retinopathy of prematurity, has become significantly less complicated as a result of the development of AI algorithms, which are currently on par with ophthalmologists in terms of their level of effectiveness. However, in the context of building AI systems for medical applications such as identifying eye diseases, addressing the challenges of safety and trustworthiness is paramount, including the emerging threat of adversarial attacks. Research has increasingly focused on understanding and mitigating these attacks, with numerous articles discussing this topic in recent years. As a starting point for our discussion, we used the paper by Ma et al. "Understanding Adversarial Attacks on Deep Learning Based Medical Image Analysis Systems". A literature review was performed for this study, which included a thorough search of open-access research papers using online sources (PubMed and Google). The research provides examples of unique attack strategies for medical images. Unfortunately, unique algorithms for attacks on the various ophthalmic image types have yet to be developed. It is a task that needs to be performed. As a result, it is necessary to build algorithms that validate the computation and explain the findings of artificial intelligence models. In this article, we focus on adversarial attacks, one of the most well-known attack methods, which provide evidence (i.e., adversarial examples) of the lack of resilience of decision models that do not include provable guarantees. Adversarial attacks have the potential to provide inaccurate findings in deep learning systems and can have catastrophic effects in the healthcare industry, such as healthcare financing fraud and wrong diagnosis.

Keywords: adversarial attacks; ophthalmology; artificial intelligence

Citation: Zbrzezny, A.M.; Grzybowski, A.E. Deceptive Tricks in Artificial Intelligence: Adversarial Attacks in Ophthalmology. *J. Clin. Med.* **2023**, *12*, 3266. https://doi.org/10.3390/jcm12093266

Academic Editors: Vito Romano, Yalin Zheng and Mariantonia Ferrara

Received: 16 March 2023
Revised: 20 April 2023
Accepted: 26 April 2023
Published: 4 May 2023

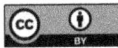

Copyright: © 2023 by the authors. Licensee MDPI, Basel, Switzerland. This article is an open access article distributed under the terms and conditions of the Creative Commons Attribution (CC BY) license (https://creativecommons.org/licenses/by/4.0/).

1. Introduction

In many areas of artificial intelligence, machine learning algorithms based on big data (Wang et al. [1] and Ching-Yu et al. [2]) and deep learning have facilitated extraordinary progress, with many applications in ophthalmology (Keenan et al. [3], Papadopoulos et al. [4], Rampasek et al. [5], Ishii et al. [6], Kermany et al. [7], Liu Y. et al. [8], Liu T. et al. [9], Burlina et al. [10], Cen et al. [11], Zheng et al. [12], Shekar et al. [13], and by Zhao et al. [14]).

Advances in artificial intelligence (AI) algorithms and easy access to large public datasets have made AI models ubiquitous, from funny filters on Instagram to automatic translators that help us perform our work to specialised models that solve complicated problems such as analysing and classifying medical photos.

With the help of artificial intelligence algorithms, we can solve complex image classification problems in different areas of life. The development of big data has given us access to millions of correctly classified images. This allows the algorithms to learn better. The latest models can achieve up to 98% accuracy, which can be misleading. Suppose we consider even minor perturbations to the image, such as the change in colour of just one pixel. Then, such models are uncertain for small perturbations. A disturbance of the image, which does not change in termsof human perception, makes it a completely different image for the AI model (Figure 1).

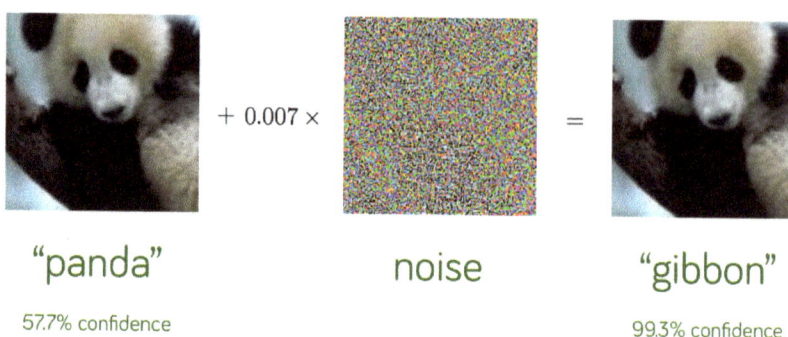

Figure 1. A classical example of an adversarial attack (Goodfellow et al. [15]).

The figure above demonstrates that the model first correctly categorised the panda image. After the perturbation was applied to this image, the model's prediction shifted to a gibbon, and the likelihood that it was a gibbon was extremely high. Humans interpret both photographs similarly. Nonetheless, the model views them as entirely distinct. This highlights the significance of adversarial attacks and that even modifications in the image that are imperceptible to humans can dramatically misrepresent the model's output, as described by Liu et al. [16].

Most of the attacks presented in this paper concern convolutional neural networks (CNNs). However, the relatively new approach in computer vision, adapted from natural language processing, vision transformers (ViTs), can achieve state-of-the-art or near-state-of-the-art performance on various image classification tasks, as demonstrated by recent advances in attention-based networks. It distinguishes transformers as a promising alternative to conventional convolutional neural networks. Mahmood et al. [17] demonstrated that white-box attacks are highly effective at producing vision transformer examples. They concluded that vision transformers are as susceptible to white-box adversaries as their CNN counterparts. Nonetheless, transferability can be utilised to achieve robustness against a black-box adversary. They developed a SAGA attack.

Hu et al. [18] also employed attacks against CNNs and ViTs. They described the IAM-UAP attack algorithm.

However, some groundbreaking studies by Naseer et al. [19] demonstrated that ViTs are more robust than CNNs against adversarial patch attacks, arguing that the dynamic, receptive field of multihead self-attention (MSA) is the reason for its superior robustness.

Wang and Ruan provided significant results [20]. The authors demonstrated that ViTs are Lipschitz continuous for vision tasks and then formally connect the local robustness of transformers to the Cauchy problem. They theoretically showed that the maximum singular value determines the local robustness of each block's Jacobian. They discovered that the initial and final layers inhibit the robustness of ViTs. In addition, contrary to existing research that suggests MSA can increase robustness, they found that the defensive power of MSA in ViT is only effective against weak adversarial attacks for large models. MSA compromises adversary robustness even against solid attacks.

Unfortunately, research using ViT to classify medical images is relatively new, and there are no presented attacks on such models for classifying medical images. It could be an interesting step in the development of specialised adversarial attacks.

In recent years, more research has been undertaken on applying artificial intelligence algorithms to solve medical problems, i.e., studies on various eye diseases. The resulting models are highly efficient. Nevertheless, we typically do not receive any information on model checking. One such difficulty may arise from the adversarial attacks presented by Goodfellow et al. [15]. They are relatively easy attacks to develop and are expected when working with images.

This study covered adversarial and specific adversarial attacks for images used in ophthalmology. In this paper, we highlight the different attacks and describe their influence on models that receive ophthalmic images as input. We also address the necessity of designing novel attack algorithms for specific sorts of pictures, such as fundus or anterior segment images.

2. Adversarial Attacks

The tendency of classifiers to overfit has led many to assume that adversarial attacks only occur in deep neural networks. All decision models have an adversarial attack as a fundamental property. Here we will explore the fundamentals of adversarial attacks to better understand attacks on ophthalmic image classification models.

Suppose d represents the number of dimensions of the input object. Consider a data point representing an image $x_0 \in \mathbb{R}^d$ of class C_i, where $0 < i \leq j$, and j is the number of classes. An adversarial attack is a malicious attempt to insert x_0 into a new data point $x \in \mathbb{R}^d$ such that the classifier misclassifies x, i.e., x belongs to a particularly hostile target class.

There are two categories of attacks: targeted and untargeted attacks. Let us consider a binary classification. In a targeted attack, a certain class C_1 is given, and with this attack, we want a given model $\mathcal{M}$ to classify an image of a given image $\mathcal{I}$ into class C_1, although its correct class is C_2. An untargeted attack aims to deceive the model $\mathcal{M}$ by giving it a distorted image $\mathcal{I}$ so that it is assigned to a class other than C_1. Untargeted attacks are not as good as targeted attacks and take much less time. Targeted attacks are more effective at changing the model's predictions, but they come at a price: time.

Problem Formulation

An adversarial attack is a malicious attempt to perturb a data point $x_0 \in \mathbb{R}^d$ to another point $x \in \mathbb{R}^d$ so that x belongs to a particular adversarial target class.

Suppose a binary classifier classifies photographs of the anterior segment of the eye for cataracts.

For example, if x_0 is a feature vector of an anterior eye segment photograph with a correct classification of cataract. With an adversarial attack, we want to create another feature vector x classified as healthy (or another class specified by the attacker). In some scenarios, the goal may not be to assign x_0 to a particular target class C_t, but to push it away from its original class C_i.

Let us define a data set as $\mathbb{D} = \{x_i, y_i\}_{i=1}^N$, where x_i is a data sample labelled y_i, and N is the size of the data set. A trained model is denoted as $\mathcal{M}$ with input x and prediction $\mathcal{M}(x)$. A loss function is denoted by ℓ. In a soft machine learning system, training attempts to minimise the loss between the target label and the predicted label:

Definition 1. *Given data $\mathcal{X} = \{x_1, x_2, \ldots, x_n\}$ and target labels $\mathcal{Y} = \{y_1, y_2, \ldots, y_n\}$ find a hypothesis $\mathcal{H}$ such that*

$$\arg\min_{\mathcal{H}} \sum_{x_i, y_i \in \mathbb{D}} \ell(\mathcal{H}(x_i), y_i).$$

The trained model is tested to see how well it can predict the predicted label. One of the methods is to calculate the error by summing the losses between the target label and the predicted label.

Let us define a test dataset as $\mathbb{D}' = \{x_i, y_i\}_{i=1}^M$, where x_i is a data sample with label y_i, and M is the size of the dataset.

Definition 2. *Given test data* $\mathcal{X}' = \{x_1, x_2, \ldots, x_m\}$ *and test labels* $\mathcal{Y}' = \{y_1, y_2, \ldots, y_m\}$, *the error is*

$$\sum_{x_i, y_i \in \mathbb{D}'} \ell(\mathcal{H}(x_i), y_i).$$

The adversarial attack algorithm is divided into two main parts:
1. The query input is changed from the benign input x to x'.
2. An attack target is set so that the prediction result $\mathcal{H}(x)$ is no longer y. The loss is changed from $\ell(\mathcal{H}(x_i), y_i)$ to $\ell(\mathcal{H}(x_i), y'_i)$, where $y'_i \neq y_i$.

Definition 3 (Adversarial Attack (AA)). *Let* $x_0 \in \mathbb{R}^d$ *be a data point belonging to class* $\mathcal{C}_i$. *Define a target class* $\mathcal{C}_t$. *An adversarial attack is a mapping* $\mathcal{A} : \mathbb{R}^d \to \mathbb{R}^d$ *such that the perturbed data*

$$x = \mathcal{A}(x_0)$$

3. Methodology

As a starting point for our discussion, we used the study by Ma et al. [21].

We began our search of open-access research papers available in Google Scholar's primary search. We searched for papers that consisted of entering various terms in three types of search engines, including "ophthalmology", "ophthalmic image", "retina", and "retinal image", "fundus", and "fundus image", along with the words "adversarial attacks" and "attacks". The exact search was performed in the Google search and PubMed engines. We considered papers published after 2018.

4. Challenges in Adversarial Attacks in Medicine

Before the paper by Ma et al. [21], adversarial machine learning analysis focused on natural images, and medical image AAs were still unclear. Unlike natural images, medical images may contain domain-specific features. AAs can affect medical deep-learning systems. AAs can arbitrarily change diagnoses and outcomes. Ma et al. emphasised the importance of the fact that the healthcare system is heavily resourced. It inevitably creates risks where potential attackers can attempt to profit from manipulating the healthcare system. They gave an example of an attacker who can manipulate the health system's investigative reports to commit insurance fraud or submit a fraudulent claim for medical reimbursement, as first presented by Paschali et al. [22].

In addition, an attacker may attempt to make a misdiagnosis by manipulating an image without detection. It may significantly affect patient decisions. DNNs operate on the black box principle, so such misclassification would be nearly impossible to detect. Other techniques can explain the DNNs' decision, but consulting an expert/doctor is necessary for the diagnosis to be certain. This was shown by Avramidis et al. [23], Kind et al. [24], Chetoui et al. [25], and Ribeiro et al. [26].

Decision models and medical imaging techniques are increasingly used in medical diagnostics. Safe and robust medical deep-learning systems have become essential, as shown by by Finlayson et al. [27] and Paschali et al. [22]. The work by Ma et al. [21] was an essential step toward developing a comprehensive understanding of AAs in this field. It provides a broad knowledge of AAs in medical images, from the perspectives of both generating and detecting these attacks. However, Finlayson et al. [27] and Paschali et al. [22] have studied AAs on medical images, primarily focusing on testing the robustness of the deep models developed for medical image analysis.

The authors emphasised that AAs can succeed faster on medical images than natural ones. It means that fewer perturbations are required to execute a successful attack. They then pointed to two main reasons why deep neural networks that classify medical images are more exposed to AAs:

1. Typically, medical images have complex biological textures, leading to areas with stronger gradients that are sensitive to small perturbations from attackers.
2. State-of-the-art deep neural networks designed for large-scale natural image processing can be reparameterised for medical imaging tasks, resulting in a severe loss of landscape and high susceptibility to AAs.

According to the analysis by Ma et al. [21], medical imaging AAs generated using attack methods developed from natural images are not really "detrimental" in the medical sense. The authors noted that caution should be used when using these AAs to evaluate the performance of DNN models for medical images. Their study also shed light on the future development of more effective attacks on medical images. Future research should focus on developing specific AAs for different types of ophthalmic images.

The Danger of Adversarial Attacks in the Healthcare System

According to Finlayson et al. [28], the U.S. healthcare system favours AAs. They summarised parts of the healthcare system that can give an attacker a reason and opportunity to perform an AA.

The paper also discusses the technical reasons why medical machine-learning systems are accessible to AAs. The authors noted that the truth must often be clarified and id more contentious. End users change images that are difficult to diagnose. In this case, they can make it very hard for medical experts to figure out how much influence they have. Deep learning is most useful in edge cases.

They also noted that medical imaging is highly standardised. They found that medical AA attacks do not require invariance. Medical AA attacks are not immune to lighting or position changes.

They also considered the fact that standard network architectures are frequently used. Most of the best-published methods in medical computer vision have the same basic structure. This lack of architectural variety makes it easier for attackers to attack multiple medical systems. Models should be made public to provide transparency and enable more targeted attacks.

Finlayson et al. [28] provided a hypothetical but intriguing example of adversarial examples in ophthalmology. According to the authors, government agencies often issue diagnostic guidelines requiring coverage for specific procedures, if requirements are met. One of the criteria could be that a patient with diabetic retinopathy should undergo a specific surgery from an insurance company. Even if the insurer cannot control the policy, it can control surgery frequency using noise instead of slightly positive photos. On the other hand, an ophthalmologist may place a universal enemy image on the lens of its image capture system. A third-party image processing system would mistakenly label all images as positive cases without changing the image in the information system.

5. Adversarial Attacks in Ophthalmology

Artificial intelligence has a significant role to play in the field of ophthalmic imaging. Colour fundus imaging and optical coherence tomography play a substantial role in ophthalmology in terms of their diagnostic accuracy and usefulness in segmenting disorders.

This section provides a summary of AAs on ophthalmology-related models. However, the original issue is partitioned into two separate ones. The first is the usage of classical adversarial algorithms, and the second, given in the following section, is the application of ophthalmology-specific adversarial algorithms. In chronological order, we began our examination in 2018.

Shah et al. [29] studied the effect of AAs on retinal imaging. To detect diabetic retinopathy, they evaluated image-based CNN-0, closely influenced by Alexnet by Krizhevsky et al. [30]; CNN-1, inspired by Enet by Paszke et al. [31]; and hybrid-lesion-based medical image analysis models by Abràmoff et al. [32]. The CNN-1 and hybrid-lesion-based models were evaluated using CNN-0 and the iterative fast gradient sign method (I-FGSM) by Kurakin et al. [33] to produce adversarial images. According to the experimental results,

CNN models performed rather poorly, but hybrid-lesion-based models were more robust and achieved 45% and 0.6% reductions in accuracy, respectively (Figure 2). They collected the image from the Eyepacs dataset by Cuadros and Bresnick [34]. The authors noted that the explainability of the decision process underlying medical-image-based diagnostic tasks is of utmost importance.

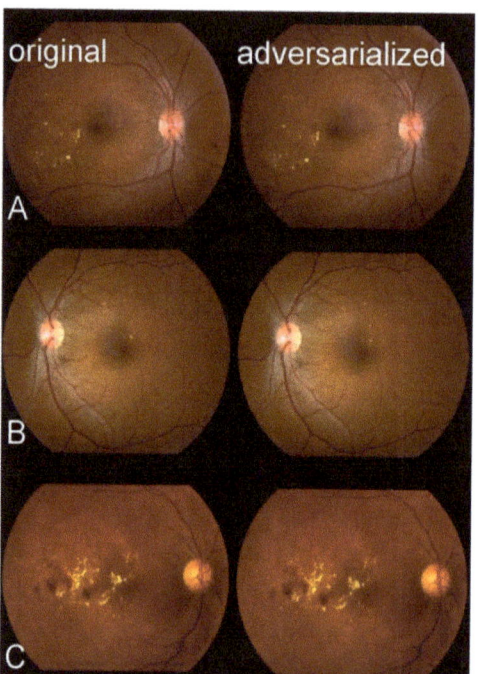

Figure 2. The AAs of three different patients (**A–C**) images that had previously been classified as a disease (referable diabetic retinopathy). The original images containing the disease are in the left column, while the right column displays the AA variants. Pixel differences are difficult to distinguish, even at high magnification (Shah et al. [29]).

Medical AAs were demonstrated to be feasible by Finlayson et al. [28]. The authors created a set of medical classifiers based on state-of-the-art clinical deep-learning algorithms. White- and black-box attacks against each other were the two types of AAs they carried out.

They created classification models for referable diabetic retinopathy based on fundoscopy images of the retina (similar to Gulshan et al. [35]). Data from the Kaggle Diabetic Retinopathy Dataset were used to train the models. Instead of the retinopathy grade, the Kaggle dataset sought to predict referable (grade 2 or worse) diabetic retinopathy using the model by Gulshan et al. [35].

Two different sorts of attacks, human undetected and patch attacks, were used to show how vulnerable their models were to AAs under various threat models. The white- and black-box projected gradient descent (PGD) attack methods were used in the undetectable by human attacks. The FGSM attack, first presented by Madry et al. [36], has evolved into the PGD attack, an iterative evolution of the FGSM attack. They adapted the approach outlined by Buckman et al. [37] for adversarial patch attacks.

The experimental results (Figure 3) showed that even very accurate medical classifiers can produce AAs, regardless of whether potential attackers have direct access to the model or must attack humans invisibly. PGD attacks require digital access to specific photographs provided to the model, while adversarial patch attacks can be used on any image, according to the research. They described realistic AAs against their systems.

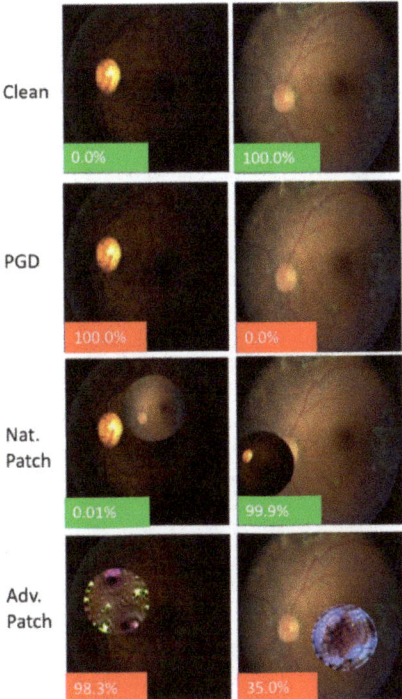

Figure 3. A demonstration that AAs can be feasible even for extremely accurate medical classifiers (Finlayson et al. [28]).

Ma et al. [21] examined four attacks on DNNs trained on five medical image datasets. They presented attack parameters, results, and analyses. FGSM, BIM, PGD, and the strongest optimisation-based Carlini and Wagner attack (L_∞ version) were performed. These attacks were limited by a maximum perturbation ϵ in the L_∞ norm on each input pixel.

They benchmarked the difficulty of classifying diabetic retinopathy fundus images. They initially categorised the image dataset into 'no DR' and 'referable'. They focused on medical photos' AA difficulty, which matched ImageNet's nature images. Medical photos were easier to attack than ImageNet photos, the findings showed. This unexpected finding was clarified by a saliency map for two ImageNet and medical images from different classes. Based on classification loss gradients, the saliency map of an input picture shows the regions that change model output most from classification loss gradients. However, comparing the model procedures with the explanations of ImageNet and medical image output from different classes would be interesting, valuable, and intriguing.

As a result, we concluded that we require explainable models in addition to unique AAs for characteristic medical images.

Yoo and Choi [38] investigated whether AAs can confound deep-learning systems based on imaging techniques such as fundus photography (FP), ultra-widefield photography (FP), and optical coherence tomography (OCT). Based on the basic FGSM algorithm, they developed a binary classifier to identify cases of diabetic retinopathy and diabetic macular oedema. Again, the unique qualities of medical imagery were ignored in this study.

The results exhibited the same characteristics as those reported by Ma et al. [21]. Using FGSM attacks helps deep learning models perform better.

Nonetheless, the authors adopted the same stance on attacks as Ma et al. [21]. Attackers may disrupt hospitals' and insurance firms' medical billing and reimbursement systems. Defensive approaches, including adversarial training, denoising filters, and generative adversarial networks, can successfully decrease the impact of AAs.

Lal et al. [39] worked on establishing a framework for diabetic retinopathy detection-specific attack detection and defence. Keeping algorithms safe and reliable is a major concern in the fast-paced growth of artificial intelligence (AI) and deep learning (DL) techniques. The main conclusion of the study was a framework that provides a protective model against the adversarial speckle-noise attack and adversarial training. The authors then proposed a feature fusion technique that maintains categorisation with correct labelling. They assessed and studied the AAs and defences created by their framework on retinal fundus images for the problem of diabetic retinopathy identification. However, the authors concentrated on only two types of attacks: FGSM and speckle-noise attack (SN). The most significant disadvantage is that these attacks are detectable at first glance. The authors correctly noted that medical images are significantly degraded because, for example, noise is unavoidable in data acquisition, contrast is low due to illumination variations, and various other factors can produce random pixel values for individual pixels in an image by multiplying speckle noise (Figure 4).

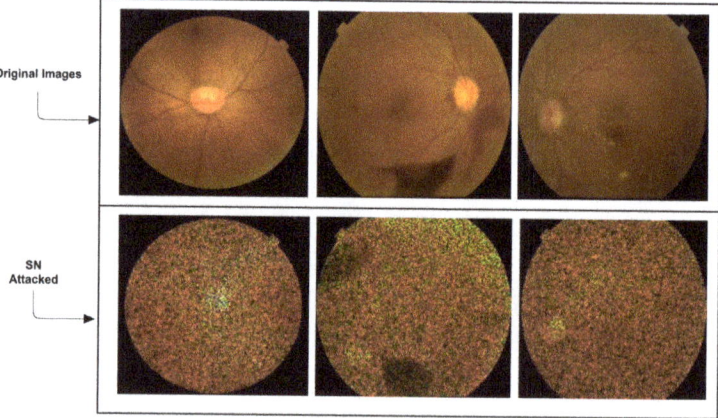

Figure 4. An example of the SN attacked images from [39] by Lal et al.

Hirano et al. [40] emphasised the need for more concentrated research on the vulnerability of DNNs to AAs. They focused on a single, modest, image-agnostic perturbation known as a universal adversarial perturbation (UAP), which can cause DNN failure in the majority of image classification tasks. Because such minute changes have little effect on data distributions, UAPs are challenging to find. Nonetheless, the authors found that UAP-based AAs are more accurate for adversaries to implement in real-world contexts. In medical imaging diagnostics, UAPs are prone to security risks.

Nonetheless, defence tactics against UAPs in DNN-based medical image classification still need to be studied, despite the sensitivity of DNNs to AAs, demonstrating the need for solutions to address security concerns.

Researchers focused on a representative medical image classification: the classification of diabetic retinopathy based on OCT images. Based on previous research, they built DNN models with different topologies for medical image recognition and investigated their susceptibility to untargeted and targeted attacks based on UAPs. They also studied the defence against attackers. They used adversarial training to test the increased resistance of DNNs to untargeted and targeted UAPs.

6. Specified Adversarial Attacks in Ophthalmology

The studies presented in the previous section have indicated a need to build algorithms for deception attacks explicitly targeted at medical images. In this section, we concentrate on attacks specifically designed for ophthalmic images in this area.

6.1. Adaptive Segmentation Mask Attack

Ozbulak et al. [41] demonstrated that deep-learning-based medical image segmentation models are susceptible to AAs. They concentrated on optic disc segmentation in glaucoma and targeted attacks. They employed the U-Net model, one of the best-recognised models for medical image segmentation. They introduced the adaptive mask segmentation attack (AMSA), a unique approach to creating AAs with realistic prediction masks. When misclassified, the algorithm modifies the masks in largely imperceptible ways to human sight. The authors posted the AA's source code on GitHub at https://github.com/utkuozbulak/adaptive-segmentation-mask-attack/ (accessed on 25 April 2023).

6.2. HFC

Yao et al. [42] presented a novel hierarchical feature constraint (HFC) to supplement current white-box attacks, allowing the adversarial representation to be concealed within the normal feature distribution. They examined the proposed approach using a fundoscopy image dataset. Their investigations revealed that the increased susceptibility of medical representations gives an adversary more opportunities for malevolent manipulation. Their premise was that medical AAs are easily detectable. They specified the HFC that can be used in attacks to evade detection. They performed comprehensive tests to determine the efficacy of the HFC. The experimental results demonstrated that HFC significantly outperformed other adaptive attacks, highlighting the inadequacies of existing approaches for identifying medical attacks in feature space.

6.3. MSA

Shao et al. [43] reported a targeted attack against a biomedical image segmentation model built on multiscale gradients. Their approach integrates the attack on the adaptive segmentation mask with a perturbation of the feature space. They suggested a targeted attack approach employing multiscale gradients and applied the binary cross-entropy loss function for semantic image segmentation. The MSA approach introduces the gradient information of the loss functions to repeatedly calculate the adversarial perturbation. The original image is fitted with the adversarial perturbation and is subsequently transformed to an AA when the predicted mask of AA is close to the target mask. They conducted glaucoma-related studies utilising U-Net and an optic disc segmentation dataset. They demonstrated that their MSA method outperformed the standard method (ASMA).

6.4. SMIA

In order to diagnose pre-existing medical systems, Qi et al. [44] presented a method for medical image AA. By maximising the deviation loss term and minimising the loss stabilisation term, the approach iteratively builds AAs. The current iteration increases the difference between the CNN prediction and the matching ground truth label for AA. In comparison, the CNN predictions for the smoothed input are similar. Similar predictions ensure that the perturbations are created in a relatively flat region in the CNN feature space. The perturbations are updated from one flat region to another throughout subsequent iterations. Hence, the suggested approach cab explore perturbation space to smooth a single point and obtain a local optimum. Compared with the perturbation movement between single locations induced just by the loss deviation term, the loss stabilisation term enhances attack performance by stabilising the perturbation movement.

They used two datasets for diabetic retinopathy evaluation: APTOS-2019 and Kaggle-DR, and they used the ResNet-50 model combined with a graph convolutional network to classify fundus images. Under the same medical analytic settings, they compared the proposed SMIA technique with existing AA methods. In addition to the commonly utilised FGSM and PGD algorithms, they included DAG, which was proposed for natural image identification and segmentation, and DeepFool, which was designed for disease classification. The visualisation and experimental results proved the attack approach's success in determining the limitations of medical diagnostic systems and further enhancing them (Figure 5).

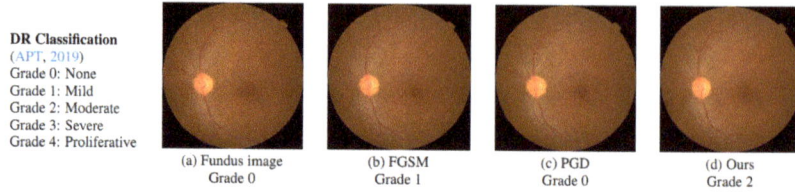

Figure 5. An example of SMIA effectiveness (Qi et al. [44]).

6.5. Remarks

The aforementioned studies have illustrated specific attack tactics for medical images. However, no novel algorithms for attacks on various ophthalmic image types have yet to be developed, which is a task that must be accomplished. As a result, algorithms that explain the results of artificial intelligence models and that validate the computation of artificial intelligence models must be developed.

7. Regulations

7.1. The European Union

In April 2021, the European Commission has proposed REGULATION OF THE EUROPEAN PARLIAMENT AND OF THE COUNCIL LAYING DOWN HARMONISED RULES ON ARTIFICIAL INTELLIGENCE (ARTIFICIAL INTELLIGENCE ACT) AND AMENDING CERTAIN UNION LEGISLATIVE ACTS [45].

Note 51 says:

"Cybersecurity plays a crucial role in ensuring that AI systems are resilient against attempts to alter their use, behaviour, performance or compromise their security properties by malicious third parties exploiting the system's vulnerabilities. Cyberattacks against AI systems can leverage AI specific assets, such as training data sets (e.g., data poisoning) or trained models (e.g., adversarial attacks), or exploit vulnerabilities in the AI system's digital assets or the underlying ICT infrastructure. To ensure a level of cybersecurity appropriate to the risks, suitable measures should therefore be taken by the providers of high-risk AI systems, also taking into account as appropriate the underlying ICT infrastructure."

Chapter 2, Article 15, point 4 says:

"High-risk AI systems shall be resilient as regards attempts by unauthorised third parties to alter their use or performance by exploiting the system vulnerabilities.

The technical solutions aimed at ensuring the cybersecurity of high-risk AI systems shall be appropriate to the relevant circumstances and the risks.

The technical solutions to address AI specific vulnerabilities shall include, where appropriate, measures to prevent and control for attacks trying to manipulate the training dataset ('data poisoning'), inputs designed to cause the model to make a mistake ('adversarial examples'), or model flaws."

7.2. The United States of America

In January 2021, the U.S. Food and Drug Administration (FDA) presented "Artificial Intelligence/Machine Learning (AI/ML)-Based Software as a Medical Device (SaMD)

Action Plan" [46]. Point 4 "4. Regulatory Science Methods Related to Algorithm Bias & Robustness" says:

> "Support regulatory science efforts to develop methodology for the evaluation and improvement of machine learning algorithms, including for the identification and elimination of bias, and for the evaluation and promotion of algorithm robustness."

7.3. Discussion

We could not find real-life adversarial attacks in the medicine descriptions in the literature. This shows how complicated and delicate the problem is. In the previous sections, we showed that two famous institutions are aware of the possibility of attacks and the lack of robustness of the models.

During our previous research, we used several commercial models. We proposed the algorithms' owners' joint research and the possibility of testing models using attacks several times. We also explained to companies that successful attacks will not discredit their product but show how their model can be improved. None of the companies expressed willingness to cooperate. .

Testing the models by sending perturbed images via the interface provided by the companies is possible. However, such attacking could be noticed by the fact that we would send a dozen or so, at first glance, photos for classification that did not differ in any way. This alsod involve high costs. The results obtained in this way could not be made available and published.

We are currently working on attacks against a model provided to us by another research group. However, again, this is not a commercially used model.

Soon, legal regulations requiring the verification of models and their explainability will come into force in the European Union. However, we should be aware that such a process may take a long time, and many misdiagnoses will occur before the law comes into force. Similar problems occurred with the rapid development of information systems in the 2000s. Many errors in the operation of the systems were detected after implementation, costing human lives and financial losses. Legal regulations regarding formal verification were introduced over time and in a few countries worldwide mainly because the cost of formal verification often exceeded the cost of software development.

8. Conclusions

Artificial intelligence algorithms may advance ophthalmic image processing and become a vital tool for clinicians and hospitals. However, AAs present a significant risk to patients as well as a barrier to the correct operation of AI models. The purpose of this study was to provide a summary of the studies focused on the use of AAs in ophthalmic image analysis. The analyses have demonstrated that these attacks can also mislead ophthalmic imaging models. Several researchers have presented novel attacks that have been created specifically for the field of ophthalmic image processing and have a very high level of accuracy. We provide a brief summary of the described attacks in Tables 1 and 2.

We think that computer scientists and the ophthalmology communities should closely cooperate and concentrate on tackling AAs to integrate AI algorithms into real-world problems.

Table 1. The standard AAs.

Type of the Attack	Characteristics
I-FGSM [29,33]	FGSM iteratively adds the noise (not random noise) whose direction is the same as the gradient of the cost function concerning the data.
PGD [28,36]	Initialises the attack to a random point in the ball of interest and performs random restarts.

Table 1. *Cont.*

Type of the Attack	Characteristics
FGSM [21,36,38]	Adds the noise (not random noise) whose direction is the same as the gradient of the cost function concerning the data.
BIM [21,33]	A simple extension of the FGSM where, rather than taking one significant step, it performs an iterative procedure by using FGSM numerous times on an image.
C&W [21,47]	A regularisation-based attack with some necessary modifications that can resolve the unboundedness issue.
SN [39]	The gritty salt-and-pepper pattern seen in radar imaging or a granular 'noise' that appears fundamentally in ultrasound.
UAP [40,48]	Leads to DNN failure in most image classification tasks.

Table 2. Specialised AAs.

Type of the Attack	Characteristics
AMSA [41]	Can produce AAs with realistic prediction masks.
HFC [42]	Enables hiding the adversarial representation in normal feature distribution.
SMIA [44]	The method iteratively generates AAs by maximising the deviation loss term and minimising the loss stabilisation term.
MSA [43]	Based on AMSA and multi-scale gradients.

In future work, we would like to compare all these attacks on a common database to conclude which attack is the strongest and evaluate the detection/defence methods, i.e., adversarial training, or explain the model susceptible to attacks using explainable methods.

Author Contributions: Conceptualisation, A.M.Z.; methodology, A.M.Z.; validation, A.M.Z. and A.E.G.; formal analysis, A.M.Z.; investigation, A.M.Z.; writing—original draft preparation, A.M.Z.; writing—review and editing, A.M.Z. and A.E.G.; supervision, A.E.G.; project administration, A.E.G., All authors have read and agreed to the published version of the manuscript.

Funding: This research received no external funding.

Institutional Review Board Statement: Not applicable.

Informed Consent Statement: Not applicable.

Data Availability Statement: Data sharing not applicable No new data were created or analyzed in this study. Data sharing is not applicable to this article.

Conflicts of Interest: The authors declare no conflict of interest.

References

1. Wang, S.Y.; Pershing, S.; Lee, A.Y. Big data requirements for artificial intelligence. *Curr. Opin. Ophthalmol.* **2020**, *31*, 318–323. [CrossRef]
2. Cheng, C.Y.; Soh, Z.D.; Majithia, S.; Thakur, S.; Rim, T.H.; Chung, T.Y.; Wong, T.Y. Big Data in Ophthalmology. *Asia-Pac. J. Ophthalmol.* **2020**, *9*, 291–298. [CrossRef] [PubMed]
3. Keenan, T.D.; Chen, Q.; Agrón, E.; Tham, Y.C.; Goh, J.H.L.; Lei, X.; Ng, Y.P.; Liu, Y.; Xu, X.; Cheng, C.Y.; et al. DeepLensNet: Deep Learning Automated Diagnosis and Quantitative Classification of Cataract Type and Severity. *Ophthalmology* **2022**, *129*, 571–584. [CrossRef] [PubMed]
4. Papadopoulos, A.; Topouzis, F.; Delopoulos, A. An Interpretable Multiple-Instance Approach for the Detection of referable Diabetic Retinopathy from Fundus Images. *Sci. Rep.* **2021**, *11*, 14326. [CrossRef]

5. Rampasek, L.; Goldenberg, A. Learning from Everyday Images Enables Expert-like Diagnosis of Retinal Diseases. *Cell* **2018**, *172*, 893–895. [CrossRef] [PubMed]
6. Ishii, K.; Asaoka, R.; Omoto, T.; Mitaki, S.; Fujino, Y.; Murata, H.; Onoda, K.; Nagai, A.; Yamaguchi, S.; Obana, A.; et al. Predicting intraocular pressure using systemic variables or fundus photography with deep learning in a health examination cohort. *Sci. Rep.* **2021**, *11*, 3687. [CrossRef]
7. Kermany, D.; Goldbaum, M.; Cai, W.; Valentim, C.; Liang, H.Y.; Baxter, S.; McKeown, A.; Yang, G.; Wu, X.; Yan, F.; et al. Identifying Medical Diagnoses and Treatable Diseases by Image-Based Deep Learning. *Cell* **2018**, *172*, 1122–1131.e9. [CrossRef]
8. Liu, Y.; Yang, J.; Zhou, Y.; Wang, W.; Zhao, J.; Yu, W.; Zhang, D.; Ding, D.; Li, X.; Chen, Y. Prediction of OCT images of short-term response to anti-VEGF treatment for neovascular age-related macular degeneration using generative adversarial network. *Br. J. Ophthalmol.* **2020**, *104*, 1735–1740. [CrossRef]
9. Liu, T.; Farsiu, S.; Ting, D. Generative adversarial networks to predict treatment response for neovascular age-related macular degeneration: Interesting, but is it useful? *Br. J. Ophthalmol.* **2020**, *104*, 1629–1630. [CrossRef]
10. Burlina, P.; Paul, W.; Mathew, P.; Joshi, N.; Pacheco, K.; Bressler, N. Low-Shot Deep Learning of Diabetic Retinopathy With Potential Applications to Address Artificial Intelligence Bias in Retinal Diagnostics and Rare Ophthalmic Diseases. *JAMA Ophthalmol.* **2020**, *138*, 1070–1077. [CrossRef]
11. Cen, L.P.; Ji, J.; Lin, J.W.; Ju, S.; Lin, H.J.; Li, T.P.; Wang, Y.; Yang, J.F.; Liu, Y.F.; Tan, S.; et al. Automatic detection of 39 fundus diseases and conditions in retinal photographs using deep neural networks. *Nat. Commun.* **2021**, *12*, 4828. [CrossRef]
12. Zheng, C.; Xie, X.; Zhou, K.; Chen, B.; Chen, J.; Ye, H.; Li, W.; Qiao, T.; Gao, S.; Yang, J.; et al. Assessment of Generative Adversarial Networks Model for Synthetic Optical Coherence Tomography Images of Retinal Disorders. *Transl. Vis. Sci. Technol.* **2020**, *9*, 29. [CrossRef]
13. Shekar, S.; Satpute, N.; Gupta, A. Review on diabetic retinopathy with deep learning methods. *J. Med. Imaging* **2021**, *8*, 060901. [CrossRef]
14. Zhao, X.; Lv, B.; Meng, L.; Xia, Z.; Wang, D.; Zhang, W.; Wang, E.; Lv, C.; Xie, G.; Chen, Y. Development and quantitative assessment of deep learning-based image enhancement for optical coherence tomography. *BMC Ophthalmol.* **2022**, *22*, 139. [CrossRef] [PubMed]
15. Goodfellow, I.J.; Shlens, J.; Szegedy, C. Explaining and Harnessing Adversarial Examples. In Proceedings of the 3rd International Conference on Learning Representations, ICLR 2015, San Diego, CA, USA, 7–9 May 2015.
16. Liu, X.; Glocker, B.; McCradden, M.M.; Ghassemi, M.; Denniston, A.K.; Oakden-Rayner, L. The medical algorithmic audit. *Lancet Digit. Health* **2022**, *4*, e384–e397. [CrossRef]
17. Mahmood, K.; Mahmood, R.; van Dijk, M. On the Robustness of Vision Transformers to Adversarial Examples. 2021. Available online: https://openaccess.thecvf.com/content/ICCV2021/papers/Mahmood_On_the_Robustness_of_Vision_Transformers_to_Adversarial_Examples_ICCV_2021_paper.pdf (accessed on 25 April 2023).
18. Hu, H.; Lu, X.; Zhang, X.; Zhang, T.; Sun, G. Inheritance Attention Matrix-Based Universal Adversarial Perturbations on Vision Transformers. *IEEE Signal Process. Lett.* **2021**, *28*, 1923–1927. [CrossRef]
19. Naseer, M.; Ranasinghe, K.; Khan, S.; Hayat, M.; Khan, F.S.; Yang, M.H. Intriguing Properties of Vision Transformers. 2021. Available online: https://proceedings.neurips.cc/paper/2021/file/c404a5adbf90e09631678b13b05d9d7a-Paper.pdf (accessed on 25 April 2023).
20. Wang, Z.; Ruan, W. Understanding Adversarial Robustness of Vision Transformers via Cauchy Problem. 2022. Available online: https://arxiv.org/abs/2208.00906 (accessed on 22 April 2023).
21. Ma, X.; Niu, Y.; Gu, L.; Wang, Y.; Zhao, Y.; Bailey, J.; Lu, F. Understanding Adversarial Attacks on Deep Learning Based Medical Image Analysis Systems. *Pattern Recognit.* **2020**, *110*, 107332. [CrossRef]
22. Paschali, M.; Conjeti, S.; Navarro, F.; Navab, N. Generalizability vs. Robustness: Adversarial Examples for Medical Imaging. *arXiv* **2018**, arXiv:1804.00504.
23. Avramidis, K.; Rostami, M.; Chang, M.; Narayanan, S. Automating Detection of Papilledema in Pediatric Fundus Images with Explainable Machine Learning. In Proceedings of the 2022 IEEE International Conference on Image Processing (ICIP), Bordeaux, France, 16–19 October 2022. [CrossRef]
24. Kind, A.; Azzopardi, G. An Explainable AI-Based Computer Aided Detection System for Diabetic Retinopathy Using Retinal Fundus Images. In *Proceedings of the Computer Analysis of Images and Patterns*; Vento, M., Percannella, G., Eds.; Springer International Publishing: Cham, Switzerland, 2019; pp. 457–468.
25. Chetoui, M.; Akhloufi, M.A. Explainable Diabetic Retinopathy using EfficientNET. In Proceedings of the 2020 42nd Annual International Conference of the IEEE Engineering in Medicine & Biology Society (EMBC), Montréal, QC, Canada, 20–24 July 2020; pp. 1966–1969. [CrossRef]
26. Ribeiro, M.T.; Singh, S.; Guestrin, C. "Why Should I Trust You?": Explaining the Predictions of Any Classifier. In Proceedings of the 22nd ACM SIGKDD International Conference on Knowledge Discovery and Data Mining, San Francisco, CA, USA, 13–17 August 2016; pp. 1135–1144.
27. Finlayson, S.G.; Bowers, J.D.; Ito, J.; Zittrain, J.L.; Beam, A.L.; Kohane, I.S. Adversarial attacks on medical machine learning. *Science* **2019**, *363*, 1287–1289. [CrossRef]
28. Finlayson, S.G.; Kohane, I.S.; Beam, A.L. Adversarial Attacks Against Medical Deep Learning Systems. *arXiv* **2018**, arXiv:1804.05296.

29. Shah, A.; Lynch, S.; Niemeijer, M.; Amelon, R.; Clarida, W.; Folk, J.; Russell, S.; Wu, X.; Abràmoff, M.D. Susceptibility to misdiagnosis of adversarial images by deep learning based retinal image analysis algorithms. In Proceedings of the 2018 IEEE 15th International Symposium on Biomedical Imaging (ISBI 2018), Washington, DC, USA, 4–7 April 2018; pp. 1454–1457. [CrossRef]
30. Krizhevsky, A.; Sutskever, I.; Hinton, G.E. ImageNet Classification with Deep Convolutional Neural Networks. In *Proceedings of the Advances in Neural Information Processing Systems*; Pereira, F., Burges, C., Bottou, L., Weinberger, K., Eds.; Curran Associates, Inc.: Red Hook, NY, USA, 2012; Volume 25.
31. Paszke, A.; Chaurasia, A.; Kim, S.; Culurciello, E. ENet: A Deep Neural Network Architecture for Real-Time Semantic Segmentation. *arXiv* **2016**, arXiv:1606.02147.
32. Abràmoff, M.D.; Lou, Y.; Erginay, A.; Clarida, W.; Amelon, R.; Folk, J.C.; Niemeijer, M. Improved Automated Detection of Diabetic Retinopathy on a Publicly Available Dataset Through Integration of Deep Learning. *Investig. Ophthalmol. Vis. Sci.* **2016**, *57*, 5200–5206. [CrossRef]
33. Kurakin, A.; Goodfellow, I.J.; Bengio, S. Adversarial examples in the physical world. In Proceedings of the 5th International Conference on Learning Representations, ICLR 2017, Toulon, France, 24–26 April 2017.
34. Cuadros, J.; Bresnick, G. EyePACS: An Adaptable Telemedicine System for Diabetic Retinopathy Screening. *J. Diabetes Sci. Technol.* **2009**, *3*, 509–516. [CrossRef]
35. Gulshan, V.; Peng, L.; Coram, M.; Stumpe, M.C.; Wu, D.; Narayanaswamy, A.; Venugopalan, S.; Widner, K.; Madams, T.; Cuadros, J.; et al. Development and Validation of a Deep Learning Algorithm for Detection of Diabetic Retinopathy in Retinal Fundus Photographs. *JAMA* **2016**, *316*, 2402–2410. [CrossRef]
36. Madry, A.; Makelov, A.; Schmidt, L.; Tsipras, D.; Vladu, A. Towards Deep Learning Models Resistant to Adversarial Attacks. In Proceedings of the 6th International Conference on Learning Representations, ICLR 2018, Vancouver, BC, Canada, 30 April–3 May 2018.
37. Buckman, J.; Roy, A.; Raffel, C.; Goodfellow, I. Thermometer Encoding: One Hot Way To Resist Adversarial Examples. In Proceedings of the International Conference on Learning Representations, Vancouver, BC, Canada, 30 April–3 May 2018.
38. Yoo, T.K.; Choi, J.Y. Outcomes of Adversarial Attacks on Deep Learning Models for Ophthalmology Imaging Domains. *JAMA Ophthalmol.* **2020**, *138*, 1213–1215. [CrossRef] [PubMed]
39. Lal, S.; Rehman, S.U.; Shah, J.H.; Meraj, T.; Rauf, H.T.; Damaševičius, R.; Mohammed, M.A.; Abdulkareem, K.H. Adversarial Attack and Defence through Adversarial Training and Feature Fusion for Diabetic Retinopathy Recognition. *Sensors* **2021**, *21*, 3922. [CrossRef]
40. Hirano, H.; Minagi, A.; Takemoto, K. Universal adversarial attacks on deep neural networks for medical image classification. *BMC Med. Imaging* **2020**, *21*, 9. [CrossRef]
41. Ozbulak, U.; Van Messem, A.; De Neve, W. Impact of Adversarial Examples on Deep Learning Models for Biomedical Image Segmentation. *arXiv* **2019**, arXiv:1907.13124. https://doi.org/10.48550/ARXIV.1907.13124.
42. Yao, Q.; He, Z.; Lin, Y.; Ma, K.; Zheng, Y.; Zhou, S.K. A Hierarchical Feature Constraint to Camouflage Medical Adversarial Attacks. In *Proceedings of the Medical Image Computing and Computer Assisted Intervention—MICCAI 2021*; de Bruijne, M., Cattin, P.C., Cotin, S., Padoy, N., Speidel, S., Zheng, Y., Essert, C., Eds.; Springer International Publishing: Cham, Switzerland, 2021; pp. 36–47.
43. Shao, M.; Zhang, G.; Zuo, W.; Meng, D. Target attack on biomedical image segmentation model based on multi-scale gradients. *Inf. Sci.* **2021**, *554*, 33–46. [CrossRef]
44. Qi, G.; Gong, L.; Song, Y.; Ma, K.; Zheng, Y. Stabilized Medical Image Attacks. 2021. Available online: https://arxiv.org/abs/2103.05232 (accessed on 25 April 2023).
45. Commision, E. Regulation of the European Parliament and of the Council Laying Down Harmonised Rules on Artificial Intelligence (Artificial Intelligence Act) and Amending Certain Union Legislative Acts. 2021. Available online: https://eur-lex.europa.eu/legal-content/EN/TXT/HTML/?uri=CELEX:52021PC0206&from=EN (accessed on 22 April 2023).
46. Food and Drug Administration Artificial Intelligence/Machine Learning (AI/ML)-Based Software as a Medical Device (SaMD) Action Plan. 2021. Available online: https://www.fda.gov/media/145022/download (accessed on 25 April 2023).
47. Carlini, N.; Wagner, D.A. Towards Evaluating the Robustness of Neural Networks. In Proceedings of the 2017 IEEE Symposium on Security and Privacy, SP 2017, San Jose, CA, USA, 22–26 May 2017; pp. 39–57. [CrossRef]
48. Moosavi-Dezfooli, S.; Fawzi, A.; Fawzi, O.; Frossard, P. Universal adversarial perturbations. In Proceedings of the IEEE Conference on Computer Vision and Pattern Recognition, Honolulu, HI, USA, 21–26 July 2017.

Disclaimer/Publisher's Note: The statements, opinions and data contained in all publications are solely those of the individual author(s) and contributor(s) and not of MDPI and/or the editor(s). MDPI and/or the editor(s) disclaim responsibility for any injury to people or property resulting from any ideas, methods, instructions or products referred to in the content.

MDPI
St. Alban-Anlage 66
4052 Basel
Switzerland
www.mdpi.com

Journal of Clinical Medicine Editorial Office
E-mail: jcm@mdpi.com
www.mdpi.com/journal/jcm

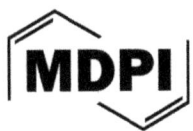

Disclaimer/Publisher's Note: The statements, opinions and data contained in all publications are solely those of the individual author(s) and contributor(s) and not of MDPI and/or the editor(s). MDPI and/or the editor(s) disclaim responsibility for any injury to people or property resulting from any ideas, methods, instructions or products referred to in the content.

www.ingramcontent.com/pod-product-compliance
Lightning Source LLC
LaVergne TN
LVHW070229100526
838202LV00015B/2109